Delmar's NCLEX-PN® Review

Delmar's NCLEX-PN® Review

Judith C. Miller
MS, RN
President, Nursing Tutorial and
Consulting Services

THOMSON

DELMAR LEARNING

Australia Canada Mexico Singapore Spain United Kingdom United States

THOMSON

DELMAR LEARNING

Delmar's NCLEX-PN® Review
Judith C. Miller

Executive Director Health Care Business Unit: William Brottmiller	**Acquisitions Editor:** Matthew Kane	**Project Editor:** Mary Ellen Cox
Executive Editor: Cathy L. Esperti	**Editorial Assistant:** Shelley Esposito	**Production Editor:** James Zayicek
Developmental Editor: Patricia A. Gaworecki	**Executive Marketing Manager:** Dawn F. Gerrain	**Art and Design Coordinator:** Jay Purcell
	Channel Manager: Jennifer McAvey	

COPYRIGHT © 2003 by Delmar Learning, a division of Thomson Learning, Inc. Thomson Learning™ is a trademark used herein under license.

Printed in the United States of America
1 2 3 4 5 XXX 06 05 04 03 02

For more information, contact Delmar Learning,
5 Maxwell Drive,
Clifton Park, NY 12065

Or you can visit our Internet site at http://www.delmarhealthcare.com

For permission to use material from this text or product, contact us by
Tel   (800) 730-2214
Fax   (800) 730-2215
www.thomsonrights.com

Library of Congress Cataloging-in-Publication Data
Miller, Judith C.
    Delmar's NCLEX-PN review / Judith C. Miller.
        p. ; cm.
Includes bibliographical references and index.
    ISBN 0-7668-0299-X (alk. paper)
    1. Practical nursing—Examinations, questions, etc.
    [DNLM: 1. Nursing, Practical—Examination Questions. 2. Nursing Care—Examination Questions. WX 18.2 M648d 2003]
I. Title: NCLEX-PN review. II. Title.
    RT62 .M555 2003
    610.73'076—dc21   20020256041

NOTICE TO THE READER

Publisher does not warrant or guarantee any of the products described herein or perform any independent analysis in connection with any of the production information contained herein. Publisher does not assume, and expressly disclaims, any obligation to obtain and include information other than that provided to it by the manufacturer.

The reader is expressly warned to consider and adopt all safety precautions that might be indicated by the activities and to avoid all potential hazards. By following the instructions contained herein, the reader willingly assumes all risk in connection with such instructions.

The Publisher makes no representation or warranties of any kind, including but not limited to, the warranties of fitness for particular purpose or merchantability, nor are any such representations implied with respect to the material set forth herein, and the publisher takes no responsibility with respect to such material. The publisher shall not be liable for any special, consequential, or exemplary damages resulting, in whole or part, from the readers' use of, or reliance upon, this material.

Contents

CHAPTER 1	HOW TO PREPARE FOR NCLEX-PN® 1

CHAPTER 2	ESSENTIAL CONCEPTS 9

CHAPTER 3	THE OLDER ADULT CLIENT 35

CHAPTER 4	THE PERIOPERATIVE CLIENT 43

CHAPTER 5	ONCOLOGY 53

CHAPTER 10   THE GASTROINTESTINAL SYSTEM   139

CHAPTER 11   THE GENITOURINARY SYSTEM   165

CHAPTER 12   THE MUSCULOSKELETAL SYSTEM   183

CHAPTER 13   THE ENDOCRINE SYSTEM   203

CHAPTER 14   THE INTEGUMENTARY SYSTEM   221

Index of Tables

Preface

This review book was expressly developed and written to help the licensed/vocational nurse graduate to study and prepare for the all-important NCLEX-PN® examination. Taking this exam can be a stressful experience since it constitutes a major career milestone, and success on the NCLEX is the key to begin a successful practice as a licensed practical/vocational nurse. The role the new LPN/LVN is expected to play in the current healthcare system has expanded enormously. This book was written with respect and a keen appreciation for this level of nursing.

ORGANIZATION, CONTENT, AND FEATURES

The content and design of this new text has been carefully constructed to reflect the NCLEX-PN® test plan effective April 2002, beginning with an introductory chapter on how to prepare for the NCLEX-PN®. Chapter 1, How to Prepare for NCLEX-PN®, includes:

- Detailed explanation of the current test plan
- Information on how the test is constructed
- How to apply to take the exam
- Data on scoring and notification of results
- Tips on how to plan your study and prepare successfully

Chapter 2, Essential Concepts, covers general care measures and is designed to help the student review basic nursing care measures commonly asked on the licensure exam. These measures apply across disease boundaries; in short, the type of care measures that apply to most clients, no matter what the actual diagnosis may be.

The chapters that follow are organized so concepts that apply across the spectrum of body systems are discussed first to lay a foundation and reduce unnecessary repetition. The Nursing Process as it applies to the LPN/LVN is an integral focal point in the design of this book. NANDA 2001–2002 diagnoses are in every chapter in table format for easy reference.

Individual chapters for the older adult client, perioperative client, oncology, nutrition/special diets and pharmacology address concepts applicable across the broad spectrum of diseases. Conceptual discussion is then followed by the review of the practical application of related nursing care measures.

All the body systems are addressed in individual chapters, as are the more specialized areas of female reproductive/maternity, mental health, and pediatrics.

Each chapter concludes with a number of sample questions that are written to mimic the NCLEX style and test the reader's mastery of the subject. Following each set of questions are the answers and rationales for those questions giving the reader a powerful learning experience.

There are 5 comprehensive practice tests at the end of this text comprised of 100 questions similar in content and style to the types of questions asked on the actual licensure exam. Each question has been "coded" for the student in the areas of Nursing Process, Category of Client Need (from the NCLEX Test Plan), and subject area. This allows the student to identify individual strengths and weaknesses allowing for maximum focus and efficient use of study time. Answers and rationales for each question follow each test.

The CD-ROM included with this book holds an additional five 100-question tests that allow the student to test their knowledge and test-taking skills in 2 different ways: learning or test mode. In learning mode, immediate feedback is given after each question is answered. The feedback consists of an explanation for the correct answer as well as incorrect answers. If the test mode option is chosen, the student will receive a score after the test is completed. Questions answered incorrectly may be reviewed at this time.

In either mode, once the practice test is completed, the student has the ability to view and print the results broken down into bar graphs that represent the areas of the test plan, subject area, and nursing process. This element gives the student clear and concise presentation for enormous amounts of information that further enhance and maximize study time.

The concept, scope, and design of this text represent a commitment, through continuing education, to help the graduate LPN/LVN reach a full professional potential. Good luck on your NCLEX-PN® Examination!

Acknowledgments

I have conducted LPN/VN review classes for many years. Thank you to each and every one of the participants in these classes. You have been an inspiration to me. You have shared with me things that have been helpful in passing the licensure exam. This book would not have been written without your feedback.

Judith C. Miller, MS, RN

Contributors

TEST ITEM WRITERS

Lenore Boris, RN, BSN, MS, JD
New York State Public Employees Federation Organizer
Albany, New York

Teresa Burkhalter, RN, BS, MSN
Nursing Faculty
Technical College of the Lowcountry
Beaufort, South Carolina

Judith M. Hall, RNC, MSN, IBCLC, ICCE, FACCE
Lactation Consultant and Childbirth Educator
Fredericksberg, Virginia

Carol Nelson, RN, BSN, MSN
Spokane Community College
Spokane, Washington

REVIEWERS

Terry Ardoin, RN, CCM
Louisiana Technical College
Charles B. Coreil Campus
Ville Platte, Louisiana

Mary E. Arnold, RN, BSN, MA
Director VOCN Program
Blinn College Bryan Campus
Bryan, Texas

Gyl Ann Burkhard, RN, BSN, MS
Instructor
OCM BOCES
Syracuse, New York

Teresa Burkhalter, RN, BS, MSN
Nursing Faculty
Technical College of the Lowcountry
Beaufort, South Carolina

Esther Gonzales, RN, MSN, MSEd.
Del Mar College
Corpus Christi, Texas

Bonnie Grusk, RN, MSN
Continuing Education Coordinator for Health Professions
Illinois Valley Community College
Oglesby, Illinois

Sheila Guidry, RN, LPN, BSN, DSN, PhD.
Wallace Community College
Dothan, Alabama

Carol Nelson, RN, BSN, MSN
Spokane Community College
Spokane, Washington

Linda Walline
Associate Dean of Instruction
Central Community College
Grand Island, Nebraska

Chapter 1

How to Prepare for NCLEX-PN®

QUESTIONS YOU MIGHT HAVE ABOUT THE EXAMINATION

The practice of nursing is regulated by the states to assure the public that only those nurses who have the necessary knowledge and skills are licensed to practice. One requirement for becoming a *licensed practical/vocational nurse* (LPN/LVN) is graduation from an approved school of practical/vocational nursing. Another requirement is passing an examination. All of the states have agreed to use the same examination, NCLEX-PN®. The NCLEX-PN® is designed to assess the candidate's ability to apply the knowledge needed for entry-level practical/vocational nursing. Once a candidate passes NCLEX-PN® and meets any other requirements the individual state might have, he or she can become licensed as an LPN/LVN.

WHAT IS THE NATIONAL COUNCIL OF STATE BOARDS OF NURSING?

The National Council of State Boards of Nursing is a council made up of state boards of nursing from all of the states and territories of the United States. The members of this group have decided to use the same examination as one of the requirements for state licensure. The examination is developed by nurses who are experts in nursing and item writing and who have an in-depth understanding of what practical/vocational nurses need to know.

Every three years, the National Council of State Boards of Nursing studies LPN/LVNs who are newly licensed to see what tasks they are doing and what knowledge and skills are required for them to do their jobs. The blueprint or outline for the licensure examination is developed after analyzing the results of the study. The examination is developed to ensure that new graduates have the knowledge and judgment-making ability that is necessary to function in the workplace as an LPN/LVN.

WHAT IS THE CURRENT TEST PLAN?

The current test plan went into effect in April 2002. The test plan that will go into effect April 1, 2002, has the same structure and the same percentage of questions in each area as the previous test plan. The test plan, or blueprint, for the examination determines what percent of questions will be in what area. The test plans are available to the public and can be obtained from the National Council of State Boards of Nursing. The framework for the test plan revolves around *client needs* because it provides a universal structure for nursing competencies and actions for a variety of clients in a variety of settings. Integrated concepts and processes are threaded throughout the categories of client needs because they are basic to the practice of nursing. Table 1.1 lists the basic categories, subcategories, and integrated concepts and processes.

The first category, Safe, Effective Care Environment has been divided into two sections. The first is called coordinated care and includes items related to legal and ethical concerns such as informed consent, client rights, confidentiality, advance directives, ethical practice, and organ donation. Coordinated care also includes practice concerns such as case management, setting priorities, consultation with health care team members, referral process, resource management (making client care assignments), supervision, incident/irregular occurrence reports, and continuous quality improvement. The second section under Safe, Effective Care Environment is called safety and infection control and includes such topics as accident and error prevention, medical and surgical asepsis, standard (universal) and other precautions, handling hazardous and infectious materials, proper use of restraints, and disaster planning.

The Health Promotion and Maintenance category is also divided into two sections. The first is growth and development through the life span and contains questions relating to growth and development from the fetus to older adult including pregnancy, labor and delivery, post-partum and newborn care. It also includes normal growth and development of infants, children, and adults, including the elderly. Family planning and human sexuality are included. The second section under health promotion and maintenance is prevention and early detection of disease. Questions related to disease prevention may include immunization and health promotion efforts such as life style changes and health screening such as self-breast examination and self-testicular exam. Also included are questions on techniques for collecting physical data.

The third category, psychosocial integrity, has two sections. The first is coping and adaptation. This category includes questions that relate to the client's ability to cope with and adapt to illness or stressful events. Questions might be related to grief and loss, situational role changes, unexpected body image changes (such as amputation, mastectomy, or colostomy). Therapeutic communication, mental health concepts, and behavior management are included. End-of-life issues and religious and spiritual influences on health are also included in this section. The second section under psychosocial integrity is psychosocial adaptation. This section includes concepts related to the care of clients with acute or chronic mental illness and cognitive psychosocial disturbances. Questions may relate to the care of clients who have been victims of elder or child abuse/neglect or sexual abuse. There also might be questions related to chemical dependency. Crisis intervention and therapeutic environment can also be included.

Table 1.1 NCLEX-PN® Test Plan

A. Safe, effective care environment
   1. Coordinated care (6–12% of total questions)
   2. Safety and infection control (7–13% of total questions)
B. Health promotion and maintenance
   3. Growth and development through the life span (4–10% of total questions)
   4. Prevention and early detection of disease (4–10% of total questions)
C. Psychosocial integrity
   5. Coping and adaptation (6–12% of total questions)
   6. Psychosocial adaptation (4–10% of total questions)
D. Physiological integrity
   7. Basic care and comfort (10–16%) of total questions
   8. Pharmacological and parenteral therapies (5–11% of total questions)
   9. Reduction of risk potential (11–17% of total questions)
  10. Physiological adaptation (13–19% of total questions)

Integrated concepts and processes include:

clinical problem solving (nursing process)	caring
communication and documentation	cultural awareness
teaching/learning	self-care

Adapted from the NCLEX-PN® Test Plan for the National Council Licensure Examination for Practical/Vocational Nurses, April 2001.

The fourth and largest category is physiological integrity (four sections). The first is basic care and comfort. Questions might relate to helping clients with activities of daily living, using assistive devices (canes, crutches, walkers, or a Hoyer lift); caring for clients who have contact lenses, hearing aids, or artificial eyes; providing personal hygiene; providing for rest and sleep; positioning clients; and transfer techniques, body mechanics, and concepts related to mobility and immobility. Also included are questions on nutrition, oral hydration and tube feedings, and elimination including catheters and enemas. There might be questions on palliative care, nonpharmacological pain interventions, and teaching self-care, such as ostomy care and pain management techniques. The second section under physiological integrity is pharmacological and parenteral therapies. This section includes administering medications and monitoring clients who are receiving parenteral therapies. Questions might relate to the actions of medications as well as expected effects, side effects, and untoward effects. The third section is reduction of risk potential. These questions relate to reducing the client's potential for developing complications or health problems related to treatments, procedures, or existing conditions. In order to answer these questions correctly, you need to understand basic pathophysiology. This knowledge includes topics such as diagnostic tests, therapeutic procedures, surgery, health alterations, how to prevent related complications, lab values, and the care of clients with drainage tubes, closed wound drainage, and water seal systems. The fourth and final section is physiological adaptation. Questions relate to caring for clients with acute, chronic, or life-threatening physical health conditions. In order to correctly answer questions in this area, you need to understand alterations in body systems, basic pathophysiology, fluid and electrolyte imbalances, radiation therapy, and hemodynamics. There might be questions relating to respiratory care, suctioning, oxygen, infectious diseases, an unexpected response to therapies, medical emergencies, and CPR. Other topics that might be included are heat and cold, dialysis, wound and pressure ulcer care, newborn phototherapy, the application of dressings, and vital signs.

Concepts and processes integrated throughout the exam questions include the clinical problem-solving process (nursing process), caring, communication and documentation, cultural awareness, self-care, and teaching/learning.

HOW DO I APPLY TO TAKE THE EXAMINATION?

You will need to apply to the state board of nursing in the state in which you wish to be licensed. This process involves completing the application forms, having your school of nursing send transcripts, and sending the required fees to the state board and the testing service. One fingerprint currently is required. Starting October 1, 2002, the new test service vendor will require two fingerprints. A passport photograph is usually required, as well. When the State Board of Nursing gives approval, the testing service will be notified. If you have paid your fees to the testing service, they will send you an "Authorization to Test" (ATT) notice along with your identification number and a list of test sites. Your Authorization to Test is valid for several months. The exact amount of time varies from state to state, so check your notice very carefully. If you do not test within the authorization period, you must apply and pay fees all over again.

The exam is administered at selected Sylvan Learning Centers through September 30, 2002. Starting October 1, 2002, the test will be administered at Pearson Professional Centers. It is your responsibility to call the desired testing center and schedule the exam. Note that you do not need to take the exam at a testing center in the state in which you wish to be licensed. The computer sends the results to the state where you have sent your credentials. The first-time candidate is guaranteed to be given a testing date within 30 days. Those who are repeating the exam might have to wait longer to be scheduled. During peak testing times, most test centers will be open evenings and weekends. If after you have scheduled the exam you find that you need to change the date, you can do so without penalty up to three business days before the scheduled appointment.

WHAT TYPES OF QUESTIONS ARE ON THE EXAM?

All questions are multiple-choice questions with only one correct answer. There is no credit for the second-best answer. Each item stands alone. The scenario that describes the client situation and the answer choices all appear on one computer screen (see Figure 1.1).

DO I HAVE TO KNOW A LOT ABOUT COMPUTERS TO TAKE THE TEST?

It is not necessary to be a computer expert to take the exam. There is a tutorial before the exam starts to help you become comfortable with the computer. You can also go to the National Council of State Boards of Nursing Web site (*www.ncsbn.org*) and do a tutorial before going to take the test. A mouse is used to select the correct answer. You have a chance to change your answer, if necessary, before going on to the next question. Once you confirm

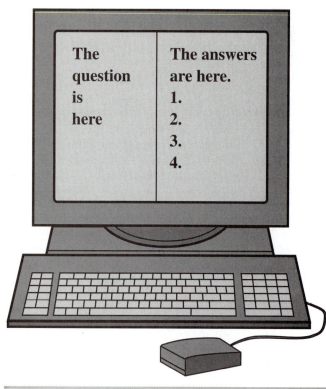

FIGURE 1.1 NCLEX-PN® computer screen

clearly that you cannot answer questions at the "passing" level. If you can successfully answer questions that are well above the passing level, you will answer fewer questions; conversely, if you cannot successfully answer questions that are well below the passing level, you will also answer fewer questions.

You will answer between 85 and 205 questions depending on how well you perform, which includes 25 experimental ("try out") questions. The purpose of the experimental questions is to be sure that all questions that count for your license are good questions that are accurate and statistically correct. These experimental questions are mixed in with real questions. You have no way of knowing which questions are experimental and which questions are real, so you must do your best on all of the questions.

The minimum number of questions that a candidate can take is 85. There is no minimum amount of time. The exam can take a maximum of five hours or 205 questions. Most candidates will not take the maximum time or the maximum number of questions. If you are answering questions that are close to the passing level, either just above or just below, you will answer more questions until you prove that you can consistently answer questions well above or well below the passing level or until you run out of questions or time.

your answer and it is recorded, you cannot go back to that question. You may use the drop-down calculator on the computer for math problems. You do not have to use the calculator. You may not bring your own calculator to the testing center.

HOW IS THE EXAM SCORED?

The exam is administered on a computer using a program called *computerized adaptive testing*. You will get questions that are tailored to how you are performing. Each candidate, therefore, takes a unique test. The questions, however, are drawn from the same test pool and conform to the test plan as described earlier.

The specific questions you are given depend upon the answers you gave to the previous question. As you answer questions correctly, you are given more difficult questions to determine your ability level. When you can successfully answer questions at the "passing" level, the test terminates. The test also terminates if you show

CAN I TAKE A BREAK?

After two hours, there is an automatic 10-minute break. You can go to the bathroom, walk outside the building, and eat a snack. At the end of $3\frac{1}{2}$ hours, you will be given an option to take another break. You can choose to take it or not, depending on how you feel. If necessary during the test, you can take a break. The clock keeps running during your breaks, however.

WHEN WILL I KNOW IF I PASSED?

The State Board of Nursing should receive notification of your results within three business days of the day you take the test. You are notified by the State Board of Nursing, usually within two to three weeks. You will not know if you passed when you leave the testing center. Most candidates feel very unsure after taking the test. This reaction is normal.

Tips for Test Taking

Read and review the tips that follow to help you do your best on the examination.

LOOK FOR KEY CONCEPTS

Read the question carefully to determine the key concepts. Key concepts include determining who the client is, what the problem is, what specifically is asked about the problem, and what the time frame is.

An elderly woman who has senile dementia is admitted to the long-term care facility by her son. During the admission process, the son says to the nurse, "Did I do the right thing to bring my mother here?" Which initial response by the nurse will be most helpful?
1. Say to the woman, "You will like it here. We will take very good care of you."
2. Ask the woman if she is comfortable or if there is anything that can be done to make her feel more at home.
3. Tell the son, "You made the right decision. We will take good care of her."
4. Say to the son, "It must have been very difficult to make this decision."

In this question, *the client is the son* of the elderly woman. *The problem is the son's concern* about whether he should have brought his mother to the long-term care facility. What is *asked about the problem is which initial response by the nurse is most helpful*. The *time frame is the day of admission*. All of these factors must be considered when choosing the correct answer.

Look at the answer choices in light of the key concepts in the question. The client is the son; therefore, answers 1 and 2 cannot be correct. The time is during the admission process. The questions asks for an initial response. Initially, the goal is to open communication. Choice 3 does not open communication. Choice 4 is an empathic answer that will open communication.

LOOK FOR KEY WORDS

Look for words in the question that focus on the issue. There might be words such as *early* or *late* symptoms; *most* or *least* likely to occur. These words are critical to understanding the question and are very easy to miss unless you practice looking for them.

When the question asks for the *initial* nursing action, remember that initial means first—and think of the first step in the nursing process, which is assessment. Assess before acting. Sometimes you will have been given enough assessment data that you can take an action. When the question asks for an initial action, always ask yourself whether there is any relevant assessment data needed. Then, ask whether there is an emergency action you should take.

When the question asks what action is *essential* for the nurse to take, think safety. Essential means that you must do it, and it cannot be left undone. When setting priorities, remember Maslow's hierarchy of needs (Figure 1.2). Remember, "Keep them breathing, keep them safe." It is also

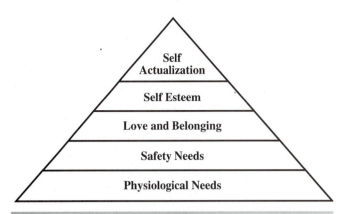

FIGURE 1.2 Maslow's Hierarchy of Needs

important to consider which actions will help prevent complications.

UTILIZE TEST-TAKING STRATEGIES

Using the following test-taking strategies will also maximize your success.

The Odd Man Wins

The option that is most different in length, style, or content is usually correct. The correct answer is often the longest or the shortest. Remember also that if two or three answers say the same thing in different words, they cannot both be correct—so neither one is correct (poor appetite and anorexia, for example).

Opposites

When two answers are opposites, such as hypotension and hypertension or tachycardia and bradycardia, the answer is usually one of the two.

An adult is admitted in shock. Which assessment finding would the nurse most expect to find in this client?
1. Elevated blood pressure
2. Blood pressure below normal
3. Slow pulse
4. Flushed color

Note that choices 1 and 2 are opposites. The answer will most likely be one of these. The answer is 2.

Repeated Words

Words from the question are repeated in the answer. Frequently, the same word or a synonym will be in both the question and the answer.

An adult client is to have a liver scan. Which explanation is most appropriate for the nurse to give the client?

---

1. You will be given a radiopaque substance to swallow before x-rays are taken.
2. You will be given a laxative the night before the x-rays are taken.
3. You will be given a radioisotope that will be picked up by the liver and can be measured by a scanner.
4. An iodine dye will be injected into your vein and will outline the liver.

Note that the question asks about a liver *scan,* and the third choice talks about a *scanner.* Also note that the correct answer is the longest. It takes more words to make the answer correct.

Absolutes

Absolutes tend to make answers wrong. Always, never, all, and none are usually not correct statements. Qualified answers such as usually, frequently, and often are usually correct statements.

A 65-year-old man stopped taking high blood pressure medication because he no longer had headaches. What is most important for the nurse to teach him about the symptoms of hypertension?
The symptoms
1. occur only when there is danger of a stroke.
2. are sometimes not evident.
3. occur only when there is kidney involvement.
4. occur only with malignant hypertension.

In the question, answers 1, 3, and 4 are absolutes and 2 is much more qualified. The correct answer is 2. You might also note that 2 is the shortest answer.

Becoming aware of the structure of questions and utilizing these test-taking strategies can help you answer questions more accurately. You will still need to study, however, and you should still understand the material. These test-taking strategies are not a substitute for knowing the material.

Read the Question Carefully

Read the entire question and all of the answers carefully before selecting the correct response. If the answer does not appear obvious to you, note the key words and use these test-taking strategies. Eliminate answers that cannot be correct. From the responses left, look at the data in the question and see which answer most correctly relates to the data. Remember, the answer must relate to the question. If you really do not know the answer, make an educated guess and move on to the next question. You cannot go back to any question.

You will be given something to write on during the test—most likely a dry erase board. When you get into the exam room, write on the board any things you are trying to remember, such as lab values, conversion facts (lbs to Kg; oz to ml, and so on). Use the writing board for any calculations and to write down key words for a question if necessary.

Tips on How to Prepare for NCLEX-PN®

You have completed a nursing program, so you should already be familiar with the material. You will need to review the material and practice many multiple choice questions before you are ready to take the exam, however.

REVIEW CONTENT

You will need to review content in an organized fashion. This book will help you do that. As you review the material in the book, note any areas that are particularly difficult for you or that you do not remember well. You will need to put more effort into these topics. As you are reviewing, remember to relate pathophysiology to nursing care. Be sure to understand the "whys" of procedures, treatments, and nursing actions. Consider priorities when reviewing nursing care. Ask yourself which of the actions listed is of highest priority.

Prepare a calendar and schedule for review. On a calendar, schedule which content areas you will review on which days. Allow time for both content review and multiple-choice questions.

Try to study in an environment where you can concentrate. If you cannot study in your home, go to the public library. You need uninterrupted study time.

PRACTICE MULTIPLE-CHOICE QUESTIONS

The examination consists of multiple-choice questions. You need two things to pass the examination. One is knowledge of nursing care. The second is the ability to answer multiple-choice questions concerning that knowledge.

You should plan to practice several thousand multiple-choice questions as part of your preparation before taking the examination. You should be consistently answering correctly 75 percent of the questions in the review books. Answering many multiple-choice questions not only increases your skill in answering multiple-choice questions, but it also helps you review the content and look at the same information from different perspectives. Be sure to read all the answers and rationales, even for the questions you answered correctly. You need to be sure that you chose the correct answer for the right reasons. You can learn a lot from reading the rationales. If you notice that you are missing several questions on the same subject, then you should review the subject again, clarifying any areas about which you are confused.

If you have a computer available, you might want to practice at least a few questions on the computer. Answering questions on the computer might make you more comfortable with the computer and the screen. It is not essential to practice on a computer, however. The key point is that you practice thousands of questions before you go to the exam. You want to be well prepared.

PRACTICE STRESS-REDUCTION STRATEGIES

When taking the exam, you might find that you become anxious. You should practice a stress-reduction technique to use during the exam. Some candidates find that closing their eyes and taking several slow, deep breaths helps clear the mind when stress is rising. Some candidates have found that closing the eyes and taking a "mini vacation" to the beach or the mountains or to their favorite rose garden might help reduce anxiety during the exam. Another technique that candidates have found helpful is getting up and taking a short walk when stress is building and the mind does not seem to function well.

The key to implementing these stress-reduction techniques is first learning to recognize the signs of anxiety that will keep you from thinking well and

secondly to practice whatever technique you choose during your study sessions. As with any skill, you need to practice it before you become good at it.

When you are practicing multiple-choice questions, note when you start to miss a lot of questions. What sensations are you experiencing at this time? How many questions have you done already? How long have you been sitting? Learn to recognize the clues that your body and mind are giving you that suggest you need to take a brief break. Utilize a stress-reduction strategy. Practice several techniques and see which one works best for you and then use that one when your mind starts to wander during study.

Do not use alcohol and sedatives as a way to reduce stress before or during the exam. These substances might reduce stress, but they also interfere with thinking and problem solving.

EXAM DAY

Plan to spend all five hours at the exam. If you do not take the maximum time, consider it a gift and do something special for yourself. Do not have someone waiting for you outside the testing center because it might make you feel as if you have to hurry during the test. You want to be able to take as much time as you need to read the questions carefully before answering them.

Eat breakfast. Remember that your brain needs fuel. You cannot think well if your brain cells do not have any fuel.

Dress in layers. The room might be cooler or warmer than you like, and the temperature might change. Dress comfortably.

Bring two forms of identification with you to the testing center—one of which is a picture ID. Also bring your authorization to test letter from the testing service.

When you get to the testing center, you will be asked for a picture ID. They will take your thumb print and your picture. This picture goes with your exam results (it does not go on your license).

Chapter 2

Essential Concepts

CLINICAL PROBLEM SOLVING (NURSING PROCESS) OVERVIEW

The nursing process is a series of interrelated steps that help the nurse provide care to clients. This process has been defined in several different ways with different labels applied to the steps, but all describe essentially the same process.

STEPS OF THE NURSING PROCESS (FIGURE 2.1)

A. Assessment (data collection)
1. Subjective data
a. Data from the client's perspective: "My incision hurts."
b. Data obtained by interviewing and listening to the client
2. Objective data
a. Observable and measurable data from the health care worker's perspective: blood pressure, weight, skin lesions, and so on
b. Data obtained from physical examination, laboratory reports, and so on
3. Nurse must determine if more data is needed
4. Nurse should distinguish between relevant and irrelevant data
B. Diagnosis (analysis and data interpretation)
1. Nursing diagnosis different from medical diagnosis
2. The nursing diagnosis is focused on the client's responses to actual or potential health problems; the medical diagnosis is focused on the illness or disease process.
3. Interpretation of data to identify problems and potential problems
a. The actual nursing diagnosis relates to problems that exist now.
b. The risk nursing diagnosis identifies problems the client is at risk for if some preventive action is not taken.
4. In many facilities, the LPN/LVN collaborates with the *registered nurse* (RN) to develop the nursing diagnoses.
C. Planning
1. Putting the nursing diagnoses in priority order
2. Determining the short- and long-term goals for the client
3. Identifying outcome measurements to determine whether the goals are met
a. Outcome criteria should be measurable; for example, "The client will report that the pain is less than 2 on a pain scale of 1 to 10," not "The client will feel better."

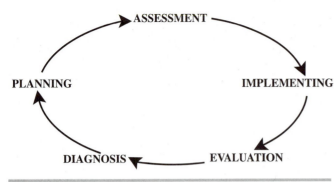

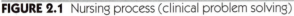

FIGURE 2.1 Nursing process (clinical problem solving)

    b. Outcome criteria should have a time limit and be realistic; for example, "The client will walk the length of the hall twice by Friday," or "The client will gain two pounds within the next week."

    4. Developing specific interventions to meet the goals

    5. Recording the plan of care in the client's record

D. Implementing
    1. Putting the plan of care into effect
    2. Involves performing many skills and procedures
    3. Reporting of activities and findings
    4. Documentation of activities
      a. Client's condition prior to intervention
      b. Intervention performed
      c. Client's response to intervention

E. Evaluation
    1. Determining if the client's goals are met, not met, or partially met
    2. If the goal is met, determine whether there is a need for continued nursing action.
    3. If the goal was not met or only partially met, determine why it was not met.
    4. Evaluation is an ongoing process; the nurse should continually be evaluating data during all steps of the nursing process.

Management of Care

CLIENT RIGHTS

A. The client has rights, according to the Patient's Bill of Rights as set forth by the American Hospital Association.
    1. Right to considerate and respectful care
    2. Right to understandable information about diagnosis, treatment, and prognosis
    3. Right to know who is caring for him or her and to know if any persons caring for him or her are students or other trainees
    4. Right to make decisions about the plan of care prior to and during the course of treatment and the right to refuse treatment
    5. Right to have advanced directives
    6. Right to privacy
    7. Right to expect that all communications and records will be kept confidential
    8. Right to review records pertaining to his or her medical care and to have the information explained and interpreted where necessary
    9. Right to be made aware of business relationships among the hospital, educational institutions, and other health care providers or payers that might influence treatment and care
    10. Right to consent or refuse to consent to participation in proposed research studies and to have those studies fully explained prior to consent
    11. Right to expect reasonable continuity of care both while in the hospital and after hospital care is no longer appropriate
    12. Right to be informed of hospital policies related to patient care, including the right to be informed of resources available for resolving disputes, grievances, and conflicts
    13. Right to be informed of the hospital's charges and available payment options

B. Nurses have an obligation to be sure that the client's rights are not violated.

DELEGATION AND SUPERVISION

A. Delegation is the process of transferring a selected nursing task to an individual who is competent to perform that task.
B. The Nurse Practice Act in every state defines what tasks can be delegated.
C. When delegating, the nurse should:
    1. Be sure the task is one that can be delegated.
    2. Match the task to the delegatee.
      a. Is the delegatee able to perform the task?
      b. Can the delegatee legally perform the task?
    3. Be specific in instructions, especially when delegating to unlicensed assistive personnel.

D. Although a task has been delegated to someone else, the nurse maintains accountability for the nursing care given to the client.
E. The nurse has an obligation to follow through and to be sure that the delegated tasks were performed.
F. When supervising other personnel, the nurse should clearly communicate the tasks to be done.
G. If the nurse observes a problem, it is usually best to communicate directly to the person involved first; if the problem is not resolved, then notify the person next in the chain of command.

INCIDENT REPORTS

A. Incident reports should be filed whenever a situation arises that could or did cause client harm, such as medication errors, client falls, and so on.

B. Purposes of incident reports
  1. Inform the facility's administration of the incident so that risk-management personnel can consider changes that might be needed to prevent future incidents.
  2. Alert the facility's insurance company to a potential claim and the need for investigation of the incident.
C. Incident reports are not part of the client record.
D. Reports should include the facts about what happened.
  1. Who was present
  2. What happened in the exact time sequence
  3. What was done about the incident
E. Incident reports should not include the nurse's opinions about the cause of the incident or the response to the incident; incident reports are factual accounts only.

Basic Hygienic Care

BATHING

A. Not all clients need a bath every day. Elderly persons who have dry, thin skin who do not perspire profusely and do not get dirty might not need a complete bath daily. Nurses use judgment to determine how frequently to give a bath.
B. Types of baths
  1. A bed bath: given to persons who must remain in bed and/or are unable to bathe themselves
  2. An assisted bath: the persons can perform part of the bath; the nurse assists with what the client cannot do.
  3. A tub bath or shower: might be ordered if the client is able and the condition allows
C. Procedure
  1. Use warm water.
  2. Start with the eyes and face.
  3. Change the water when cool.
  4. Bathe the perineal area last; wear sterile clothes while giving perineal care.
  5. Inspect skin during the bath.
  6. Do range of motion (ROM) exercises as appropriate during the bath.
  7. Use bath time as an opportunity to communicate with the client.
D. Skin care
  1. Use soap sparingly and rinse well with warm water; soap dries skin.
  2. Lotions prevent dry skin; powders tend to cake and should be used sparingly.

  3. Gentle massage of pressure areas increases circulation to the area and keeps skin healthy.
  4. Pat dry, do not rub; rubbing might cause damage to delicate skin.
E. Mouth care
  1. Routine mouth care: brush and floss teeth, use mouthwash
  2. Special mouth care
    a. Routine care more frequently
    b. Glycerin and lemon swabs or hydrogen peroxide
    c. Viscous lidocaine mouthwash for persons with stomatitis (lidocaine is a local anesthetic)
  3. Dentures
    a. Hold dentures over a basin lined with a towel and filled with water to lessen the chance of breakage if dropped.
    b. Hold dentures with gauze or a washcloth to prevent dropping.
    c. Clean with tepid, not hot, water using the client's choice of dentrifice.
    d. Store dentures in a denture cup with tepid water; place in the drawer of bedside stand.
F. Foot care
  1. Wash and dry feet carefully, especially between the toes.
  2. Apply cotton between the toes if indicated to keep area dry (diabetic client).
  3. Order needed to cut nails; cut straight across

Measurement of Vital Signs

TEMPERATURE
(see Table 2.1)

A. Oral
   1. Mercury thermometer (seldom used because of the danger of mercury toxicity): leave in place 2 to 5 minutes
   2. Electronic thermometer: leave in place until reading indicated
   3. If the client is eating, drinking, or smoking, wait 10 minutes before taking temperature.
   4. Contraindications
      a. Client receiving oxygen
      b. Client irrational or unconscious or having seizures
      c. Client less than 5 years old
      d. Client is breathing through mouth
      e. Recent oral surgery or mouth trauma
B. Rectal
   1. Mercury thermometer held in place 3 to 4 minutes
   2. Electronic thermometer held in place until reading indicated
   3. Lubricate with water-soluble lubricant before inserting; insert $1\frac{1}{2}$ inches.
   4. Contraindications
      a. Perineal or rectal surgery
      b. Diseases of the rectum; severe hemorrhoids
      c. Diarrhea
C. Axillary
   1. Mercury thermometer held in place 10 minutes
   2. Electronic thermometer held in place until reading indicated
   3. Pat the axilla dry before inserting; hold the arm close to the client's side.

PULSE

A. The pulse measures the beat of the heart; note the rate, rhythm, and strength of the heart beat.
B. Sites
   1. Apical: over the apex of the heart; listen with stethoscope; count one full minute
   2. Radial artery: feel with fingertips
   3. Temporal artery: feel with fingertips
   4. Carotid artery: feel with fingertips
   5. Femoral artery: feel with fingertips
   6. Popliteal artery: feel with fingertips
   7. Pedal: feel with fingertips
C. Apical-radial pulse
   1. One person takes the apical pulse while a second person takes the radial pulse at

same time; count one full minute.
   2. Radial is never more than apical.

RESPIRATION

A. Process of inhaling and exhaling or moving air in and out of lungs; one inhalation and one exhalation is one respiration
B. Note the rate, rhythm, and depth of respirations; count for one full minute if an irregular or abnormal rate is present.
C. Respirations are best measured when the client is not aware that respirations are being counted.
D. Variations
   1. Apnea: absence of breathing
   2. Tachypnea: rapid breathing
   3. Bradypnea: slow breathing
   4. Stertorous: noisy breathing
   5. Hyperpnea: deep respirations
   6. Cheyne-Stokes: periods of apnea alternating with hyperpnea; often precedes death
   7. Dyspnea: difficulty breathing
   8. Orthopnea: must sit up to breathe
   9. Kussmaul's: paroxysms of deep breathing; seen in metabolic acidosis

BLOOD PRESSURE

A. Force exerted against the walls of the arteries
   1. Systolic is force exerted against the arterial walls while the heart is beating.
   2. Diastolic is the force exerted against the arterial walls while the heart is at rest.
B. Measured at the brachial artery or popliteal artery
C. Cuff must be proper size for individual
   1. Cuff should occupy two-thirds of upper arm
   2. A cuff that is too small causes the reading to be higher than it actually is.
   3. A cuff that is too large causes the reading to be lower that it actually is.
D. Variations
   1. Hypotension: blood pressure lower than normal
   2. Hypertension: blood pressure higher than 140/90 in an adult
E. Pulse pressure: the difference between systolic and diastolic pressures
   1. Pulse pressure increased in intracranial pressure
   2. Pulse pressure decreased in shock

Table 2.1 Normal Vital Signs

Age	Temperature	Pulse	Respiration	Blood Pressure
Infant	Oral: 98.6°F 37°C 97°–99°F Rectal: 99.2°F 7.3°C 98°–100°F Axillary: 96°–98°F	110–160 irregular	32–60 irregular	75/49 Younger than one year, arm and thigh the same; older than 1 year, systolic in leg higher than arm by 10–40 mm Hg
Child (2–6 years)	see above	90–110	20–30	85/60 to 100/70
Child (6–12 years)	see above	70–100	18–30	95/56 to 108/68
Adult	see above	60–100	12–18	90/60 to 140/90

Prevention of Infection

CHAIN OF EVENTS LEADING TO INFECTION

A. For infection to occur, all of the following must be in place (Figure 2.2):
  1. Causative agent
  2. Reservoir
  3. Portal of exit
  4. Mode of transmission
  5. Portal of entry
  6. Susceptible host
B. To prevent infection, the nurse must interfere with one or more of the links in the chain of events.

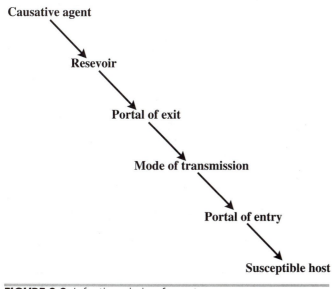

FIGURE 2.2 Infection chain of events

ASEPSIS

A. Medical asepsis
  1. Clean technique
  2. Reduces microorganisms
  3. Hand washing (Table 2.2)
    a. Most important nursing action to prevent nosocomial (hospital-acquired) infection
    b. Hands should be washed before and after ALL client contacts.
  4. Universal precautions for all clients at all times (Table 2.3)
  5. Isolation when indicated
B. Surgical asepsis
  1. Sterile technique
  2. Destroys pathological organisms
  3. Physical barriers
  4. Sterile fields (Table 2.4)
C. Universal precautions break the chain by preventing the mode of transmission (Table 2.3)

Table 2.2 Handwashing

- Remove jewelry; watch can be pushed up above the wrist to mid-forearm level.
- Assess hands for breaks in the skin, hangnails, and heavily soiled areas.
- Turn on the water and adjust the flow and temperature; temperature should be warm, not hot.
- Wet hands and lower arms by holding under running water; keep hands and forearms in the down position.
- Apply about 5 ml of liquid soap and lather thoroughly.
- Thoroughly rub hands together for 10-15 seconds; interlace fingers to clean between fingers; be sure to scrub under and around fingernails and knuckles.
- Rinse with hands in the down position.
- Blot hands and wrists and forearms with a paper towel to dry thoroughly; discard paper towel in a waste receptacle.
- Turn off the faucet with a clean, dry paper towel.

Table 2.3 Standard (Universal) Precautions

- Dispose of sharp items in puncture-resistant containers.
- Do not recap needles.
- Wear protective barriers (gloves, gowns, masks, and eye wear) when at risk for exposure to body fluids.
- Clean blood spills with soap and water or household bleach (1:10 dilution).
- Wash hands before and after every client contact.
- Use barriers when performing CPR.

Table 2.4 Guidelines for a Sterile Field

- Never turn your back on a sterile field.
- Avoid talking over a sterile field
- Keep all sterile objects within view.
- Objects below the waist are not sterile.
- Moisture carries organisms through a barrier.
- Open sterile packages away from, not over, a sterile field.

Table 2.5 Transmission-Based Precautions

Category	Private Room	Gloves	Gown	Mask
Contact	If possible; might be with someone with the same condition	Yes	If any drainage of any kind	Not needed
Droplet	If possible; separation of 3 feet always needed	Not needed	Not needed	Yes.
Airborne	Yes. Negative air pressure with 6-12 air changes per hour; door must be kept closed and air must be discharged outdoors or must use a HEPA filter	Not needed	Not needed	N95 respirator required for known or suspected tuberculosis and measles or varicella if not immune

D. Transmission-based precautions (Table 2.5)
   1. Used in addition to universal precautions
   2. Based on routes of transmission
E. Reverse or protective isolation
   1. Term used to denote isolation precautions used to protect the client
   2. Used when the client is immunocompromised, such as when receiving cancer chemotherapy, steroids, immunosuppressants, or in persons who have *acquired immunodeficiency syndrome* (AIDS)

Immobility

A. Problems resulting from immobility (Table 2.6)
   1. Muscle atrophy (decrease in muscle strength and size) due to a lack of exercise
   2. Joint contractures due to a lack of joint movement
   3. Osteoporosis due to not enough weight bearing on bones
   4. Urinary tract stones due to osteoporosis and dehydration
   5. Orthostatic hypotension due to a prolonged recumbent position causing vessels to lose tone
   6. Venous thrombosis due to slowed venous return from little movement of legs
   7. Hypostatic pneumonia due to not fully expanding the lungs and maintaining one position, allowing fluid to accumulate in the lungs
   8. Pressure sores (decubitus ulcers): localized areas in which necrosis of skin and subcutaneous tissues have been produced by pressure on bony prominences; pressure causes the compression of small vessels leading to tissue anoxia, ischemia, and necrosis; sloughing and ulceration is followed by invasion of microorganisms causing infection and sepsis, which can invade fascia, muscle, and bone. Common sites include ischial tuberosities if the client sits; trochanters in persons who lie on their sides; sacrum in persons who lie on their backs; knees; malleoli; heels; and elbows.
   9. Urinary incontinence due to a lack of opportunity to void in a normal position
   10. Bowel incontinence and constipation due to decreased activity, diet, and inability to assume normal position for defecation
   11. Psychological deterioration due to isolation and inactivity
   12. External rotation of the hip due to a lack of voluntary muscle control; prolonged supine position
   13. Footdrop (plantar flexion): deformity caused by contraction of both the gastrocnemius and soleus muscles; might be produced by loss of flexibility of the Achilles tendon; if allowed to continue, client will walk on toes without heels touching floor

Table 2.6 Immobility

Problem	Cause	Prevention
Muscle atrophy	Lack of exercise	Active exercise
Joint contracture	Lack of joint motion	Passive range of motion; positioning
Osteoporosis	Insufficient weight bearing; post-menopause	Weight bearing
Urinary tract stones	Immobility; dehydration	Increase fluids; do not give excessive vitamins and minerals; treat *urinary tract infection* (UTI) promptly
Orthostatic hypotension	Recumbent position	Stand-up exercises; tilt table
Venous thrombosis	Slowed venous return; little movement of legs	Exercises; elastic stockings
Hypostatic pneumonia	Maintaining one position; decreased thoracic expansion	Turn, cough, deep breathe
Pressure sores	Pressure; immobility; poor circulation; friction; shearing force; sensory and motor deficits; poor nutrition; edema; infection; aging and debilitation; equipment (casts, traction, and restraints)	Frequent position changes (turn q 2 hours); relieve pressure by using devices such as a gel-type flotation pad; fleeces; waterbeds; alternating pressure mattresses; avoid shearing forces by using a turning sheet and not raising the head of the bed above 30 degrees; proper positioning to relieve pressure on bony prominences; maintain healthy skin; maintain good nutrition
Urinary incontinence	Lack of opportunity	Push fluids; bedpan q 2 hours.; avoid a catheter
Bowel incontinence; constipation	Diet; decreased activity	Fluids; fiber; activity; toilet after meals
Psychological deterioration	Inactivity; isolation	Activity; participation in own care; increase sensory input
External rotation of the hip	Loss of voluntary muscle control; supine position	Place a trochanter roll extending from the crest of the ilium to the mid thigh when the client is lying on his or her back; the trochanter roll serves as a mechanical wedge under the projection of the greater trochanter.
Footdrop (plantar flexion)	Prolonged bed rest and lack of exercise; incorrect positioning in bed; weight of bedding forcing toes into plantar flexion	Keep foot at right angles to the legs by the use of a foot board, pillows, or high-top sneakers; encourage client to flex and extend his or her feet and toes frequently; encourage the client to rotate his or her ankles clockwise and counterclockwise several times every hour.

B. Nursing interventions
  1. Exercises
     a. Purposes
        1) maintain and build muscle strength
        2) maintain joint function
        3) prevent deformity
        4) retrain for neuromuscular coordination
        5) stimulate circulation
        6) build tolerance and endurance
     b. Types of exercises (Table 2.7)
        1) passive
        2) active assistive
        3) active
        4) resistive
        5) isometric or muscle-setting
     c. Types of movements (Table 2.8)
        1) Joints need to be put through a full range of motion, including all types of movement.
        2) Exercises should be done during the bath and several times a day.
        3) Stop exercises if the motion causes pain.

Table 2.7 Types of Exercises

Type	Definition	Purpose
Passive	Exercise carried out by the nurse without assistance from the client	Prevent deformities; maintain circulation
Active-assistive	Exercise carried out by the patient with the assistance of the nurse	Increase muscle strength
Active	Exercise done by the patient without the help of the nurse	Increase muscle strength
Resistive	Active exercise carried out by the patient working against resistance produced by manual or mechanical means	Provide resistance in order to increase muscle power
Isometric or muscle-setting	Performed by client; alternately contracting and relaxing a muscle while keeping the part in a fixed position (Kegel's, quadriceps setting)	Maintain strength when a joint is immobilized; improve muscle tone

Table 2.8 Types of Movement

Abduction:	movement away from the midline of the body
Adduction:	movement toward the midline of the body
Flexion:	bending of the joint so that the angle of the joint diminishes
Extension:	the return movement from flexion; the angle of the joint is increased
Inversion:	movement that turns the sole of the foot inward
Eversion:	movement that turns the sole of the foot outward
Dorsiflexion:	flexing or bending the foot toward the leg
Plantar flexion:	flexing or bending the foot in the direction of the sole
Pronation:	rotating the forearm so that the palm of the hand is down
Supination:	rotating the forearm so that the palm of the hand is up
Rotation:	turning or movement of a part around its axis
internal:	turning inward toward the center
external:	turning outward away from the center

2. Change position every two hours to promote circulation, prevent skin breakdown, and promote respiratory function.
3. Cough, and deep breathe every two hours to promote respiratory function and prevent atelectasis.
4. Sit up if allowed to prevent orthostatic hypotension.
5. Leg exercises and antiembolism stockings to prevent venous stasis and possible thrombosis
6. Encourage fluids if allowed to promote bladder and bowel function.
7. Use the trochanter roll to prevent external rotation of the hip.
8. Provide support to feet to prevent foot drop.

PRESSURE ULCER (DECUBITUS ULCER, OR BEDSORE)

A. Ulcer caused by local interference with the circulation
B. Risk factors
   1. Immobility
   2. Incontinence
   3. Poor nutrition
   4. Poor circulation
   5. Weakened physical condition
   6. Diabetes, neuropathy, peripheral vascular disease, anemia, cortisone therapy

C. Prevention
   1. Keep skin clean and dry; clean soiled skin and urine-contaminated skin.
   2. Use moisturizers on skin.
   3. Massage around bony prominences but not over bony prominences.
   4. Change position frequently; every two hours is usually recommended, but more often might be indicated.
   5. Lift rather than sliding or dragging the client when moving him or her up in bed
   6. Use turning sheets; do not slide clients (sliding causes friction)
   7. ROM exercises and ambulation if possible to promote circulation
   8. Avoid pressure from appliances such as braces.
   9. Do not use donut rings because they cut off circulation.
D. Staging of pressure ulcers
   1. Stage I: changes in color (red, blue, or purple); changes in temperature (warm or cool); changes in skin stiffness
   2. Stage II: partial-thickness loss of skin involving epidermis and/or part of dermis
   3. Stage III: full-thickness skin loss involving subcutaneous damage or necrosis
   4. Stage IV: full-thickness skin loss with severe destruction, necrosis, or damage to muscle, bone, or supporting structures
E. Care of pressure ulcer
   1. Goals of treatment
      a. Allow for moist wound healing.
      b. Prevent infection.
      c. Prevent trauma and injury to surrounding skin.
      d. Promote the client's comfort.
   2. Procedures
      a. Damp to dry dressings (gauze dressing applied damp and removed when dry) to debride slough and eschar
      b. Dry to wet dressing impregnated with sodium chloride to draw in wound exudate and decrease bacteria
      c. Apply commercial dressings and preparations as ordered to keep the wound moist, to prevent infection, to promote healing, and to debride the wound.
   3. Record assessment of wound
      a. Note the stage of the pressure ulcer.
      b. Record undermining, pockets, or tracts.
      c. Condition of tissue
      d. Drainage

Positioning

A. General principles
   1. Provide for privacy.
   2. Keep the body in good alignment.
   3. Consider the client's diagnosis and condition when positioning the client, supporting body parts as needed.
   4. Use supports such as pillows, foam wedges, and so on as needed.
   5. Change position often, usually every two hours.
B. Dorsal, supine, horizontal recumbent (on the back)
   1. Head and shoulders usually slightly elevated on pillow
   2. May have small pillow in lumbar curve
   3. Trochanter rolls prevent the external rotation of hips.
   4. Prevent footdrop with a foot board or high-topped sneakers.
C. Prone (on the stomach)
   1. Position provides for extension of the hips and helps prevent hip flexion contractures
   2. Client lies on abdomen with head turned laterally; may have small pillow
   3. May have small pillow just below diaphragm to support lumbar curve, support female breasts, and make breathing easier
   4. Pillow under lower legs flexes knees and reduces plantar flexion; might be contraindicated if client is a lower-leg amputee or has had CVA and is at high risk for hip flexion contracture
D. Side-lying or lateral
   1. Client on side
   2. Pillow under head
   3. Arms should be slightly flexed in front of the body; use a pillow to provide support to the upper arm and shoulder; promotes better chest expansion.
   4. Pillow under upper leg and thigh to provide support and prevent internal rotation and adduction of hip
   5. Pillow behind client's back for additional support
E. Sims position, semiprone (Figure 2.3)
   1. Useful for enemas, vaginal and rectal exams, and drainage of oral secretions from the unconscious client; comfortable position in last trimester of pregnancy
   2. Client lies on the left side with the left thigh slightly flexed and right knee and thigh drawn up
   3. The left arm is drawn behind the body along the back.

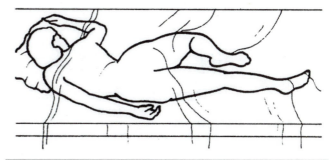

FIGURE 2.3 Sims position

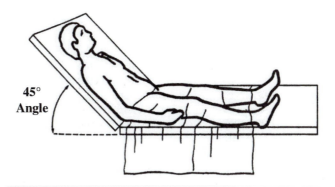

FIGURE 2.4 Semi-Fowler's position

F. Low-Fowler's (semi-reclining)
   1. Useful following head injuries and after craniotomy to decrease intracranial pressure and also following cervical laminectomy to decrease edema formation
   2. Head of the bed is elevated 15 to 30 degrees
   3. Pillows can be placed at the small of the back, under the ankles, under the arms, and under the head of the client if desired.
G. Semi-Fowler's (semi-sitting) (Figure 2.4)
   1. Used post operatively when client has drains (remember the law of gravity); for persons with cardiac conditions; and for persons with respiratory conditions such as pneumonia
   2. Head elevated 45 to 60 degrees
   3. Knees supported in slight flexion
   4. Arms rest at sides
H. High-Fowler's (Figure 2.5)
   1. Used to increase thoracic expansion in conditions such as asthma, *chronic obstructive pulmonary disease* (COPD), or respiratory conditions
   2. Head elevated nearly 90 degrees

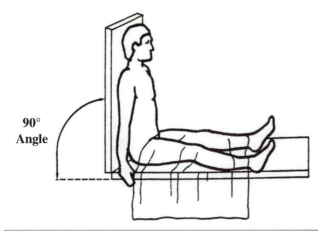

FIGURE 2.5 High Fowler's position

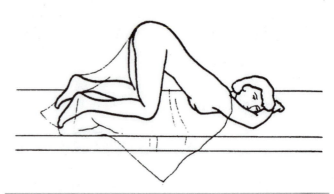

FIGURE 2.6 Knee-chest position

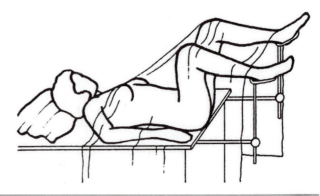

FIGURE 2.7 Lithotomy position

3. Knees slightly flexed
4. Arms supported on pillows or over bed table

I. Shock position
   1. Used for persons in shock to quickly increase circulating volume without compromising respirations
   2. Legs elevated to increase venous return; trunk flat; head on a small pillow

J. Trendelenburg
   1. Traditionally used to treat shock; seldom used now because the abdominal viscera press on the diaphragm and heart
   2. Supine on a surface inclined 45 degrees with the head at the lower end

K. Knee chest (Figure 2.6)
   1. Used for vaginal and rectal exams and rectal procedures such as proctoscopy and sigmoidoscopy
   2. Client lies on abdomen with head turned to one side
   3. Arms are flexed on either side of the head.
   4. Client draws knees up to meet chest; bottom is up in the air
   5. Chest and knees on table with bottom up in the air
   6. Difficult position for client to maintain; client should not be left alone

L. Lithotomy (Figure 2.7)
   1. Used for gynecological exams, childbirth, and perineal surgery
   2. Client lies on back, legs flexed on the thighs, thighs flexed on the abdomen and abducted
   3. Stirrups often used to support the feet and legs
   4. Bring both legs down slowly to prevent hypovolemic shock from blood flowing rapidly into the legs.
   5. If stirrups are used for a prolonged period, as in surgery or delivery, observe for clot formation in the legs.

BODY MECHANICS, TRANSFER, AND AMBULATION TECHNIQUES

A. Principles of body mechanics
   1. Keep your back straight to prevent injury.
   2. Keep your feet separated to provide a wide base of support.
   3. Bend from the hip and knees, not the waist.
   4. Use the longest and strongest muscles.
   5. Use your body weight to help push or pull.
   6. Turn with the whole body; do not twist.
   7. Hold heavy objects close to your body.
   8. Push or pull objects when possible instead of lifting.
   9. Ask for help when needed.
   10. Use turning sheets and mechanical devices when possible.

B. Transfer from bed to chair
   1. Place chair beside the bed on the client's strongest side, facing the foot of the bed.
   2. Stabilize chair and lock wheels on wheel chair
   3. Lower bed, lock wheels of bed, and raise head of bed
   4. If the client needs help:
      a. Place one arm under the client's shoulders and the other arm over and around the client's knees.

b. Bring legs over the side of the bed while raising the client's shoulders off the bed.

c. Dangle the client until the client is no longer dizzy or faint; stand in front of the client.

d. Protect paralyzed arm during transfer if necessary; use sling or clothing for support

e. Place the client's feet flat on the floor; if the client has a weak leg, use your leg and foot to brace the weak leg.

f. Face the client; place your arms under the arm pits and grasp firmly; have the client lean forward so you can stabilize the upper body.

g. Use a wide base of support, bend your knees, and stand the client upright by pivoting the feet, legs, and hips to a standing position.

h. Continue to pivot until the client is positioned over a chair; lower the client gently into the chair.

i. Place client's feet on pedals and secure client in chair using safety belt.

j. Encourage client to assist with the procedure as able.

C. Log rolling with turning sheet
1. Used when spinal column must be kept straight (after surgery on the spinal column)
2. Two or more persons are needed to log roll a client.
3. Elevate bed to highest position.
4. Place turning sheet under client.
5. One person stands on each side of the bed.
6. Person on the side of the bed in the direction of the move holds the turning sheet to guide the move.
7. The person on the other side of the bed provides gentle pressure on the client's back toward the direction of the move, assisting the client to roll.
8. Position pillows at client's back and abdomen.
9. Assess the client for proper alignment and comfort.
10. Raise the side rails and lower the bed for safety.

D. Log rolling without turning sheet
1. Used when spinal column must be kept straight (after surgery on the spinal column)
2. Two or more persons are needed to log roll a client.
3. Elevate bed to highest position.
4. Both persons on side opposite to where client will be turned
5. One person places hands under client's head and shoulders; second person places hands under client's hips and legs.

6. Move client as a unit toward you.
7. Cross client's arms on chest and put pillow between client's legs.
8. Both persons move to other side of bed; the side toward which client is being turned
9. One person keeps client's shoulders and head straight, second person keeps client's hips and legs straight.
10. Moving together at the same time, both persons draw the client toward them in a single, unified motion; the client's head, spine, and legs are kept in a straight position.
11. Position with pillows for support.
12. Raise the side rail.

E. Assisting client with ambulation
1. Elevate head of bed and wait until client is adjusted (no dizziness or fainting and pulse is normal)
2. Lower the bed height.
3. Place one arm under the client's back and one arm under the client's legs and move the client into a dangling position.
4. Dangle the client for several minutes.
5. Assist client to a standing position; give client time to balance
6. Place hand under client's forearm and stay close to client during ambulation

F. Assisting client with drainage tubes (catheters, chest tubes, and so on) to ambulate
1. Assist out of bed as described previously
2. Keep drainage containers below level of body cavity being drained
3. Nurse or client can hold drainage container during ambulation
4. Upon return to bed, position the drainage tubes and containers appropriately.

G. Ambulating a client who is weak
1. Assist the client to a dangling position.
2. Place a gait or transfer belt around the client.
3. Nurse holds back of belt during ambulation
4. Two nurses, one on each side of the client, can assist a weak client during ambulation.

H. Assisting a client who becomes dizzy or faints during ambulation
1. If client becomes faint or dizzy while dangling, return to lying position in bed and lower head of bed
2. If the client becomes dizzy during ambulation, seat the client in a chair and ask for assistance to get a wheelchair to take the client back to bed; do not leave the client.
3. If client starts to faint while walking, gently lower to floor, protecting head; allow client to slide down your body

Care of Client Needing Restraints

A. Restraints are protective devices used to limit the physical activity of the client or to immobilize a client or extremity.
B. Purposes of restraints
   1. Protect the client
   2. Allow procedures to be performed safely
   3. Reduce risk of injury to others
C. Restraints require a physician's order.
D. Use the least-restrictive form of restraint that will provide for client safety.
E. Guidelines for using restraints
   1. Document the rationale for restraint, other measures tried before restraints were used, the type of restraint, the client's response to the restraint, and preventive care.
   2. Use a clove hitch knot so restraints can be changed and released easily (Figure 2.8).
   3. Restraints should not interfere with treatments or aggravate the client's condition.
   4. There should be enough slack so that the client can move his or her arms and legs for ROM.
   5. Restraints must be removed for 10 minutes every two hours for ROM, repositioning, or ambulation.
   6. Only one type of restraint should be used.
F. Types of restraints (Figure 2.9)
   1. Jacket (body) restraint: a sleeveless vest with straps that cross in front or back of the client and are tied to the bed frame or chair legs
   2. Belt: straps or belts applied across the client to secure them to the stretcher, bed, or wheelchair
   3. Mitten or hand: enclosed cloth material applied over the client's hand to prevent injury scratching
   4. Elbow: a combination of fabric and plastic or wooden tongue blades that immobilize the elbow to prevent flexion
   5. Limb or extremity: cloth devices that immobilize one or all limbs by securely tying the restraint to the bed frame or chair
   6. Mummy: a blanket or sheet that is folded around the child to limit movement; used to perform procedures on children

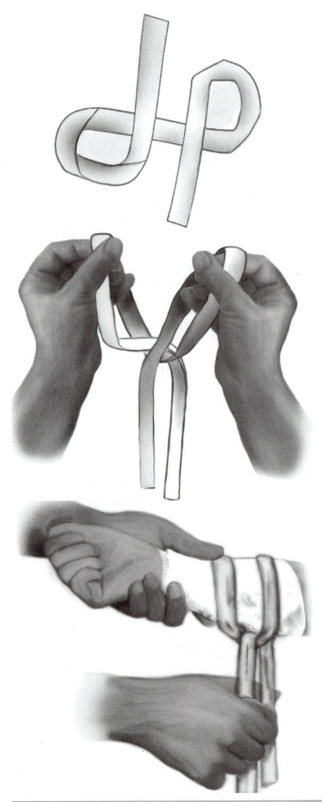

FIGURE 2.8 Clove hitch knot

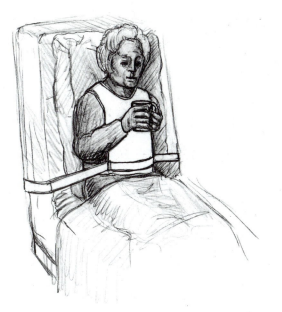

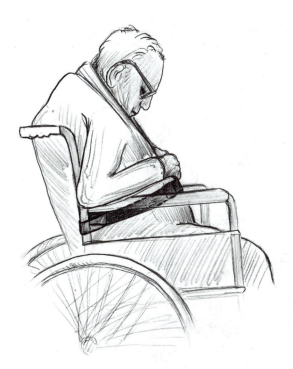

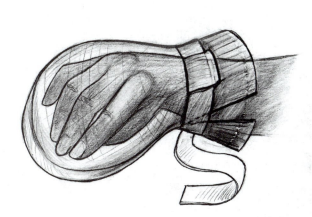

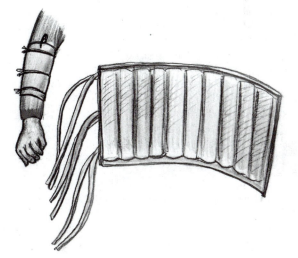

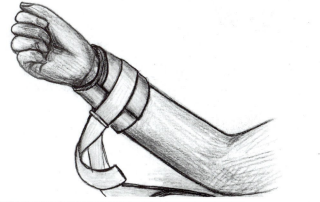

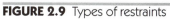

FIGURE 2.9 Types of restraints

Care of the Client Needing Application of Heat or Cold

APPLICATION OF COLD

A. Purposes
   1. Lower metabolic rate
   2. Promotes vasoconstriction and decreases bleeding and swelling following an injury
   3. Anesthetic effect
B. General principles
   1. Reduce the metabolic rate and body temperature without inducing shivering (shivering raises body temperature).
   2. Prevent tissue damage.
   3. Be very careful when applying cold to elderly clients and clients with impaired circulation because they have a decreased tolerance to cold and are susceptible to tissue damage.
   4. Moist application of cold penetrates better than dry application.
B. Systemic application of cold
   1. Lowers metabolic rate and lowers body temperature
   2. Used during some types of surgery and for high fevers
   3. Cooling blanket
      a. Client lies on or between cooling blankets.
      b. Always have a sheet between the client and the source of cold.
      c. Monitor vital signs frequently.
      d. Assess skin frequently; protect with oil if indicated
      e. Assess for signs of tissue damage and frostbite (pale areas).
      f. Reposition every two hours.
      g. Thorazine can be ordered if the client is shivering.
      h. Identify the temperature at which cooling blanket is to be turned off; usually 1-2 degrees above target temperature because temperature continues to drift downward.
      i. Monitor temperature frequently for 72 hours after treatment is discontinued.
   4. Sponge baths
      a. Used when temperature is dangerously high
      b. Use tepid water, not cold, to reduce the chance of shivering.
      c. Sponge large areas at a time; arms, legs, abdomen, and so on to allow for greatest heat loss

   d. Apply cool compresses to forehead, ankles, wrist, arm pits, and groin to increase heat loss.
   e. Monitor vital signs and discontinue treatment if the client is shivering, has a rapid, weak pulse, or develops cyanosis of the lips or nails.
   5. Local cold application
      a. Used to control bleeding, reduce inflammation, and decrease pain
      b. Should be done as soon after injury as possible (cold for the first 24 hours, then heat is often applied to promote healing)
      c. Always have cloth or towel between source of cold and client
      d. Ice cap or collar applied for no more than one hour
      e. Cold compresses
         1) If the wound is open, use sterile technique.
         2) Remove after 20 minutes.

APPLICATION OF HEAT

A. Purposes
   1. Relaxes muscle spasm
   2. Softens exudate for removal
   3. Vasodilates and hastens healing
   4. Localizes infection
   5. Reduces congestion
   6. Relaxes and comforts
   7. Increases peristalsis
B. General principles
   1. Prevent tissue damage.
   2. Be very careful when applying heat to the very young and the very old and clients with impaired circulation because they might have a decreased tolerance to heat and are susceptible to tissue damage.
   3. Moist heat penetrates deeper than dry and is better tolerated as a rule.
C. Dry heat
   1. Hot water bottle, heating pad, aquathermia pads
   2. Ultrasound and diathermy might be administered in the physical therapy department; these modes give deeper penetration.
   3. Check temperature carefully and stay within agency guidelines; an aquathermia pad is usually set at 45°C for adults.

4. Cover source of heat with a thin cloth or pillowcase prior to application
5. Do not have client lie on aquathermia pads or heating pads because of danger of burning.
6. Apply treatment as ordered, usually 20-30 minutes; repeat at scheduled intervals.
7. Assess the site for color changes and bleeding.

D. Moist heat
   1. Soaks, compresses, and hot packs
   2. Use sterile technique for open wounds.
   3. Assess skin after five minutes for increased swelling, redness, blistering, maceration, and pronounced pallor or if the client reports pain or discomfort.
   4. Remove after 15-25 minutes.

Managing Pain

A. Assessment findings in the client with pain
   1. Acute pain
      a. Relatively short duration; serves as a warning that something is wrong
      b. Subsides as healing occurs
      c. Sympathetic nervous system response ("fight or flight") due to adrenalin
         1) elevated BP, P, R
         2) perspiration
         3) skeletal muscle tension
      d. Psychological response
         1) irritability, apprehension, anxiety
         2) focuses on pain
   2. Chronic pain
      a. Pain lasts longer than six months
      b. Serves no useful purpose
      c. Persists after the injury heals
      d. No sympathetic nervous system response

   3. Assess the onset, nature, duration, and location of pain before medicating the client for pain.
   4. A pain scale is useful: on a scale of 1 to 10, rate your pain.
B. Nursing diagnosis: altered comfort
C. Interventions
   1. Administer analgesics as ordered (Narcotic analgesics page 000 and nonnarcotic analgesics page 000)
   2. Administer tranquilizers and muscle relaxants as ordered.
   3. Provide comfort measures.
   4. Relieve localized pain.
   5. *Patient controlled analgesia* (PCA)
      a. Monitor the client for complications and pain relief.
      b. Check the infusion system for accuracy and amount.
   6. Diversion

Care of the Client in Shock

A. Shock is a decrease in the circulating volume, causing an inadequate blood supply to vital organs (brain, heart, and kidneys).
B. Types of shock
   1. Cardiogenic: decrease in heart pumping action
   2. Hypovolemic: loss of blood or plasma (occurs when 10% of blood volume is lost)
   3. Neurogenic (vasogenic): marked vasodilation
   4. Septic: change in the capillary endothelium, allowing the loss of blood and plasma through capillary walls into surrounding tissues
C. Assessment findings
   1. Decrease in circulating blood volume
   2. Increased pulse and respiration

   3. Decreased pulse pressure, blood pressure
   4. Decreased urine output
   5. Apprehension, restlessness
   6. Cold, moist, pale skin
D. Nursing diagnoses related to shock (Table 2.9). Is it ineffective or altered?
E. Interventions
   1. Maintain a patent airway.
   2. Stop hemorrhages if bleeding.
   3. Shock position: head on small pillow, legs elevated 20 to 30 degrees (see page 000) to promote adequate venous return
   4. *Central venous pressure* (CVP) might be ordered; shock causes a decrease in CVP.
   5. Plasma expanders, whole blood for hypovolemic shock
   6. Monitor blood gases.

Table 2.9 Nursing Diagnoses Related to Shock

1. Ineffective tissue perfusion related to changes in circulating volume and/or vascular tone
2. Anxiety related to change in health status and threat of death
3. Cardiogenic shock: decreased cardiac output related to structural damage to heart, decreased myocardial contractility, and presence of dysrhythmias
4. Hemorrhagic shock: fluid volume deficit related to excessive vascular loss, inadequate intake/replacement

7. Indwelling urinary catheter to monitor hourly output; maintain above 30 ml/hr (preferably above 50 ml/hr)
8. Administer vasoconstrictors as ordered to increase blood pressure.
9. Cardiac drugs for cardiac shock
10. Antibiotics for septic shock

Fluid and Electrolyte Balance

BODY FLUIDS

A. Adults
  1. Women: 50–55% body weight is water
  2. Men: 60–70% body weight is water
  3. Elderly: 47% body weight is water
B. Infants: 75–80% body weight is water
C. Intracellular: 70% of total body fluid
D. Extracellular: 30% of total body fluid
  1. Interstitial: 24% of total body fluid
  2. Intravascular: 6% of total body fluid

MECHANISMS OF FLUID BALANCE

A. Kidneys: major route of fluid excretion
B. Lungs: route of fluid loss
C. Skin: route of fluid loss
D. Hormonal control
  1. *Antidiuretic Hormone* (ADH)
    a. Made in the hypothalamus and stored and secreted in the posterior pituitary
    b. Tells the kidneys to retain sodium and water
  2. Aldosterone
    a. Made in the adrenal cortex
    b. Tells the kidneys to retain sodium and excrete potassium

Fluid Imbalances (see Table 2.10)

A. Dehydration: extracellular fluid volume deficit
B. Circulatory overload: extracellular volume excess

ELECTROLYTES

A. Extracellular
  1. Na^+: 135–145 mEq/l
  2. K^+: 3.5–5.5 mEq/l
  3. Cl^-: 85–115 mEq/l
  4. HCO_3^-: 22–29 mEq/l
B. Movement of Electrolytes
  1. Diffusion: movement of particles (electrolytes) from higher to lower concentration
  2. Osmosis: movement of fluid from lower to higher concentration
  3. Osmotic pressure: the pressure demonstrated when a solvent moves through the semipermeable membrane from weaker to stronger concentrations
C. Types of solutions (Table 2.11)
  1. Hypotonic: less osmotic pressure than blood serum
  2. Isotonic: same osmotic pressure as in the cell
  3. Hypertonic: higher osmotic pressure than blood serum; causes cells to shrink

Table 2.10 Fluid Imbalances

Imbalance	Causes	Assessment Findings	Interventions
Dehydration (extracellular fluid volume deficit)	Hemorrhage, vomiting, diarrhea, diuretics, increased respirations, draining wounds, insufficient I.V. fluid replacement	Weight loss, poor skin turgor, dry, warm, feverish, oliguria, dark, odorous urine, decreased CVP, increased respirations, anorexia, hypotension	Replace fluid: p.o. or I.V.; weigh daily; intake and output; monitor BP lying down, sitting, and standing; report urine output less than 30 ml/hr; assess skin and mucous membranes
Circulatory overload (extracellular volume excess)	Too many I.V. fluids, decreased kidney function, cardiac or liver disease	Weight gain, cough, dyspnea, crackles, tachypnea, increased blood pressure, increased CVP, neck vein distention, tachycardia, flushed skin, headache	Intake and output, Diuretics (furosemide [Lasix]), fluid restriction, measure abdominal girth, assess for pitting edema, daily weight

Electrolyte Imbalances (see Table 2.12)

A. Potassium
  1. Hypokalemia: serum potassium less than 3.5 mEq/l
  2. Hyperkalemia: serum potassium greater than 5.5 mEq/l

B. Sodium
  1. Hyponatremia: serum sodium less than 135 mEq/l
  2. Hypernatremia: serum sodium greater than 145 mEq/l
C. Calcium
  1. Hypocalcemia: serum calcium less than 4.5 mEq/l
  2. Hypercalcemia: serum calcium greater than 5.8 mEq/l

Table 2.11 Types of Solutions

Hypotonic (less osmotic pressure than blood serum; expands cells)	Isotonic (same osmotic pressure as in the cell)	Hypertonic (higher osmotic pressure than blood serum; causes cells to shrink; expands blood volume)
Sodium chloride 0.45%; Tap water	Normal saline (0.9% NaCl); dextrose 5% in water; Lactated Ringer's; balanced isotonic	Dextrose 5% in saline Dextrose 10% in saline Dextrose 10% in water Dextrose 5% in ½ strength saline Dextrose 20% in water Albumin Dextran

Intravenous Infusion Therapy

A. Purposes
  1. Maintain or replace fluid, electrolytes, calories, vitamins.
  2. Restore acid-base balance.
  3. Replenish blood volume.
  4. Administer medications.
B. Composition of fluids (Table 2.13)
C. Interventions during IV infusions
  1. Assess for signs of circulatory overload.
  2. Assess urinary output to determine renal function.
  3. Assess the infusion site for signs of infiltration.
  4. Assess the flow rate.
  5. Assess the IV container and tubing.
  6. Assess the armboard, if used, for comfort and to be sure that circulation is not occluded.

Table 2.12 Electrolyte Imbalances

Imbalance	Causes	Assessment Findings	Interventions
Hypokalemia	Diuretics, burns, colitis, diarrhea, vomiting, gastric and intestinal suction, laxative abuse, thiazide and loop diuretics, steroid therapy, alkalosis	Muscle weakness; rapid, weak, thready pulse; ECG changes; mental changes; decreased or absent reflexes; shallow respirations; anorexia; vomiting; weight loss	Potassium supplements to replace losses; monitor acid-base balance; monitor pulse, blood pressure, and ECG
Hyperkalemia	Renal failure; Addison's disease; burns; infection; acidosis; potassium-sparing diuretics	Thready, slow pulse; shallow breathing; nausea and vomiting; diarrhea; intestinal colic; muscle weakness; numbness; flaccid paralysis; tingling	Kayexalate enema or PO to remove potassium through GI tract; IV infusion of glucose and insulin to drive potassium into cells; discontinue potassium IV and PO; provide adequate calories and carbohydrates
Hyponatremia	Excessive sodium loss through perspiration, GI suction, or diuretics; adrenal insufficiency; or decreased sodium intake	Lethargy; postural hypotension; rapid, thready pulse; oliguria; apprehension; muscle weakness; abdominal cramps; nausea and vomiting; headaches; confusion; convulsions	Increase sodium intake with high-sodium foods; normal saline IV; assess BP frequently (lying down, sitting, and standing)
Hypernatremia	Decreased water intake; increased sodium intake; impaired renal function	Edema; hypertonicity; dry, sticky mucous membranes; elevated temperature; flushed skin; thirst; oliguria to anuria	Weigh daily; assess edema frequently; I&O; assess skin frequently; prevent skin breakdown; sodium-restricted diet
Hypocalcemia	Hypoparathyroidism (sometimes occurs after thyroidectomy); diarrhea; acute pancreatitis; lack of vitamin D in diet; long-term steroid therapy	Tetany (painful tonic muscle spasms); facial spasms; laryngospasm; Trousseau's and Chovstek's signs; convulsions; dyspnea	Calcium either PO or IV; pad side rails for safety; dietary sources of calcium; quiet environment
Hypercalcemia	Hyperparathyroidism; immobility; osteoporosis	Nausea and vomiting; anorexia; constipation; headache; confusion; stupor; poor muscle tone; deep bone pain	Mobilize client; limit vitamin D and calcium intake; diuretics; protect from injury

Table 2.13 Composition of IV Fluids

Fluid	Composition
Saline	Fluid, Na+, Cl–
Dextrose	Fluid, calories (1000 ml = 200 calories)
Lactated Ringer's	Fluid, Na+, K+, Cl–, Ca++, lactate
Balanced isotonic	Fluid, some calories, Na+, K, Mg++, Cl–, HCO_3–, gluconate
Plasma expanders	Albumin, dextran, and plasminate

D. Complications of IV therapy
  1. Infection
     a. A local reaction due to contamination; might spread systemically
     b. Prevention
        1) Use aseptic technique
        2) Solution should be changed every 24 hours and tubing changed every 48–72 hours.
  2. Mechanical failures: solution slowing down or stopping
     a. Causes
        1) Needle against side of the vein
        2) IV fluid too low slows flow rate; too high speeds up flow rate
        3) Needle clogged by clot
        4) Faulty regulator
     b. Interventions
        1) Assess for swelling and coolness at the needle site; suggests infiltration.
        2) Remove tape and check for kinking of tubing.
        3) Pull the cannula back from the edge of the vein; raise or lower the needle; and move the needle back a little.
        4) Change position of client's arm
        5) If above steps are unsuccessful, needle should be removed by RN and infusion restarted
  3. Bacteremia: a generalized reaction to contaminated equipment or solutions
     a. Assessment findings
        1) chills and fever 30-60 minutes after start of infusion
        2) flushing, sudden pulse increase
        3) backache, headache
        4) nausea, vomiting
        5) hypotension, vascular collapse, cyanosis
     b. Interventions
        1) Notify the RN immediately so the infusion and IV cannula can be discontinued.
        2) Monitor vital signs.
        3) Save all equipment for a culture.
        4) Record pertinent information: solution name, lot number, manufacturer, and any medications added.

  4. Infiltration: dislodging of needle causes fluid to infiltrate tissues
     a. Assessment findings
        1) edema, blanching, puffiness on under surface of arm
        2) discomfort
        3) slow drip rate
        4) cool to the touch
        5) necrosis and sloughing of tissue with certain drugs (Levophed)
     b. Interventions
        1) Stop the infusion.
        2) Notify the RN or physician.
        3) Apply warm compresses to increase fluid absorption.
        4) Infusion will be restarted in another site.
  5. Circulatory overload
     a. Assessment findings
        1) headache, flushed skin, tachycardia
        2) venous distention
        3) increased venous pressure
        4) coughing, dyspnea, cyanosis
        5) pulmonary edema
     b. Prevention
        1) Check for a preexisting heart condition.
        2) Monitor the flow rate of the solution.
        3) Place in a semi-Fowler's position during infusion
        4) Monitor the elderly and infants very carefully.
     c. Interventions
        1) Slow IV to keep open rate
        2) Notify the RN or physician.
        3) Put the client in a semi-Fowler's position.
  6. Superficial thrombophlebitis
     a. Assessment findings
        1) tenderness and pain in vein
        2) edema and redness at site
        3) warmth
     b. Interventions
        1) Notify the RN or physician.
        2) cold compresses immediately to relieve pain and inflammation
        3) Follow with moist warm compresses to stimulate circulation and promote absorption.
  7. Air embolism
     a. Assessment findings
        1) hypotension
        2) cyanosis
        3) tachycardia
        4) increased venous pressure
        5) loss of consciousness
     b. Prevention
        1) Run fluid through the tubing and needle or catheter to force air out before starting the infusion.

2) Replace the bottle before it is completely empty.

3) In "Y" sets, tightly clamp the nearly empty bottle.

c. Interventions

1) Immediately turn client on left side in Trendelenburg position so air will rise and not enter the pulmonary artery (trapped air will slowly be absorbed).

2) Quickly fatal if no action taken.

3) Notify the RN or physician.

Acid Base Balance

GENERAL CONCEPTS

A. The body is constantly making acid.

B. The body gets rid of acids in several ways (Table 2.14).

  1. Respiratory: blowing off acid; CO_2 is acid; we excrete acid with every exhalation

  2. Kidneys: urine is normally acid; urine contains H^+, which is acid

  3. Stomach is acid; vomiting depletes acid

  4. Buffering systems neutralize acids.

C. Measuring acid base balance

  1. Arterial blood gases (ABGs) measure pH; bicarbonate levels and partial pressure of oxygen and carbon dioxide

  2. ABG studies helpful in diagnosis and treatment of

    a. Unexplained tachypnea and dyspnea

    b. Unexplained restlessness and anxiety

    c. Drowsiness in clients receiving oxygen

    d. Before and after oxygen therapy

    e. Cardiopulmonary disease

    f. Chronic lung disease

  3. Procedure

    a. Arterial puncture is performed by qualified personnel.

    b. Following puncture, pressure must be applied to site for five minutes to stop the bleeding.

    c. Specimen is placed in ice and taken immediately to the lab to prevent metabolism and changes in values.

  4. Normal values (Table 2.15)

Table 2.15 Blood Gas Values

pH	= 7.35–7.45
pCO_2	= 35–45
pO_2	= 80–100
HCO_3	= 22–26

INTERPRETING BLOOD GASES

A. Compare client values to the norms (Table 2.16).

B. Determine the cause if the pH is abnormal.

  1. Ask these questions:

    a. What is the pH: acid, alkaline, or normal?

    b. What is the CO_2: high or low; could it cause the pH? If yes, the problem is respiratory.

    c. What is the HCO_3^-: high or low; could it cause the pH? If yes, the problem is metabolic.

    d. What is the O_2: if abnormal, probably a respiratory problem?

C. Remember, it is not the value that is abnormal that determines the cause of the problem (sometimes all values are abnormal); rather, it is the value that is consistent with the pH (the other value is compensating or trying to correct the problem).

D. Major acid-base alterations (Table 2.17)

  1. Respiratory acidosis is caused by retention of CO_2, as in COPD.

  2. Respiratory alkalosis is caused by blowing off CO_2, as in hyperventilation.

Table 2.14 Acid Base Facts

Facts	Ways to Remove Acid	Ways to Remove Alkaline
• CO_2 is acid.	• Blow it off.	
• Urine is acid (usually).	• Urinate it off.	
• The stomach is acid.	• Vomit it off.	
• Intestines are alkaline.		• Diarrhea
• Buffering systems exist.	• Buffer it (neutralize).	

Table 2.16 Helpful Hints for Interpreting Blood Gases

- Always start with the pH.
- Determine if the pH is normal, acid, or alkaline.
- Look at other values to see which one could cause the pH.
- If the CO_2 value is consistent with, agrees with, or matches the pH, the problem is respiratory.
- If the HCO_3 (bicarbonate) value is consistent with, agrees with, or matches the pH, the problem is metabolic.

Table 2.17 Major Acid-Base Alterations

	Respiratory Acidosis	Respiratory Alkalosis	Metabolic Acidosis	Metabolic Alkalosis
pH	7.32	7.51	7.32	7.52
pCO_2	58	30	30	52
HCO_3	32	22	16	34
pO_2	60	80–100	80–100	80–100

3. Metabolic acidosis is caused by a decrease in HCO_3, as in diarrhea when HCO_3 is lost, in renal failure when acid is retained, or in diabetic ketoacidosis when excessive acids are produced.
4. Metabolic alkalosis is caused by an increase in HCO_3, as in vomiting when acid is lost or diuresis when acid urine is lost.

E. Compensation
   1. When the metabolic system is causing the problem, the respiratory system attempts to correct the problem or compensate.
      a. Compensation for metabolic acidosis is known as Kussmaul or "air hunger" respirations in which the person breathes deeply and blows off acid (CO_2).
      b. Compensation for metabolic alkalosis is shallow breathing to conserve CO_2.
   2. When the respiratory system is causing the problem, the metabolic system attempts to correct the problem or compensate.
      a. Compensation for respiratory acidosis is a rise in HCO_3.
      b. Respiratory alkalosis is such that a rapid process there might not be significant compensation.

Death

A. Death is a normal part of life. Many people fear death and try to stop the process. Nurses must care for persons who are dying and for those who are grieving the loss of a loved one.
B. Care for a dying client might be in an acute care setting, in the home with or without hospice, or at a hospice center.
C. Stages of dying and death (Table 2.18)
D. Nursing diagnoses (Table 2.19)
E. Interventions
   1. Assess the client's understanding of his or her illness and pending death.
   2. Determine if client has advance directives (who is responsible for making decisions if/when the client is unable to do so).
   3. Encourage communication between the client and family and among family members.
   4. Remember, a "do not resuscitate" order does not mean do not treat.
   5. Attend to the physical needs of a dying client:
      a. Nutrition and fluids
      b. Hygiene and grooming
      c. Pain management/comfort
      d. Bowel and bladder

Table 2.18 Stages of Dying and Death According to Kubler-Ross

Denial	"Oh no, not me!" A client who is diagnosed with heart disease continues to smoke and eat fatty foods.
Anger	"Why me?" The client becomes angry and yells at family and caregivers.
Bargaining	"God, if only I can live long enough to see my daughter get married."
Depression	"Woe is me." "It's hopeless, what's the use?" The client withdraws and just lies in bed.
Acceptance	"I am ready for whatever happens." The client gets his or her affairs in order and does the things that need to be done, including saying goodbye to loved ones. The client exhibits a sense of peace.

(Information from Kubler-Ross, E. (1969), *On Death and Dying*. New York: Macmillan.)

Table 2.19 Nursing Diagnoses Related to Dying and Death

1. Powerlessness related to diagnosis of a terminal illness, chronic pain, social isolation
2. Hopelessness related to diagnosis of a terminal illness, chronic pain, deterioration of his or her health status, altered body image, and inability to care for self.
3. Acute pain related to effects of illness
4. Altered nutrition: less than body requirements related to nausea and vomiting from illness or medications, effects of disease process
5. Activity intolerance related to physiological effects of an illness
6. Fatigue related to the disease process
7. Disturbed body image related to the effects of illness and treatment
8. Ineffective individual coping
9. Anticipatory grieving related to the diagnosis of a terminal illness
10. Spiritual distress related to impending death
11. Impaired skin integrity related to wasting disease and prolonged bedrest
12. Ineffective family coping related to effects of prolonged illness on the family; diagnoses related to the underling illness also exist.

6. Prepare the family for signs of impending death; explain that these signs do not predict an exact time frame of death.
    a. General slowing of body functions
    b. Loss of control of bowel and bladder functions
    c. Labored breathing and Cheyne-Stokes respirations (periods of apnea alternating with periods of dyspnea)
    d. Fluid accumulates in the lungs and causes "death rattle."
    e. The skin becomes moist and cool with mottled coloring.
    f. Blood pressure and temperature drop.
    g. The pulse becomes rapid and weak.
    h. Pupils do not respond to light.
    i. Verbal response is weak or absent.
    j. The client reports seeing angels or hearing beautiful music.
7. The final process:
    a. When the client takes his or her last breath, the heart stops beating very quickly.
    b. Brain death occurs within minutes.
    c. Rigor mortis, a temporary stiffening of the body, occurs several hours after death and disappears after 24 hours.
8. Care of the body:
    a. If family is present at the client's death, allow family time to be with the client; they might prefer your company or might want to be left alone.
    b. If an autopsy is to be performed, catheters, feeding tubes, and intravenous devices are usually left in place; if an autopsy is not to be done, remove external devices.
    c. Treat the body gently and with respect.
    d. Bathe the body and put on a clean gown; put an incontinent pad under the hips because body fluids might drain.
    e. Place the body in good alignment with extremities straight.
    f. Put dentures in mouth if the client normally wore them.
    g. Comb the hair.
    h. After the family has completed time with the client, place identification tags on the body, put the chin strap in place, and place in a shroud.
    i. Give belongings to the family or place in a labeled plastic bag and send with the body.

Sample Questions

1. When caring for a client in hemorrhagic shock, how should the nurse position the person?
    1. Flat in bed with legs elevated
    2. Flat in bed
    3. Trendelenburg position
    4. Semi-Fowler's position
2. An adult woman has been in an automobile accident. She sustained numerous lacerations, a fractured tibia set by closed reduction, and a mild concussion. She has no apparent renal injuries and is conscious. An indwelling catheter is inserted for which of the following purposes?
    1. To measure urine flow as an indicator of shock
    2. To prevent contamination of her cast
    3. For her comfort
    4. To prevent renal complications
3. An adult is admitted with chronic renal failure. Strict intake and output is ordered. The client is sometimes incontinent, so it is impossible to obtain an accurate record of output. How can the nurse best assess the client's fluid status?
    1. Estimate the amount voided each time.
    2. Observe her skin turgor.
    3. Weigh the client daily.
    4. Record the number of voidings.
4. A client has Crohn's disease with chronic diarrhea. Which nursing diagnosis is most likely to be appropriate for this client?
    1. Alteration in acid-base balance (metabolic acidosis) related to loss of intestinal fluids
    2. Alteration in potassium balance (hyperkalemia) related to renal potassium retention with bicarbonate
    3. Alteration in acid-base balance (metabolic alkalosis) related to excessive chloride losses in diarrhea
    4. Alteration in calcium balance (hypercalcemia) related to loss of phosphorus in diarrhea
5. The nurse is assessing a woman upon admission. Which data should be recorded as subjective data?
    1. Her weight is 142 pounds.
    2. She has a red rash covering the backs of her hands.
    3. She states, "My hands itch so bad, I can hardly stand it."
    4. Her temperature is 99.8°F.
6. The LPN/LVN working in a long-term care facility is supervising a CNA. Which observation indicates that the CNA needs further instruction in performing hygienic care?
    1. The CNA washes the client's face before washing the rest of the body.
    2. The CNA puts one foot at a time into the basin of warm water when bathing the client's feet.
    3. The CNA applies lotion and powder liberally after bathing the client.
    4. The bath water contains only a small amount of soap.

7. The nurse is taking vital signs on a very obese individual and uses an extra-wide cuff. What is the primary reason for using an extra-wide cuff?
    1. A regular-size cuff is not going to be long enough to go around the client's arm.
    2. Blood pressure taken with a cuff that is too narrow gives an artificially high reading.
    3. A regular cuff is too tight and causes discomfort to the client.
    4. A narrow cuff causes the client's pulse to be elevated.

8. The LPN/LVN notes that an apical-radial pulse is ordered for a client. Which is the correct way to obtain this reading?
    1. Have another nurse take the radial pulse while the LPN takes the apical pulse.
    2. Take the apical pulse and immediately take the radial pulse.
    3. The LPN should listen to the apical pulse and ask the client to take the radial pulse.
    4. Take the radial pulse and then take the apical pulse.

9. Which behavior by a CNA in a long-term care facility indicates a need for further instruction?
    1. Placing bed linens at the bedside prior to giving morning care.
    2. Using the same wash basin for both residents in the semi-private room.
    3. Washing hands after caring for one resident and before starting care for the next.
    4. Wearing unsterile gloves to clean a resident who is soiled with feces.

10. There is blood on the floor. How should the nurse clean up the spill?
    1. Wipe up the spill, then clean the area with alcohol.
    2. Use a 1:10 solution of chlorine bleach to clean the spill.
    3. Wipe up the spill and clean the area with water.
    4. Use an iodine solution to clean up the spill.

11. The nurse is changing a dressing. Which behavior, if observed, would indicate a break in technique?
    1. The nurse opens a package of 4 × 4s away from the sterile field and then drops them onto the sterile field.
    2. The sterile field is at waist height.
    3. The nurse opens the first flap of a sterile package away from his or her body.
    4. While pouring sterile saline into a sterile basin on the sterile field, the saline splatters onto the cloth backing.

12. The nurse is caring for a woman who had a CVA and has right-sided hemiplegia. Which action is least appropriate?
    1. Performing ROM exercises when bathing her
    2. Changing her position every two hours
    3. Positioning the client supine and pulling the bed sheets tightly across her feet

    4. Placing her in the prone position for one hour three times a day

13. The nurse is caring for an adult who had abdominal surgery this morning. Which action will do the most to prevent vascular complications?
    1. Turn the client every two hours.
    2. Encourage deep breathing and coughing every two hours.
    3. Have the client move her legs and make circles with her toes every two hours.
    4. Dangle the client as soon as she is awake and alert.

14. The nurse observes that an elderly man who is bedridden has a reddened area on his coccyx. The skin is not broken. The nurse most correctly interprets this pressure ulcer to be which stage?
    1. Pre-ulcer
    2. Stage one
    3. Stage two
    4. Stage three

15. An older adult who has a stage one pressure ulcer asks the nurse why a clear dressing has been put over the site when the skin is not broken. What should the nurse include when replying?
    1. This dressing is a preventive measure to protect the skin from injury.
    2. Covering it so the area is moist makes it heal faster.
    3. Covering the area makes it more comfortable for you.
    4. The clear dressing is designed to let light through and promote healing.

16. An adult is now alert and oriented following abdominal surgery. What position is most appropriate for the client?
    1. Semi-Fowler's
    2. Prone
    3. Supine
    4. Sims

17. The LPN has delegated the task of taking vital signs to an unlicensed assistive personnel (UAP). Which instruction is most appropriate?
    1. Take all the vital signs at 10 a.m.
    2. Report any abnormalities to me.
    3. Tell me if any blood pressure readings are over 140/90 or under 100/70.
    4. I am available if you have any problems.

18. The LPN/LVN delegates the task of performing hygienic care of a bedridden client to a UAP. What responsibility does the LPN/LVN have regarding the performance of the care?
    1. The LPN/LVN should check to be sure the task is performed correctly.
    2. The UAP is solely responsible for his or her own actions.
    3. The LPN/LVN should observe all of the care.
    4. The UAP has the responsibility to ask for assistance if needed.

19. Following a craniotomy, the nurse positions a client in a low-Fowler's position for which reason?
    1. To promote comfort
    2. To promote drainage from the operative area
    3. To promote thoracic expansion
    4. To prevent circulatory overload
20. The nurse is to help a client who has had a CVA and has right-sided hemiplegia get up into a wheelchair. How should the nurse place the wheelchair?
    1. On the left side of the bed facing the foot of the bed
    2. On the right side of the bed facing the head of the bed
    3. Perpendicular to the bed on the right side
    4. Facing the bed on the left side of the bed
21. The nurse is observing 2 UAPs log roll a client who had a laminectomy yesterday. Which observation indicates the procedure is being incorrectly performed?
    1. One person moves the head and shoulders and the second person moves the hips and legs at the same time.
    2. The UAPs use a turning sheet to help turn the client.
    3. One person keeps the client from falling out of bed while the other person moves first the head and shoulders and then the hips and legs.
    4. The UAPs place the bed in the highest position prior to turning the client.
22. An elderly adult has a *nasogastric* (NG) tube and an *intravenous* (IV) line. The client is confused and attempts to remove both the NG tube and the IV. How should the nurse assure the client's safety?
    1. Apply four-point restraints.
    2. Ask the physician for an order for wrist restraints.
    3. Request a sitter to stay with the client.
    4. Suggest that the family stay with the client at all times.
23. The client has just returned to the nursing care unit following a hemorrhoidectomy. What order should the nurse expect?
    1. A sitz bath stat and qid
    2. Warm compresses to the surgical area prn
    3. A hot water bottle to the surgical area prn
    4. An ice pack to surgical area
24. Warm compresses are ordered for an open wound. Which action is appropriate for the nurse?
    1. Use sterile technique when applying the compresses.
    2. Leave the compresses on continually, pouring warm solution on the area when it cools down.
    3. Alternate warm compresses with cool compresses.
    4. Apply a wet dressing to the wound and cover with a dry dressing.
25. An adult returned from the *Post Anesthesia Care Unit* (PACU) following abdominal surgery. At 2 p.m., he asks for pain medication. He has an order for meperidine (Demerol) 75 mg I.M. q 3–4 hr prn for operative site pain. He was last medicated at 10:30 a.m. What is the best initial action for the nurse?
    1. Administer 75 mg of meperidine.
    2. Ask the client to tell you where he hurts.
    3. Listen to the client's bowel sounds and breath sounds before administering the meperidine.
    4. Inform the client he has to wait a half hour before receiving pain medication.
26. The family of an adult who is terminally ill with advanced metastatic cancer asks the nurse to "let him die in peace." The client is alert and oriented and in severe pain. What response is appropriate for the nurse?
    1. Ask the family member to sign a release form for a DNR order.
    2. Encourage the family to talk with the client and the physician.
    3. Suggest that not doing all that is possible for the client is unethical.
    4. Ask the doctor for a DNR order.
27. An adult who is terminally ill says to the nurse, "Am I going to die soon?" What is the best response for the nurse to make?
    1. "No one can tell for sure when the end will come."
    2. "Are you afraid of dying?"
    3. "You are concerned about when you will die?"
    4. "Everyone has to die sometime."
28. An adult has just died. How should the nurse prepare the body for transfer to the mortuary?
    1. Leave the body as is; no preparation is necessary.
    2. Bathe the body and put identification tags on it.
    3. Remove dentures before bathing the body.
    4. Position the body with its head down and arms folded on its chest.
29. A cooling blanket is ordered for an adult who has a temperature of 106°F. Which nursing action is appropriate?
    1. Place a sheet over the cooling blanket before putting the client on the blanket.
    2. Maintain the client in a supine position on the blanket.
    3. Apply powder to the skin that is in contact with the blanket.
    4. Turn the client every 10 minutes and assess for frostbite.
30. An adult is admitted to the hospital after several days of vomiting. Her breathing is now slow and shallow. What acid-base imbalance does the nurse suspect?
    1. Respiratory acidosis with metabolic compensation
    2. Respiratory alkalosis with little metabolic compensation

3. Metabolic alkalosis with respiratory compensation
4. Metabolic acidosis with little respiratory compensation.

Answers and Rationales

1. (1) The shock position is flat in bed with the legs elevated to increase venous return. The head can be placed on a pillow. The Trendelenburg position, with the head lower than the chest, is no longer the recommended position because the abdominal organs can put pressure on the diaphragm and interfere with breathing and heart function. The semi-Fowler's position would make the client worse by increasing venous return.

2. (1) 25% of the cardiac output goes to the kidneys. If cardiac output goes down, as it will in shock, the kidneys will produce less urine. Most trauma victims will be catheterized to help determine if there is shock caused by possible internal bleeding. A urinary catheter does not prevent kidney damage; it merely measures urine output.

3. (3) Daily weights are the best way to assess fluid balance. Estimations of the amount voided are usually not accurate. Skin turgor can give some information about fluid status but is not the best way to assess it. Recording the number of voidings gives some indication of fluid status but does not indicate how much urine is in each voiding. When unable to measure output, the best assessment measure is daily weights.

4. (1) Loss of alkaline intestinal fluid causes metabolic acidosis. Hyperkalemia is unlikely because intestinal fluids are high in potassium. Sodium, not potassium, is resorbed with bicarbonate. Chloride is retained as bicarbonate is lost, contributing to metabolic acidosis. Calcium levels do increase as phosphorus is lost, but diarrhea does not cause a loss of large amounts of phosphorus.

5. (3) Subjective data is data from the client's perspective, something that the client tells you. Weight and temperature are measured and are objective data. A rash is observed and is objective data.

6. (3) Powder tends to cake and dry the client's skin. Powder applied following the application of lotion makes a sticky mess. The bath should start with the eyes and face first. Putting the feet into warm water when bathing the feet is a very good thing to do. It is comforting and soothing to the client and helps soften any tough skin on the feet. The bath water should contain only small amounts of soap; too much soap dries the skin.

7. (2) A too-narrow cuff gives an artificially high reading. A cuff that is too wide will give a reading that is too low. The pulse will not be affected. It is not the length of the cuff that is the concern, it is the width of the cuff.

8. (1) When an apical radial pulse is taken, two nurses are needed. One listens to the apical pulse while the other nurse takes the radial pulse. The nurse should not ask the client to take his or her own radial pulse.

9. (2) Each person should have their own wash basin which is used exclusively for them. Bed linens can be placed at the bedside prior to morning care so that the needed materials are close at hand. Hands should be washed before and after all client contact. Feces are full of bacteria. Protective barriers should be working when the health care worker is at risk for exposure to body fluids. Gloves are appropriate when cleaning up feces.

10. (2) Blood should be cleaned with a solution of bleach at a 1:10 dilution. Alcohol and iodine are not appropriate because they do not kill HIV, which might be in the blood. Sometimes soap and water are used, but just plain water does not kill microorganisms.

11. (4) Moisture carries organisms through a barrier. If moisture spills on a cloth or paper sterile field, the field is no longer sterile. Sterile packages should be opened away from the sterile field. Items below the waist on a sterile field are not considered sterile. The first flap of a sterile package should be opened away from the nurse so that the last flap will come toward the nurse. Reaching across a sterile field is not appropriate.

12. (3) The bed sheets should not be drawn tightly over the feet, because this action might cause foot drop—especially with the client in the supine position. ROM exercises should be performed during the bath and several other times during the day. The client's position should be changed every two hours. Placing a person who has had a CVA in the prone position for an hour three times a day will help prevent hip flexion contractures. Note that the question asked which action is LEAST appropriate.

13. (3) Moving the legs and drawing circles with the toes promotes venous return and helps prevent venous stasis and thrombophlebitis. Turning the client every two hours will help prevent respiratory complications and skin breakdown. Deep breathing and coughing help to prevent respiratory complications. Dangling the client is not related to preventing vascular complications. In fact, it promotes venous stasis. Not enough information is given as to whether dangling the client as soon as she is alert is appropriate.

14. (2) Pressure areas that have color changes and changes in skin texture with no break in the skin are assessed as stage one pressure ulcers. Stage two ulcers have a break in the skin with

involvement of the dermis. Stage three pressure ulcers involve the subcutaneous tissue. Pressure ulcers are not classed as pre-ulcers.

15. (2) Moist skin will heal better than skin that is dried out. There is some truth to the idea that covering the area helps to prevent further injury, but answer 2 is more correct. Comfort is not the primary reason for covering the area. The dressing is not primarily designed to let light in.

16. (1) The semi-Fowler's position is the position of choice following abdominal surgery. This position allows for greater thoracic expansion and puts less pressure on the suture line. Supine puts pressure on the suture line and is very uncomfortable for persons who have had abdominal surgery. Prone is contraindicated for someone who has abdominal surgery. The Sims position is a semi-lateral, semi-prone position and would put too much pressure on the suture line.

17. (3) The nurse should give specific instruction to the UAP. This answer choice is the most specific of the instructions. The other choices are all very vague. The UAP might not know the norms.

18. (1) The LPN/LVN can delegate tasks that are delegatable to the UAP. The responsibility for making sure that the task is correctly performed, however, rests with the LPN/LVN. The UAP has responsibility, but the delegator also retains responsibility for the care given by those to whom it has been delegated. It is not necessary to directly observe all care given by the UAP. While the UAP should ask for help if needed, it is the responsibility of the delegator to be sure that assistance is not needed.

19. (2) The low-Fowler's position will promote drainage from the operative area and prevent cerebral edema without putting undue pressure on the cerebral structures. The major goal post-craniotomy is to prevent cerebral edema and increased intracranial pressure. The position might or might not promote comfort. That is not the major reason for placing the client in the low-Fowler's position, however. Low-Fowler's allows for moderate thoracic expansion (not as much as semi-Fowler's), but that is not the reason for using low-Fowler's in a client who had a craniotomy. Low-Fowler's will help a little in preventing circulatory overload (not as much as semi-Fowler's), but that is not the reason for using low-Fowler's in a client who has had a craniotomy.

20. (1) The wheelchair should be placed on the unaffected side of the bed, facing the foot of the bed. The client can then stand on the unaffected leg and pivot and sit in the chair.

21. (3) Log rolling is used when the spine must be kept straight. The head and shoulders and hips and legs should be moved as a unit at the same time. Log rolling can be correctly performed by using a turning sheet. The bed should be placed in the highest position before turning the client to protect the backs of the personnel.

22. (2) The client is at risk for injuring himself or herself, so restraints are indicated. The nurse should ask the physician for an order for wrist restraints. The least restraint possible should be used. Four-point restraints are not indicated by the data in the question. A sitter does not appear to be necessary in this situation. There is no data to support that need. The nurse and the staff should be able to assure the client's safety without requiring the family to be present at ALL times.

23. (4) The client will have an ice pack applied to the surgical area on the day of surgery. Sitz baths will probably be ordered for the following day. The rule is cold for the first 24 hours to prevent edema followed by warmth to promote healing. The day after surgery, the client will start taking sitz baths.

24. (1) The nurse should use sterile technique when applying compresses to an open wound. Warm compresses are not left in place continually. Moist heat is left on for 15-25 minutes at a time. Alternating warm compresses and cool compresses is not what is ordered for the client. Option 4 describes a wet to dry dressing.

25. (2) The question states that the client asks for pain medication. There is no indication of where the pain is. The nurse cannot assume that the pain is in the operative area. The time frame is adequate, so if the client's pain is in the operative area, the nurse should administer the medication. Listening to bowel and breath sounds is not a criteria for administering pain medication.

26. (2) Because the client is alert, he should be involved in making the decision. This matter should be discussed with the client and with the physician who will need to write any orders. Suggesting that such a request is unethical is not appropriate. Clients have the right to refuse treatment and shave advance directives. The alert client should be involved in the process.

27. (3) This response is the most therapeutic. It focuses on what the client asked and opens the lines of communication. The first answer might be true but does not encourage the client to discuss his concerns. The second choice is not appropriate because it focuses on fear, which is not in the client's questions. The third response is much better than choice 2. Choice 4 closes communication and is not appropriate.

28. (2) The body should be bathed, a clean gown put on and it should have identification tags placed on it. Dentures, if normally used by the client, should be placed in the mouth. The body should be flat with extremities straight. If the head is down, the blood will go to the head and discolor the skin, making viewing difficult.

29. (1) There should always be a sheet between the client and the cooling blanket to protect from frostbite. The position of the client should be changed every two hours. Powder is not applied to the skin; it will cause the skin to be dry. If necessary oil could be applied to the skin. The client should be checked for frostbite and should be turned every two hours, not every 10 minutes.

30. (3) A client who is vomiting is losing acid and will go into metabolic alkalosis. The slow, shallow breathing is evidence of trying to hold on to CO_2, which is acid, thus compensating for the alkalosis.

Chapter 3

The Older Adult Client

GENERAL CONCEPTS

A. Terms
1. Gerontology: concerned with normal aging
2. Geriatrics: concerned with older adults who have a disease process
3. Old age: young old—60 to 75 years; old—75 to 84 years; and old-old—85 to 94 years
4. Frail elderly: usually older than 75 with health problems that make them vulnerable to physical and psychosocial problems and loss of independence
5. Ageism: negative attitudes toward the elderly that affect how they are treated

B. Aging is a natural process that begins at birth and results in a gradual decrease in cellular, organ, and system functioning and a loss of reserve capacity.

C. Profiles of the aged in the United States:
1. Approximately 12% of the population is older than 65.
2. Those older than 75 years are the fastest-growing segment.
3. The aging population is growing in numbers, proportion, and years.
4. Approximately 5% of the aged are in nursing homes at any one time.
5. Many have one or more chronic diseases.
6. Many take numerous over-the-counter (OTC) and prescription drugs.

Theories of Aging

BIOLOGICAL

A. Immunological: immune functions decrease, resulting in an increase in infections and an inability of the body to recognize its own cells—resulting in antibodies being produced that work against the body
B. Genetic programming: normal cells have a built-in limit on reproducing
C. Stress: "wear and tear," overexertion, and stress cause cells to wear out.

PSYCHOSOCIAL

A. Disengagement: the individual and society withdraw from each other
B. Activity: the best aging occurs when the activity level of middle age is continued
C. Continuity: basic personality and behavior are maintained with aging

DEVELOPMENTAL TASKS

Erikson: ego integrity versus despair

A. Ego integrity: acceptance of one's lifestyle; believing that one lived well under the circumstances
B. Despair: looking at one's past with dissatisfaction and a sense of despair and fear of death
C. Nursing interventions
   1. Assess for expressions of decreased life satisfaction, depression, and apathy.
   2. Nursing diagnoses (Table 3.1)
   3. Promote achievement of ego integrity by encouraging reminiscing about the person's life ("life review").
   4. Develop a relationship with the person.
   5. Accept positive and negative feelings that the person expresses by being empathetic.
   6. Ask open-ended questions about the past.
   7. Obtain old photos and objects from the past.
   8. Play music from the past.

Table 3.1 Nursing Diagnoses Related to Aging

1. Ineffective coping
2. Fear
3. Ineffective family coping
4. Social isolation
5. Risk for altered thought processes
6. Disturbed sleep patterns
7. Altered sensory perception (specify)
8. Risk for injury
9. Impaired verbal communication
10. Anticipatory grieving related to diminished senses and loss of spouse or friends
11. Risk for ineffective airway clearance
12. Risk for ineffective breathing patterns
13. Risk for impaired gas exchange
14. Activity intolerance
15. Altered tissue perfusion related to (R/T) interruption of arterial and venous flow
16. Fatigue
17. Risk for impaired physical mobility
18. Alteration in nutrition: less than body requirements or more than body requirements
19. Risk for impaired swallowing
20. Risk for constipation
21. Risk for bowel incontinence
22. Risk for urinary incontinence
23. Alteration in sexual patterns
24. Knowledge deficit: normal physical changes due to aging
25. Knowledge deficit: normal changes and related skin care
26. Risk for impaired skin integrity
27. Risk for distrubed body image
28. Risk for situational low self-esteem R/T changes in appearance
29. Risk for impaired oral mucus membrane
30. Risk for hypothermia R/T exposure to cold environment
31. Risk for hyperthermia R/T exposure to extreme high temperature

Havighurst

A. Tasks to be accomplished:
   1. Adjust to the decreased physical strength.
   2. Adjust to retirement.
   3. Adjust to less income.
   4. Establish ties with one's age group.
   5. Adopt changing social roles.
   6. Establish satisfactory living arrangements.
B. Nursing diagnoses (Table 3.1)
C. Nursing interventions
   1. Facilitate the expression of feelings.
   2. Provide anticipatory guidance.
   3. Provide information on resources.

CHANGES OF NORMAL AGING

Neurologic

A. Changes
   1. Decrease in number and size of brain cells and amount of neurotransmitters
   2. Prolonged reaction time
B. Nursing implications
   1. Assess sleep, memory, response, and reaction time.
   2. Nursing diagnoses (Table 3.1)
   3. Nursing interventions
      a. Provide more time to perform tasks.
      b. Give client time to answer/respond.
      c. Maintain nighttime routines.
      d. Promote reality orientation with calendars, clocks, and visits.

Neurosensory

A. Changes related to the ears:
   1. Presbycusis: progressive hearing loss related to aging
   2. High-frequency tones are lost first.
   3. Sounds might be distorted; might have difficulty understanding words when there is background noise
B. Changes related to the eyes:
   1. Lens might become opaque (cataract; see Chapter 9)
   2. Decreased visual field
   3. Decreased color discrimination
   4. Presbyopia: farsightedness due to decreased accommodation
   5. Pupillary changes with loss of light responsiveness so they adapt to darkness more slowly and have difficulty seeing in dim light
C. The number of taste buds declines, resulting in a dulled taste sensation (especially for bitter, sour, and salty flavors)
D. Sense of smell decreases

E. Touch (tactile) changes:
1. Sense of touch dulled
2. Pain threshold higher
3. Sense of vibration decreased
F. Vestibular/Kinesthetic changes:
1. Decreased proprioception
2. Decreased coordination and equilibrium
G. Nursing implications:
1. Assess for normal physiological changes.
2. Nursing diagnoses (Table 3.1)
3. Nursing interventions
    a. Lower your tone of voice when speaking to an older person with hearing loss.
    b. Reduce background noise before speaking.
    c. Determine if the client uses a hearing aid and if it is working.
    d. Determine if the client uses eyeglasses/lenses.
    e. Provide increased lighting.
    f. Provide night lights.
    g. Provide hand rails.
    h. Promote the expression of feelings.
    i. Touch the person.

Respiratory

A. Decrease in respiratory muscle tone, functional alveoli, ciliary action, force of cough, pO_2, response to increased O_2 demand
B. Nursing interventions:
1. Assess for respiratory problems.
2. Nursing diagnoses (Table 3.1)
3. Teach relaxation exercises, deep breathing, correct positions, adequate fluid, and smoking cessation.
4. Encourage the client to take preventive vaccines (influenza and pneumococcal).
5. Provide rest periods.

Cardiovascular

A. Changes
1. Decreased elasticity of the heart and arteries; efficiency of heart and peripheral valves; maximum heart rate with exercise
2. Increased peripheral resistance and formation of atherosclerotic plaques
3. Takes longer to recover following exercise
B. Nursing implications:
1. Assess cardiovascular (CV) functioning.
2. Nursing diagnoses (Table 3.1)
3. Nursing interventions:
    a. Provide for rest periods.
    b. Teach the client about low salt, low fat, and high-fiber diets and about having regular health checkups, including blood pressure checks.
    c. Monitor for orthostatic hypertension; suggest a slow position change from lying to sitting to standing.

Musculoskeletal

A. Changes
1. Decreased height; loss of muscle mass, tone, and strength; and loss of bone mass and mineralization
2. Increased joint and cartilage erosion and thinning of vertebrae
B. Nursing implications:
1. Assess the strength and ability to walk.
2. Nursing diagnoses (Table 3.1)
3. Nursing interventions:
    a. Teach the need for aerobic exercises, walking, and swimming.
    b. Environmental safety
    c. Need for calcium intake

Gastrointestinal

A. Changes
1. Decreased esophageal peristalsis; external sphincter reflexes; saliva production; liver size, weight, and efficiency; gastric acid secretion; intestinal motility
2. Decreased metabolic and caloric needs
B. Nursing implications:
1. Assess swallowing, weight, and bowel functioning.
2. Nursing diagnosis (Table 3.1)
3. If the client is overweight, teach him or her to reduce caloric intake by decreasing fat and simple carbohydrates.
4. Encourage the client to maintain protein in his or her diet.
5. Teach the client about the need for adequate calcium, iron, and vitamins.
6. Teach the client about the need for increased fluids, fiber, roughage, and exercise to prevent constipation.
7. If the client has impaired swallowing, teach the use of thickened fluids to facilitate swallowing and prevent choking.

Genitourinary

A. Changes:
1. Decreased kidney function, bladder muscle tone, and sphincter tone
2. Decrease in vaginal secretions
3. Decrease in size of testes and speed and force of ejaculation
B. Nursing implications:
1. Assess urinary output and continence, vaginal itching/discomfort, and sexual functioning.
2. Nursing diagnoses (Table 3.1)
3. Encourage 2000–3000 ml of fluid daily.
4. Assess for drug toxicity related to a decrease in renal function.
5. Provide for toileting.
6. Administer ordered diuretics by 4 p.m.
7. Teach Kegel exercises for incontinence.
8. Provide privacy for intimacy.

Integumentary

A. Changes:
   1. Decrease in circulation, number of cells, and elastic collagen fibers
   2. Decrease in pressure and light-touch sensation
   3. Decreased production of sweat, sebum, and vitamin D
   4. Decreased cell replacement resulting in thinning of the skin
   5. Decreased hair color and pigment
   6. Skin dry and wrinkled and often itches
   7. Uneven pigmentation and appearance of age spots, skin tags, and other skin lesions
B. Nursing implications:
   1. Assess the skin condition and discomfort.
   2. Nursing diagnoses (Table 3.1)
   3. Teach monitoring of skin condition, skin care, cleansing, and protection from the sun.
   4. Check skin turgor over the sternum.
   5. Facilitate the expression of feelings regarding changes in appearance.
   6. Handle the client gently to prevent skin tears.

Regulation: Endocrine, Temperature and Infection

A. Changes
   1. Decreased secretion of growth hormone and thyroid hormone
   2. Decreased ovarian function with female menopause
   3. Decreased glucose tolerance
   4. Decreased shivering and decreased function of sweat glands
   5. Temperature does not rise as readily in response to infection.
   6. Decreased tolerance to cold
B. Nursing implications:
   1. Assess for activity tolerance and signs of infection other than temperature elevation.
   2. Nursing diagnoses (Table 3.1)
   3. Teach appropriate care during hot or cold weather.
   4. Monitor temperature and observe for other signs and symptoms of infection.
   5. Provide rest periods.

Medication Problems

A. Multiple medications: prescription and *over-the-counter* (OTC)
   1. Danger of drug interactions with multiple medications
   2. Assess for drug toxicity and side effects

B. Decreased liver and kidney functioning related to aging
   1. Half life might be increased
   2. Danger of overdose
C. Self-administration
   1. Might have difficulty taking the right drug and the right dose at the right time
   2. Color code to facilitate proper administration if necessary.
   3. Determine if client can open the container.
   4. Oral medications:
      a. Check swallowing.
      b. If swallowing difficulties exist:
         (1) Suggest a liquid preparation if unable to swallow pills or capsules.
         (2) Crush large, non-enteric coated tablets.
         (3) Give a drink of water prior to medication to ensure moist mucous membranes.
         (4) Give with pudding, applesauce, or ice cream.
D. Parenteral medications
   1. Do not use an immobile limb.
   2. Closely monitor the IV rate to avoid overhydration and the onset of pulmonary edema

Elder Abuse

A. Definitions:
   1. Abuse: willful, active actions resulting in physical, psychosocial, or material harm
   2. Neglect: failure to meet physical, psychosocial, or material needs
B. Incidence occurs in homes and in long-term and acute care institutions.
C. Characteristics of abused persons:
   1. Female more than male
   2. Caucasians most frequently abused
   3. Physical and/or cognitive impairments that make the person dependent on others for daily care
   4. Display dependency characteristics
   5. Exhibit problematic behavior
      a. Bossy, demanding
      b. Incontinent
      c. Wandering
      d. Nighttime shouting
D. Characteristics of an abuser:
   1. Is ill-prepared or reluctant to provide care
   2. Has unrealistic expectations of the older person
   3. Lacks knowledge/skills required to provide care
   4. Has ineffective coping patterns
   5. Personal life in disarray
      a. Problems with own children
      b. Marital conflict

c. Personal physical/emotional problems
d. Alcohol or drug abuser
e. Lacks communication skills
6. Absence of support system
E. Nursing implications:
 1. Need for self awareness
  a. Evaluate the client's personal feelings toward aging and toward older people.
  b. Become aware of personal attitudes toward neglect/abuse.
  c. Acknowledge that every person is capable of being an abuser.
 2. Assess for potential/active abuse.
  a. Does the client have high-risk characteristics?
  b. Does the caregiver have high-risk characteristics?
  c. Signs of abuse:
   (1) Frequent visits to the *emergency department* (ED)
   (2) Multiple bruising, fractures, lacerations, and abrasions in various stages of healing
   (3) Evidence of burns or rope burns
   (4) A head injury due to hair pulling
   (5) Appearing over-medicated
  d. Behaviors indicting possible abuse:
   (1) Wariness of contact with adults
   (2) Very aggressive or infantile behavior
   (3) Withdrawn
   (4) Expresses ambivalent feelings toward caregivers
  e. Signs of neglect:
   (1) dehydration
   (2) malnourishment
   (3) poor hygiene
   (4) inappropriate clothing
F. Nursing Diagnoses (Table 3.2)
G. Nursing Interventions
 1. Promote safety:
  a. Report to the appropriate supervisor/social agency.
  b. Determine if person needs to be removed.
 2. Develop a relationship with the abused.
 3. Promote trust with consistency and caring.
 4. Promote self-esteem by providing affection and caring.
 5. Ensure that basic needs are met.
 6. Develop a relationship with the abuser.
 7. Promote the expression of feelings.
 8. Communicate empathy with the abuser.
 9. Explore resources available to the abuser.
 10. Refer to community resources:
  a. Daycare
  b. Respite care
  c. Self-help groups
  d. Counseling services
 11. Teach the abuser realistic expectations for the abused and how to provide care.
 12. Document findings, interventions, and evaluations.

Table 3.2 Nursing Diagnoses Related to Abuse of an Older Adult Client

1. Risk for violence
2. Ineffective individual coping
3. Compromised/disabled
4. Hopelessness
5. Knowledge deficit
6. Spiritual distress—guilt
7. Risk for situational low self-esteem
8. Risk for injury
9. Social isolation
10. Risk for imbalanced nutrition
11. Risk for imbalanced fluid volume

Sample Questions

1. A 75-year-old man is brought to the auditory clinic by his son, who tells the nurse that his father is having trouble hearing and seems to be a little depressed. The man says, "There's no point in getting a hearing aid. I don't have much time left and didn't use the time I had very good anyway." The nurse recognizes that this behavior indicates that the client might be
   1. actively suicidal.
   2. suffering bipolar depression.
   3. struggling with generativity versus stagnation.
   4. struggling with development of integrity versus despair.
2. An 88-year-old woman in a long-term care facility is having difficulty remembering where her room is. Which of the following solutions would best help her?
   1. Put a light-blue painting on the door to her room.
   2. Assign her a buddy who will help her when she gets lost.
   3. Put her picture and her name in large letters on the door to her room.
   4. Assigning her the room next to the nurses' station so that the staff can assist her
3. The family of an elderly client asks why their father puts so much salt on his food. The nurse should include which information in the response?
   1. The taste buds become dulled as a person ages.
   2. The body is attempting to compensate for lost fluids during the aging process.
   3. Elderly clients need more sodium to ensure adequate kidney function.
   4. The client is confused and does not remember putting salt on the food.
4. A 65-year-old client is seen in an urgent care center for a sprained ankle. The client also tells the nurse, "I don't know what the problem is. I'm tired all the time. I guess it's just a sign I'm getting old." What is the best response for the nurse to make?

1. "Sixty-five isn't that old. Do you have enough activities to keep you from getting bored?"
        2. "It's normal for someone your age to feel tired like that. Try taking a two-hour nap during the day."
        3. "It's not normal for someone your age to be tired all the time. Have you had a physical exam recently?"
        4. "You sound depressed. Would you like the name of a psychiatrist?"

5. A 64-year-old woman tells the nurse she has vaginal itching and dryness and that she has pain "down there" at times. What should the nurse do?
        1. Reassure the client that these are normal changes that come with aging.
        2. Explain to the client that this situation is of little importance because sexual activity is not likely at this age.
        3. Suggest to the client that she use a vaginal cream for the itching and dryness.
        4. Encourage the client to see her physician.

6. An elderly woman is admitted to the hospital with a productive cough, progressive forgetfulness, an inability to concentrate, and disinterest in her personal hygiene. What should be of greatest priority as the nurse assesses this client?
        1. Her progressive forgetfulness
        2. Her inability to concentrate
        3. Her disinterest in her personal hygiene
        4. Her productive cough

7. The nurse in a retirement home has noticed that Mr. A. and Ms. C. have been holding hands frequently. One day, the nurse enters Mr. A.'s room and finds Mr. A. and Ms. C. having sexual intercourse. Both residents are alert and oriented. What is the most appropriate action for the nurse to take?
        1. Interrupt the couple and send Ms. C. to her room.
        2. Leave the room and close the door.
        3. Notify the relatives of both residents.
        4. Ask Ms. C. if she is all right.

8. A 45-year-old tells the nurse that she is having difficulty reading the newspaper. She states that she holds it away from her but still cannot see it. What is the best response for the nurse to make?
        1. Reassure her that this situation is normal and encourage her to use a magnifying glass.
        2. Ask her if any of her relatives have had this problem.
        3. Suggest that she see an eye doctor for a prescription for reading glasses.
        4. Explain that she can try on reading glasses at the drugstore.

9. An elderly man tells the nurse that all his family members mumble when they talk. How should the nurse respond to this statement?
        1. Refer the family members to speech therapy.
        2. Suggest that the client have his hearing tested.
        3. Discuss with the family how to speak more clearly.
        4. Ask the client if his parents had difficulty hearing.

10. The nurse is discussing the care of a client who has a hearing deficit. Which suggestion is most appropriate to make to those around him?
        1. Speak in a higher tone of voice.
        2. Raise your voice when speaking.
        3. Be sure to stand so there are no bright lights behind you.
        4. Keep the television or radio on when having a conversation.

Answers and Rationales

1. (4) Integrity versus despair is the developmental task of the elderly. This concept includes looking at one's life with some satisfaction for what has been accomplished. This client indicates he is not satisfied with his life. There are no data to suggest that the client is suicidal or bipolar. Generativity versus stagnation is the developmental task for the middle adult.

2. (3) The behavior suggests short-term memory loss. Identifying her room with her picture, probably a picture of her as a younger woman, and her name in large letters so she can easily read it will help her find her room. Older persons are apt to have difficulty with blue, green, and pastel colors. It is not necessary to assign her a buddy, nor is it necessary to put her next to the nurse's station.

3. (1) As people age, the taste buds diminish and become dulled. Many elderly persons put large amounts of salt on food. The other answers do not make sense. If the client loses fluids, thirst is the response, not a desire for more salt. Elderly clients do not need more sodium for renal function or anything else. Confusion could play a role, but the more likely reason is a loss of taste sensation.

4. (3) It is not normal for a 65-year-old to be tired all the time. Chronic fatigue can be a sign of many things, including anemia, diabetes, and so on. The client should be thoroughly evaluated by a physician. Fatigue could be related to boredom or depression, but the nurse should not make that assumption. The client should be evaluated for physical illness first.

5. (4) Dryness is normal for a post-menopausal woman. Itching and pain are not normal, however. The client needs to be seen by a physician. She might have an infection or another problem.

6. (4) The highest priority has to be the productive cough. It could signify a problem that needs immediate treatment. The other concerns are longer term and should be addressed after the cough.

7. (2) Both residents are alert and oriented. A relationship has existed. There is no evidence of force being used. It would appear to be a mutually consenting act. Leave the room and close the door. There is no need to notify the relatives of this alert and oriented couple.

8. (3) The data suggest presbyopia—the normal loss of accommodation that occurs with aging. The best response is to suggest that the client see an eyedoctor for reading glasses. Reading glasses can be purchased at the drugstore. There are other eye conditions that occur with aging, however, so the client should be seen by an eyedoctor.

9. (2) When a person says that everyone is mumbling, the problem is usually with the person's hearing. The most appropriate response is to suggest that his hearing be tested. It is doubtful that the family needs speech therapy or instruction in speaking more clearly. Asking the client about a family history of hearing problems is not particularly relevant. Hearing difficulties might or might not be hereditary.

10. (3) Persons with hearing impairments tend to read lips and faces. Standing with a bright light behind the speaker makes it very difficult to read lips. Persons with hearing impairments usually hear lower tones better, so speaking in a higher tone of voice makes it more difficult to hear. Raising the voice tends to raise the pitch and make it more difficult to hear. Background noise makes hearing more difficult.

Chapter 4

The Perioperative Client

LEGAL ASPECTS: INFORMED CONSENT

A. Operative permit: a form signed by the client and witness, granting permission for a specific surgery to be performed
B. Informed consent is necessary for any invasive procedure
C. Before signing the permit, the client must be told:
   1. What is to be done
   2. Risks and possible complications
   3. Alternatives to surgery
   4. Expected idea of early and late postoperative periods
   5. Must have the opportunity to ask questions
   6. Detailed information about surgery, complications, alternatives, and expected postoperative care needs is the responsibility of the surgeon
D. Adult (18 and older) signs own permit unless unconscious or mentally incompetent
   1. If unable to sign the permit, spouse, next-of-kin, or guardian can sign
   2. Telephone or telegram permission can be given; telephone consent must be witnessed by second nurse listening on the line
   3. Consent must be obtained before the client is medicated for surgery
E. Criteria for Treatment without Consent
   1. There is an immediate threat to life.
   2. Experts agree that it is an emergency situation.
   3. The client is unable to consent.
   4. A legally authorized person cannot be reached.
F. Emancipated minor
   1. Married minor
   2. Military service
   3. Person who is under age but not subject to parental control and regulation
   4. The age of majority is 18.
G. Witness
   1. A witness can be a nurse, another physician, or a clerk.
   2. Nurses should state whether they are witnessing the signature only or the explanation of the surgery.

Preoperative Period

SURGICAL RISK FACTORS

A. Obesity
  1. Problems:
     a. Surgery—technically more difficult
     b. Greater danger of dehiscence
     c. Lessened resistance to infection
     d. Postop turning more difficult, increasing the likelihood of respiratory problems
     e. Increased demands on heart
     f. Increased possibility of renal, biliary, hepatic, and endocrine disorders
  2. Nursing care
     a. Encourage weight loss if there is time.
     b. Be sure that the client turns and does deep breathing and coughing exercises every two hours to prevent respiratory complications.
     c. Encourage leg exercises to prevent thrombophlebitis.
     d. Encourage splinting of the incision when turning, coughing, and so on to prevent dehiscence.
B. Fluid and Electrolyte Imbalance; Malnutrition
  1. Problems:
     a. Anesthesia and surgery can cause further imbalances.
     b. Poor wound healing occurs.
  2. Nursing care:
     a. Assess imbalances.
     b. Monitor intake and output.
     c. Encourage a diet high in protein and vitamin C.
     d. Assist with parenteral fluids and hyperalimentation as ordered.
C. Aging
  1. Problems:
     a. Reactions to the injury are not as obvious and appear more slowly.
     b. A greater cumulative effect of medications occurs.
     c. Sedative and analgesic medications might cause confusion and respiratory depression in lower doses.
  2. Nursing care:
     a. Monitor the dosage of medication.
     b. Anticipate problems resulting from chronic conditions.
D. Presence of Other Diseases
  1. Cardiovascular:
     a. Danger of congestive failure; avoid fluid overload
     b. Avoid prolonged immobilization because it might cause venous stasis.
     c. Encourage change of position; avoid sudden exertion.
  2. Diabetes Mellitus:
     a. Hypoglycemia and ketoacidosis can be life threatening; pick up on the early signs.
     b. Healing might be delayed.
     c. Infections occur more easily.
  3. Alcoholism:
     a. Malnutrition might be present.
     b. Find out the time of the client's last drink to anticipate possible withdrawal symptoms.
     c. Lavage might be indicated to reduce the risk of vomiting and aspiration if emergency surgery is necessary.
     d. Cross-addiction to narcotics and sedative/ hypnotic drugs might occur.
  4. Pulmonary and upper-respiratory disease:
     a. Upper Respiratory Infection (URI) might predispose to pneumonia; surgery might be canceled
     b. Chronic lung problems predispose to difficulty with anesthesia induction and postop respiratory complications
  5. Medications:
     a. Anticoagulants, including aspirin and NSAIDs, predispose to a hemorrhage; discontinue before surgery.
     b. Central nervous system depressants such as phenothiazines and monoamine oxidase inhibitor (MAOI) antidepressants increase the hypotensive action of anesthetics.
     c. Diuretics might cause electrolyte imbalances and respiratory depression during anesthesia.
     d. Notify the physician of all drugs that the client is taking, including over-the-counter medications.
  6. Excessive fear or anxiety:
     a. Might increase anesthesia needs
     b. Might make recovery more difficult
     c. Report to the charge nurse or physician

PREOPERATIVE TEACHING

A. Assess the client's knowledge of the surgery and required care.
B. Explain the nursing procedures and answer questions.
C. Encourage the expression of fears.
D. Teach measures to prevent frequently occurring postoperative complications.

1. Deep breathing and coughing
2. Leg exercises
3. Splinting of incision
E. Reassure the client that pain medication will be available postoperatively.

PHYSICAL PREPARATION FOR SURGERY

A. Nursing history including:
  1. Past medical conditions
  2. Surgical procedures
  3. Allergies
  4. Dietary restrictions
  5. Medications
B. Baseline nursing assessment:
  1. Head to toe assessment
  2. Vital signs
  3. Height and weight
C. Diagnostic procedures as ordered:
  1. *Complete blood count* (CBC)
  2. Electrolytes
  3. Clotting studies (PT/PTT) as ordered
  4. Urinalysis
  5. *Electrocardiogram* (ECG) for clients older than 40 and those who have a history of cardiac problems
  6. Type and crossmatch if ordered
D. Skin preparation
  1. Shower with antibacterial soap if ordered.
  2. Teach the client that shaving will take place in the operating room on the day of the surgery.
E. Bowel preparation
  1. Enema as ordered; usually for clients having gastrointestinal or gynecological surgery
  2. Antibiotics and enemas for lower bowel surgery as ordered

F. Bedtime sedation to promote relaxation if ordered
G. Nothing by mouth (NPO) after midnight to prevent vomiting and aspiration during surgery

IMMEDIATE PREOPERATIVE CARE

A. Vital signs: report temperature elevation and any other abnormality to the charge nurse or physician.
B. Remove dentures, contact lenses, hair pins, and prostheses.
C. Remove nail polish and cosmetics so that skin and nails can be observed for color changes.
D. Put on a clean gown.
E. Have the client empty his or her bladder.
F. Check the identification band.
G. Check the client's chart for a signed operative permit.
H. Administer ordered preoperative medications.
  1. Narcotic analgesics (meperidine HCl [Demerol] and morphine sulfate) to relax the client, relieve anxiety, and enhance the effectiveness of general anesthesia
  2. Sedatives (secobarbital sodium [Seconal] and sodium pentobarbital [Nembutal]) to decrease anxiety and reduce the amount of general anesthesia needed
  3. Anticholinergics (atropine sulfate and scopolamine [Hyoscine]) to decrease tracheobronchial secretions to minimize the danger of aspiration and to decrease the client's vagal response to general anesthesia (bradycardia)
I. Put up the side rails.
J. Complete the preoperative checklist.

Anesthesia

GENERAL ANESTHESIA

A. Central nervous system (CNS) depression induced by medications causes a decrease in muscle reflex activity and loss of consciousness.
B. Stages of general anesthesia (Table 4.1):
  1. The client goes through these stages when general anesthesia is administered.
  2. When recovering from general anesthesia, the client goes through the stages in reverse.

C. Types of general anesthesia:
  1. Inhalation anesthesia: both gas and liquid anesthetic agents are available
  2. IV anesthetics: methohexital (Brevital); sodium thiopental (Pentothal)
    a. Used to give rapid, smooth induction
    b. Can cause respiratory and myocardial depression in high doses
  3. Dissociative anesthetics: Ketamine (Ketalar)
    a. Produce state of profound analgesia and amnesia without loss of consciousness

Table 4.1 Stages of General Anesthesia

Stage	Begins with	Ends with	Client Response
Stage I (induction)	Administration of anesthetic agent	Loss of consciousness	Euphoric, drowsy, dizzy
Stage II (excitement or delirium)	Loss of consciousness	Relaxation	Breathing irregular, blood pressure and pulse may increase, very susceptible to external stimuli
Stage III (operative)	Relaxation	Loss of reflexes and depression of vital functions	Regular breathing; absence of corneal reflexes; pupils constricted
Stage IV (danger stage)	Depression of vital functions	Respiratory and possible cardiac arrest	No respirations; absent or minimal heartbeat; dilated pupils; death if prolonged
		Not part of normal anesthesia	

b. Used alone for short procedures or for induction prior to the administration of general anesthetics

c. Decrease verbal, tactile, and visual stimulation during recovery period

4. Neuroleptic: fentanyl and droperidol (Innovar)
   a. Cause decreased motor activity, decreased anxiety, and analgesia without loss of consciousness
   b. Can be used alone for short surgical and diagnostic procedures or as premedication or in combination with other anesthetics for longer procedures
   c. Side effects: hypotension, bradycardia, respiratory depression, twitching, and skeletal muscle rigidity
   d. Decrease narcotic doses by 1/3 to 1/2 for at least eight hours after anesthesia.

5. Neuromuscular blocking agents: gallamine (Flaxedil), pancuronium (Pavulon), succinylcholine (Anectine), tubocurarine, and Atracurium bromide (Norcuron)
   a. Used as adjuncts to general anesthesia to enhance skeletal relaxation
   b. Monitor respirations for one hour after the drug's effects are worn off.

REGIONAL ANESTHESIA

A. Causes loss of pain sensation in one area of the body; does not alter consciousness
B. Used for biopsies, endoscopies, surgery on extremities, and childbirth
C. Lidocaine (Xylocaine); procaine (Novocain); and tetracaine (Pontocaine)
D. Topical: cream, spray, drops, or ointment applied externally directly to the desired area
E. Local infiltration: injected into subcutaneous tissue of surgical area
F. Nerve block: injection into a nerve plexus
G. Spinal
   1. Anesthetic agent is introduced into subarachnoid space of spinal cord, causing loss of cerebrospinal fluid.
   2. Keep the client flat and hydrate postoperatively due to the loss of cerebrospinal fluid.
H. Epidural
   1. Anesthetic agent is injected extradurally, so no loss of cerebrospinal fluid occurs.
   2. Once sensation and motion return, the client can be up.

Postoperative Period

IMMEDIATE POSTOPERATIVE CARE (RECOVERY ROOM, POST ANESTHESIA CARE UNIT)

A. Maintain a patent airway.
   1. Position an unconscious or semiconscious client on his or her side or back with the head to the side and the chin extended forward.
   2. Check for the gag reflex.
   3. Keep the airway in place until the gag and swallowing reflex is returned.
B. Oxygen as ordered
C. Assess:
   1. Respirations: rate, depth, and quality

2. Vital signs every 15 minutes until stable; then every 30 minutes
3. Level of consciousness: reorient to time and place; sound is first sense to return
4. Color and temperature of skin, nail beds, and lips
5. IV infusions: site and flow rate
6. All drainage tubes: connect to suction or gravity drainage; assess color, amount, and type of drainage
7. Dressings for intactness, drainage, hemorrhage
8. Temperature: might need blankets, especially following epidural anesthesia
D. Cough and deep breathe after the airway is removed.

NURSING CARE ON SURGICAL UNIT

Preventing respiratory complications

A. Risk factors:
1. Thoracic or high abdominal surgery
2. History of respiratory problems
3. Older than age 40
4. Obesity
5. History of smoking
6. Administration of narcotics
7. Severe pain
8. Immobility
B. Complications
1. Atelectasis: collapse of pulmonary alveoli caused by a mucus plug
2. Bronchitis: inflammation of bronchi, causing a cough and mucus secretion
3. Pneumonia
   a. Hypostatic pulmonary congestion
   b. More common in the debilitated or elderly
C. Preventive nursing care
1. Deep breathe q 1-2 h; cough if secretions
2. Splint incision while coughing
3. Turn q 2 hours
4. Incentive spirometer q 2 hrs to inflate alveoli
5. Ambulation
6. Auscultate lungs q 4 hours; report crackles to charge nurse or physician.

Preventing Gastrointestinal Tract Complications

A. Nausea and vomiting
1. Causes
   a. Food or fluid in the stomach before the return of peristalsis
   b. Abdominal distention caused by manipulation of organs during surgery
   c. Anesthesia

d. Expectation
e. Narcotics
2. Management
   a. Pre-op NG tube to prevent abdominal distention as ordered
   b. Deep breaths when the client feels nausea
   c. Support wound during vomiting
   d. Mouth care
   e. Antiemetics as ordered: prochlorperazine (Compazine)
   f. Hot tea with lemon or sips of carbonated beverage, such as ginger ale
   g. Assess for abdominal distention and a paralytic ileus.
B. Thirst
1. Causes include the effect of preoperative anticholinergics, fluid loss, and dehydration due to NPO status pre-op
2. Nursing care
   a. Fluids IV or PO as ordered
   b. Sips of hot tea with lemon juice to dissolve mucus
   c. Moistened gauze square to lips
   d. Mouthwash (not one with alcohol)
   e. Hard candies or chewing gum to stimulate saliva flow
C. Singultus (Hiccups)
1. Spasms of diaphragm caused by irritation of the phrenic nerve
2. Risk factors:
   a. Distended stomach or abdomen, peritonitis, or surgery near the diaphragm
   b. Reflex stimulation caused by exposure to cold, drinking very hot or cold liquids, or intestinal obstruction
3. Management
   a. Remove the cause if possible.
   b. Pressure on the eyeballs, holding breath, inhaling carbon dioxide
   c. Chlorpromazine (Thorazine) and barbiturates as ordered
   d. The physician can interrupt the impulses from the vagus nerve by putting a catheter 3–4 inches (7-10 cm) in the client's pharynx.
   e. Surgical crush of phrenic nerve if intractable hiccups
D. Intestinal function
1. Check for the return of peristalsis: assess bowel sounds every four hours; and check for the passage of flatus.
2. Dietary progression following the return of peristalsis:
   a. Clear liquids (tea, gelatin, water, broth, and sometimes cranberry juice)
   b. Full liquids (a clear liquid diet plus milk products)
   c. Soft (solid foods added to the full liquid diet; no fried or hard-to-digest foods)
   d. Regular

3. Promotion of intestinal function:
    a. Fluid
    b. Fiber makes the stool have more bulk and stimulates evacuation.
    c. Activity stimulates peristalsis.
    d. Opportunity:
        (1) Teach clients to obey the urge.
        (2) Gastrocolic reflex: when client eats, peristalsis occurs throughout the GI tract; offer client bedpan or take to bathroom following a meal
4. Intestinal obstruction:
    a. Risk factors:
        (1) surgery on lower abdomen and pelvis, especially if there is drainage
        (2) adhesions
    b. Manifestations
        (1) occurs 3-5 days postop
        (2) intermittent, sharp abdominal pain
        (3) vomiting of intestinal contents
        (4) no feces; diarrhea if partial obstruction
        (5) abdominal distention
        (6) hypoactive bowel sounds distal to obstruction; hyperactive bowel sounds proximal to obstruction
        (7) shock and death
    c. Management:
        (1) NG tube as ordered to relieve distention
        (2) IVs with electrolytes
        (3) Surgery might be necessary.

Managing Pain

A. Manifestations of pain caused by tissue damage
    1. Severe pain for 12-36 hours; less after 48 hours
    2. Sympathetic nervous system response (adrenalin): "fight or flight," elevated blood pressure, pulse, respiration; perspiration
    3. Skeletal muscle tension
    4. Psychological: irritable, apprehensive, anxious; focuses on pain
B. Nursing care:
    1. Provide comfort measures
    2. Diversion
    3. Relieve localized pain
    4. Administer analgesics as ordered (page 000))
        a. Monitor the respiratory rate when giving narcotics.
        b. Administer tranquilizers and muscle relaxants as ordered.
    5. *Patient-controlled analgesia* (PCA)
        a. Monitor the client for pain, pain relief, and side effects.
        b. Check the infusion system for accuracy and amount.

Care of a Client with Vascular Problems

A. Femoral phlebitis or deep thrombophlebitis
    1. Risk factors:
        a. Surgery on the lower abdomen or pelvis
        b. Septic conditions such as rupture, ulcer, or peritonitis
        c. Injury to vein
        d. Hemoconcentration due to dehydration
    2. Manifestations:
        a. Pain or cramp in calf, progressing to painful swelling of the entire leg
        b. Low-grade fever
        c. Tenderness
        d. Positive Homan's sign (pain in calf when the ankle is dorsiflexed)
    3. Prevention:
        a. Antiembolism stockings
        b. Leg exercises every two hours
        c. Ambulation
        d. Check vital signs, skin color, and temperature q 4h.
    4. Treatment:
        a. Bedrest
        b. Anticoagulant therapy: heparin followed by coumadin
B. Client with pulmonary embolism
    1. An embolus (foreign body, usually a blood clot that has become dislodged from the original site) that is carried to the heart and forced into the pulmonary artery or one of its branches
    2. Manifestations:
        a. Sudden onset of sharp chest pain
        b. Anxiety
        c. Cyanosis
        d. Profuse perspiration
        e. Rapid and irregular pulse
        f. Death often occurs rapidly
    3. Immediate treatment:
        a. Oxygen
        b. Place in upright position
        c. Morphine or Demerol for pain
        d. Thrombolytics (streptokinase, tissue plasminogen activase), anticoagulants (heparin, coumadin)

Urinary Tract

A. Urinary retention
    1. Occurs most often after surgery on the rectum, anus, vagina, or lower abdomen; caused by spasm of sphincter
    2. Nursing care:
        a. Monitor the intake and output.
        b. The client should void within eight hours following surgery if not catheterized; frequent (q 15-30 min.) voiding of small amounts (30-60 cc) suggests an over-distended bladder.

     c. Check for bladder distention.
     d. Promote urination: sitting, warm water on perineum, standing (male).
  B. Urinary incontinence
     1. Caused by loss of tone of bladder sphincter; can occur in the elderly after surgery or injury
     2. Management:
        a. Offer bedpan q 1 hour
        b. Skin care
        c. Fluids: cannot bladder train an empty bladder

Wound care

  A. Types of wounds:
     1. Incision: made by a clean cut with a sharp instrument such as a scalpel
     2. Contusion: made by a blunt force that does not break the skin but causes soft tissue damage
     3. Laceration: made by an object that breaks tissue, causing jagged and irregular edges
     4. Puncture: made by a pointed instrument such as an ice pick, knife, or nail
     5. Clean: made aseptically
     6. Contaminated: exposed to excessive amounts of bacteria, such as in colon surgery
     7. Infected
     8. Dehiscence: separation of layers of a surgical wound
     9. Evisceration: extrusion of viscera (intestines) outside the body through a surgical incision
        a. Risk factors:
           (1) aging
           (2) Pulmonary and cardiovascular diseases interfere with delivery of nutrients to wound
           (3) abdominal distention; obesity
           (4) poor nutrition
           (5) diabetes
        b. Manifestations:
           (1) The client says that something gave way in his or her wound.
           (2) Intestines might protrude from the intestinal wound.
        c. Management:
           (1) Apply abdominal binders for heavy or elderly clients to prevent rupture.
           (2) Stay with the client if dehiscence or evisceration occurs.
           (3) Notify the charge nurse or surgeon stat.
           (4) If intestines are exposed, cover with sterile, moist saline dressings.
           (5) Order bed rest; have the client bend his or her knees to relieve tension on the abdomen.
           (6) Prepare the client for surgery for the repair of the wound.

Wound infection

  A. Common organisms include *staphylococcus aureus, escherichia coli, proteus vulgaris, pseudomonas aeruginosa*, and anaerobic bacteria.
  B. Assessment findings:
     1. Redness, swelling, and tenderness
     2. Red streaks near wound
     3. Pus or discharge from wound
     4. Tender lymph nodes near wound
     5. Foul smell
     6. Chills and fever
     7. Tachycardia
  C. Prevention:
     1. Cleanliness in environment
     2. Aseptic technique
     3. Good nutritional status pre-op
  D. Treatment:
     1. Culture wound
     2. Wound irrigation
     3. Rubber or gauze drain
     4. Antibiotics
     5. Hot, wet dressings

Sample Questions

  1. When informed consent is obtained for surgery, who must explain the surgical procedure to the client?
     1. Physician
     2. Nurse on the surgical unit
     3. Anesthesiologist
     4. Operating room nurse
  2. A 19-year-old unmarried college student is admitted unconscious following a car accident. He is hemorrhaging from severe internal injuries. Which statement is true concerning obtaining informed consent for treating him?
     1. Emergency care can be given because his injuries are life threatening.
     2. He can sign his own consent form because he is older than 18.
     3. Parental consent must be obtained before treatment is started.
     4. The hospital must obtain a court order before treating him.
  3. An adult is to have abdominal surgery this morning. Immediately, preoperatively the nurse must assure that he:
     1. is comfortable.
     2. has an empty bowel.
     3. practices coughing.
     4. voids.
  4. A woman who is to have surgery tomorrow denies any fears or worries about the upcoming surgery. She talks incessantly about trivial matters and is constantly rearranging the items on her bedside stand, however. What is the most appropriate action for the nurse to take?
     1. Listen to her trivial talk.

2. During preoperative teaching, encourage her to ask questions and express concerns.
3. Assume that she is well prepared for surgery and discuss it very little.
4. Probe deeply to find out what is bothering her.

5. What is the primary reason that surface hair is removed from the skin prior to surgery?
   1. To enhance vision of the surgical field
   2. To reduce the chance of infection as the skin is opened
   3. To prevent postoperative discomfort from adhesive tape
   4. To prevent itching in the postoperative period

6. Preoperative orders for an adult client include pentobarbital. This drug is administered primarily to:
   1. control secretions.
   2. control pain.
   3. promote sedation.
   4. provide anesthesia.

7. An adult was given meperidine HCl (Demerol) 75 mg and Atropine Sulfate 0.4 mg as a preoperative medication. On her arrival in the operating room, she says to the nurse, "My mouth is very dry." What is the best response for the nurse to make?
   1. "I will tell the doctor about that."
   2. "That is a normal response to your medication."
   3. "Have you ever had an allergic reaction to any other drugs?"
   4. "Everything is going to be all right."

8. What is the primary problem that can occur as a result of vomiting in the immediate postoperative period?
   1. electrolyte imbalance
   2. dehiscence
   3. aspiration
   4. wound contamination

9. An adult has returned to the surgical floor following an abdominal cholecystectomy and an uneventful stay in the post-anesthesia room. Which nursing action should be the highest priority?
   1. Encourage her to take deep breaths.
   2. Ask her to flex and extend her feet.
   3. Assist her in performing range-of-motion exercises.
   4. Irrigate her T-tube with normal saline.

10. A young man had an emergency appendectomy for a ruptured appendix. He is in the post-anesthesia care unit. He has not yet awakened. An IV is running. A penrose drain is in place. How should the nurse position this client?
    1. Semi-Fowler's position
    2. Supine with head turned to the side
    3. Prone with head and neck extended
    4. Right Sims

11. A young man had an emergency appendectomy for a ruptured appendix and is in the post-anesthesia care unit. A penrose drain is in place. After he recovers from anesthesia, how should he be positioned?
    1. Right Sims
    2. Dorsal
    3. Trendelenburg
    4. Semi-Fowler's

12. The nurse is planning care for a woman who had an abdominal hysterectomy and bilateral salpingectomy and oophorectomy. The nurse knows that because of the location of her surgery, the client is at risk for the development of:
    1. thrombophlebitis.
    2. pneumonia.
    3. stress ulcers.
    4. wound infection.

13. An adult client is admitted to the post-anesthesia care unit following an abdominoperineal resection. Which action should the nurse take initially?
    1. Assess respiratory function.
    2. Monitor IV fluids.
    3. Check abdominal and perineal dressings.
    4. Apply antithromboembolic stockings.

14. The nurse is caring for a woman who just delivered a healthy baby. She received a saddle block anesthesia during delivery. She is admitted to the post-partum unit. Which nursing action is most appropriate?
    1. Encourage her to ambulate as soon as sensation and motion have returned.
    2. Keep her flat and quiet for eight hours.
    3. Keep her NPO for four hours.
    4. Position her in the semi-Fowler's position as soon as she is alert.

15. A man who is recovering from a prostatectomy complains of pain in his left calf. The nurse observes slight ankle swelling and elicits Homan's sign. What is the best action for the nurse to take at this time?
    1. Tell him to stay in bed and notify the charge nurse.
    2. Massage his leg to relieve the pain.
    3. Place a blanket roll under his left knee.
    4. Encourage active ambulation.

Answers and Rationales

1. (1) Explaining the surgical procedure is the physician's responsibility. The nurse teaches about deep breathing, coughing, turning, pain management, and so on.
2. (1) Emergency care can be given without informed consent when there is a life-threatening emergency. He is older than 18 and could sign a consent form if he were conscious. The hospital will attempt to get consent from

his parents for continuing medical care if he remains unconscious after the emergency care is rendered.

3. (4) The key word is *immediately*. An enema can be given the evening before surgery to assure an empty bowel. Comfort is not the highest priority. Neither is coughing immediately preoperatively. The client should go to surgery with an empty bladder.

4. (2) The nurse should open communication with this client who is exhibiting anxious behavior. The nurse never assumes and should not probe deeply. Listening is appropriate, but trivial means unimportant.

5. (2) While there is some controversy about the need to shave a client prior to surgery, the primary reason that it is done is to reduce the chance of infection.

6. (3) Pentobarbital is a barbiturate and promotes sedation. Atropine is given to control secretions. Demerol will control pain. Scopolamine in large doses promotes anesthesia.

7. (2) Atropine is an anticholinergic drug given for the purpose of reducing secretions to prevent the possibility of aspiration.

8. (3) The key word is *immediate*. Aspiration is the primary problem associated with vomiting before the client is alert. Electrolyte imbalance could occur as the result of prolonged vomiting. Dehiscence might occur after violent vomiting.

9. (1) Persons who have a cholecystectomy are especially prone to the development of respiratory complications, because the incision is located under the ribcage.

10. (2) Before clients have awakened from anesthesia, they should be positioned either on their back with their head turned to the side or semi-side lying.

11. (4) The semi-Fowler's position promotes drainage. The client has a penrose drain.

12. (1) Pelvic surgery is a significant risk factor in the development of thrombophlebitis.

13. (1) Assessing airway function is of prime importance immediately following surgery and anesthesia. The other actions will all be done but only after the nurse is assured that the client has an adequate airway.

14. (2) A saddle block is a spinal anesthesia. Because of the loss of cerebrospinal fluid (CSF) during this procedure, it is necessary to keep the client flat for eight hours to prevent the development of a spinal headache. Choice 1 is appropriate for a client who has had an epidural anesthesia. Fluids should be encouraged to promote the formation of CSF.

15. (1) Homan's sign (pain in the calf when the ankle is dorsiflexed) and ankle swelling are suggestive of thrombophlebitis. The client should be placed on bedrest, and the physician should be notified. Massaging and ambulating are contraindicated because these activities might cause a thrombus to become an embolus. Placing a blanket roll under a knee causes venous stasis and clot formation.

Chapter 5

Oncology

CHARACTERISTICS AND PATHOPHYSIOLOGY

Characteristics:

A. Cancer is an umbrella term used to define more than 250 types of neoplastic diseases.
B. Healthy cells are transformed into malignant cells upon exposure to certain etiologic agents such as viruses, bacteria, and chemical and physical agents.
C. Causes:
  1. Genetic predisposition
  2. Chemical carcinogens
  3. Radiation
  4. Tobacco and alcohol
  5. Diet
  6. Viruses and bacteria
  7. Failure of immune response

Pathophysiology:

A. It begins with mutation of a single cell.
B. Mutated cells do not reproduce like normal cells; instead, they grow very rapidly.
C. Malignant cells metastasize (spread) by:
  1. extending directly into adjacent tissue.
  2. permeating along lymphatic vessels.
  3. traveling through the lymph system to nodes.
  4. entering blood circulation.
  5. diffusing into a body cavity.
D. Classification of Tumors (classification according to type of tissue from which they evolve)
  1. Carcinomas:
    a. Arise from epithelial tissues (lung, breast, uterus, or gastrointestinal tract [GI] lining)
    b. Solid tumors originating from a single cell
    c. Can metastasize to distant sites
  2. Sarcomas:
    a. Arise from connective tissue (bone and muscle)
    b. Solid tumors originating from a single cell
    c. Can metastasize to distant sites
  3. Leukemias:
    a. Arise from the blood-forming organs (bone marrow)
    b. Are disseminated throughout the bone marrow
  4. Lymphomas:
    a. Originate in the lymphoreticular system (for example, Hodgkin's disease)
    b. Might be confined initially
    c. If not arrested early, will disseminate throughout the body via the lymphatic system

Assessment

STAGING

A. Describes the extent and anatomic spread of a tumor at a given time, usually at diagnosis, and serves as a guide for prognosis and treatment
B. TNM system:
1. T refers to primary tumor site:
   a. T_0 indicates no evidence of a primary tumor.
   b. T IS means carcinoma in situ (no invasion of lymph nodes or venous metastasis).
   c. T_1, T_2, T_3, or T_4 describes a progressive increase in the tumor, size, and regional tissue involvement; the higher the number, the larger the tumor.
2. N refers to regional node involvement:
   a. N_0 means that regional lymph nodes are not abnormal.
   b. N_1, N_2, N_3, or N_4 indicates an increasing degree of abnormal regional lymph nodes.
3. M refers to distant metastasis:
   a. M_0 means no evidence of distant metastasis.
   b. M_1 indicates distant metastasis.

GRADING

A. Classifies a tumor as to the degree of differentiation or lack of differentiation (anaplasia) from the normal cells
1. The less a cancer cell resembles the normal cell of tissue origin, the greater its degree of anaplasia and the higher its numerical grade (1–4).
2. The higher the grade, the poorer the prognosis.
   a. G_1 = well differentiated, resembles the normal cell
   b. G_2 = moderately well differentiated, some anaplasia
   c. G_3 = poorly differentiated, more anaplasia
   d. G_4 = very poorly differentiated to undifferentiated, highly anaplastic

ASSESSMENT

A. Manifestations suggestive of malignant disease:
1. Change in bowel or bladder habits
2. A sore that does not heal
3. Unusual bleeding or discharge
4. Thickening or lumps in breast or elsewhere
5. Indigestion or difficulty in swallowing
6. Obvious change in wart, mole, or freckle
7. Nagging cough or hoarseness
8. Unexplained weight loss
B. *Complete Blood Count* (CBC):
1. *White Blood Count* (WBC):
   a. Increased levels seen in leukemia
   b. Decreased levels can occur with chemotherapy and radiation therapy
2. *Red Blood Count* (RBC):
   a. Decreased levels seen with some cancers
   b. Decreased levels can occur with chemotherapy and radiation therapy
3. Hematocrit
4. Hemoglobin
5. Platelet count (Thrombocytes):
   a. Decreased levels seen with some cancer
   b. Decreased levels can occur with chemotherapy and radiation therapy.
C. *Carcinoembryonic Antigen* (CEA) test:
1. High titers are found in carcinomas of the stomach, colon, liver, and pancreas.
2. The test is relatively nonspecific; not used for a definitive diagnosis. Following surgery for cancer, rising levels can indicate the recurrence of cancer.
D. Radiographic and imaging tests:
1. *Computerized Axial Tomography* scanning (CT scan or CAT scan):
   a. Helps to detect and localize cancer but does not confirm the diagnosis
   b. Check for an allergy to shellfish or iodine.
   c. Client's diet might or might not be nothing by mouth (NPO), depending on the area of body to be scanned and the type of contrast media used (oral or IV contrast)
   d. When an IV contrast is used, check that the blood urea nitrogen (BUN) and serum creatinine are within normal limits
2. Nuclear studies (for example, bone scan):
   a. It uses radioisotopes to study the internal physiologic processes of the body.
   b. Explain that radioisotopes are given in very small amounts, have a very short life span, and are not considered radioactive
   c. Ask about allergies to shellfish or iodine
3. *Magnetic Resonance Imaging* (MRI):
   a. Assess for claustrophobia.

b. Ask about metal in the patient (head plates, joints, pacemakers, and so on); these are contraindications for MRI

E. Histologic tests (biopsies):
1. Establishes a definitive diagnosis
2. Done under local or general anesthesia depending on the type of biopsy and location of tumor

Interventions

GOALS OF TREATMENT

A. To destroy or eliminate malignant cells while minimizing damage to normal cells
B. To cure the patient and to ensure that minimal functional and structural impairment results from the disease
C. If a cure is not possible:
1. Prevent further metastasis.
2. Relieve symptoms.
3. Maintain a high-quality life as long as possible.

SURGERY

A. Curative removes the entire tumor along with a small margin of regional tissue or lymph nodes
B. Preventive removes noncancerous growths that would probably become cancerous if left in place
C. Palliative is performed to relieve symptoms such as pain or dyspnea

CHEMOTHERAPY

A. Most drugs interfere with cell division; affect any rapidly growing cells, not just cancer cells
B. Classification of drugs (see Table 5.1):
1. Alkylating agents
2. Antimetabolites
3. Antitumor antibiotics
4. Vinca (plant) alkaloids
5. Antihormonal therapy
6. Hormonal therapy
7. Miscellaneous
8. Corticosteroids (prednisone, cortisone, dexamethasone, and hydrocortisone) used as adjuncts to other chemotherapeutic agents
C. Major side effects and nursing interventions:
1. Bone marrow depression causing a decrease in RBC, WBC, and platelets
   a. Assess for signs and symptoms of anemia, leukopenia, and thrombocytopenia.

   b. Administer Epogen to increase RBC production and Neupogen to increase WBC production if indicated.
   c. Place the client on neutropenic or bleeding precautions if indicated (see Tables 5.2 and 5.3).
   d. Monitor CBC studies.
   e. Allow periods of rest and give oxygen if indicated.
2. Gastrointestinal tract/mucous membranes:
   a. Stomatitis and esophagitis: client has difficulty eating and swallowing because of ulcers; prone to mouth thrush
      (1) Give meticulous mouth care
      (2) Might need local anesthesia for pain
      (3) Viscous lidocaine mouthwash; no mouthwash containing alcohol
   b. Taste alterations:
      (1) Food tastes bitter
      (2) Increased threshold for sugar (takes more sugar to taste sweet)
      (3) Metallic taste
      (4) Room temperature and cold foods better than hot foods
      (5) Encourage snacking
   c. Nausea, vomiting, and anorexia causes decreased nutrition, weight loss, and electrolyte imbalance.
      (1) Give chemotherapy in the late afternoon or night to decrease nausea and vomiting at meal times.
      (2) Provide antiemetics as ordered: prochlorperazine (Compazine), promethazine (Phenergan), metoclopramide (Reglan), ondansetron (Zofran), diphenhydramine (Benadryl), and lorazepam (Ativan).
      (3) Maintain adequate hydration and nutrition.
      (4) Monitor intake and output.
   d. Constipation caused by neurotoxicity of Vinca alkaloids:
      (1) Encourage fluids.
      (2) Give stool softeners as indicated.

Table 5.1 Cancer Chemotherapeutic Agents

Type	Action	Examples	Uses
Alkylating agents	Produces breaks and cross-linking in the DNA strands, interfering with cell reproduction	cyclophosphamide (Cytoxan)	Cancer of ovary, breast, malignant lymphomas, retinoblastoma, multiple myeloma, leukemias, and neuroblastoma
		mechlorethamine (Mustargen)	Polycythemia vera, Hodgkin's disease, chronic leukemia, and bronchogenic cancer
		busulfan (Myleran)	Chronic myelogenous leukemia
Antimetabolites	Substances bearing close resemblance to one required for normal physiologic functioning; exerts effect by interfering with the utilization of the essential metabolite, causing cell death	fluorouracil (Adrucil)	Cancer of colon, rectum, breast, stomach, and pancreas
		methotrexate (Folex)	Acute lymphocytic leukemia
		Cytarabine (Cytosar-U or Ara -c)	Leukemias
Antitumor antibiotics	Kills the host cell as well as the organism	doxorubicin (Adriamycin)	Leukemias, Wilm's tumor, neuroblastoma, sarcomas, lymphomas; bronchogenic, gastric, thyroid, breast, and ovarian cancers
		bleomycin (Blenoxane)	Squamous cell carcinoma, lymphomas, and testicular cancer
		dactinomycin (Cosmegen)	Wilm's tumor, testicular cancer, and Ewing's sarcoma
Vinca (plant) alkaloids	Alkaloids extracted from the periwinkle plant; arrests cell division by disrupting the microtubules that form the spindle apparatus	vincristine sulfate (Oncovin)	Leukemias, lymphomas, and Wilm's tumor
		vinblastine (Velban)	Leukemias, lymphomas, testicular cancer, Kaposi's sarcoma, and breast cancer
		etoposide (VP-16)	testicular tumor, small cell lung cancer
Antihormonal therapy	Inhibits natural hormones and stops the growth of tumors dependent on that hormone	tamoxifen (Nolvadex)	Breast cancer
		flutamide (Eulexin)	Prostate cancer
		goserelin acetate (Zoladex)	Prostate cancer
Hormonal therapy	Manipulation of hormones to stop cancer cell growth	Estrogens (diethylstilbestrol [DES])	Breast and prostate cancer
		medroxyprogesterone (DepoProvera)	Endometrial and renal carcinoma
		megestrol (Megase)	Breast and endometrial carcinoma
		testolactone (Teslac)	Breast carcinoma
Miscellaneous	Works by different methods	L-asparaginase (Elspar)	Acute lymphocytic leukemia
		procarbazine hydrochloride (Matulane)	Hodgkin's disease

e. Diarrhea caused by destruction of epithelium of the intestines:
   (1) Monitor electrolytes.
   (2) Hydrate the patient.
   (3) Medicate as indicated with Imodium or Lomotil.

3. Integumentary system:
   a. Skin reactions:
      (1) rashes, redness, photosensitivity
      (2) requires good skin care
   b. Alopecia
      (1) Wash hair gently.
      (2) Get a short haircut.
      (3) Buy a hairpiece before hair loss begins.

Table 5.2 Bleeding Precautions

Bleeding Precautions

- Use a soft toothbrush and brush gently.
- If the platelet count is extremely low, foam swabs should be used instead of a toothbrush.
- Report any bleeding of the gums.
- Use only electric razors.
- Minimize lab draws and IM injections; apply pressure to all needle sticks for 3–5 minutes.
- Report any bruising, rashes, or bleeding.
- Check urine and stool for hidden blood.
- Avoid constipation.
- Do not allow drugs containing aspirin or anticoagulants.

Table 5.3 Neutropenic Precautions

Neutropenic Precautions

- No fresh fruit or vegetables allowed (causes intestinal bacteria growth).
- No flowers allowed.
- Limit visitors (absolutely no one with a cold or infection).
- Enforce strict hand washing; visitors can wear mask and gloves.
- Watch for signs of infection.
- Assess lab values and temperature.
- No rectal temperatures, suppositories, or enemas allowed.
- Avoid urinary catheters.
- Use onlt soft toothbrush (the mouth is the most frequent site of infection).

4. Neurotoxicity occurs most frequently with Vinca alkaloids.
5. Nephrotoxicity:
   a. Monitor electrolytes, BUN, and creatinine.
   b. Monitor hydration, intake, and output.
6. Elevated uric acid and crystal and urate stone formation:
   a. Encourage fluids.
   b. Use Allopurinol (Zyloprim) as ordered to increase uric acid excretion.

RADIATION THERAPY

A. Destroys the cancer cells' ability to grow; also destroys normal cells
B. Uses:
   1. Before surgery to shrink the tumor
   2. After surgery to stop the growth of the remaining tumor or to prevent a recurrence
   3. In conjunction with chemotherapy to shrink the tumor
C. External radiation:
   1. The client must lie still on the x-ray table.
   2. The client will be marked with water-soluble ink to define the area of treatment; do not wash the marks off.

3. Side effects:
   a. Anorexia, nausea and vomiting
   b. Skin irritation
   c. Some hair loss
4. Instruct the client:
   a. Not to apply soap, deodorant, lotion, perfume, or topical medication to skin
   b. To avoid extreme heat and cold to the skin
   c. To avoid rubbing the area
   d. To wear loose clothes
   e. To use electric shaver not safety razor
   f. To wear a sunscreen
   g. If a "wet" reaction occurs, wash with water, keep open, and can use antibiotic cream
D. Internal radiation:
   1. Can be implanted into a body cavity or directly into the tumor
   2. Might require the use of a private room with lead walls
   3. Limit number of staff/visitors and time in the room
   4. Might require body excretion precautions
   5. If the radiation source falls out:
      a. Do not touch it with bare hands.
      b. Pick it up with long forceps and place in a lead container that should be in the client's room.
   6. Limit radiation exposure.
      a. Keep your distance; radiation exposure is decreased with distance.
      b. Limit the time of exposure; radiation is cumulative.

EMOTIONAL SUPPORT

A. Coping with loss of health or body part:
   1. Denial: characterized by shock, disbelief, isolation, and detachment
   2. Anger: client might try to control the situation by becoming demanding; asks "Why me?"
   3. Bargaining: client will bargain for time by making promises, usually to God, in an attempt to postpone the inevitable
   4. Depression: sadness overwhelms as the impact of the loss becomes real
   5. Acceptance: characterized by a void in feeling and by diminished communication or disengagement from worldly concerns; loved ones need support at this time
B. Encourage clients and families to verbalize feelings
C. Support services:
   1. National groups:
      a. American Cancer Society
      b. Leukemia Society of America
      c. National Cancer Institute

  d. Make Today Count, Inc.
  e. American Lung Association
 2. Local groups:
  a. Ostomates for ostomy clients
  b. Lost chord for laryngectomies
  c. Reach for Recovery for mastectomy
  d. Hospital support groups
 3. Hospice:
  a. Provides palliative and supportive care to terminally ill persons and their families
  b. Primary medical concern is pain control and comfort measures
  c. Emphasis on emotional support

Sample Questions

1. The nurse is caring for a client who is being treated for cancer. Which question by the client indicates that the client is not ready for teaching?
   1. "Am I going to lose my hair?"
   2. "Should I get a second opinion?"
   3. "Will this make me really sick?"
   4. "Will I have to stop exercising at the gym?"
2. The nurse caring for a client who is receiving chemotherapy is concerned about the client's nutritional status. What should the nurse encourage the client to do?
   1. Increase the amount of spices in the food.
   2. Avoid red meats.
   3. Medicate with Compazine before meals.
   4. Eat foods that are hot in temperature.
3. In planning care for a client with a platelet count of 8,000, and a WBC of 8,000 the nurse can expect to:
   1. remove flowers from the room.
   2. encourage fresh fruit and vegetables.
   3. use a strict hand-washing technique.
   4. take the client's temperature frequently.
4. The nurse is teaching a client with a WBC of 1,400. Which statement made by the client indicates an understanding of the teaching?
   1. "I will eat fresh fruits and vegetables to avoid constipation."
   2. "I will stay away from my cat."
   3. "I will avoid crowded places."
   4. "I will wash all my fruits and vegetables before I eat them."
5. In evaluating the client with cancer what best indicates that the nutritional status is adequate?
   1. calorie intake
   2. stable weight
   3. amount of nausea and vomiting
   4. serum protein levels
6. An adult client with newly diagnosed cancer says, "I'm really afraid of dying. Who's going to take care of my children?" What is the best initial response for the nurse to make?
   1. "What makes you think you are going to die?"
   2. "How old are your children?"
   3. "This must be a difficult time for you."
   4. "Most people with your kind of cancer live a long time."
7. A client with terminal cancer yells at the nurse and says "I don't need your help, I can bathe myself." Which stage of grief is the client most likely experiencing?
   1. Projection
   2. Denial
   3. Anger
   4. Depression
8. The nurse can expect a client with a platelet count of 8,000 and a WBC count of 8,000 to be placed:
   1. in a private room.
   2. on protective isolation.
   3. on bleeding precautions.
   4. on neutropenic precautions.
9. Which statement made by the client indicates understanding of the needs related to external radiation therapy?
   1. "I'll stay away from small children since I am radioactive."
   2. "I won't wash these marks off until after my therapy."
   3. "I'll put lotion on my skin to keep it moist."
   4. "I'll flush the toilet twice each time I use the bathroom."
10. When teaching and preparing a client for a bone marrow biopsy, the nurse should:
    1. check for an iodine allergy.
    2. position the client in the fetal position with his or her back curved.
    3. have the client sign the consent form.
    4. have the client remain NPO.
11. An adult says to the nurse, "The doctor said I have a carcinoma and my friend has a sarcoma. What is the difference?" What should the nurse include in the response?
    1. Carcinoma is usually more serious than a sarcoma.
    2. Carcinoma indicates that the tissue involved is epithelial, such as the GI tract or breast; sarcoma indicates that the tissue involved is connective tissue, such as the bone.
    3. Carcinoma is a malignancy that usually appears early in life, while individuals who develop a sarcoma of any type are usually older.
    4. Carcinomas are not as likely to metastasize to distant sites as sarcomas are.
12. The nurse is teaching a group of persons in the community about risk factors for cancer. Which is not a risk factor and should not be included in the teaching?
    1. A change in bowel habits
    2. Difficulty in swallowing
    3. Unexplained weight gain
    4. Nagging hoarseness

13. A woman who has had surgery for colon cancer asks the nurse why the doctor has her come back for a blood test called CEA. What is the best response for the nurse to make?
    1. "You should ask your physician about specific tests."
    2. "High levels of CEA are found in cancers of the colon; continued low levels after surgery indicate there is probably not a recurrence."
    3. "CEA is used to monitor your blood to be sure you are not getting side effects from the treatment."
    4. "CEA levels should increase as your general health increases."

14. An adult is undergoing diagnostic tests for possible cancer. A liver scan is scheduled. The client asks whether she will need to stay away from people because she is radioactive following the test. What should be included in the nurse's response?
    1. She will be radioactive after the scan and should avoid small children and pregnant women.
    2. The radioisotope doses used in the scan are very small, and she will not be a hazard to others.
    3. Radioopaque substances are used, not radioisotopes, so there is no radioactivity.
    4. Because the liver is being scanned, the breakdown of the substances will be delayed, so caution is needed.

15. The client has been receiving chemotherapy for cancer and has stomatitis. What nursing care is indicated because the client has stomatitis?
    1. Have the client rinse his or her mouth well with Listerine or other mouthwash before and after eating.
    2. Use meticulous care when cleaning the stoma and applying the drainage bag.
    3. Maintain NPO status until the condition improves.
    4. Encourage the client to use viscous lidocaine mouthwash as needed.

16. An adult woman is scheduled to start chemotherapy next week. In anticipation of alopecia, which recommendation is appropriate?
    1. Encourage the client to cut her hair and buy a wig.
    2. Recommend the client wash her hair carefully daily to prevent hair loss.
    3. Suggest that the client have a color photograph taken before starting chemotherapy so that hair color can be matched if necessary.
    4. Explain to the client that she should plan to have a hair transplant following chemotherapy.

17. The client is receiving cancer chemotherapy. Metoclopramide (Reglan) is also ordered. She asks the nurse why she is receiving Reglan. What nursing response is most accurate?
    1. Reglan is a stool softener and will help with the constipation the chemotherapy might cause.
    2. Reglan will help prevent alopecia.
    3. Reglan helps prevent diarrhea.
    4. Reglan will help control nausea and vomiting.

18. Allopurinol (Zyloprim) is ordered for the client who is receiving cancer chemotherapy. What instruction should the nurse give the client because allopurinol is ordered?
    1. Drink several additional glasses of water each day.
    2. Avoid foods containing folic acid.
    3. When you get up from lying down, sit on the edge of the bed for a few minutes before standing up.
    4. Avoid caffeine-containing products.

19. Which instruction is appropriate for the nurse to give the client who is undergoing external radiation therapy?
    1. Avoid gas-forming foods such as beans and cabbage.
    2. Be sure to get outdoors in the sun for a few minutes each day.
    3. Do not apply powders, deodorants, or ointments to your skin.
    4. Tight-fitting clothes will give you the most support.

20. The nurse is caring for a person who has radiation pellets inserted in the mouth to treat oral cancer. One of the pellets falls out. What should the nurse do initially?
    1. Put on rubber gloves and pick up the pellet and place it in the utility room.
    2. Use long-handled forceps to pick up the pellet and place it in a lead-lined container.
    3. Call the Nuclear Medicine Department.
    4. Replace the pellet in the mouth.

Answers and Rationales

1. (2) This statement indicates denial of his illness. The question states that he has cancer. All of the other comments indicate an interest in what is going to happen to him.
2. (1) Because taste buds are affected, increasing the spices will improve flavor.
3. (2) Fresh fruits and vegetables will help the client prevent constipation, which could cause bleeding. All of the other choices are appropriate for a low WBC, but this WBC is normal. The problem for this client is a low platelet count.
4. (3) Crowded places predispose to client infection. Choice 1 is related to low platelet count. The client should not eat fresh fruits and vegetables even if they are washed.

5. (2) Stable weight indicates adequate nutritional status.
6. (3) This empathetic response will open communication. Choice 1 is really a "why" question, which would put the client on the defensive. Choices 2 and 4 do not focus on the client's feelings.
7. (3) Yelling at the nurse would be typical of anger. Projection is putting his feelings on the nurse: "You are angry at me." Denial would be denying that he was terminally ill or that he had cancer. A client who is depressed would be apathetic and would probably not have the energy to yell at the nurse.
8. (3) The platelet count is very low. Normal is 150,000–500,000. Platelets clot the blood. The client must be on bleeding precautions. A WBC of 8,000 is within the normal range, so neutropenic precautions, protective isolation, and a private room are not indicated.
9. (2) It is important that the client not wash off the marks until after therapy is finished. The marks outline the tumor and show where the radiation should be concentrated. The client who is receiving external radiation is not radioactive and should not put anything on the skin. While flushing the toilet after each use is good hygiene, it is not related to external radiation. There is no radioactivity in the waste of a person who is receiving external radiation.
10. (3) A bone marrow biopsy is an invasive procedure that requires a legal consent form to be signed. No iodine dye is used. The usual site is the iliac crest; the client will not be placed in the fetal position. That is the position for a lumbar puncture. There is no need for the client to be NPO. Only a local anesthetic is used.
11. (2) Carcinoma indicates that the tissue involved is epithelial, such as the GI tract or breast; sarcoma indicates that the tissue involved is connective tissue, such as the bone. No general statement about the difference in severity or age of onset can be made because the terms indicate the type of tissue involved. Both types of cancers can metastasize.
12. (3) An unexplained weight loss is a possible sign of cancer. Unexplained weight gain is not usually associated with undetected cancer. A change in bowel habits, difficulty in swallowing, and nagging hoarseness are all possible warning signs of cancer.
13. (2) High levels of CEA are found in cancers of the colon; continued low levels after surgery indicate that there is probably not a recurrence. When cancers of the GI tract are present or when they have been removed and recur, the *Carcinoembryonic Antigen* (CEA) levels rise. CEA levels are monitored following surgery to pick up a possible spread or recurrence early. The nurse should know this information and should not have to refer to the physician for general information about this test. CEA tests do not monitor the side effects of cancer treatment; a *complete blood count* (CBC) would pick up bone marrow depression. CEA levels do not increase with improvement in general health.
14. (2) Radioisotopes are used when most scans (except CT scans) are performed. The doses are so small, however, that the client is not considered radioactive—and no special precautions need to be taken.
15. (4) Stomatitis is a sore mouth and is commonly seen in persons who are receiving cancer chemotherapy. Lidocaine is a local anesthetic and will help relieve the pain of stomatitis. Listerine mouthwash contains alcohol and is contraindicated for a person who has mouth sores. Stomatitis refers to mouth sores, not a colostomy stoma. There is no need to maintain NPO status.
16. (1) The client should be encouraged to cut her hair and buy a wig if desired before starting chemotherapy. Alternatively, she could purchase scarves and use them to cover her head. When the hair falls out, it is easier to manage the loss of short hair than long hair. Washing hair will not prevent hair loss from chemotherapy. Having a color photograph taken before chemotherapy to match hair color is not the best answer. It would be better to match hair color in a wig before starting chemotherapy than waiting until after the hair is gone. Hair usually grows back following chemotherapy. It might not be the same color or have the same characteristics, however. A hair transplant is not indicated.
17. (4) Reglan is an antiemetic and will help control nausea and vomiting caused by the chemotherapy. It is not a stool softener and does not prevent alopecia or diarrhea.
18. (1) Allopurinol is given to help the client excrete uric acid, which might accumulate when cancer chemotherapeutic agents are given. The client should drink several additional glasses of water each day to help the kidneys flush the uric acid out of the system. There is no need to avoid foods containing folic acid because the client is taking allopurinol. This measure might be indicated depending on the chemotherapeutic agent the client is taking. Allopurinol does not cause orthostatic hypotension. Antiemetics might cause orthostatic hypotension. There is no need to avoid caffeine-containing products because the client is taking allopurinol.
19. (3) The client should put nothing on the skin. Deodorants and powders usually contain heavy metals, such as aluminum or zinc, and block radiation rays. Lotions and ointments should not be applied to the skin because they might further irritate the skin. There is no major

reason to avoid gas-forming foods. That instruction is more appropriate for a person who has had a colostomy. If the client becomes nauseated, she should avoid any irritating food. Sun will irritate the client's sensitive skin. The person should wear loose-fitting clothes to avoid skin irritation, not tight-fitting clothes.

20. (2) The nurse should use long-handled forceps to pick up the pellet and place it in a lead-lined container. Afterward, the nurse should call the Nuclear Medicine Department. The nurse should never touch the pellet directly. Rubber gloves give no protection from radiation.

Chapter 6

Cardiovascular System

ANATOMY AND PHYSIOLOGY OF THE CARDIOVASCULAR SYSTEM

Heart (Figure 6.1)

A. A muscular pump that propels blood into the arterial system and receives blood from the venous system
B. Heart wall:
1. Pericardium: outermost layer
2. Epicardium: covers the surface of the heart
3. Myocardium: middle, muscular layer
4. Endocardium: thin, inner layer lining the chambers of the heart
5. Papillary muscles: arise from the endocardial and myocardial surface of the ventricles and attach to the chordae tendinae
6. Chordae tendinae: attach to the tricuspid and mitral valves and prevent eversion during systole
C. Chambers
1. Atria:
   a. Two upper chambers; function as receiving chambers
   b. Right atrium receives systemic venous blood through the superior and inferior vena cava and coronary sinus
   c. Left atrium receives oxygenated blood returning to the heart from the lungs through the pulmonary veins
2. Ventricles:
   a. Two lower chambers; function as pumping chambers
   b. Right ventricle pumps deoxygenated blood into the pulmonary circulation
   c. Left ventricle pumps blood into the systemic circulation
D. Valves
1. Atrioventricular valves
   a. Mitral valve:
      (1) Located between the left atrium and left ventricle
      (2) Contains two leaflets attached to the chordae tendinae
   b. Tricuspid valve:
      (1) Located between the right atrium and right ventricle
      (2) Contains three leaflets attached to the chordae tendinae
   c. Functions:
      (1) Permits unidirectional flow of blood during ventricular diastole
      (2) Prevents reflux during ventricular systole

(3) First heart sound (S₁) is leaflets closing during ventricular systole

2. Semilunar valves:
  a. Pulmonary valve located between the right ventricle and pulmonary artery
  b. Aortic valve located between left ventricle and aorta

c. Functions:
  (1) Permit unidirectional flow of blood during ventricular systole
  (2) Prevent reflux during ventricular diastole
  (3) Valves open when ventricles contract and close during ventricular diastole
  (4) Valve closure produces second heart sound (S₂)

E. Conduction System (Figure 6.2)
  1. Sinoatrial (SA) node: pacemaker of the heart. Initiates cardiac impulse that spreads across the atria and into the AV node.
  2. Atrioventricular (AV) node: delays the impulse from the atria while the ventricles fill
  3. Bundle of His: Arises from the AV node and conducts impulse to the bundle branch system
  4. Purkinje fibers: Transmit impulses to the ventricles and provide for depolarization after ventricular contraction
  5. ECG is the visualization of electrical activity of the heart.

F. Coronary circulation
  1. Coronary arteries:
    a. Branch off at the base of the aorta
    b. Supply blood to the myocardium
  2. Coronary veins return blood from the myocardium back to the right atrium via the coronary sinus.

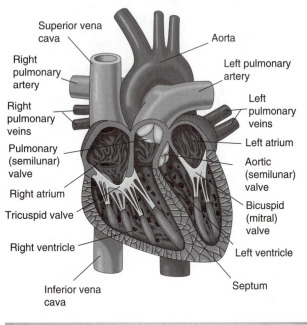

Figure 6.1 Internal view of the heart.

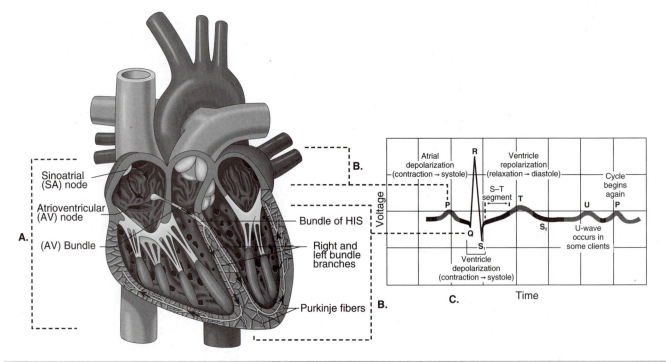

Figure 6.2 A. Conduction system of the heart; B. Relationship of the conduction system to an EKG strip; C. Relationship of S₁ and S₂ heart sounds to an EKG strip.

Vascular System

A. Major function is to supply the tissues with blood, remove wastes, and carry unoxygenated blood back to the heart
B. Arteries:
1. Elastic walled vessels that can stretch during systole and recoil after diastole
2. Carry blood away from the heart
3. Distribute oxygenated blood throughout the body
C. Arterioles:
1. Small arteries that distribute blood to the capillaries
2. Function in controlling systemic vascular resistance and arterial pressure
D. Capillaries:
1. Exchange oxygen and carbon dioxide at the cellular level
2. Exchange solutes between the blood and tissues
3. Fluid volume transfer between the plasma and interstitial spaces
E. Venules:
1. Small veins that receive blood from the capillaries
2. Function as collecting channels between the capillaries and the veins
F. Veins:
1. Low-pressure vessels with thin walls
2. Most contain valves that prevent backward blood flow
3. Carry deoxygenated blood flow back to the heart
4. When skeletal muscles around veins contract, veins are compressed—pushing blood back to the heart.

Diagnostic Procedures

LABORATORY TESTS

A. Serum electrolytes
1. Sodium (Na$^+$)
a. 136–142 mEq/L
b. Hyponatremia associated with excessive fluid intake or chronic diuretic use with sodium restriction
2. Potassium (K$^+$)
a. 3.5–5.0 mEq/L
b. Both high and low values affect the electrical activity of heart muscle and cause dysrhythmias.
c. Diuretics can be potassium-depleting (thiazides, Lasix) or potassium-sparing (Aldactone).
3. Calcium (Ca^{++})
a. 8.5–10.5 mg/dl
b. Imbalances directly affect the strength of myocardial contraction and impulse formation
B. Sedimentation rate (ESR): Nonspecific test indicating inflammatory response somewhere in the body
1. Measures speed with which RBCs settle in uncoagulated blood
2. Elevated in acute MI, bacterial endocarditis, and rheumatic fever

C. Blood coagulation tests
1. Prothrombin Time (PT, ProTime)
a. Prothrombin (Factor II) is produced by the liver; vitamin K is required for synthesis; prothrombin is converted to thrombin by the action of thromboplastin, which is needed to form a clot
b. Normal: 11–15 seconds or 7–100%
c. For clients on anticoagulant therapy [Warfarin (Coumadin)] normal is 2–2.5 times the control in seconds (or 20–30%)
d. May be reported as International Normalized Ratio (INR); INR of 2–3 times on Warfarin (Coumadin) therapy
e. Decreased level caused by thrombo-phlebitis, barbiturates, digitalis, oral contraceptives, Rifampin, or vitamin K
f. Increased level
(1) Causes include liver diseases, deficiency of clotting factors II, V, VII, X; leukemias, drug toxicity
(2) Assess alcohol consumption; PT may be prolonged with regular high alcohol consumption.
(3) Observe for signs of bleeding
(4) Vitamin K is the antidote for coumadin; vitamin K is given when PT is over 40 seconds

2. Partial Thromboplastin Time (PTT)
   a. Can detect deficiencies in all clotting factors except VII and XIII; used to monitor heparin dosage
   b. Normal: 60–70 seconds; clients on heparin therapy should have a PTT value of 1.5 to 3 times normal
   c. Increased level
      (1) Causes include deficiency of factors V, VIII, IX, X, XI, XII; liver diseases, vitamin K deficiency, DIC, excessive heparin, and salicylates
      (2) Observe for bleeding
      (3) Decreased level caused by extensive cancer
3. Coagulation Time (Lee White Clotting Time)
   a. Clotting time determines the time it takes for venous blood to clot in a glass test tube; used to monitor and regulate patients receiving heparin therapy
   b. Normal: 5–15 minutes; clients receiving heparin should be 20 minutes
   c. Decreased time may be caused by cortisone or adrenaline
   d. Prolonged (increased) time
      (1) Desired with heparin therapy
      (2) Indicative of severe clotting disorder in client not on heparin
      (3) Observe for bleeding
D. Serum lipids: cholesterol, triglycerides, phospholipids, high-density lipids, low-density lipids, very low-density lipids
   1. Serum cholesterol should be < 200 mg/dL
   2. High density lipoproteins (HDL); Male: > 45 mg/dL; Female: > 55 mg/dL
   3. Low-density lipoproteins (LDL) 60–180 mg/dL
   4. Very low-density lipoproteins (VLDL) 25%–50%
   5. Client must be fasting
   6. High-density lipids carry fat out of vessels; low-density lipids carry fat into vessels
   7. Clients with low HDL and high LDL levels are at high risk for coronary artery disease and myocardial infarction.
E. Blood cultures: crucial in the diagnosis of infective endocarditis
F. Drug levels: monitoring of blood levels of cardiac drugs is essential for successful and safe treatment
G. Enzymes: CPK, LDH, AST (SGOT); troponin valuable in diagnosis of MI
   1. CPK (Creatinine phosphokinase) Male: 12–70 U/mL or 55–170 U/L (SI units); Female: 10–55 U/mL or 30–135 U/L (SI units)
   2. LDH: 45–90 U/L or 115–225 IU/L or 0.4–1.7 µmol/ l (SI units)
3. AST (SGOT): 8–2 U/L or 5–40 IU/L or 8–20 U/L (SI units)
4. Troponin: negative

NONINVASIVE TESTS

A. Electrocardiogram (ECG or EKG)
   1. Recording of electrical activity of the heart (Figure 6.2B)
   2. Useful in all types of heart disease; ischemia, infarct, CAD, valvular heart disease, and arrhythmias
   3. No client preparation required
B. Ambulatory electrocardiography (Holter Monitor)
   1. A portable recorder is worn and a continuous ECG is obtained
   2. Diaries of activity and episodes of client perception of irregular heart beats are kept
C. Exercise stress test
   1. ECG is monitored during exercise on a treadmill or a bicycle-like device
   2. Purposes
      a. Identify ischemic heart disease
      b. Evaluate patients with chest pain
      c. Assess results of therapy
      d. Develop individual fitness programs
   3. Nursing care
      a. No smoking, eating, or drinking for four hours before the test; sometimes a light meal is allowed
      b. Avoid stimulants or extreme temperature changes after the test
D. Chest X-ray
   1. Provides information about the size, shape, and location of the heart
   2. Can detect enlarged heart or chambers of the heart
E. Echocardiogram (Ultrasound cardiography)
   1. Used to locate and study the movements and dimensions of the various cardiac structures
   2. Evaluates valvular function, chamber size, and filling and ejection defects
   3. Can also detect endocarditis and effusions
   4. No client preparation is needed
F. Myocardial nuclear scanning (Thallium stress test)
   1. Involves injection of radioactive technetium or Thallium during exercise
   2. Useful in evaluation of the size of infarct, diagnosis of CAD, and evaluation of patency or occlusion of vein bypass grafts
   3. Preparation is the same as for a normal stress test.
G. Doppler ultrasonography
   1. Evaluates the circulation in the blood vessels

2. Useful in diagnosis of deep vein thrombosis
3. Requires no client preparation

INVASIVE PROCEDURES

A. Central venous pressure
   1. Monitors pressure within the right atrium and assesses right-sided heart function
   2. Zero level of the manometer is at the level of the patient's heart
   3. Serial CVP readings should be made with the patient in the same position
B. Swan Ganz Catheter
   1. A flow-directed, balloon-tipped, four-lumen catheter allowing for right heart catheterization at the bedside
   2. Provides continuous monitoring of:
      a. Right and left ventricular function
      b. Pulmonary artery pressures
      c. Cardiac output
      d. Arterial venous oxygen difference
C. Arteriogram
   1. Injection of contrast medium into the vascular system to outline the heart and arteries
   2. NPO before procedure sometimes
   3. Nursing care after procedure
      a. Vital signs q 15 minutes until stable
      b. Check for bleeding at puncture or cutdown site
      c. Pressure dressing and/or sandbag on puncture site for several hours post procedure to prevent bleeding at puncture site

   d. Check distal extremity for color and pulses to monitor for clot obstructing circulation
D. Cardiac catheterization
   1. An arteriogram of the coronary arteries and structures of the heart
   2. Used to assess:
      a. Patency of coronary arteries
      b. Cardiac function and output
      c. Oxygen levels in chambers of the heart
      d. Valves
   3. Procedure
      a. Right heart catheterization: venous approach (antecubital or femoral) to vena cava to right atrium to right ventricle to pulmonary artery
      b. Left heart catheterization: arterial approach (brachial or femoral) to aorta to left ventricle
   4. Pre-procedure nursing care
      a. Assess for iodine allergy because iodine dye is used to visualize arteries
      b. Baseline vital signs
      c. Have client void
      d. Administer sedatives if ordered
      e. Mark distal pulses
   5. Post-procedure nursing care
      a. Check peripheral pulses to monitor for clot obstructing circulation
      b. Assess puncture site for hemorrhage or clot
      c. Immobilize punctured extremity
      d. Monitor vital signs and ECG
      e. Push fluids (IV or PO) to help dilute contrast media and rid body of dye

Cardiovascular Conditions

HYPERTENSION

A. General Information
   1. Persistent blood pressure above 140 systolic and 90 diastolic
   2. Known as the "silent killer" because there are few early signs and symptoms
   3. 90% of hypertension is known as essential hypertension (hypertension not caused by renal or adrenal problems)
B. Factors associated with development of hypertension (risk factors)
   1. Heredity
   2. High incidence among African Americans, Hispanic Amercians, Native Americans
   3. Medications such as estrogen and progesterone

   4. High-fat diet and obesity
   5. Smoking
   6. Stress
   7. High-sodium diet in some individuals
   8. Lack of exercise
C. Nursing Diagnoses (Table 6.1)
D. Interventions: Antihypertensive medications as prescribed
   1. Potassium-depleting diuretics: thiazides, furosemide (Lasix)
      a. Monitor for hypokalemia and deficiencies of other electrolytes
      b. Potassium supplement may be ordered
      c. Teach dietary sources of potassium (Table 6.2)
      d. Monitor blood pressure and pulse
      e. Monitor blood sugar levels in diabetics

Table 6.1 Nursing Diagnoses Related to Hypertension

- Risk for noncompliance related to negative side effects of prescribed therapy versus the belief that no treatment is needed unless symptoms are present
- Risk for ineffective sexuality patterns related to decreased libido or erectile dysfunction secondary to medication side effects
- Risk for ineffective health maintenance related to insufficient knowledge of diet restriction, medications, signs of complications, risk factors, follow-up care, and stress reduction activities

Table 6.2 Dietary Sources of Potassium

• citrus fruits (oranges, grapefruit)	• apricots
• melons	• bananas
• dried lima beans	• winter squash
• dried prunes	• soybeans
• dried white beans	• baked potato
• broiled meat	• milk

2. Potassium-sparing diuretics: Spironolactone (Aldactone) Amiloride Hydrochloride (Midamor)
   a. Monitor potassium level for hyperkalemia.
   b. Maximum hypotensive effect may not be seen for two weeks.
   c. Give with meals to improve absorption.
3. Antihypertensives: Cause peripheral vasodilation, reducing blood pressure
   a. Beta Adrenergic Blockers
      (1) Nadolol (Corgard); Acebutolol (Sectral); Propranolol HCl (Inderal); Metoprolol (Lopressor); Atenolol (Tenormin); Labetalol (Mormodyne, Trandate)
      (2) Block action of epinephrine and lower heart rate and blood pressure
      (3) May cause increased airway resistance; should not be given to clients with asthma
   b. Central Acting Drugs: Alpha Agonists
      (1) Clonidine (Catapres); Methyldopa (Aldomet)
      (2) Depress the activity of the sympathetic nervous system
   c. Angiotensin Converting Enzyme (ACE) Inhibitors: captopril (Capoten); enalapril, enalaprilat (Vasotec); benazepril (Lotensin); fosinopril (Monopril); Lisinopril (Prinivil, Zestril); Ramipril (Altace)
      (1) Vasoconstrictor and also decreases aldosterone secretion. Aldosterone causes sodium and fluid retention.
      (2) Monitor heart rate, because drugs can cause bradycardia.
      (3) Monitor blood pressure, because drugs can cause severe hypotension.
      (4) Teach client to change positions slowly because orthostatic hypotension is common.
      (5) Teach client to avoid alcohol because alcohol also causes vasodilation.
      (6) Teach the client not to take over-the-counter medications, especially cold medications, without physician approval because interactions may occur with antihypertensives.
      (7) Teach the client not to stop drugs suddenly because rebound hypertension may occur.
      (8) Adverse effects include blood dyscrasias, angioedema, renal failure, hyperkalemia, rash, and fever.
      (9) Because of the serious side effects, these drugs are usually given to patients whose blood pressure has not been controlled with less toxic medications.
     (10) Capoten should be taken one hour before meals because food decreases absorption.
   d. Vasodilator: hydralazine (Apresoline)
      (1) Acts directly on the smooth muscle to lower blood pressure
      (2) Adverse effects include headache, tachycardia, angina, palpitations, and sodium retention
      (3) Give with meals to increase absorption.
   e. Alpha Adrenergic Blockers
      (1) Block alpha adrenergic receptors causing peripheral vascular dilation resulting in decrease in blood pressure and relaxation of muscles of bladder and prostate
      (2) Doxazosin (Cardura), Prazosin (Minipres), Terazosin (Hytrin)
      (3) First dose is given at bedtime to decrease hypotension
E. Interventions: Teach patient
   1. Lose weight if overweight
   2. Avoid stimulants such as coffee, tea, and chocolate because they constrict blood vessels
   3. Avoid nicotine because it is a potent vasoconstrictor
   4. Regular physical exercise to tone cardiovascular system
   5. Learn more constructive ways of adapting to stresses in life
   6. Dietary modifications: restrict sodium and fat and lose weight if overweight

ANGINA

A. Transient chest pain caused by insufficient blood flow to myocardium resulting in myocardial ischemia
B. Causes and precipitating events:
   1. Atherosclerosis is a primary cause.
   2. Precipitating events:
      a. Exertion (vigorous exercise done very sporadically)
      b. Emotions (excitement, sexual activity)
      c. Eating (after heavy meal)
      d. Environment (very cold or very hot)
C. Nursing Diagnoses (Table 6.3)
D. Interventions
   1. Oxygen
   2. Nitrates (nitroglycerine)
      a. sublingual q 5 min. x 3; store in cool, dark, glass, or metal container
      b. paste or patch
   3. Monitor vital signs, ECG monitoring
   4. Position in semi/high Fowler's
   5. Emotional support
   6. Teach low sodium, low-fat diet, no smoking, stress management
   7. Medications
      a. Calcium blocking agents: Nifedipine (Procardia); Verapamil (Isoptine, Calan)
         (1) Used to treat angina and supraventricular arrhythmias; decrease myocardial need for oxygen
         (2) Side effects:
            (a) hypotension
            (b) headache
            (c) pulse changes
            (d) AV block

   b. Beta adrenergic blockers: Nadolol (Corgard); Propranolol HCl (Inderal)

MYOCARDIAL INFARCTION

A. Death of myocardial cells from inadequate oxygenation (Figure 6.3)
B. Causes:
   1. Atherosclerotic heart disease
   2. Coronary artery embolism
   3. Decreased blood flow with shock and/or hemorrhage
C. Assessment findings
   1. Pain: substernal, heavy, vise-like, radiating down left arm
   2. Nausea, vomiting
   3. Sweating, dizziness
   4. Cool, clammy, ashen skin
   5. Low-grade fever for first three days following MI
   6. B.P. up at first from pain, then may decrease
   7. ECG changes (ST segment changes may indicate ischemia)
   8. Elevated ESR, cholesterol
   9. Serum enzyme changes (Table 6.4)

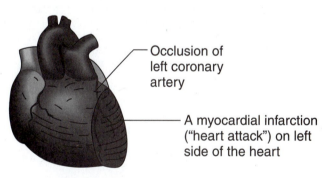

Occlusion of left coronary artery

A myocardial infarction ("heart attack") on left side of the heart

Severe acute myocardial ischemia and infarction

Figure 6.3 Myocardial infarction.

Table 6.3 Nursing Diagnoses Related to Angina

- Anxiety related to chest pain secondary to effects of cardiac ischemia.
- Acute pain related to decreased oxygen supply to the myocardium.
- Activity intolerance related to fear of recurrent angina.
- Risk for ineffective sexuality patterns related to fear of angina and altered self concept.
- Risk for ineffective health maintenance related to insufficient knowledge of condition, home activities, diet, and medications.
- Deficient knowledge related to disease process, medications, and treatment regimen.

Table 6.4 Serum Enzyme Changes Following a Myocardial Infarction

Enzyme	Rises	Peaks	Return to Normal
Creatine Kinase (CK) Creatine Phosphokinase (CPK)	3–6 hrs	12–18 hrs	3 days
Aspartate Aminotransferase (AST)	6 hrs	12–14 hrs	3–4 days
Lactic Dehydrogenase (LDH)		72 hrs	11–14 days
CK-MB fraction	3–6 hrs	18–24 hrs	3 days
Troponin	within 6 hours		

D. Nursing diagnoses (Table 6.5)
E. Interventions
1. Patent IV line for administration of medications
2. Pain relief: morphine
3. Oxygen via nasal cannula or mask
4. ECG monitoring for dysrhythmias
5. Drugs used to treat ventricular arrhythmias
   a. All of the drugs except Bretylium are well absorbed from the GI tract and can be given p.o. Most can also be given I.M. or I.V.
   b. Because they are designed to treat ventricular tachycardia and ventricular fibrillation (fast rates), the nurse should watch for bradycardia as a side effect. Other dysrhythmias may occur.
   c. Isuprel or atropine (drugs used to speed up the heart) should be available.
   d. Give antiarrhythmic drugs at equal intervals.
   e. Monitor vital signs and ECG for dysrhythmias.

Table 6.5 Nursing Diagnoses Related to Myocardial Infarction

- Acute chest pain related to decreased oxygenation of myocardial tissue.
- Decreased cardiac output related to damaged heart tissue.
- Anxiety related to chest pain secondary to effects of cardiac ischemia
- Fear related to pain secondary to cardiac tissue ischemia
- Activity intolerance related to impaired oxygen transport secondary to decreased cardiac output and fear of recurrent angina
- Risk for constipation related to decreased peristalsis secondary to effects of narcotic analgesics, decreased activity, and change in diet
- Risk for disturbed self-concept related to perceived or actual role changes
- Risk for ineffective sexuality patterns related to fear of angina and altered self-concept
- Deficient knowledge related to disease process, medications, diet, and plan for recovery.
- Risk for ineffective health maintenance related to insufficient knowledge of condition, home activities, diet, and medications

f. Side effects include postural hypotension for most of the antiarrhythmics.
g. Antiarrhymic drugs:
   (1) Quinidine (Cardioquin, Quinaglute, Quinidex)
   (2) Disopyramide (Norpace)
   (3) Lidocaine (Xylocaine) used to treat acute ventricular dysrhythmias; usually given IV bolus followed by IV drip for cardiovascular clients
   (4) Phenytoin Sodium (Dilantin)
   (5) Procainamide (Pronestyl)
   (6) Bretylium (Bretylol)
   (7) Adenoside (Adenocard)
   (8) Amiodarone (Cardarone)
h. Cardiac Stimulants:
   (1) Atropine: anticholinergic, increases heart rate
   (2) Isoproteronol (Isuprel): adrenergic
6. Reduce oxygen demand
   a. Bed rest in semi-Fowler's position
   b. Bedside commode
   c. Self feed
7. Monitor intake and output
8. Thrombolytic drugs may be ordered
   a. Alteplase (tissue plasminogen activator recombinant, tPA, Activase); Streptokinase
   b. Should be given within six hours of myocardial episode
   c. Monitor for bleeding.
   d. Heparin therapy may be started following treatment.
9. Administer anticoagulants as ordered
   a. Heparin (Table 6.6)
      (1) PTT (partial thromboplastin time) or aPTT (activated partial thromboplastin time) done to monitor heparin administration. Therapeutic levels are considered to be 1 1/2 to 2 times control values.
      (2) Observe for bleeding.
   b. Warfarin (Coumadin, Dicumarol) (Table 6.6)
      (1) Prothrombin time should be monitored. When warfarin is being administered, the PT should be 1 1/2 to 2 times the control. Results may

Table 6.6 Anticoagulants

Drug	Route	Action	Monitoring Tests	Normal Value	Value when on Medication	Antidote
Heparin	Parenteral IV or SC (Can't be given orally because it is destroyed by gastric juices)	Blocks the conversion of prothrombin to thrombin and prolongs clotting time	PTT (partial thromboplastin time) aPTT (activated partial thromboplastin clotting time)	60–70 seconds 30–40 seconds	1 1/2 to 2 times normal; 1 1/2 to 2 times normal	Protamine sulfate
Warfarin (Coumadin)	Oral	Blocks prothrombin synthesis	Prothrombin time (PT) INR	11–12.5 seconds	1 1/2 to 2 times normal; 2–3	Vitamin K

Table 6.7 High Sodium Foods

- Soups
- Canned vegetables
- Carrots, spinach, and celery
- Bread (200 mg per slice)
- Corn flakes (260 mg/oz)
- Ocean fish, clams, shrimp
- Bologna (226 mg/slice)
- Beef (190 mg/4 oz)
- Instant pudding
- Dill pickle (1137 mg/large)
- Milk (130 mg/8 oz)
- American cheese (238 mg/L)
- Cottage cheese (435 mg/4 oz)

be reproduced as International Normalized Ratio (INR); should be 2–3.
    (2) Observe for bleeding.
    (3) Client should be taught not to take aspirin or NSAIDs while taking warfarin unless prescribed by physician
10. Administer stool softeners as ordered
11. Provide low-fat, low-sodium, low-cholesterol diet
    a. Avoid high sodium foods (Table 6.7)
    b. Chicken is low in sodium (57 mg/2 pieces)
    c. Avoid saturated fats: animal fats and coconut oil and palm oil
    d. Use unsaturated fats (vegetable sources) when using fats or oils
12. Plan for rehabilitation
    a. Exercise program
    b. Stress management
13. Long-term drug therapy:
    a. Antiarrhythmics
    b. Antihypertensives
    c. Anticoagulants
    d. Antilipemics

PERCUTANEOUS TRANSLUMINAL CORONARY ANGIOPLASTY (PTCA)

A. PTCA is performed to revascularize the myocardium and decrease angina symptoms. A balloon catheter is inserted through the skin and into the appropriate artery and is passed through the vessel until the lesion is reached; the balloon is then inflated to flatten plaque against the artery wall.
B. Interventions
    1. Procedure usually performed in the cardiac catheterization lab
    2. Nursing care before and after the procedure is similar to that for a client having a cardiac catheterization.

3. Teach the client about necessary lifestyle changes:
    a. High fiber, low-fat diet
    b. Regular exercise program with doctor's approval

CORONARY ARTERY BYPASS GRAFT (CABG)

A. Coronary Artery Bypass Graft (CABG) done for client with severe coronary artery disease. Obstruction in coronary artery is bypassed with a graft that is attached to the aorta and to a coronary artery distal to the point of obstruction. Client may have one or more bypasses during the surgical procedure, depending on how many blockages exist.
B. Procedure requires extracorporeal circulation (heart-lung machine, cardiopulmonary bypass)
C. Nursing Interventions
    1. Preoperative:
        a. Explain that the client will be in a critical care unit following surgery.
        b. Explain nursing care to client and family; deep breathing and coughing exercises, ROM exercises, turning procedures
        c. Reassure the client that pain medication will be available after surgery
    2. Postoperative
        a. Maintain airway
        b. Promote lung reexpansion by:
            (1) Monitoring chest drainage system
            (2) Assisting client with turning, coughing, and deep breathing
        c. Monitor vital signs for rhythm disturbances, breathing difficulties, and temperature elevation
        d. Administer anticoagulants as ordered
        e. Maintain intake and output record; report if less than 30 ml/hour urine
        f. Daily weights
        g. Administer pain medications as ordered
        h. Leg exercises to prevent thrombophlebitis
        i. Discharge teaching regarding:
            (1) Gradual increase in exercise regimen; avoid heavy lifting and activities requiring continuous arm movements such as vacuuming, playing golf, or bowling until well healed
            (2) Sexual intercourse: can usually be resumed safely 3 or 4 weeks after surgery
            (3) Medications as ordered by physician

(4) Dietary modifications: usually a high-fiber, low-fat diet with possible restriction of sodium and carbohydrates

(5) Wound care: cleanse daily with mild soap and water and report signs of infection

CARDIAC FAILURE

A. Left ventricular failure
   1. Left ventricle cannot pump enough blood into the systemic circulation; may occur in client with long-standing hypertension or client who has had heart damage from a myocardial infarction
   2. Assessment findings
      a. Dyspnea
      b. Moist cough
      c. Crackles, wheezing
   3. Pulmonary edema results causing:
      a. Excessive quantities of fluid in pulmonary interstitial spaces or alveoli
      b. Moist rales
      c. Pink, frothy sputum
      d. Severe anxiety
      e. Marked dyspnea
      f. Cyanosis
B. Right ventricular failure
   1. Right ventricle unable to pump blood out of the heart into the lungs; blood backs up into vena cava; may follow left-sided failure; occurs in chronic obstructive lung disease
   2. Assessment findings
      a. Peripheral edema
      b. Distended neck veins
      c. Weight gain
      d. Hepatomegaly
C. Nursing diagnoses (Table 6.8)
D. Interventions:
   1. Oxygen
   2. Diuretics (hydrochlorothiazide or furosemide [Lasix]) to reduce fluid buildup
      a. Monitor serum potassium (3.5–5.5 mEq normal)
      b. Potassium supplement may be indicated; never give potassium on an empty stomach because it may cause GI irritation
      c. Encourage dietary potassium (Table 6.2)
   3. Digitalis (Lanoxin) to improve myocardial contraction
      a. Observe for signs of digitalis toxicity (Table 6.9)
      b. Nursing care:
         (1) Withhold digoxin if apical pulse < 60 in adult
         (2) Check for toxicity
         (3) Check K levels

Table 6.8 Nursing Diagnoses Related to Heart Failure

- Decreased cardiac output related to mechanical failure of heart muscle.
- Impaired gas exchange related to decreased cardiac output and pulmonary edema.
- Fluid volume excess related to decreased cardiac output and decreased renal output.
- Risk for impaired skin integrity related to edema, inactivity, and poor tissue perfusion.
- Activity intolerance related to insufficient oxygen to perform activities of daily living.
- Imbalanced nutrition: less than body requirements related to nausea; anorexia secondary to venous congestion of gastrointestinal tract and fatigue.
- Ineffective peripheral tissue perfusion related to venous congestion
- Self-care deficit related to dyspnea and fatigue.
- Powerlessness related to progressive nature of condition.
- Anxiety related to change in health status, lifestyle changes, or fear of death.
- Deficient knowledge related to disease process, medications, diet, and plan for recovery.

Table 6.9 Signs of Digitalis Toxicity

Nausea and vomiting
Bradycardia
Dysrhythmias
Visual disturbances (green and yellow)

      c. Antidote for severe, life-threatening digitalis toxicity is digoxin immune FAB (Digibind) given IV
   4. Low-sodium diet may be ordered due to fluid retention
   5. Teach client to live within cardiac reserve; reduce activities that cause shortness of breath

Valvular Disease

A. Stenosis (narrowing of valvular opening); insufficiency (incomplete closure of valve); mitral and aortic valves may be affected; may be congenital or caused by infections such as rheumatic fever
B. Assessment findings:
   1. Left or right heart failure
   2. Murmurs
   3. Decreased cardiac output
C. Nursing diagnoses (see Table 6.8, Nursing diagnoses related to heart failure)
D. Interventions:
   1. Same as heart failure diuretics, digitalis, diet, and activity modification
   2. Antibiotic therapy especially if caused by rheumatic fever
   3. Surgery often indicated as symptoms progress
      a. Heart valve replacement
      b. Mitral commisurotomy (valvulotomy)

Dysrhythmias

A. Bradycardia
1. Heart rate of 60 beats per minute or less
2. May be caused by myocardial ischemia, electrolyte disturbances, vagal stimulation, heart blocks, drug toxicity, increased intracranial pressure, sleep, and vomiting
3. Treatment may include atropine to increase heart rate or a permanent pacemaker
B. Tachycardia
1. Heart rate of 100 to 150 beats per minute
2. Causes may include emotional stress, fever, medications, pain, anemia, hyperthyroidism, heart failure, or excessive caffeine and tobacco
3. Treatment includes medications such as beta blockers, calcium channel blockers, and digitalis
4. Treatment may include having client perform Valsalva maneuver
C. Atrial dysrhythmias
1. Premature atrial contraction (PAC): an impulse starting in the atria outside the sinoatrial node
a. Infrequent PACs may not cause many symptoms.
b. Causes include myocardial ischemia, digitalis toxicity, hypokalemia, stress, too much caffeine, or too much nicotine
c. Treatment
(1) Occasional PACs may not be treated.
(2) Quinidine or procainamide hydrochloride
2. Atrial tachycardia
a. An ectopic impulse that causes the ventricles to contract at the rate of 140 to 250 beats per minute
b. Causes include hypokalemia, digitalis toxicity, and ischemia.
c. Treatment:
(1) Correcting the cause (giving potassium supplements or withholding digitalis)
(2) Antiarrhythmic drugs such as phenytoin sodium (Dilantin sodium)
(3) Pacemaker

PACEMAKER

A. Electronic device that provides electrical stimuli to the heart muscle for the control of heart rate in conditions such as heart block
B. Types of pacemakers:
1. Demand: if patient's heart rate falls below a predetermined level, the heart is electrically stimulated
2. Fixed: an electrical stimulus delivered to the patient's heart at a preset rate
3. External:
a. Power source remains outside of body
b. Nursing care
(1) Prevent dislodgment
(2) Limit activity of extremity
(3) Secure wires to chest
(4) Do NOT defibrillate over insertion site
(5) Prevent infection when external invasive pacemaker in place
(6) Maintain electrical safety
4. Internal:
a. Power source implanted under skin; usually for long-term use
b. Nursing care:
(1) Limit activity of shoulder for 48–72 hours
(2) Passive ROM every shift after 48 hours
(3) Health teaching
(a) Wear identification indicating pacemaker in place
(b) No contact sports
(c) Daily pulse
(d) Avoid sources of electricity such as microwaves and cell phones next to pacemaker

DEFIBRILLATION (COUNTERSHOCK)

A. The passing of an electrical shock of short duration through the heart to terminate ventricular fibrillation
B. Procedure:
1. Start CPR immediately to maintain perfusion.
2. Apply interface material (gel, paste, saline pads) to the paddles so they will be in firm contact with the client's skin.
3. Disconnect the oxygen to prevent fire.
4. Position paddles so one electrode is just to the right of the upper sternum below the clavicle and the other electrode is just to the left of the cardiac apex or left nipple; about 20–25 lbs of pressure is applied to paddles to ensure good contact with the client's skin.
5. Grasp the paddles only by the insulated handles.
6. Instruct all personnel to stand clear of the client and the bed.
7. Second person turns on the defibrillator to 200–300 watt seconds of delivered energy.
8. Second shock may be delivered at the same level; level can be increased if shocks are unsuccessful.
9. Push the discharge buttons in both paddles simultaneously.
10. Remove the paddles from the client immediately after the shock is administered.
11. Resume CPR until stable rhythm, spontaneous respirations, pulse and blood pressure return, or treatment is to be terminated.

Peripheral Vascular Disorders

A. Reduction of blood flow due to arterial obstruction from arteriosclerosis (thickening and loss of elasticity of the arterial walls) or atherosclerosis (cholesterol or fat plaques in the artery)

B. Assessment findings:
1. Intermittent claudication progressing to severe, unrelenting pain
2. Tingling and numbness of toes
3. Decreased or absent pulses in lower extremities
4. Feet and legs become red when dependent, pale when elevated
5. Thickened nails, dry, shiny skin, cool to cold temperature in lower extremities
6. Bruits (the sound produced by turbulent flow of blood through an irregular stenotic vessel) may be ausculatated with a stethoscope
7. Doppler ultrasonic flow studies show decreased blood flow in extremities
8. Angiogram shows narrowing of blood vessels

C. Nursing Diagnoses (Table 6.10)

Table 6.10 Nursing Diagnoses Related to Peripheral Vascular Disease

- High risk for impaired tissue integrity related to compromised circulation
- Chronic pain related to muscle ischemia during prolonged activity
- Risk for injury related to decreased sensation secondary to chronic atherosclerosis
- Risk for infection related to compromised circulation
- Risk for injury related to effects of orthostatic hypotension
- Activity intolerance related to claudication
- Risk for ineffective health maintenance related to insufficient knowledge of condition, risk factors, signs and symptoms of complications, prevention of complications, exercise program, foot care, and diet

D. Interventions:
1. Prevent injury to client's extremities
2. Assess pulses in lower extremities
3. Administer antilipemics as ordered (Table 6.11)
4. Teach client to:
   a. Avoid smoking because nicotine is a potent vasoconstrictor
   b. Follow a low-fat diet to reduce atherosclerotic plaque formation
   c. Avoid stress (stress stimulates sympathetic nervous system and causes vasoconstriction)
   d. Avoid constricting garments to improve circulation
   e. Keep legs in straight plane or down to promote arterial blood flow to the extremities; may be necessary to elevate legs if client also has venous insufficiency
5. Assist client with Buerger-Allen exercises as ordered:
   a. Client lies on back with legs above level of heart for three minutes
   b. Client sits on edge of bed with legs relaxed and dependent and exercises feet and toes (upward and downward, inward and outward) for three minutes
   c. Client lies on back with legs straight for three minutes
   d. Repeat the above series six times, four times a day
6. Surgery:
   a. Percutaneous transluminal angioplasty: balloon catheter inserted into vessel and maneuvered across the occluded area; balloon is inflated and cracks lesion, compressing it back up against the vessel wall

Table 6.11 Antilipemic Agents

Medication	Actions	Nursing Care
Cholestyramine (Questran)	Binds bile acids in the intestine causing increased fecal excretion, which causes increased production of bile acids from cholesterol. Lowers LDL cholesterol.	Give fat-soluble Vitamins (A, D, K) and folic acid in a water-soluble form; observe for bleeding tendencies. Should not be taken at the same time as other medications; take other medications 1 hour before or 4 hours after Questran. Monitor liver function tests. Monitor cholesterol and serum triglyceride levels.
Gemfibrozil (Lopid)	Acts by inhibiting lipolysis and triglyceride synthesis.	Monitor liver function tests. Monitor cholesterol and serum triglyceride levels.
Lovastatin (Mevacor) Atorvastin (Lipitor) Simvastin (Zocor)	Acts by inhibiting HMG-CoA reductase, the enzyme that initiates cholesterol synthesis. Lowers LDL, VLDL, and triglycerides and raises HDL.	Monitor liver function tests. Monitor cholesterol and serum triglyceride levels. Encourage regular eye exams for cataracts for persons taking lovastatin. Examine for myalgia.

b. Grafting: connecting two vessels with good blood flow to each other
c. Endartarectomy: incision into occluded artery and removal of obstruction
d. Post-operative nursing care
   (1) Assess peripheral pulses
   (2) Check extremities for color and temperature and sensation
   (3) Intake and output
   (4) Central venous pressure
   (5) Mini doses of heparin to prevent clotting at graft sites
   (6) Do not bend extremity for 24 hours to prevent bleeding

ARTERIOSCLEROSIS OBLITERANS (ASO)

A. Complete obstruction of lumen of arteries affecting the aorta or the arteries of the lower extremities; commonly associated with diabetes mellitus
B. Assessment findings and interventions as above

BUERGER'S DISEASE

A. Recurring inflammation of the arteries and veins of lower and upper extremities, resulting in thrombus and occlusion occurring most frequently in men aged 30 to 50
B. Assessment findings and interventions as above

RAYNAUD'S DISEASE

A. Vasospastic condition of arteries that occurs with exposure to cold or stress; affecting primarily the hands and occurring most often in women aged 16 to 40
B. Assessment findings:
   1. Extreme sensitivity to cold, especially in fingertips, toes, and tip of nose
   2. Upon exposure to cold, hands become pale and then blue as small amounts of blood enter the capillaries and finally turn red as vessels dilate (white, blue, and red).
C. Interventions:
   1. Teach to avoid cold
   2. No smoking (nicotine is a strong vasoconstrictor)
   3. Vasodilators or calcium channel blockers as ordered
   4. Antilipemics as ordered
   5. Teach client to change positions slowly because medications may cause orthostatic hypotension

Aortic Aneurysm

A. Local distention of the artery wall, usually thoracic or abdominal, caused by atherosclerosis
B. Assessment findings:
   1. Thoracic aneurysm: pain, dyspnea, and/or hoarseness
   2. Abdominal aneurysm: abdominal pain, persistent or intermittent low back pain, pulsating abdominal mass
C. Interventions:
   1. Surgical repair
      a. Monitor carefully before surgery for signs of rupture of aneurysm.
      b. Postoperative nursing care
         (1) Care as for abdominal or thoracic surgery
         (2) Monitor peripheral pulses and blood pressure carefully
         (3) Monitor output carefully

Vein Disorders

THROMBOPHLEBITIS; DEEP VEIN THROMBOSIS

A. Thrombophlebitis: inflammation of the vein wall may result in a clot in the superficial or deep veins. Deep vein thrombosis (DVT) is very serious and can result in pulmonary embolus.
B. Risk factors:
   1. Prolonged bed rest
   2. Pelvic surgery
C. Assessment findings:
   1. Local swelling, bumpy, knotty

Table 6.12 Nursing Diagnoses Related to Thrombophlebitis

- Risk for impaired skin integrity related to chronic ankle edema
- Pain related to impaired circulation
- Risk for impaired respiratory function related to immobility
- Risk for constipation related to decreased peristalsis secondary to immobility

2. Red, tender, local induration
3. Homan's sign
4. Warmth in affected area
5. Many cases have no early symptoms

D. Nursing diagnoses (Table 6.12)
E. Interventions
1. Elastic support hose and leg exercises to prevent clots from forming
2. Bed rest and elevation of affected extremity once clots have formed
3. Continuous, warm, moist soaks
4. Control of discomfort
5. Administration of thrombolytics and anticoagulants:
   a. Thrombolytics (t-PA, streptokinase) dissolve clots; watch for bleeding
   b. Heparin for 10 to 12 days; watch for bleeding (Table 6.6)
      (1) Do not give aspirin-containing products
      (2) Monitor PTT while client on heparin
   c. Coumadin derivatives following heparin administration (Table 6.6):
      (1) Monitor PT while client on coumadin
      (2) Teach the client to avoid drugs that inhibit coumadin: barbiturates, Doriden, and Placidyl
      (3) Teach the client to avoid drugs that potentiate coumadin: ASA, anabolic steroids, chloral hydrate, neomycin, phenylbutazone, and quinidine
6. Surgery (thrombectomy and possibly a vena cava filter to trap large emboli [Figure 6.4]) is indicated when thrombolytic or anticoagulant therapy contraindicated, danger of pulmonary embolus is extreme, or there is danger of permanent damage to veins.

VARICOSE VEINS

A. Swollen, distended, and knotted veins usually in the subcutaneous tissues of the leg
B. Risk factors: situations that promote venous stasis
   1. Prolonged standing
   2. Obesity
   3. Pregnancy
   4. Heredity

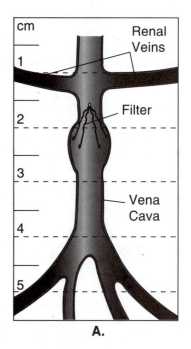

A.

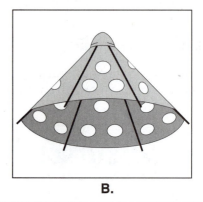

B.

Figure 6.4 Vena caval filters to prevent embolus from traveling to the lungs, heart, or brain. A. Greenfield; B. Unbrella

C. Interventions:
   1. Activities to promote venous return
      a. Rest periods with legs elevated above heart level
      b. Walking
      c. Weight loss
   2. Injection of veins
   3. Surgery: ligation and stripping of affected vein in the legs—usually saphenous
      a. Postoperative nursing interventions:
         (1) Ace bandages
         (2) Elevate legs
         (3) Observe feet for edema, warmth, and color
         (4) Patient may lay down or walk; should not sit or stand
         (5) Teach lifestyle changes to prevent recurrence

Sample Questions

1. The nurse counts an adult's apical heart beat at 110 beats per minute. The nurse describes this as:
   1. asystole
   2. bigeminy
   3. tachycardia
   4. bradycardia

2. A client has an elevated AST 24 hours following chest pain and shortness of breath. This is suggestive of which of the following?
   1. Gall bladder disease
   2. Liver disease
   3. Myocardial infarction
   4. Skeletal muscle injury

3. An adult has a coagulation time of 20 minutes. The nurse should observe the client for:
   1. Blood clots
   2. Ecchymotic areas
   3. Jaundice
   4. Infection

4. A prothrombin time test should be performed regularly on persons who are taking which medication?
   1. Heparin
   2. Warfarin
   3. Phenobarbital
   4. Digoxin

5. Which prothrombin time value would be considered normal for a client who is receiving warfarin (coumadin)?
   1. 12 seconds
   2. 20 seconds
   3. 60 seconds
   4. 98 seconds

6. The nurse is caring for a client who is receiving heparin. What drug should be readily available?
   1. Vitamin K
   2. Caffeine
   3. Calcium gluconate
   4. Protamine sulfate

7. An adult who is receiving heparin asks the nurse why it cannot be given by mouth. The nurse responds that heparin is given parenterally because:
   1. It is destroyed by gastric secretions.
   2. It irritates the gastric mucosa.
   3. It irritates the intestinal lining.
   4. Therapeutic levels can be achieved more quickly.

8. An adult who is admitted for a cardiac catheterization asks the nurse if she will be asleep during the cardiac catheterization. What is the best initial response for the nurse to make?
   1. "You will be given a general anesthesia."
   2. "You will be sedated but not asleep."
   3. "The doctor will give you an anesthetic if you are having too much pain."
   4. "Why do you want to be asleep?"

9. During the admission interview, a client who is admitted for a cardiac catheterization says, "Every time I eat shrimp I get a rash." What action is essential for the nurse to take at this time?
   1. Notify the physician.
   2. Ask the client if she gets a rash from any other foods.
   3. Instruct the dietary department not to give the client shrimp.
   4. Teach the client the dangers of eating shrimp and other shell fish.

10. The nurse is preparing a client for a cardiac catheterization. Which action would the nurse expect to take?
    1. Administer a radioisotope as ordered.
    2. Give the client a cleansing enema.
    3. Locate and mark peripheral pulses.
    4. Encourage high fluid intake before the test.

11. A young adult with a history of rheumatic fever as a child is to have a cardiac catheterization. She asks the nurse why she must have a cardiac catheterization. The nurse's response is based on the understanding that cardiac catheterization can accomplish all of the following EXCEPT:
    1. Assessing heart structures
    2. Determining oxygen levels in the heart chambers
    3. Evaluating cardiac output
    4. Obtaining a biopsy specimen

12. When a client returns from undergoing a cardiac catheterization, it is most essential for the nurse to:
    1. Check peripheral pulses.
    2. Maintain NPO.
    3. Apply heat to the insertion site.
    4. Start range of motion exercises immediately.

13. A male client with angina pectoris has been having an increased number of episodes of pain recently. He is admitted for observation. During the admission interview, he tells the nurse that he has been having chest pain during the last week. Which statement by the client would be of greatest concern to the nurse?
    1. "I had chest pain while I was walking in the snow on Thursday."
    2. "We went out for a big dinner to celebrate my wife's birthday, but I couldn't enjoy it because I got the pain before we got home from the restaurant."
    3. "I had chest pain yesterday while I was sitting in the living room watching television."
    4. "I felt pain all the way down my left arm after I was playing with my grandson on Monday."

14. The nurse responds to the call light of a client who has a history of angina pectoris. He tells the nurse that he has just taken a nitroglycerin

tablet sublingually for anginal pain. What action should the nurse take next?
1. If the pain does not subside within five minutes, place a second tablet under his tongue.
2. Position him in the Trendelenburg position.
3. Administer a prn narcotic for pain if he still has pain in 10 minutes.
4. Call his physician and alert the code team for possible intervention.

15. The nurse is teaching an adult who has angina about taking nitroglycerine. The nurse tells him he will know the nitroglycerine is effective when:
1. He experiences tingling under the tongue.
2. His pulse rate increases.
3. His pain subsides.
4. His activity tolerance increases.

16. A client with angina will have to make lifestyle modifications. Which of the following statements by the client would indicate that he understands the necessary modifications in lifestyle to prevent angina attacks?
1. "I know that I will need to eat less, so I will only eat one meal a day."
2. "I will need to stay in bed all the time so I won't have the pain."
3. "I'll stop what I'm doing whenever I have pain and take a pill."
4. "I will need to walk more slowly and rest frequently to avoid the angina."

17. A client who has been treated for angina is discharged in stable condition. On a clinic visit, he tells the nurse he has anginal pain when he has sexual intercourse with his wife. The best response for the nurse to make is:
1. "Do you have ambivalent feelings toward your wife?"
2. "Many persons with angina have less pain when their partner assumes the top position."
3. "Be sure that you attempt intercourse only when you are well rested and relaxed."
4. "You might try having a cocktail before sexual activity to help you relax."

18. A low-sodium, low-cholesterol weight-reducing diet is prescribed for an adult with heart disease. The nurse knows that he understands his diet when he chooses which of the following meals?
1. Baked chicken and mashed potatoes
2. Stir-fried Chinese vegetables and rice
3. Tuna fish salad with celery sticks
4. Lean steak with carrots

19. An adult client is admitted with a diagnosis of left-sided congestive heart failure. Which assessment finding would most likely be present?
1. Distended neck veins
2. Dyspnea
3. Hepatomegaly
4. Pitting edema

20. Digoxin (Lanoxin) and Lasix (Furosemide) are ordered for a client who has congestive heart failure. Which of the following would the nurse also expect to be ordered for this client?
1. Potassium
2. Calcium
3. Aspirin
4. Coumadin

21. When the nurse is about to administer digoxin to a client, the client says, "I think I need to see the eye doctor. Things seem to look kind of green today." The nurse takes his vital signs which are B.P. 150/94; P 60; R. 28. What is the most appropriate initial action for the nurse to take?
1. Administer the medication and record the findings on his chart.
2. Withhold the digoxin and report to the charge nurse.
3. Request an appointment with the ophthalmologist.
4. Reassure the client that he is having a normal reaction to his medication.

22. An adult client is admitted to the hospital with peripheral vascular disease of the lower extremities. He has several ischemic ulcers on each ankle and lower leg area. Other parts of his skin are shiny and taut with loss of hair. A primary nursing goal for this client should be to:
1. Increase activity tolerance
2. Relieve anxiety
3. Protect from injury
4. Help build a positive body image

23. An adult client who has peripheral vascular disease of the lower extremities was observed smoking in the waiting area. What is the most appropriate response for the nurse to make in regards to the client's smoking?
1. "Smoking is not allowed for patients with blood diseases."
2. "Smoking causes the blood vessels in your legs to constrict and reduces the blood supply."
3. "Smoking increases your blood pressure and strains your heart."
4. "Smoking causes your body to be under greater stress."

24. An adult client with peripheral vascular disease tells the nurse he is afraid his left leg is not improving and may need to be amputated. How should the nurse respond?
1. "You and your wife should discuss your feelings before surgery."
2. "You sound concerned about your leg and possible surgery."
3. "It is better to have an amputation when the ulcers are not improving."
4. "You don't need to be afraid of surgery."

25. An adult is diagnosed with hypertension. He is prescribed chlorothiazide (Diuril) 500 mg po. What nursing instruction is essential for him?

1. Drink at least two quarts of liquid daily.
2. Avoid hard cheeses.
3. Drink orange juice or eat a banana daily.
4. Do not take aspirin.

26. A low-sodium diet has been ordered for an adult client. The nurse knows that the client understands his low-sodium diet when the client selects which menu?
    1. Tossed salad, carrot sticks, and steak
    2. Baked chicken, mashed potatoes, and green beans
    3. Hot dog, roll, and coleslaw
    4. Chicken noodle soup, applesauce, and cottage cheese

27. A female client is admitted to the hospital with obesity and deep vein thrombophlebitis (DVT) of the right leg. She weighs 275 pounds. Which of the following factors is least related to her diagnosis?
    1. She has been taking oral estrogens for the last three years.
    2. She smokes two packs of cigarettes daily.
    3. Her right femur was fractured recently.
    4. She is 30 years old.

28. Which assessment finding would most likely indicate the client has thrombophlebitis in the leg?
    1. Diminished pedal pulses
    2. Color changes in the extremities when elevated
    3. Red, shiny skin
    4. Pain when climbing stairs

29. What should be included in the teaching plan for an adult who has hypertension?
    1. Reduce dietary calcium.
    2. Avoid aerobic exercise.
    3. Reduce alcohol intake.
    4. Limit fluid intake.

30. The nurse is caring for an elderly client who has congestive heart failure and is taking digoxin. The client should be monitored for which of the following signs of toxicity?
    1. Disorientation
    2. Weight gain
    3. Constipation
    4. Dyspnea

31. The LPN is assisting the RN in developing the nursing care plan for an older adult who has congestive heart failure. Which nursing diagnosis is most likely to be included?
    1. Fluid volume deficit
    2. Impaired verbal communication
    3. Chronic pain
    4. Activity intolerance

32. The nurse is caring for a client who is being evaluated for arteriosclerosis obliterans. Which complaint is the client most likely to have?
    1. Burning pain in the legs that wakens him/her at night
    2. Numbness of the feet and ankles with exercise

3. Leg pain while walking that becomes severe enough to force him/her to stop
4. Increasing warmth and redness of the legs when they are elevated

33. An adult is admitted with venous thromboembolism. What treatment should the nurse expect during the acute stage?
    1. Application of an elastic stocking
    2. Ambulation three times a day
    3. Passive range of motion exercises to the legs
    4. Use of ice packs to control pain

34. The nurse is observing a client who is learning to perform Buerger-Allen exercises. The nurse knows that the client is performing these exercises correctly when the client is observed:
    1. Alternately dorsiflexing and plantar flexing the feet while the legs are elevated
    2. Massaging the legs beginning at the feet and moving toward the heart
    3. Alternately walking short distances and resting with the legs elevated
    4. Elevating the legs, then dangling them, then lying flat for three minutes

35. What should be included in foot care for the client who has a peripheral vascular disorder?
    1. Soaking the feet for 20 minutes before washing them
    2. Walking barefoot only on carpeted floors
    3. Applying lotion between the toes to avoid cracking of the skin
    4. Avoiding exposure of the legs and feet to the sun

36. An adult male is being evaluated for possible dysrhythmia and is to be placed on a Holter monitor. What instructions should the nurse give him to ensure that this test provides a comprehensive picture of his cardiac status?
    1. Remove the electrodes intermittently for hygiene measures.
    2. Exercise frequently while the monitor is in place.
    3. Keep a diary of all your activities while being monitored.
    4. Refrain from activities that precipitate symptoms.

37. An older adult is scheduled for coronary arteriography during a cardiac catheterization. Which nursing intervention will be essential as she recovers from the diagnostic procedure on the hospital unit?
    1. Encouraging frequent ambulation to prevent deep vein thrombosis.
    2. Limiting fluid intake to prevent fluid overload.
    3. Evaluating cardiac status via continuous ECG monitoring.
    4. Assessing the arterial puncture site when taking vital signs.

38. An older adult is admitted to the hospital with symptoms of severe dyspnea, orthopnea, diaphoresis, bubbling respirations, and cyanosis.

He states that he is afraid "something bad is about to happen." How should the nurse position this client?
1. High-Fowler's
2. Trendelenburg
3. Supine
4. Prone

39. An adult male has a high level of high-density lipoproteins (HDL) in proportion to low-density lipoproteins (LDL) level. How does this relate to his risk of developing coronary artery disease (CAD)?
1. His risk for CAD is low.
2. There is no direct correlation.
3. His risk may increase with exercise.
4. His risk will increase with age.

40. A 72-year-old man had a total hip arthroplasty eight days ago. He suddenly develops tenderness in his left calf, a slight temperature elevation, and a positive Homan's sign. Which of the following will be included in the initial care of this man?
1. Warm packs to the left leg
2. Vigorous massage of the left leg
3. Placing the left leg in a dependent position
4. Performing range of motion exercises to the left leg

Answers and Rationales

1. (3) Tachycardia in an adult is defined as a heart rate above 100 beats per minute. Asystole is cardiac arrest. There is no heart beat. Bigeminy means that the heart beats are coming in pairs. Bradycardia in an adult is defined at a heart rate of 60 beats or less per minute.

2. (3) AST is an enzyme released in response to tissue damage. The symptoms are suggestive of myocardial damage. AST rises 24 hours after a myocardial infarction. It will also rise when there is liver damage and skeletal muscle injury. This client has symptoms typical of myocardial infarction; however, gall bladder disease may present with pain in the right scapula (shoulder blade) region but would not have an elevated AST.

3. (2) The normal clotting time is 9–12 minutes. A prolonged clotting time would suggest a bleeding tendency; the client should be observed for signs of bleeding, such as ecchymotic areas. Blood clots would occur with a clotting time of less than normal. Jaundice occurs with liver damage or rapid breakdown of red blood cells, such as is seen in sickle cell anemia. Infection occurs when there are too few white blood cells.

4. (2) A prothrombin time test is done to determine the effectiveness of warfarin. A partial thromboplastin time test is done for persons taking heparin. Phenobarbital and digoxin do not require regular clotting tests.

Serum levels of these drugs may be done if the client is on long-term therapy.

5. (2) When a client is receiving coumadin, the prothrombin time should be 1 1/2 to 2 times the normal value, which is 11–12.5 seconds. Twenty seconds falls within that range. Twelve seconds is normal for someone who is not receiving coumadin. Sixty seconds is normal for a PTT test. Ninety-eight seconds on a PTT would be acceptable for a client who is receiving heparin. It should be 1 1/2 to 2 times the normal range of 60 to 70 seconds.

6. (4) The antidote for heparin is protamine sulfate. Vitamin K is the antidote for coumadin. Calcium gluconate is the antidote for magnesium sulfate. Caffeine is a central nervous system stimulant and will increase alertness and heart rate.

7. (1) Heparin is a protein and is destroyed by gastric secretions. It is given either IV or subcutaneously for that reason.

8. (2) Persons who are undergoing cardiac catheterization will receive a sedative but are not put to sleep. Their cooperation is needed during the procedure. Asking "why" makes the client defensive and is not appropriate for this client at this time. Give the client the information asked for.

9. (1) Allergy to shellfish is indicative of an allergy to iodine. The dye used in a cardiac catheterization is an iodine dye. Anaphylactic reactions can occur. Because the exam is scheduled for the morning, the nurse should notify the physician immediately. The other actions might have relevance but are not essential (safety related) at this time.

10. (3) It is essential to monitor peripheral pulses after the procedure. They should be assessed before the procedure to determine location and baseline levels. An iodine dye is used during a cardiac catheterization, not a radioisotope. There is no need to give the client an enema. Fluids may be encouraged after the test. The client will be NPO for eight hours before the test.

11. (4) A biopsy specimen cannot be obtained during a cardiac catheterization. Heart structures can be assessed, oxygen levels in the heart chambers can be determined, and cardiac output can be measured during a cardiac catheterization.

12. (1) Checking peripheral pulses is of highest priority. The complications most likely to occur are hemorrhage and obstruction of the vessel. The client is NPO before the procedure, not after. Cold may be applied to the insertion site to vasoconstrict. Heat vasodilates and is contraindicated because it might cause bleeding. Range of motion exercises might cause bleeding. The extremity used for the insertion site is kept quiet immediately following a cardiac catheterization.

13. (3) This answer indicates pain at rest, which suggests a progression of the angina. The other answers all indicate pain with known causes of angina—exercise, cold environment, or eating.

14. (1) Nitroglycerine can be given at five-minute intervals for up to three doses if the pain is not relieved. The Trendelenburg position (head lower than feet) increases cardiac work load and would make the client worse. PRN narcotics are not usually ordered for clients who have anginal pain. Nitroglycerine, a vasodilator, is usually the medication of choice. At some point, the physician will need to be called, but there is no need to alert the code team for possible intervention.

15. (3) Pain relief is the expected outcome when taking nitroglycerine. Vasodilation of coronary vessels will increase the blood supply to the heart muscle, decreasing pain caused by ischemia. Tingling under the tongue and a headache indicate that the medication is potent. His pulse rate should decrease when the pain is relieved. Increase in activity tolerance is nice but nitroglycerine is given to relieve anginal pain.

16. (4) Walking more slowly and resting decreases energy expenditure and *prevents* an attack. Answer #3 *treats* an attack. By the time he has pain, he is experiencing angina. To prevent angina, he needs to walk slowly and rest frequently. He should eat small, frequent meals—not one large meal. He should exercise within his tolerance level. Staying in bed predisposes the client to the complications of immobility, such as clots and pneumonia.

17. (2) Reducing his physical activity reduces the cardiac workload. This response suggests a way he can engage in sexual activity with minimum strain on the heart. Ambivalent feelings toward his wife are unlikely to cause anginal pain. There is some truth to being well rested and relaxed, but telling him this is the only time he should have intercourse is not realistic. The nurse should not advise the client to have an alcoholic beverage before sexual activity.

18. (1) Chicken is lower in sodium than beef or seafood. Baking adds no sodium to the chicken. Barbecuing adds sodium and fat, and frying adds fat and usually sodium. Mashed potatoes contain little sodium. Chinese food is usually high in sodium. Tuna fish is high in sodium; so is celery. Steak is high in sodium; so are carrots.

19. (2) Dyspnea occurs with left-sided heart failure. Distended neck veins, hepatomegaly and pitting edema are signs of right-sided heart failure.

20. (1) Lasix is a potassium-depleting diuretic. Digoxin toxicity occurs more quickly in the presence of a low serum potassium. Potassium supplements are usually ordered when the client is on a potassium-depleting diuretic. There is no indication for supplemental calcium. Aspirin and coumadin are anticoagulants and not indicated because the client is taking Lasix and digoxin.

21. (2) Disturbance in green and yellow vision is a sign of digoxin toxicity. A pulse of 60 is borderline for digoxin toxicity. When there is any possibility of digoxin toxicity, withhold the medication and report to the charge nurse. Once a person takes digoxin, it stays in the system for nearly a week. The LPN will of course record the findings, but withholding the medication is essential. The client needs to have serum digoxin levels done, not be seen by an ophthalmologist. Visual disturbances are a sign of digoxin toxicity, but these are not normal.

22. (3) Because the client has such poor blood supply to his legs, the nurse must be very careful to protect him from injury. Increasing activity tolerance might be desirable but is certainly not the primary nursing goal. Note that the question does not indicate that he has poor exercise tolerance. There is no data in the question to indicate that the client is anxious. He may need help in building a positive body image because his legs are disfigured, but this is certainly not a high priority.

23. (2) This is an accurate answer that relates his behavior to his illness. All of the other statements are true about smoking but do not relate to his current health problem.

24. (2) This response opens communication and allows him to talk about his feelings. The other answers do not allow him to discuss his feelings with the nurse now.

25. (3) Chlorothiazide (Diuril) is a potassium-depleting diuretic. Orange juice and bananas are good sources of potassium. It is not necessary to increase fluids to two quarts when the client is taking a diuretic. Hard cheeses should be avoided when the client is taking monamine oxidase inhibitors. MAOIs are antidepressants. People who take coumadin should not take aspirin.

26. (2) Chicken is low in sodium, as are mashed potatoes and green beans. Carrot sticks, steak, hot dogs, soup, and cottage cheese are all high in sodium.

27. (4) Age is least related to DVT. Oral estrogens, smoking, and a broken leg are all risk factors for DVT.

28. (3) Red, shiny skin suggests inflammation. Diminished pedal pulses, pain when climbing stairs, and color changes in the extremities when elevated are indicative of arterial insufficiency, not a clot in the vein.

29. (3) High alcohol intake contributes to increases in blood pressure. Hypertensive clients are usually advised to limit alcohol intake to the equivalent of two glasses of wine or less per day. Dietary sodium should be limited in people

with hypertension; however, dietary calcium is not a contributing factor in hypertension. Aerobic exercise is helpful in controlling high blood pressure. It may also contribute to weight reduction, which can help decrease blood pressure. Restriction of fluid intake is a medical order and is not appropriate advice for a nurse to give. Fluid restriction is avoided unless other measures are not successful.

30. (1) Disorientation and confusion are often the first signs of digitalis toxicity in the elderly. Weight gain and dyspnea are not signs of digoxin toxicity. They might indicate exacerbation of congestive heart failure. Diarrhea, not constipation, is a sign of digoxin toxicity. Constipation could occur if the client has restricted activity.

31. (4) Dyspnea and impaired oxygenation of tissues reduce the client's ability to tolerate exercise. Fluid volume excess, manifested by edema, is much more likely to occur with CHF than fluid volume deficit. Impaired verbal communication would describe dysphasia, which occurs with CVA, not CHF. Acute pain may occur with CHF when exacerbations occur. Chronic pain does not usually occur with CHF.

32. (3) Severe leg pain while walking describes intermittent claudication, which is the most common symptom of arteriosclerosis obliterans. Pain at rest develops in the late stages of the disease. Pain is much more likely than numbness with exercise. Paresthesias (including numbness) do occur, but they are likely at rest. The legs and feet of the client with arteriosclerosis obliterans become cool and pale when elevated because there is not enough blood flow to the extremities.

33. (1) Compression bandages or stockings help prevent edema and promote adequate venous blood flow and are a major element in the treatment of venous thromboembolism. Bed rest is appropriate in the acute stage of venous thromboembolism. Any form of exercise to the legs would increase the risk of pulmonary emboli. Heat is appropriate in the treatment of venous thromboembolism. Ice causes vasoconstriction, which decreases blood flow to the extremities.

34. (4) In Buerger-Allen exercises, the feet are elevated until they blanch, then dangled until they redden, then stretched out while the client is lying flat. This promotes arterial circulation to the feet. Dorsiflexing and plantar flexing the feet help to maintain range of motion but are not Buerger-Allen exercises. The client with peripheral vascular disease should never massage the legs because of the high risk of dislodging a thrombus if one is present. Walking promotes venous circulation but is not a Buerger-Allen exercise.

35. (4) Sunburn would damage the already fragile skin, increasing the risk of ulceration and infection. Feet should not be soaked. Soaking leads to maceration, predisposing to skin breakdown or infection. The client with a peripheral vascular disorder should never walk barefoot. Small sharp objects such as pins may not be visible in carpet and could be stepped on. Lotion may be applied to dry areas of the legs and feet but must be avoided between the toes, where the excess moisture causes maceration. Ingredients in lotion provide a nutrient source for bacteria and fungi, increasing the infection risk if cracks in the skin occur.

36. (3) The client should function according to his normal daily schedule unless directed to do otherwise by the physician. Keeping a diary or log of these daily activities is necessary so that it can be correlated with the continuous ECG monitor strip to determine whether the dysrhythmia occurs during a certain activity or at a particular time of day. The Holter monitor is usually worn for only 24 hours, so it is not necessary to change the leads. Activities that precipitate symptoms may be correlated with a dysrhythmia that can be treated, preventing further symptoms from occurring. Therefore, it would be helpful if the patient were symptomatic while attached to the Holter monitor.

37. (4) Following a cardiac catheterization in which an arterial site is used for access, the puncture or cutdown site should be assessed at least as often as vital signs are monitored. The client is at risk for development of bleeding, hemorrhage, hematoma formation, and arterial insufficiency of the affected extremity. When the arterial access site is used, the client is on strict bed rest for at least several hours. Fluids are encouraged after catheterization to increase urinary output and flush out the dye used during the procedure. Clients are not routinely placed on a cardiac monitor after cardiac catheterization.

38. (1) The client's symptoms suggest pulmonary edema. Any client with severe dyspnea, orthopnea, and bubbling respirations needs to be in an upright position. High-Fowler's decreases venous return to the heart by allowing blood to pool in the extremities. Decreasing venous return lowers the output of the right ventricle and decreases lung congestion. High-Fowler's also allows the abdominal organs to fall away from the diaphragm, easing breathing. The Trendelenburg position would not promote venous pooling in the extremities and would increase venous return and pulmonary congestion. The supine position also would contribute to increased pulmonary congestion. The prone

position, lying on the abdomen, does not decrease venous return—which is what this client desperately needs.

39. (1) While elevated LDL levels in proportion to HDL levels are positively correlated with CAD, elevated HDL levels in proportion to LDL levels may decrease the risk of developing CAD. HDL levels may increase with exercise, thereby decreasing a client's risk of CAD. Age is not a predictor of HDL and LDL levels.

40. (1) Warm, moist heat applied to the extremity reduces the discomfort associated with thrombophlebitis. Vigorous massage of the leg is contraindicated in any client because it may cause a thrombus to become dislodged and possibly cause a pulmonary embolus. The leg should be elevated to prevent venous stasis. Leg exercises are used to prevent thrombophlebitis; once a client has thrombophlebitis, the leg is not exercised to prevent the thrombus from becoming an embolus.

Chapter 7

Hematologic System

ANATOMY AND PHYSIOLOGY OF THE HEMATOLOGIC SYSTEM

Bone Marrow

A. Found inside all bones in the body. Primary function is hematopoiesis (manufacture of blood cells)
B. Kinds of bone marrow
  1. Red:
     a. Carries out hematopoiesis
     b. Found in ribs, vertebral column, and other flat bones
  2. Yellow:
     a. Red marrow that has changed to fat
     b. Does not carry out hematopoiesis
  3. All blood cells start as stem cells in bone marrow.

Blood

A. Plasma:
  1. Liquid part of blood
  2. Yellow in color
  3. Consists of serum and fibrinogen
  4. Contains plasma proteins
B. Red blood cells (RBC) contain hemoglobin, which is needed to carry oxygen.
  1. Normal: male = 4.6–6.0 million; female = 4.0–5.0 million
  2. Decreased RBC may be caused by hemorrhage, anemias, chronic infections, leukemias, multiple myeloma, chronic renal failure, pregnancy, or overhydration.
  3. Increased RBC may be caused by disease, dehydration, hemoconcentration, high altitudes, COPD, or cardiovascular disease.
  4. Hematocrit: the percent of blood which is RBCs
     a. Normal: male = 40–54%; female = 36–46%
     b. Decreased level may be caused by acute blood loss, anemias, lymphomas, leukemias, multiple myeloma, malnutrition, vitamin deficiencies, pregnancy, rheumatoid arthritis, or drug toxicity.
     c. Increased level may be caused by dehydration, hypovolemia, diarrhea, polycythemia vera, diabetic acidosis, COPD, TIA, or eclampsia.
  5. Hemoglobin: a protein found in RBCs that contains iron, which carries oxygen and gives blood its red color
     a. Normal: male = 13.5–18 gm/dL; female = 12–16 gm/dL
     b. Decreased level may be caused by anemias, hemorrhage, cirrhosis, leukemias, Hodgkin's disease, cancer, pregnancy, kidney diseases, or drug toxicity.

c. Increased level may be caused by dehydration / hemoconcentration, polycythemia, high altitudes, COPD, burns, or drug toxicity.
C. Platelets (thrombocytes): necessary for clotting
    1. Normal: 150,000–500,000
    2. Thrombocytopenia may be caused by leukemias, aplastic anemia, or idiopathic thrombocytopenia purpura (ITP), liver diseases, kidney diseases, or drug toxicity.
    3. Increased levels may be caused by polycythemia vera, trauma, acute blood loss, metastatic carcinoma, high altitudes, or severe exercise.
D. White Blood Cells (WBC): part of the body's defense system to fight infections
    1. Also called neutrophil or leukocyte
    2. Normal: 5,000–10,000
    3. Leukopenia (low WBC) is a common side effect of chemotherapy treatment
    4. Leukocytosis (too many WBC) may indicate an infection
E. Blood groups:
    1. RBCs carry antigens, which determine the blood groups.
    2. ABO groups
        a. Client has A antigens (type A blood), B antigens (type B blood), both A and B antigens (type AB blood) or no antigens (type O blood)
        b. If a person receives blood with AB antigens that are not on their own, RBC antibodies are formed against them
F. Rh typing:
    1. Identifies presence (Rh positive) or absence (Rh negative) of Rh antigen
    2. Anti-Rh antibodies are not automatically formed in an Rh negative person, but if Rh positive blood is given, antibody formation starts and a second exposure to the Rh antigen will trigger a transfusion reaction.

SPLEEN

A. Largest lymphatic organ; lies beneath the diaphragm, behind and to the left of the stomach
B. Functions:
    1. Blood filtration system and reservoir
    2. Important hematopoietic site in fetus; postnatally produces monocytes and lymphocytes
    3. Important in phagocytosis; removes misshapen RBCs
    4. Involved in antibody production by plasma cells
    5. Involved in iron metabolism
    6. In an adult, functions of the spleen can be taken over by the reticuloendothelial system.

Blood Transfusions and Blood Products

A. Purpose:
    1. Improve oxygen transport—RBCs
    2. Volume expansion—whole blood, plasma, and albumin
    3. Provide proteins—Fresh frozen plasma, albumin, and plasma protein fraction
    4. Coagulation factors—cryoprecipitate, fresh frozen plasma, and fresh whole blood
    5. Platelets—platelet concentrate, and fresh whole blood
B. Types of Blood and Blood Products
    1. Whole blood:
        a. Provides all components
        b. Takes 12–24 hours for Hgb and Hct to rise
        c. Volume overload can occur from large volume
        d. Complications include hepatitis, AIDS, transfusion reaction, Na and K excess, and calcium depletion from citrate (preservative) in massive transfusions
        e. Usually administered at rate of 3–4 hours for 1 unit
    2. Red Blood Cells (Packed Red Blood Cells)
        a. RBCs provide twice the amount of Hgb as an equivalent amount of whole blood.
        b. Complications include transfusion reactions; less frequently than with whole blood because plasma proteins are not given
        c. Takes 2–4 hours to administer 1 unit
    3. Fresh Frozen Plasma
        a. Contains all coagulation factors
        b. Can be stored for 12 months
        c. Takes 20 minutes to thaw and then is hung immediately and infused quickly because it loses its coagulation factors rapidly at room temperature
    4. Platelets:
        a. Will raise the recipient's platelet count by 10,000/liter

b. One unit pooled from 4–8 units of whole blood
   c. Single donor platelet transfusions may be necessary for patients who have developed antibodies; may need compatibility testing
   d. Infused quickly
5. Factor VIII fractions (cryoprecipitate):
   a. Contains Factors VIII, fibrinogen, and XIII
   b. Used in the treatment of hemophilia
   c. Infused quickly
C. Management of Clients Receiving Blood Products:
   1. Determine a prior history of transfusions or transfusion reactions
   2. 18 or 19 gauge needle used
   3. Sodium chloride always used as IV solution; never use dextrose solution; dextrose causes agglutination of blood cells
   4. Two nurses (usually RNs) MUST verify ABO group, Rh type, patient and blood numbers, and expiration date
   5. Before starting transfusion, take baseline vital signs including temperature
   6. Initially, infusion rate is 2 cc/min
   7. Stay with patient first 15 minutes and monitor vital signs, including temperature frequently (temperature elevation suggests a transfusion reaction).

8. Monitor for transfusion reactions:
   a. Hemolytic
      (1) Causes:
         (a) ABO or Rh incompatibility (antibodies in recipient plasma react with antigen in donor cells)
         (a) Use of dextrose solutions (agglutinated cells block capillary blood flow)
      (2) Manifestations include headache, lumbar or sternal pain, nausea, vomiting, chills, flushing, jaundice, dyspnea, signs of shock, renal shutdown, or DIC
      (3) Stop IV infusion. Saline IV. Send blood unit and patient blood to the lab.
   b. Allergic
      (1) Transfer of an antigen or antibody from donor or recipient; client has immune sensitivity to foreign serum protein; allergic donors
      (2) Manifestations are allergies—urticaria, laryngeal edema, wheezing, dyspnea, bronchospasm, or anaphylaxis
      (3) Stop transfusion; give antihistamine and epinephrine as ordered
9. Document carefully. Include type of blood component, blood unit number, date and time infusion starts and ends, amount infused, patient reaction, and vital signs.

Disorders

ANEMIAS

Anemia is an insufficient number of red blood cells. Anemia can be caused by blood loss, manufacture of insufficient RBCs, or abnormal destruction of RBCs.

Iron Deficiency Anemia

A. Chronic microcytic (little cells); hypochromic (little color) anemia caused by either inadequate absorption or excessive loss of iron
B. Assessment:
   1. Fatigue, dizziness
   2. Pallor
   3. Cold sensitivity
   4. Palpitations
   5. Brittle hair and nails
   6. Decreased Hgb, Hct, and RBC
C. Nursing diagnoses (Table 7.1)

Table 7.1 Nursing Diagnoses Related to Anemia

- Activity intolerance related to impaired oxygen transport secondary to diminished red blood count
- High risk for ineffective health maintenance related to insufficient knowledge of condition, nutritional requirements, and drug therapy

D. Management:
   1. Assess for bleeding; stool for occult blood
   2. Rest
   3. Iron Administration:
      a. Intramuscular; give Z track deep IM; don't massage after IM injection; encourage walking
      b. Oral
         (1) Preferred route
         (2) Liquid stains teeth
         (3) Give WITH meals to decrease GI irritation

c. Increase intake of iron-containing foods:
  (1) Iron-containing foods include meats, egg yolks, green leafy vegetables, raisins, enriched breads, and cereals
  (2) Give iron foods with vitamin C

Pernicious Anemia

A. Chronic, progressive anemia caused by a deficiency of intrinsic factor, which is normally produced by the gastric mucosa
   1. Intrinsic factor is necessary for the absorption of Vitamin B_{12} into the blood stream.
   2. Vitamin B_{12} deficiency diminishes DNA synthesis, which results in defective maturation of RBCs and GI tract cells and poor functioning of the nervous system.
B. Assessment:
   1. Anemia and pallor
   2. Fatigue
   3. Sore mouth and beefy red tongue
   4. Decreased HCl in stomach
   5. Paresthesias and paralysis
   6. Depression, psychosis
C. Diagnosis:
   1. CBC and blood studies to detect anemia
   2. Gastric analysis to determine HCl level
   3. Schilling Test
      a. Radioactive vitamin B_{12} given PO
      b. 24-hour urine collected, decreased amount of vitamin B_{12} in urine if pernicious anemia
D. Nursing diagnoses (Table 7.1)
E. Management:
   1. Vitamin B_{12} injections regularly (usually monthly) for life
   2. Iron
   3. Transfusions if severe

Aplastic Anemia

A. Depression of white cell, red cell, and platelet production due to bone marrow destruction; can be either idiopathic or secondary. Secondary causes include chemical toxins, drugs (chloramphenicol), radiation, or immunologic therapy.
B. Assessment:
   1. Fatigue and dyspnea (due to decreased RBCs)
   2. Infections (due to decreased WBCs)
   3. Bleeding tendencies (due to decreased platelets)
   4. Bone marrow biopsy shows fatty marrow with few developing cells
C. Management:
   1. Remove offending agent
   2. Blood transfusions

Table 7.2 Nursing Diagnoses Related to Sickle Cell Anemia

- Activity intolerance related to impaired oxygen transport secondary to diminished red blood count
- High risk for ineffective health maintenance related to insufficient knowledge of condition, nutritional requirements, and drug therapy
- Impaired gas exchange related to decreased oxygen-carrying capacity of blood and reduced RBC life span
- Altered tissue perfusion related to stasis and vassocclusion
- Pain related to sickling and occlusion
- Deficient knowledge regarding disease process, genetic factors, and treatment
- Ineffective family coping related to chronic nature of illness

3. Prevent and treat infections:
   a. Protective isolation
   b. High protein, high vitamin diet
   c. Good mouth care
4. Bone marrow transplant
5. Prevent and treat bleeding episodes:
   a. Use a soft toothbrush and electric razor
   b. No IM injections
   c. Observe for bleeding

Hemolytic Anemia

A. Anemia caused by increased destruction of RBCs; can be inherited (sickle cell anemia or thalassemia), acquired (transfusion reaction), or of an unknown cause
B. Assessment:
   1. Pallor due to decreased RBC, jaundice as a result of rapid destruction of RBC
   2. Fatigue due to decreased RBC
   3. Chills, fever, and pain
   4. Hematuria
   5. Decreased Hgb and Hct
C. Nursing diagnoses (Table 7.2)
D. Management:
   1. Eliminate causative factors if possible
   2. Corticosteroids (autoimmune types)
   3. Folic acid to assist in RBC production
   4. Transfusions
   5. Splenectomy (in adults; children need spleen for antibody formation)

Sickle Cell Anemia

A. Most common inherited disorder in African American population; 10% of African Americans have sickle cell trait
B. Transmitted as autosomal recessive gene (Figure 7.1):
   1. Both parents must carry the gene for a child to develop the condition.
   2. When both parents carry the gene, there is a 25% chance with each pregnancy of having a child with the disorder; a 50% chance with each pregnancy of having a

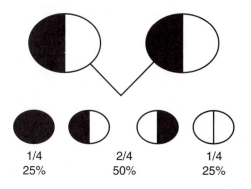

1/4 25%   2/4 50%   1/4 25%

Dark side of circle = sickle cell trait

Figure 7.1 Sickle Cell Anemia—Method of Inheritance

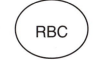

Normal Red Blood Cell

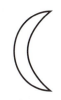

Sickled RBC

Figure 7.2 Pathophysiology of Sickle Cell Anemia

child who is a carrier; and a 25% chance with each pregnancy of having a child who will be disease and carrier free.

3. Inherited diseases transmitted as autosomal recessive include sickle cell anemia, cystic fibrosis, PKU, and Tay-Sachs.

C. Pathophysiology (Figure 7.2):
   1. Structure of Hgb changed; Hgb S contains deformed, rigid S-shaped cells and has reduced oxygen-carrying capacity; Hgb S replaces all or part of Hgb in RBCs
   2. When oxygen is released, the shape of the RBCs changes from round and pliable to crescent-shaped, rigid, and inflexible.
   3. RBCs live for 6–20 days instead of 120, causing hemolytic anemia.
   4. Local hypoxia and continued sickling lead to blockage of blood vessels.

5. No symptoms before 6–12 months of age because of high fetal hemoglobin
6. Sickling is caused by decreased oxygen saturation which is caused by high altitudes, dehydration, and acidosis.
7. Sickle cell crisis (Figure 7.3)
   a. Sickled cells clump together and obstruct blood vessels, causing increased blood viscosity, and producing more sickling and hypoxia.
   b. Symptoms occur in areas where circulation is obstructed; may be renal, joint pain, pneumonias, leg ulcers, abdominal pain, stroke, etc.
   c. Enlarged liver and spleen from rapid red cell breakdown

D. Assessment findings:
   1. Decreased Hgb
   2. Sickle cell test and Sickledex: screening tests results don't differentiate between trait and disease
   3. Hgb electrophoresis—differentiates between trait and disease

E. Management:
   1. Hydration (oral and IV)
   2. Oxygenation
   3. Correct acidosis
   4. Analgesics for pain (no aspirin; may cause acidosis which causes sickling)
   5. Antibiotics for infections
   6. Exchange transfusions
   7. Bed rest
   8. Splenectomy

CLOTTING DISORDERS

Hemophilia

A. Inherited bleeding disorder caused by a deficit of one of the clotting factors
B. Classic hemophilia (Factor VIII deficiency) most common
C. Transmission:
   1. Carried on the X chromosome
   2. Manifested in the male
   3. European Caucasians primarily affected
D. Pathophysiology of classic hemophilia: deficiency of Factor VIII affects intrinsic clotting mechanism
E. Assessment findings:
   1. Bleeding after minor injuries
   2. Hemarthrosis (bleeding into joints such as knees, ankles, elbows, or wrists)
F. Nursing diagnoses (Table 7.3)
G. Management
   1. Control acute bleeding:
      a. Ice compresses to promote vasoconstriction
      b. Immobilization of bleeding area
      c. No aspirin

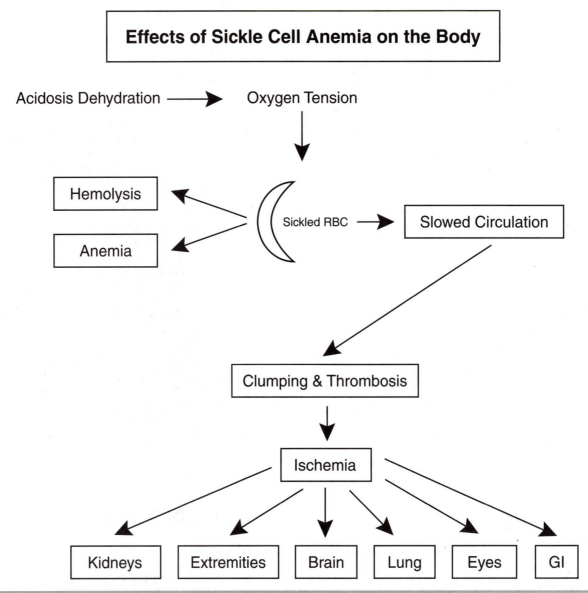

Figure 7.3 Effects of Sickle Cell Anemia on the Body

Table 7.3 Nursing Diagnoses Related to Hemophilia

- Acute pain related to joint swelling and limitations secondary to hemarthrosis
- Risk for impaired physical mobility related to joint swelling and limitations secondary to hemarthrosis
- Risk for impaired oral mucus membranes related to trauma from coarse food and insufficient dental hygiene
- Risk for ineffective health maintenance related to insufficient knowledge of condition, contraindications, genetic transmission, environmental hazards, and emergency treatment to control bleeding

    d. Fibrin foam
    e. Topical epinephrine
    f. Cryoprecipitate (frozen Factor VIII)
  2. Care for hemarthrosis:
    a. Immobilize joint

    b. Bed cradle to keep bed clothes off joint
    c. Passive ROM 48 hours after bleeding controlled; stop if there is pain

Disseminated Intravascular Coagulation (DIC)

A. Widespread formation of thromboses in the microcirculation, mainly within the capillaries, with subsequent depletion of clotting factors resulting in hemorrhage from kidneys, brain, adrenals, heart, and other organs; patients are usually critically ill with a surgical, hemolytic, obstetric, or neoplastic disease
B. Pathophysiology:
  1. Underlying disease causes release of thromboplastic substances into blood that

promote fibrin deposits throughout the microcirculation.
2. Microthrombi form in many organs, causing microinfarcts and tissue necrosis.
3. RBCs are trapped in fibrin strands and hemolysed. Platelets, prothrombin, and other clotting factors are destroyed, causing bleeding.
4. Excessive clotting activates the fibrinolytic inhibiting platelet function, causing further bleeding.
C. Assessment findings:
1. Petechiae and ecchymoses
2. Excessive bleeding from IVs, surgery, or childbirth
3. Oliguria and acute renal failure
4. PT, PTT prolonged
5. Decrease in clotting factors
D. Management:
1. Control of underlying disease process
2. Blood transfusion
3. Heparin (stops clotting in microcirculation and frees clotting materials)
4. Prevent bleeding:
   a. No injections
   b. Handle gently
   c. Nontraumatic mouth care
   d. No aspirin

WHITE CELL DISORDERS

Infectious Mononucleosis ("Kissing Disease")

A. An acute infectious disease caused by the Epstein Barr virus characterized by increased monocytes that affects primarily children and young adults
B. Assessment findings:
1. Lymphadenopathy
2. Headache, sore throat
3. Mental and physical fatigue
4. Spleen and liver enlargement
5. Heterophil antibody agglutination and Monospot tests positive
6. Incubation period of 2–6 weeks; spread by oral secretions
C. Management:
1. No specific treatment or immunization (rarely hospitalized)
2. Rest for several weeks to months
3. Treat secondary infections if they develop

Leukemia

A. A progressive, malignant disease of the blood-forming organs marked by distorted proliferation and development of leukocytes and their precursors in the blood and bone

---

Table 7.4 Nursing Diagnoses Related to Leukemia

- Risk for infection related to altered immune system secondary to leukemic process and side effects of chemotherapeutic agents
- Risk for injury related to bleeding tendencies secondary to leukemic process and side effects of chemotherapy
- Risk for delayed growth and development related to impaired ability to achieve developmental tasks secondary to limitations of disease and treatments
- Powerlessness related to inability to control situation
- Risk for social isolation related to effects of disease and treatments on appearance and fear of embarrassment

---

marrow; the most common form of childhood cancer; some forms occur in adults
B. Pathophysiology:
1. Uncontrolled proliferation of WBC precursors
2. Normal WBCs, RBCs, and platelets crowded out by leukemic cells
3. Type of leukemia is designated by the type of cell proliferating (Myelocytic leukemia, acute lymphocytic leukemia)
C. Assessment findings:
1. Anemia, pallor, dyspnea (due to decreased RBCs)
2. Ecchymoses and bleeding (due to decreased platelets)
3. Infections (due to decreased normal WBCs)
4. Lymphadenopathy
5. Enlarged liver and spleen
6. Abdominal pain, weight loss, and nausea
7. Bone pain due to expansion of marrow
D. Nursing diagnoses (Table 7.4)
E. Management:
1. Chemotherapy: side effects include bone marrow depression, nausea, vomiting, alopecia, and/or stomatitis
2. Radiation therapy
3. Support child during painful procedures: bone marrow aspirations, lumbar punctures, venipuncture
4. Help client and family cope with a possible fatal illness

OTHER MALIGNANT DISORDERS

Hodgkin's Lymphoma

A. A primary lymph node neoplastic disease characterized by painless progressive enlargement of the lymph nodes, spleen, and lymphoid tissues. Often begins in a cervical node and spreads through the body. Occurs primarily in adolescents and young adults.
B. Assessment findings:
1. Lymphadenopathy usually starting with cervical nodes

2. Sweating, weakness, fever
3. Itching
4. Staging:
   a. Stage One—only one lymph node involved (good prognosis)
   b. Stage Two—two or more nodes on same side of diaphragm (good prognosis)
   c. Stage Three—nodes on both sides of diaphragm involved (poor prognosis)
   d. Stage Four—diffuse involvement with one or more extra lymphatic organs involved (very poor prognosis)
C. Management:
   1. Radiation used alone for localized disease
   2. Chemotherapy:
      a. Used in combination with radiation for advanced disease
      b. Combination of drugs used usually
   3. Protect client from infections: Remember both the disease and the treatment reduce ability to fight infections
   4. Splenectomy in advanced disease

Non-Hodgkin's Lymphoma

A. Tumor originating in the lymphoid tissue that is diffuse, disseminates easily, and is difficult to control
B. Assessment findings: similar to Hodgkin's lymphoma
C. Management:
   1. Chemotherapy
   2. Radiation
   3. Surgery for diagnosis and staging
   4. Nursing care similar to Hodgkin's

Multiple Myeloma

A. A malignant neoplasm in which the plasma cells proliferate and invade the bone marrow, causing destruction of the bone and resulting in pathologic fractures and bone pain; affects primarily men after the age of 40
B. Pathophysiology:
   1. Bone demineralization and destruction with osteoporosis and a negative calcium balance
   2. Disruption of RBC, WBC, and thrombocyte production
C. Assessment findings:
   1. Headache and bone pain
   2. Pathologic fractures and skeletal deformities of sternum and ribs
   3. Osteoporosis and loss of height
   4. Renal calculi
   5. Anemia, infections, and bleeding tendencies
   6. Hypercalcemia
   7. Spinal cord compression and paraplegia
   8. Urine positive for Bence-Jones protein

D. Management
   1. Drug therapy:
      a. Analgesics for bone pain
      b. Cancer chemotherapy to reduce tumor mass
      c. Antibiotics to treat infections
      d. Gamma globulin to prevent infections
      e. Corticosteroids and mithramycin for severe hypercalcemia
      f. Medications such as etidronate (Didronel) or alendronate (Fosamax) to slow the loss of calcium from the bones
   2. Radiation therapy to reduce tumor mass
   3. Transfusions
   4. Comfort measures for bone pain
   5. Ambulation to slow demineralization
   6. Push fluids to prevent kidney stones from calcium overload
   7. Safety: patients prone to pathologic fractures, bleeding, and infection

Acquired Immune Deficiency Syndrome (AIDS)

A. Suppression or deficiency of the cellular immune response acquired by exposure to the human T-cell lymphocytic virus; manifested clinically by opportunistic infections and unusual neoplasms
B. Risk Factors:
   1. Sexually active homosexual and bisexual men
   2. IV drug abusers
   3. Hemophiliacs and recipients of blood transfusions
   4. Children of persons with AIDS
   5. Heterosexual partners of persons with AIDS
C. Assessment findings:
   1. Nonspecific symptoms such as weight loss, fatigue, diarrhea, fever, pallor
   2. Dyspnea and hypoxemia due to pneumonia
   3. Neurologic dysfunction secondary to acute meningitis, dementia, and encephalopathy
   4. Opportunistic infections:
      a. Pneumocystis carini pneumonia
      b. Herpes simplex, cytomegalovirus, and Epstein-Barr virus
      c. Fungal infections
   5. Neoplasms:
      a. Kaposi's sarcoma
      b. CNS lymphoma
      c. Burkitt's lymphoma
      d. Non-Hodgkin's lymphoma
   6. Leukopenia, anemia, thrombocytopenia
   7. Elevated transaminases and alkaline phosphatase
   8. Low serum albumin
D. Nursing Diagnoses (Table 7.5)

Table 7.5 Nursing Diagnoses Related to Acquired Immune Deficiency Syndrome

- Altered comfort related to headache, fever secondary to inflammation of cerebral tissue
- Fatigue related to pulmonary insufficiency, chronic infections, malnutrition secondary to chronic diarrhea and gastrointestinal malabsorption
- Risk for impaired skin integrity related to perineal and anal tissue excoriation secondary to diarrhea and chronic genital candida or herpes lesions
- Imbalanced nutrition: less than body requirements related to chronic diarrhea, gastrointestinal absorption, fatigue, anorexia and/or oral/esophageal lesions
- Risk for infection transmission related to contagious nature of blood and body excretions
- Social isolation related to rejection of others after diagnosis
- Hopelessness related to nature of the condition and poor prognosis
- Powerlessness related to unpredictable nature of condition

E. Management:
1. Antiretrovirals: interfere with the replication of the virus
   a. Didanosine (Videx) (ddl); Lamivudine (3TC) (Epivir); Stavudine (d4T) (Zerit); Zidovudine (AZT) (Retrovir)
   b. Delavirdine (DLV) (Rescriptor); Nevirapine (NVP) (Viramune)
   c. Indinavir (Crixivan); Nelfinavir (Viracept); Ritonavir (Norvir); Saquinavir (Invirase)
   d. Teach patient and family
      (1) Drugs do not cure AIDS but will control the symptoms.
      (2) Call the physician if signs of other infections occur, such as sore throat or swollen lymph nodes.
      (3) Patient is still infective and must use methods to prevent the transmission of AIDS virus: universal precautions and safer sex.
      (4) Follow-up visits important to monitor for toxicity to treatment
      (5) Avoid OTC products because of the many incompatibilities.
2. Medications for concomitant disease
3. Protective isolation if leukopenia develops
4. Universal precautions:
   a. Gowns and gloves when contact with secretions
   b. Hand washing
   c. Secretion precautions
5. Emotional support

Sample Questions

1. The nurse is discussing dietary sources of iron with a client who has iron deficiency anemia. Which menu, if selected by the client, indicates the best understanding of the diet?
   1. Milkshake, hot dog, and beets
   2. Beef steak, spinach, and grape juice
   3. Chicken salad, green peas, and coffee
   4. Macaroni and cheese, coleslaw, and lemonade

2. Ferrous Sulfate is prescribed for a client. She returns to clinic in two weeks. Which assessment by the nurse indicates that she has NOT been taking iron as ordered?
   1. The client's cheeks are flushed.
   2. The client reports having more energy.
   3. The client complains of nausea.
   4. The client's stools are light brown.

3. A Schilling test has been ordered for a client suspected of having pernicious anemia. What is the nurse's primary responsibility in relation to this test?
   1. Collect the blood samples.
   2. Collect a 24-hour urine sample.
   3. Assist the client to X-ray.
   4. Administer an enema.

4. A client who receives a diagnosis of pernicious anemia asks why she must receive vitamin shots. What is the best answer for the nurse to give?
   1. "Shots work faster than pills."
   2. "Your body cannot absorb Vitamin B12 from foods."
   3. "Vitamins are necessary to make the blood cells."
   4. "You can get more vitamins in a shot than a pill."

5. A woman who has been diagnosed as having pernicious anemia asks how long she will have to take shots. What is the best answer for the nurse to give?
   1. "Until your blood count returns to normal."
   2. "Until you are feeling better."
   3. "For the rest of your life."
   4. "That varies with each person. Ask your doctor."

6. A toddler has been treated for sickle cell crisis. The crisis subsides and the child improves. Which statement is essential for the nurse to include in the discharge teaching?
   1. Your child will bruise easily. Do not let your child bump into things.
   2. Notify the physician immediately if your child develops a fever.
   3. Your child will need special help with feeding.
   4. Observe your child frequently for difficulty breathing.

7. Which statement made by the parent of a child newly diagnosed with sickle cell anemia indicates a need for more teaching?
   1. "We are going to the mountains for our vacation this year."
   2. "It's a good thing she likes to drink juices."
   3. "If she needs something for pain, I will give her baby acetaminophen."
   4. "I will make sure that she doesn't get chilled when it is cold outside."

8. A five-year-old boy is admitted because he bled profusely when he lost his first baby tooth. After a workup, he is diagnosed as having classic hemophilia. His mother asks the nurse if his two younger sisters will also develop hemophilia. The best answer for the nurse to give is:
   1. "They will not develop the disease."
   2. "Statistically, one of them is likely to develop the disease."
   3. "They won't get the disease, but they may be carriers."
   4. "If it doesn't show up by the time they start school, they are unlikely to develop the condition."

9. The nurse has been teaching the parents of a child with hemophilia about the care he will need. Which statement by the parents indicates a need for more instruction?
   1. "If my child needs something for pain or a fever, I will give him acetaminophen instead of aspirin."
   2. "I will take my child to the dentist for regular checkups."
   3. "I will keep my child in the house most of the time."
   4. "My son's medic-alert bracelet arrived."

10. A college student who is diagnosed as having infectious mononucleosis asks how the disease is spread.
    The nurse's response is based on the knowledge that the usual mode of transmission is through:
    1. skin
    2. genital contact
    3. contaminated water
    4. intimate oral contact

11. A young man who has infectious mononucleosis asks what the treatment is for his condition. The best response for the nurse to make is:
    1. "You will receive large doses of antibiotics for the next 10 days."
    2. "Rest and good nutrition are the best things you can do."
    3. "You will be given an antiviral agent that will help to control the symptoms."
    4. "You will probably be given steroid medications for several months."

12. An 8-year-old boy is admitted to the unit with a diagnosis of acute lymphocytic leukemia. During a routine physical exam, numerous ecchymotic areas were noted on his body. The parents reported that the child had been more tired than usual lately.
    The parent says that the child has had a cold for the last several weeks and asks if this is related to the leukemia. The nurse's response is based on the knowledge that:
    1. Leukemia causes a decrease in the number of normal white blood cells in the body.

2. A chronic infection such as the child has had makes a child more likely to develop leukemia.
3. The virus responsible for colds is thought to cause leukemia.
4. Having an infection prior to the onset of leukemia is merely a coincidence.

13. A child with leukemia bruises easily. This is most likely due to:
    1. Decreased fibrinogen levels
    2. Excessive clotting elsewhere in the body
    3. Decreased platelets
    4. Decreased erythrocytes

14. A child who is being treated for leukemia develops stomatitis. Which of the following nursing care measures is essential?
    1. Using dental floss to clean the teeth
    2. Frequent cleaning of the mouth with an astringent mouth wash
    3. Use of an overbed cradle
    4. Swabbing the mouth with moistened cotton swabs.

15. When planning care for a client who is HIV positive, the nurse should:
    1. Teach persons coming in contact with the client to wear a gown and mask at all times.
    2. Teach persons to wear gloves when handling any of the client's body fluids.
    3. Restrict visitors to immediate family.
    4. Encourage the client to stay away from other persons as much as possible.

16. Which action should the nurse expect to perform after a client has a bone marrow biopsy taken from the iliac crest?
    1. Apply pressure to the site for 1 minute.
    2. Administer a narcotic analgesic.
    3. Apply an adhesive bandage to the site.
    4. Place the client in a recumbent position.

17. Which of the following would be the most appropriate snack for a client who has iron deficiency anemia?
    1. A half grapefruit
    2. A carrot raisin salad
    3. A cup of yogurt
    4. Apple slices and cheese

18. Which of the following assessment findings should alert the nurse that the elderly client should be evaluated for pernicious anemia?
    1. Clubbing of the nails
    2. Bloody stools
    3. Beefy-red tongue
    4. Enlarged lymph nodes

19. An elderly client who is being treated for pernicious anemia needs to be monitored periodically for which of the following conditions?
    1. Lactose intolerance
    2. Stomach cancer
    3. Dementia
    4. Hearing loss

20. Which of the following would be the best lunch for a client with folic acid deficiency anemia?
    1. Bologna sandwich and vegetable soup
    2. Grilled cheese sandwich and tomato soup
    3. Coleslaw and cream of mushroom soup
    4. Spinach salad and bean soup
21. The nurse administers iron using the Z track technique. What is the primary reason for administering iron via Z track?
    1. To prevent adverse reactions
    2. To prevent staining of the skin
    3. To improve the absorption rate
    4. To increase the speed of onset of action
22. The nurse is caring for a client who is thought to have pernicious anemia. What signs and symptoms would the nurse expect in this person?
    1. Easy bruising
    2. Beefy-red tongue
    3. Fine red rash on the extremities
    4. Pruritus
23. A one-year-old is admitted to the hospital with sickle cell anemia in crisis. Upon admission, which therapy will assume priority?
    1. Fluid administration
    2. Exchange transfusion
    3. Anticoagulant
    4. IM administration of iron and folic acid
24. A toddler is diagnosed with sickle cell anemia. Her mother is four months pregnant with her second child. The mother asks if there is any chance the new baby will have sickle cell anemia. She says that neither she nor her husband have sickle cell anemia. What is the best response for the nurse to make?
    1. "No. Sickle cell anemia is not inherited."
    2. "Yes. The new baby will also have sickle cell anemia."
    3. "There is a 25% chance that each child you have will have the disease."
    4. "Because neither of you have the disease, another child will not have it. You should ask your physician."
25. A child who has hemophilia is admitted to the hospital with a swollen knee joint. He is complaining of severe pain. What is the priority of nursing care for this child upon admission?
    1. Maintain joint function
    2. Use a bed cradle
    3. Administer aspirin prn for pain
    4. Encourage fluids
26. The nurse is caring for a child who has hemophilia. He is admitted with a bleeding episode. Which of the following should the nurse expect will be given to stop the bleeding?
    1. Heparin
    2. Cryoprecipitate
    3. Packed cells
    4. Whole blood
27. A 19-year old-college student reports to the health service with a sore throat, malaise, and fever of four days duration. Examination shows cervical lymphadenopathy and splenomegaly. Temperature is 103°F. Blood is positive for heterophil antibody agglutination test. Which condition does the nurse expect this student has?
    1. Streptococcal sore throat
    2. Infectious mononucleosis
    3. Rubella
    4. Influenza
28. The nurse knows that infectious mononucleosis is caused by which of the following?
    1. Cytomegalovirus
    2. Beta hemolytic streptococcus
    3. Epstein-Barr virus
    4. Herpes simplex virus I
29. A child who has leukemia is to have a bone marrow biopsy performed. How will the child be positioned for this procedure?
    1. On his side with the top knee flexed
    2. Prone
    3. Modified Trendelenburg
    4. On his back with his head elevated 30 degrees
30. A child is being evaluated for possible leukemia. Which assessment finding is most likely to be present?
    1. Numerous bruises on the child's body
    2. Ruddy complexion
    3. Diarrhea and vomiting
    4. Chest pain

Answers and Rationales

1. (2) Beef, spinach, and grape juice contain iron. Milk contains no iron.
2. (4) Iron turns stool black. The other answers all indicate compliance with the medication regime.
3. (2) The client is given radioactive Vitamin B_{12} orally, and a 24-hour urine sample is collected to see if Vitamin B_{12} is absorbed from the GI tract into the blood stream and excreted in the urine.
4. (2) Injections of Vitamin B_{12} will be necessary, because without intrinsic factor her body cannot absorb Vitamin B_{12} from foods.
5. (3) Because she is deficient in intrinsic factor and cannot absorb Vitamin B_{12} from foods, she will have to take Vitamin B_{12} shots for life.
6. (2) Fevers cause dehydration and sickling, which may result in a crisis.
7. (1) The mountains are high in altitude and have less oxygen saturation, which may precipitate an attack. Drinking juices is good because it will help to prevent dehydration. Acetaminophen is better for the child than aspirin, which may cause acidosis. The child should be protected from extremes in temperature.
8. (3) Hemophilia is carried on the X chromosome and causes disease when it appears in

combination with the Y chromosome in the male. Number 1 is a true statement, but it is not complete and, therefore, not the best answer.

9. (3) Parents of children with hemophilia tend to over-protect them. A goal is to have the child lead as normal a life as possible. Number 1 is correct. He should not receive aspirin because it is an anti-coagulant. Number 2 indicates good knowledge. Prophylactic dental care is important, so he will not need dental work or extractions. Number 4 indicates good knowledge. He should always wear a medic-alert bracelet in case he is injured.

10. (4) The virus is spread through intimate oral contact. It is called the "kissing disease." It can also be spread by sharing eating and drinking utensils and by coughing and sneezing.

11. (2) Rest and good nutrition are the hallmarks of treatment for mononucleosis. Recovery may take several months. Because it is caused by a virus, antibiotics are not indicated. He would receive antibiotics only if he develops a secondary infection. There are no effective antiviral agents for this condition. Steroids are not indicated.

12. (1) Leukemia causes a decrease in normal white cells. White blood cells are the infection fighting cells. Infections occur because of the decrease in WBCs due to leukemia. Infections do not cause leukemia.

13. (3) In leukemia, there is bone marrow failure. In addition to producing abnormal, immature WBCs, the bone marrow fails and does not produce stem cells from which RBCs and platelets develop.

14. (4) Stomatitis is a frequent complication of chemotherapy for leukemia. He has a tendency to bleed because of his decreased platelets. Dental floss might cause bleeding. An astringent mouth wash is too strong for his tender mouth. An overbed cradle does not relate to stomatitis. Moistened cotton swabs are a gentle means of cleaning the mouth.

15. (2) Universal precautions are indicated. Number 1 is not correct. It is not necessary to wear a gown and mask unless there is a risk of exposure to body fluids. Number 3 is not correct. There is no reason to limit visitors. Number 4 is not correct. The client is HIV positive. There is no indication that the client is immunocompromised and at an increased risk of infection from others. The client will not transmit the disease unless there is contact with body fluids.

16. (4) The client should lie in bed in a recumbent position on top of a pressure dressing that has been applied to the site. Hemorrhage poses a slight risk after this procedure. Pressure should be applied to the site for several minutes. A pressure dressing should then be applied for one hour to reduce the chances of bleeding or hemorrhage. An analgesic may be ordered and

administered prior to the procedure. Use of deep breathing and relaxation techniques may also be helpful. There is seldom any pain after the biopsy, although the site may ache for a few days.

17. (2) Carrots and raisins are both high in iron. Red meats and spinach are other good iron sources. Citrus fruits such as grapefruit are high in folic acid, vitamin C, and potassium but not iron. Dairy products such as yogurt and cottage cheese provide calcium but no iron. Apples are not good sources of iron.

18. (3) Early in the course of pernicious anemia, the tongue becomes beefy red and painful. Later, the tongue atrophies and becomes smooth. Nail clubbing is associated with respiratory and cardiac disorders. Numbness and tingling of the hands and feet are more common with pernicious anemia. Mild diarrhea is associated with pernicious anemia, whereas bloody stools usually are not. Colorectal bleeding is likely to lead to iron deficiency anemia. Enlarged lymph nodes are associated with leukemia, not anemia.

19. (2) The incidence of stomach cancer is increased in clients with deficiency of gastric acid. Intrinsic factor is in gastric acid. Treatment of pernicious anemia corrects the deficiency of vitamin B_{12} but does not alter the gastric acid production, so the client remains at risk for stomach cancer. Both lactose intolerance and hearing loss occur more commonly with aging, as does pernicious anemia. The presence of pernicious anemia does not alter the risk for either lactose intolerance or hearing loss, however. Dementia does occur in the late stages of untreated pernicious anemia, but for a client who is receiving treatment, there is no increased risk of dementia.

20. (4) Leafy green vegetables and dried beans are good sources of folic acid. Nuts and citrus fruits are other good sources. The other options do not contain foods high in folic acid.

21. (2) Iron is black and stains the skin. The Z track method of pulling the skin to one side before injecting the medications prevents staining of the skin. It also reduces pain from the medication. It does not prevent adverse reactions, improve the absorption rate, or increase the speed of onset of action.

22. (2) A beefy-red tongue is characteristic of pernicious anemia. Easy bruising would be seen in a clotting disorder such as hemophilia or in leukemia or in bone marrow depression. Pruritus is characteristic of Hodgkin's disease. Pernicious anemia does not present a fine, red rash on the extremities.

23. (1) Dehydration causes sickling. Sickling causes clumping and pain. First priority of care upon admission should be the administration of fluids. Exchange transfusion, if done, is not the

first priority. Anticoagulants are not the first priority. Iron and folic acid may be given but are not the first priority. They will not help stop the sickling. Folic acid and iron are necessary to make RBC.

24. (3) Sickle cell anemia is a recessive gene that is transmitted, giving a 25% chance that each child will have the disease. To have a child with the disease, both parents must be carriers for the disease even though neither one has the disease.

25. (2) Hemarthrosis (bleeding into a joint) is very painful. A bed cradle will keep the bed covers off of his sore joint. Moving a bleeding joint will increase bleeding and should not be done. Aspirin is an anticoagulant and contraindicated for a hemophiliac. Fluid administration is not the priority nursing action.

26. (2) Cryoprecipitate is frozen clotting factor and replaces the factors that the child is missing. Heparin is an anticoagulant and contraindicated for this child. Packed cells might be given after a severe hemorrhage but do not contain any clotting factors. Whole blood does not contain clotting factors.

27. (2) The findings are characteristic of infectious mononucleosis. The heterophil antibody agglutination test is diagnostic for mononucleosis. A throat culture would identify a streptococcal sore throat. Rubella (German measles) typically has a rash. The fever and sore throat are not typical of rubella. Influenza might have similar symptoms but would not have a positive heterophil agglutination test.

28. (3) The Epstein-Barr virus is the causative organism for infectious mononucleosis.

29 (1) The iliac crest is the site usually used for a bone marrow biopsy.

30. (1) The child with leukemia has a large number of immature white blood cells and not enough red blood cells and platelets. He is likely to have numerous bruises because of the low platelet count. He is likely to have a pale, not ruddy, complexion because he is deficient in red blood cells. Diarrhea and vomiting are possible if he had an intestinal virus, but bruises are much more common. Chest pain is unlikely.

Chapter 8

The Respiratory System

(FIGURE 8.1) ANATOMY AND PHYSIOLOGY

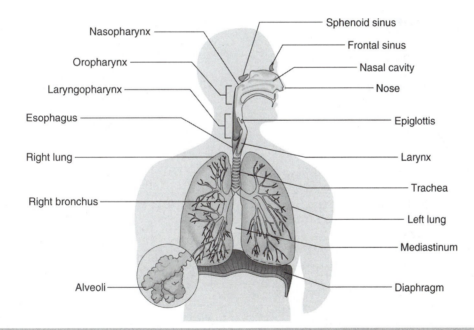

Figure 8.1 Respiratory System

NOSE

A. The external nose is a framework of bone and cartilage divided on the inside into two passages, or nares, by the nasal septum through which air enters the respiratory system.
B. The septum is covered with a mucus membrane that has olfactory (smell) receptors.
C. Turbinates located inside the nose assist in warming and moistening the air.
D. The major functions of the nose are warming, moistening, and filtering the air and the sense of smell.

PHARYNX

A. Muscular passageway called the throat
B. Air passes through the nose to the pharynx which is composed of three parts:
   1. *Nasopharynx,* located above the soft palate of the mouth and containing adenoids and openings to eustachian tubes
   2. *Oropharynx,* located directly behind the mouth and tongue and which contains the palatine tonsils
   3. *Laryngopharynx,* which starts at the epiglottis

LARYNX

A. "Voice box" connects upper and lower airways
B. Epiglottis, a flap at the base of the tongue, closes the larynx to prevent aspiration when food passes through pharynx and opens to allow respiration; larynx closes to prevent aspiration when food passes through the pharynx
C. Vocal cords are reedlike bands that produce speech and are involved in the cough reflex.

TRACHEA (WINDPIPE)

A. The air passage extending from the pharynx (throat) to the main bronchi
B. Adult trachea is 11–13 cm long and 1.5–2.5 cm in diameter

BRONCHIAL TREE

A. The trachea divides into two branches (bronchi):
   1. Right mainstem bronchus is larger and straighter than the left and divides into three lobar branches to supply the three lobes of the right lung
   2. Left mainstem bronchus divides into upper and lower lobar bronchi to supply two lobes of left lung
B. When the bronchus is 1 mm in diameter, it is called a bronchiole.
   1. Tracheobronchial tree ends at the terminal bronchioles.
   2. Beyond the terminal bronchioles, the major function is not air conduction but gas exchange between blood and alveolar air.

LUNGS

A. Main organs of respiration; lie within the thoracic cavity on either side of the heart
B. Top portion of lung is called the apex; broad area of lung that rests on the diaphragm is called the base

C. Right lung has three lobes; left lung has two lobes
D. Pleura is a two-layered membrane that covers the lungs and contains lubricating fluid between its inner and outer layers.
E. Lungs and associated structures protected by the chest wall

CHEST WALL

A. Includes rib cage, intercostal muscles, and diaphragm
B. Parietal pleura lines the chest wall and secretes small amounts of lubricating fluid into the intrapleural space; this fluid holds the lung and chest wall together as a single unit while allowing them to move separately.
C. Chest is shaped and supported by 12 pairs of ribs and costal cartilages; ribs have several attached muscles that help with respiration
D. The diaphragm is the major muscle of ventilation (exchange of air between atmosphere and alveoli). Contraction of muscle fibers causes the dome of the diaphragm to descend, increasing the volume of the thoracic cavity.

PULMONARY CIRCULATION

A. Circulation of blood to and from the lungs where it is oxygenated
B. Pulmonary arteries (right and left) carry unoxygenated blood from the right ventricle to the right and left lungs. They are the only arteries in the nonfetal circulation that carry unoxygenated blood.
C. Within the lung, the pulmonary arteries subdivide and finally become capillaries that surround the alveoli and exchange carbon dioxide for oxygen.
D. After picking up oxygen, capillaries reform to make the pulmonary veins.
E. Pulmonary veins, right and left, empty into the left atrium. They are the only veins in the nonfetal circulation that carry oxygenated blood.

GAS EXCHANGE: ALVEOLAR DUCTS AND ALVEOLI

A. Alveoli are the functional cellular units of the lungs where oxygen and carbon dioxide exchange takes place.
B. Alveoli produce surfactant, which reduces surface tension and increases stability of the alveoli and prevents their collapse.

Nursing Assessment

HEALTH HISTORY

A. Presenting Problem:
   1. Nose: Symptoms may include discharge, colds, epistaxis, or sinus congestion.
   2. Throat: Symptoms may include sore throat, hoarseness, or difficulty swallowing.
   3. Lungs: Symptoms may include:
      a. Cough: note characteristics such as duration, frequency, type, color, and amount of sputum, when cough occurs, and what client has done for cough
      b. Dyspnea: note onset, duration, severity, when it occurs, and presence of cyanosis
      c. Wheezing: note when it occurs and what causes it
      d. Chest pain
      e. Hemoptysis
B. Lifestyle
   1. Smoking: note amount per day and duration
   2. Occupation: work conditions that could cause respiratory irritation
   3. Nutrition/diet
   4. Past medical history: immunizations against influenza, tuberculosis; results of tuberculin testing; allergies; history of frequent respiratory infections

PHYSICAL EXAMINATION

A. Inspect chest for evidence of kyphosis, scoliosis, barrel chest
B. Observe for cyanosis
C. Observe tracheal position for deviation and movement of chest for symmetry
D. Percuss lung fields (should find resonance over normal lung tissue)
E. Auscultate for normal (vesicular, bronchial, bronchovesicular) and adventitious (rales or crackles, rhonchi, pleural friction rub) breath sounds (Figure 8.2)

DIAGNOSTIC STUDIES

A. Chest X-ray: no client preparation needed
B. Bronchoscopy/Bronchography :
   1. Bronchoscopy is the direct inspection and observation of the larynx, trachea, and bronchi through a flexible or rigid bronchoscope. During bronchography, a radiopaque medium is instilled directly

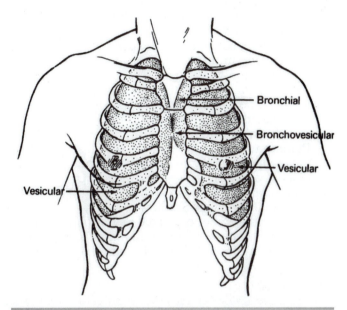

Figure 8.2 Locations for Hearing Normal Breath Sounds

into the trachea and bronchi and the entire bronchial tree or selected areas may be visualized.
   2. Purposes of bronchoscopy:
      a. Collect secretions for analysis and specimens for biopsy
      b. Remove foreign objects and excise lesions
      c. Instillation of dye and visualization of bronchial tree (bronchogram)
   3. Nursing Care
      a. Before the procedure:
         (1) Obtain informed consent and permit
         (2) Check for allergies to contrast medium (iodine) or anesthesia if indicated
         (3) Administer atropine and Valium as ordered
         (4) Maintain client as nothing by mouth (NPO) for 6 hours
         (5) Remove dentures, prostheses, contact lenses
      b. After procedure:
         (1) Check for return of cough and gag reflex before giving fluids by mouth (local anesthetic used during procedure has deadened the gag reflex)
         (2) Cough and deep-breathe client
         (3) Monitor temperature (low-grade fever common)

C. Lung Scan
   1. Radioisotope is injected, after which scans are made with a scintillation camera.
   2. Measures blood perfusion through the lungs
D. Sputum examination:
   1. Sputum examined to identify prominent organisms
   2. Collect early-morning specimen after rinsing mouth with water
E. Biopsy of lung
   1. Removal of lung tissue for examination
   2. Can be performed during bronchoscopy via a needle inserted into the lung or during surgery
F. Pulmonary function studies—Tests used to evaluate clients in the diagnosis of pulmonary disease and assessment of progress of pulmonary disease
G. Arterial Blood Gas Studies
   1. Measurement of partial pressure of oxygen and carbon dioxide in blood as well as the pH of blood and bicarbonate levels

   2. Procedure:
      a. Arterial blood taken from indwelling arterial catheter or femoral puncture
      b. Pressure to arterial puncture site for five minutes after sample drawn to prevent bleeding
      c. Put specimen on ice and transport immediately to lab
H. Thoracentesis
   1. Surgical puncture and drainage of the thoracic cavity
   2. Position client upright, leaning on overbed table or straddling chair
   3. Following procedure:
      a. Cover site with sterile, air-occlusive dressing
      b. Chest X-ray done to detect possible pneumothorax
      c. Position client on unaffected side to allow insertion site to seal itself
      d. Observe client for excessive coughing, blood-tinged sputum, or tightness of the chest

Therapies and Procedures Related to the Respiratory System

OXYGEN THERAPY

A. Indications
   1. Arterial hypoxemia caused by conditions such as apnea, cardiovascular collapse, or carbon monoxide poisoning
   2. Chronic Obstructive Pulmonary Disease (COPD)
   3. Adult Respiratory Distress Syndrome (ARDS)
   4. Cardiac conditions such as congestive heart failure and myocardial infarction
   5. Acute pulmonary diseases such as pulmonary embolism and pneumonia
B. Delivery of oxygen:
   1. Low concentrations (1–2 liters/min. via nasal cannula) indicated when client has oxygen for a long time
   2. Moderate concentrations (3–5 liters/min. via nasal cannula) indicated when client has impaired circulation of oxygen, such as congestive heart failure and pulmonary embolism
   3. High concentrations (12 liters/min. via tight face mask or endotracheal tube) indicated when client needs high levels of oxygen for a short period of time

   4. Delivery systems:
      a. Nasal cannula
         (1) Most common
         (2) 2 prongs inserted 1 cm in each nostril
         (3) Flow rates of 1–4 liters/min. 24–40% oxygen
         (4) Remove cannula and clean nares every 8 hours
         (5) Gauze pads behind ears decrease irritation
      b. Standard mask—covers nose and mouth
         (1) Flow rates of 6–12 liters/min 40–65% oxygen
         (2) Remove and clean mask every 2–3 h
         (3) Use cannula during meals
      c. Nonrebreathing mask:
         (1) Standard mask with a reservoir bag designed to deliver 90–100% oxygen; a one-way valve between reservoir bag and mask allows client to inhale only from the reservoir bag and exhale through separate valves on the side of the mask
         (2) Flow rates of 6–15 liters/min 60–90% oxygen
         (3) Bag should not collapse completely with each inspiration

(4) Remove and clean mask every 2–3 h
(5) High-flow system
(6) Client receives entire inspired air from the apparatus
d. Venturi mask:
(1) Allows precise delivery of oxygen concentrations of 24–50%
(2) Cannula during meals
(3) Remove and clean mask every 2–3 h
5. Oxygen above 2 liters should be humidified to prevent drying to the tissues of the respiratory tract.
6. Prevent sparks and fires when oxygen is in use; oxygen supports combustion.
a. Instruct the client and family that no smoking is allowed.
b. Check electrical equipment for frayed cords and so on.

TRACHEOSTOMY

A. An opening into the trachea through the neck with insertion of an indwelling tube to facilitate the passage of air or removal of secretions
B. Nursing Care:
1. Client in semi-Fowler's position if possible to promote lung expansion
2. Suction trachea as needed to clear secretions (see Table 8.1). Amount of secretions determines frequency of suctioning: every hour immediately after insertion; less frequently later
3. Nursing diagnoses (see Table 8.2)
4. Tracheostomy care:
a. Remove old tracheostomy dressing
b. Use sterile, gloved hand to cleanse area around tube
c. For double cannula tube, remove inner cannula and soak in hydrogen peroxide to remove crusted secretions
d. Cleanse stomal area
e. Cleanse and reinsert inner cannula, locking into place
f. Apply dressing and ties

CLOSED CHEST DRAINAGE

A. Purposes:
1. Remove fluid and/or air from the pleural space
2. Re-establish normal negative pressure in the pleural space
3. Promote re-expansion of the lung following thoracic surgery or pneumothorax
4. Prevent reflux of air/fluid into the pleural space from the drainage apparatus
B. Commercial water seal units (Figure 8.3)
1. Most popular is Pleur-evac®
2. Lightweight, disposable
3. May be used with or without suction

Table 8.1 Tracheobronchial Suctioning

Removal of secretions from the tracheobronchial trees using a sterile catheter inserted into the airway to prevent bacterial contamination and obstruction of tube
1. The client should be in the semi or high-Fowler's position.
2. Disconnect the ventilator before suctioning.
3. Use sterile gloves.
4. Hyperventilate the client with 100% oxygen before and after suctioning.
5. Insert the catheter with a gloved hand.
6. Do not apply suction during insertion of the catheter.
7. Place your thumb over the hole in the proximal end of catheter to establish suction.
8. When withdrawing the catheter, rotate it while applying intermittent suction for 10 seconds.
9. Reconnect the ventilator.

Table 8.2 Nursing Diagnoses Related to Tracheostomy Care

• Risk for ineffective airway clearance related to increased secretions secondary to tracheostomy, obstruction of inner cannula, or displacement of tracheostomy tube
• Risk for infection related to excessive pooling of secretions and bypassing upper respiratory defenses
• Impaired verbal communication related to inability to produce speech secondary to tracheostomy
• Risk for ineffective health maintenance related to insufficient knowledge of tracheostomy care, hazards, and signs and symptoms of complications

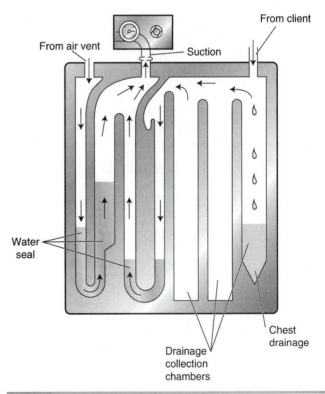

Figure 8.3 Closed Chest Drainage

4. Consist of three chambers:
   a. Air and fluid in first chamber, water seal in second chamber, suction control in third chamber
   b. Observe for intermittent bubbling and fluctuation with respiration in water seal chamber, continuous bubbling in the suction control chamber
C. Nursing care:
   1. Rubber-shod hemostats at bedside
   2. Chest X-ray is done to assess placement after tubes are inserted
   3. Assess respiratory status
   4. Turn, cough, and deep-breathe
   5. Mark the amount of drainage on drainage container at regular intervals
   6. Observe character of drainage
   7. Keep tubing without kinks

8. Keep tubing below chest level
9. Assist with removal of chest tubes by physician:
   a. Equipment needed: suture removal kit, petroleum gauze, sterile gauze, adhesive tape
   b. Place client in semi-Fowler's position
   c. Chest tube removed during expiration or at end of full inspiration (have client take a deep breath and hold it)
   d. Apply air-occlusive dressing (petrolatum gauze)
   e. Chest X-ray
   f. Assess client for complications such as subcutaneous emphysema, respiratory distress

Respiratory Tract Conditions

EPISTAXIS (NOSEBLEED)

A. Causes:
   1. Injury
   2. Diseases such as arteriosclerosis and hypertension, nasal polyps, vitamin deficiencies, and clotting disorders
B. Treatment:
   1. Sit client up with head tilted forward; grasp the soft portion of the nose firmly between thumb and forefinger for 5 to 15 minutes.
   2. Once bleeding stops, instruct the client to rest for an hour and not blow his or her nose vigorously.
   3. If not controlled by pressure, physician may insert packing.

CANCER OF THE LARYNX

A. Seen more frequently in men than women; especially men over 50 who have been smokers
B. Assessment findings:
   1. Hoarseness and persistent sore throat
   2. Cough
   3. Dysphagia, "lump" in neck
   4. Pain
   5. Enlarged cervical lymph nodes
C. Nursing diagnoses (Table 8.3)
D. Medical Management and Nursing Care:
   1. Laryngoscopy and biopsy for diagnosis
   2. Endoscopic removal of early malignancy
   3. Radiation

Table 8.3 Nursing Diagnoses Related to Cancer of the Larynx

- Risk for impaired physical mobility; shoulder, head, related to removal of muscles, nerves, flap graft reconstruction, trauma secondary to surgery
- Risk for disturbed self-concept related to change in appearance
- Risk for ineffective health maintenance related to insufficient knowledge of condition, home care, contraindications (lifting), signs and symptoms of complications (swelling, pain, difficulty swallowing, purulent sputum), follow-up care, identification card/medallion, esophageal speech, and community services
- See also tracheostomy nursing diagnoses.

4. Partial laryngectomy
   a. Temporary tracheostomy
      (1) Intravenous (IV) or Nasogastric (NG) feeding for 48 hours
      (2) Gradual resumption of speaking
5. Total laryngectomy (often with radical neck dissection)
   a. Pre-operative nursing care
      (1) Teach client about laryngectomy tube
      (2) Practice communication to be used after surgery (writing on a note pad, gestures, picture board)
      (3) Encourage client to have visit by laryngectomee
   b. Postoperative nursing care:
      (1) Laryngectomy tube for 10 days
      (2) NG tube for 7–10 days
      (3) Tube feeding or TPN for 7–10 days

(4) Start oral feedings with thick fluids such as Ensure and gelatin because they are easy to swallow

(5) Have client rinse mouth with warm water and brush teeth frequently

  c. Discharge planning:

    (1) Speech rehabilitation: esophageal speech (talk on a burp); speech devices such as artificial larynx

    (2) Stoma care:

      (a) Scarf or protective bib over opening

      (b) No swimming

      (c) Wear shield when taking shower

      (d) Mouth care

CHRONIC OBSTRUCTIVE PULMONARY DISEASE (COPD)

A. A group of conditions associated with chronic obstruction of airflow entering or leaving the lungs

B. Pulmonary Emphysema

  1. An increase in the size of the distal air spaces with loss of alveolar walls and elastic recoil of the lungs (Figure 8.4)

  2. Related to cigarette smoking and deficiency of alpha anti-trypsin in the lungs

  3. Assessment Findings:

    a. Shortness of breath with rapid, shallow respirations

    b. Difficult exhalation

    c. Pursed lip breathing

    d. Wheezing, rales

    e. Barrel chest

    f. Anorexia, weight loss

    g. Hypoxia

    h. Productive cough

    i. Respiratory acidosis

  4. Nursing diagnoses (see Table 8.4)

  5. Nursing interventions:

    a. Position in high-Fowler's or orthopneic position

    b. Chest physiotherapy

      (1) Used to help remove thick secretions

      (2) Done before meals or three hours after meals

      (3) Postural drainage: gravity and positioning used to stimulate movement of secretions (Figure 8.5)

      (4) Percussion (clapping with cupped hands on the chest wall over the segment to be drained) to loosen and remove secretions

      (5) Vibration (flattened hand pressed firmly over the appropriate segment of the chest wall and muscles of the upper arm and shoulder tensed) to loosen and remove secretions

    c. Frequent rest

    d. Nebulization

    e. Respiratory therapy

    f. Oxygen at 1–2 liters per minute; higher levels may stop respiratory drive

    g. Teaching:

      (1) Necessity of stopping smoking

      (2) Management of disease

C. Chronic Bronchitis

  1. Excessive mucous secretions within the airways block air intake and cause recurrent cough (Figure 8.6)

  2. Related to heavy cigarette smoking, pollution, and infection

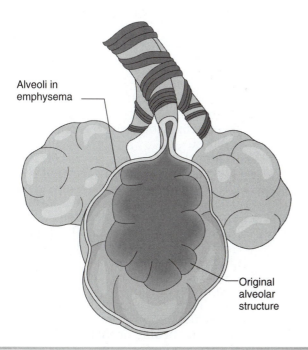

Alveoli in emphysema

Original alveolar structure

Figure 8.4 Alveoli Changes in Emphysema

Table 8.4 Nursing Diagnoses Related to COPD

- Ineffective airway clearance related to excessive and tenacious mucus secretions
- Risk for unbalanced nutrition: less than body requirements related to anorexia secondary to dyspnea, halitosis, and fatigue
- Activity intolerance related to insufficient oxygenation for activities of daily living
- Impaired verbal communication related to dyspnea
- Anxiety related to breathlessness and fear of suffocation
- Powerlessness related to loss of control and the restrictions this condition places on lifestyle
- Disturbed sleep pattern disturbance related to cough, inability to assume recumbent position, and environmental stimuli
- Risk for altered health maintenance related to insufficient knowledge of condition, pharmacologic therapy, nutritional therapy, prevention of infection, rest versus activity, breathing exercises, and home care (equipment)

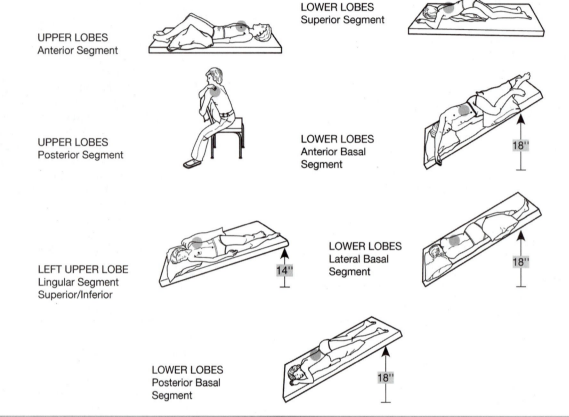

UPPER LOBES
Apical Segment

RIGHT MIDDLE LOBE
Lateral Segment
Medial Segment

14"

UPPER LOBES
Anterior Segment

LOWER LOBES
Superior Segment

UPPER LOBES
Posterior Segment

LOWER LOBES
Anterior Basal
Segment

18"

LEFT UPPER LOBE
Lingular Segment
Superior/Inferior

14"

LOWER LOBES
Lateral Basal
Segment

18"

LOWER LOBES
Posterior Basal
Segment

18"

Figure 8.5 Positions to Facilitate Postural Drainage

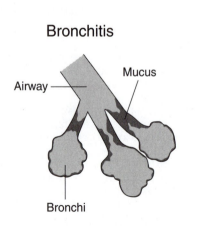

Bronchitis

Airway

Mucus

Bronchi

Figure 8.6 Chronic Bronchitis

3. Assessment findings:
   a. Productive cough with large amount of sputum
   b. Rales, rhonchi
   c. Dyspnea on exertion at first; at rest as disease progresses
   d. Hypoxemia resulting in increased production of red blood cells
   e. Pulmonary hypertension leading to cor pulmonale (right-sided heart failure) and peripheral edema
4. Nursing diagnoses (see Table 8.4)
5. Nursing interventions:
   a. Teach clients about risk of smoking and untreated respiratory infections to prevent chronic bronchitis
   b. Reduce irritants in the client's environment

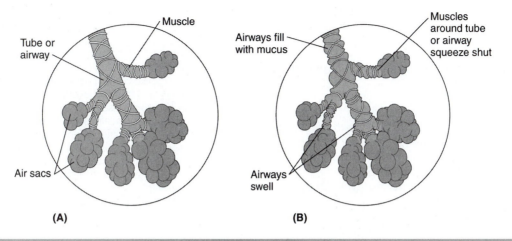

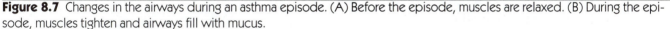

Figure 8.7 Changes in the airways during an asthma episode. (A) Before the episode, muscles are relaxed. (B) During the episode, muscles tighten and airways fill with mucus.

c. Relieve bronchospasm by administering bronchodilators as ordered

d. Increase humidity to loosen secretions

e. Chest physiotherapy to loosen and remove secretions

f. Postural drainage to remove secretions

g. Teach client pursed-lip and diaphragmatic breathing techniques

D. Asthma

1. A condition in which the bronchi constrict and excessive mucus is produced, causing dyspnea (Figure 8.7)

2. Can be an allergic reaction to food, drugs, or inhaled particles or by pathophysiologic conditions within the respiratory tract

3. Assessment findings:
   a. Severe, sudden dyspnea with wheezing and sometimes cyanosis
   b. Use of accessory muscles for respiration
   c. Orthopnea
   d. Diaphoresis
   e. Anxiety, apprehension

4. Nursing diagnoses (see Table 8.4)

5. Nursing interventions:
   a. Bronchodilators such as Epinephrine and Aminophylline as ordered to relieve bronchospasm
   b. Inhaler
   c. Hydration to loosen secretions
   d. Oxygen therapy as ordered
   e. Emotional support
   f. High-Fowler's position to ease breathing
   g. Monitor respiratory status and blood gases

6. Status asthmaticus:
   a. Asthma attack lasting more than 24 hours
   b. Medical emergency

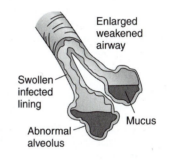

Figure 8.8 In Bronchiectasis, the brochi widen and lose elasticity. Drawing by J. Miller.

c. High-Fowler's position to promote air exchange

d. Monitor vital signs

e. Aminophylline as ordered (may be given IV)

f. Emotional support

E. Bronchiectasis

1. Disorder of medium-sized bronchi characterized by chronic dilation of the bronchi and destruction of the bronchial elastic and muscular structures (Figure 8.8)

2. Usually no single cause; begins in childhood secondary to a lower respiratory tract infection that develops as a complication of measles, whooping cough, or flu

3. Assessment findings:
   a. Severe, often paroxysmal cough with large amounts of thick, purulent sputum
   b. Fetid breath
   c. Hemoptysis

4. Nursing diagnoses (see Table 8.4)

5. Nursing interventions:
   a. Postural drainage to remove secretions
   b. Nebulization to loosen secretions

c. Rest to conserve oxygen
d. Oral hygiene
e. Good nutrition
f. Antimicrobials
g. Care of lung resection if surgery necessary
F. Cor Pulmonale
1. Complication of COPD
2. Right ventricular hypertrophy secondary to disease of the lungs; may or may not be accompanied by heart failure
   a. Assessment findings:
      (1) Dyspnea and cough with cyanosis
      (2) Substernal pain
      (3) Fainting on exertion
      (4) Symptoms of heart failure: orthopnea, peripheral edema, jugular vein distention
   b. Nursing interventions:
      (1) Bed rest to reduce oxygen need
      (2) Monitor oxygen therapy
      (3) Low-sodium diet because client has peripheral edema
      (4) Monitor for side effects of digitalis and diuretics

PNEUMONIA

A. Inflammation of the lung parenchyma caused by infectious agents, aspiration, or inhalation of irritating fumes
B. Persons at risk for pneumonia
1. Elderly
2. Infants
3. Alcoholics
4. Postoperative clients
5. Clients with chronic respiratory disease
6. Clients with viral infections
7. Clients with impaired immune systems
C. Assessment findings:
1. Sudden onset of chills, fever
2. Cough: dry and painful at first; later productive of rusty sputum
3. Dyspnea
4. Pallor, cyanosis
5. Pleuritic pain (worse on inspiration)
6. Tachypnea, tachycardia
D. Nursing diagnoses (see Table 8.5)
E. Nursing interventions:
1. Administer medications as prescribed:
   a. Cough suppressants
   b. Expectorants
   c. Antibiotics such as penicillin, cephalosporins, tetracyclines, or erythromycin
2. Bed rest
3. Oral hygiene
4. Maintain fluid and electrolyte balance
5. Pulmonary care
6. Skin care
7. Nutrition
8. Teaching and emotional support

Table 8.5 Nursing Diagnoses Related to Pneumonia

- Ineffective airway clearance related to pain, increased tracheobronchial secretions, and fatigue
- Activity intolerance related to insufficient oxygenation for activities of daily living
- Risk for impaired oral mucus membrane related to mouth breathing and frequent expectoration and decreased fluid intake secondary to malaise
- Risk for hyperthermia related to infectious process
- Risk for deficient fluid volume related to increased insensible fluid loss secondary to fever and hyperventilation
- Risk for imbalanced nutrition: less than body requirements related to anorexia, dyspnea, and abdominal distention secondary to air swallowing
- Risk for infection transmission related to the communicable nature of the disease
- Impaired comfort related to hyperthermia, malaise, secondary to pulmonary pathology
- Risk for impaired skin integrity related to prescribed bed rest
- Risk for ineffective health maintenance related to insufficient knowledge of fluid requirements, caloric requirements, spread of infection, signs and symptoms of recurrence, prevention of recurrence, and medication regimen

PNEUMOTHORAX

A. Collection of air in the pleural space from trauma, thoracic surgery, positive pressure ventilation, or thoracentesis
B. Assessment findings:
1. Spontaneous pneumothorax:
   a. Sudden, sharp chest pain
   b. Sudden shortness of breath with violent attempts to breathe
   c. Hypotension; weak and rapid pulse
   d. Tachycardia
   e. Hyperresonance and decreased breath sounds over the affected lung
   f. Anxiety, diaphoresis, restlessness
2. Tension pneumothorax (air escapes into the pleural cavity from a bronchus but cannot regain entry into the bronchus)
   a. Subcutaneous emphysema
   b. Cyanosis
   c. Acute chest pain
   d. Tympany on percussion
3. Mediastinal shift: contents of mediastinum shift to unaffected side as a result of air in thoracic cavity
   a. Cyanosis
   b. Tracheal deviation
C. Nursing diagnoses (Table 8.6)
D. Nursing interventions:
1. Remain with client and stay calm
2. Position in high-Fowler's
3. Take vital signs and monitor for shock
4. Notify physician
5. Client will need chest X-ray and blood gases
6. Assist physician with insertion of chest tubes

Table 8.6 Nursing Diagnoses Related to Pneumothorax

- Ineffective breathing pattern related to decreased lung expansion
- Risk for decreased cardiac output
- Acute pain related to irritation of nerve endings within pleural space

Table 8.7 Nursing Diagnoses Related to Thoracic Surgery

- Ineffective airway clearance related to difficulty in coughing secondary to pain
- Activity intolerance related to reduction in exercise capacity secondary to loss of alveolar ventilation
- Acute pain related to incision, drainage tubes, and the surgical procedure
- Impaired physical mobility related to arm/shoulder muscle trauma secondary to surgery, position restrictions, and drainage tubes
- Grieving related to loss of body part and its perceived effects on lifestyle
- Risk for ineffective health maintenance related to insufficient knowledge of condition, pain management, shoulder/arm exercises, incisional care, breathing exercises, splinting, prevention of infection, nutritional needs, rest versus activity, respiratory toilet, and follow-up care

THORACIC SURGERY

A. Performed for lung conditions requiring surgery and for surgery of the esophagus
B. Nursing diagnoses (Table 8.7)
C. Post-op positioning:
   1. Pneumonectomy: position in semi-Fowler's and observe for mediastinal shift
   2. Other procedures: position in semi-Fowler's on unaffected side to allow expansion of the affected lung
D. Medicate for pain before coughing and deep breathing
E. Range of motion exercises to arm on affected side: passive on day of surgery, then active

TUBERCULOSIS

A. Reportable, communicable, infectious, inflammatory disease that occurs most frequently in the lungs; caused by the mycobacterium tuberculosis
B. Risk factors:
   1. Poor, overcrowded living conditions
   2. Poor nutritional status
   3. Prolonged exposure to someone with active tuberculosis
   4. Alcohol abuse
C. Assessment findings:
   1. Productive cough
   2. Rales
   3. Dyspnea
   4. Hemoptysis
   5. Malaise
   6. Low-grade afternoon fever followed by night sweats
   7. Weight loss
   8. Indigestion, anorexia, vomiting
D. Diagnostic Tests
   1. Tuberculin Skin Test (Mantoux, Putrified Protein Derivative [PPD])
      a. 0.1 ml PPD tuberculin injected intradermally into forearm
      b. Read 48–72 hours after injection
      c. 10 mm or more induration indicates positive reaction; redness does not indicate a positive reaction
   2. Chest X-ray
   3. Sputum for acid-fast bacillus
   4. Gastric analysis to identify acid-fast bacilli
E. Medical Interventions
   1. Chemoprophylaxis:
      a. Indicated for persons (who have never received antituberculosis [BCG] vaccine) who have positive skin test and negative chest X-ray
      b. Isoniazid (INH) and pyridoxine for one year
   2. Isoniazid (INH)
      a. Usually administered with at least one other drug
      b. Major side effects include peripheral neuritis and hepatotoxicity
      c. Pyridoxine (Vitamin B$_6$) prevents peripheral neuritis caused by INH
      d. Liver function tests before starting INH therapy and periodically when client is receiving INH
   3. Streptomycin:
      a. Administered intramuscularly one to three times a week
      b. Side effects: eighth cranial (auditory) nerve damage and renal toxicity
   4. Rifampin:
      a. Side effects: red-orange color to urine and feces, hepatotoxicity, nausea and vomiting, thrombocytopenia
      b. Negates action of birth control pills and other drugs
   5. Ethambutol: side effects include optic neuritis, color blindness, and skin rash
   6. Kanamycin: side effects include eighth cranial (auditory) nerve damage and renal toxicity
   7. Viomycin: side effects include eighth cranial nerve damage and renal toxicity
   8. Para Amino Salicylic (PAS) acid
      a. Side effects: gastrointestinal, renal toxicity
      b. Give with food to decrease gastrointestinal side effects
   9. Surgery if disease can not be controlled with medications
F. Nursing diagnoses (Table 8.8)

Table 8.8 Nursing Diagnoses Related to Tuberculosis

- Risk for infection transmission
- Ineffective airway clearance related to thick, viscous, or bloody secretions
- Risk for impaired gas exchange
- Activity intolerance related to imbalance between oxygen supply and demand
- Imbalanced nutrition, less than body requirements, related to inability to ingest adequate nutrients
- Risk for ineffective management of therapeutic regimen

G. Nursing Interventions
   1. Teaching:
      a. Tuberculosis can be controlled, not cured.
      b. Drugs must be taken in combination to avoid bacterial resistance.
      c. Drugs are to be taken once a day on an empty stomach except PAS.
      d. Drugs are taken for 18–24 months even though X-ray and sputum specimens are normal.
      e. Avoid upper respiratory infections.
      f. Yearly checkups
   2. During hospitalization:
      a. Infection control:
         (1) Respiratory isolation until sputum specimens negative for tuberculosis
         (2) Teach good handwashing
      b. Emotional support
      c. Prevent complications

HISTOPLASMOSIS

A. A systemic fungal disease caused by inhalation of dust contaminated by Histoplasma capsulatum, which is transmitted through bird manure
B. Assessment Findings
   1. Symptoms similar to tuberculosis or pneumonia:
      a. Cough
      b. Fever
      c. Joint pain
      d. Malaise
   2. Sometimes asymptomatic
C. Diagnostic Tests
   1. Chest X-ray (often appears similar to tuberculosis)
   2. Histoplasmin skin test (read the same as PPD)
D. Medical Management: Antifungal agent Amphotericin B
   1. Very toxic: toxicity includes anorexia, chills, fever, headache, and renal failure
   2. Acetaminophen, Benadryl, and steroids given with Amphotericin B to prevent reactions

Sample Questions

1. An adult client is to have a sputum for culture. When is the best time for the nurse to collect the specimen?
   1. In the morning right after he awakens
   2. Immediately after breakfast
   3. Two hours after eating
   4. Shortly before he retires for the evening
2. A thoracentesis was performed on an adult client. After the procedure, the client has hemoptysis and a pulse of 80, respirations of 28 and temperature of 99°F. Which of these is of greatest concern to the nurse?
   1. Hemoptysis
   2. Respirations of 28
   3. Pulse of 80
   4. Temperature of 99
3. An adult client is to have postural drainage qid. In developing the care plan, the nurse should schedule this for:
   1. 7 A.M.; 11 A.M.; 4 P.M.; 10 P.M.
   2. 10 A.M.; 2 P.M.; 6 P.M.; 10 P.M.
   3. 6 A.M.; 12 noon; 6 P.M.; 12 mid.
   4. 6 A.M.; 10 A.M.; 2 P.M.; 6 P.M.
4. An adult man has a tracheostomy tube in place. Which of the following actions is most appropriate for the nurse to take when suctioning the tracheostomy?
   1. Use a sterile tube each time and suction for 30 seconds
   2. Use sterile technique and turn the suction off as the catheter is introduced
   3. Use clean technique and suction for 10 seconds
   4. Discard the catheter at the end of every shift
5. During suctioning of a tracheostomy tube, the catheter appears to attach to the tracheal wall and creates a pulling sensation. What is the best action for the nurse to take?
   1. Release the suction by opening the vent
   2. Continue suctioning to remove the obstruction
   3. Increase the pressure
   4. Suction deeper
6. A client comes to the clinic with a bloody nose. Which instruction is most appropriate?
   1. "Sit up with your head tilted forward. Grasp the soft part of your nose firmly between your thumb and forefinger."
   2. "Lay down and tilt your head backward. Grasp the end of your nose between your fingers."
   3. "Sit up and lean backwards. Put pressure on the side of your nose with your hand."
   4. "Lie down with your head lower than your feet. Grasp as much of your nose as possible between your fingers."
7. A client is admitted with a diagnosis of cancer of the larynx. Which statement made by the

client is most likely related to the cause of his illness?

1. "I have always enjoyed hot Mexican-style food."
2. "I have smoked three packs of cigarettes a day for the last 40 years."
3. "I used to work in a factory that burned coal."
4. "I sang in the church choir every Sunday until my voice got hoarse last year."

8. During the preoperative period, which nursing action will be of greatest priority for a person who is to have a laryngectomy?
   1. Establish a means of communication.
   2. Prepare the bowel by administering enemas until clear.
   3. Teach the client to use an artificial larynx.
   4. Demonstrate the technique for suctioning a laryngectomy tube.

9. A 62-year-old man is admitted with emphysema and acute upper-respiratory infection. Oxygen is ordered at 2 liters per minute. The reason for low-flow oxygen is to:
   1. Prevent excessive drying of secretions
   2. Facilitate oxygen diffusion of the blood
   3. Prevent depression of the respiratory drive
   4. Compensate for increased airway resistance

10. An adult is admitted with COPD. The nurse notes that he has neck vein distention and slight peripheral edema. The practical nurse notifies the registered nurse and continues frequent assessments because the nurse knows that these signs signal the onset of:
    1. Pneumothorax
    2. Cor pulmonale
    3. Cardiogenic shock
    4. Left-sided heart failure

11. A 79-year-old is admitted to the hospital with a diagnosis of pneumococcal pneumonia. The client has dyspnea. The client's temperature is 102°F; respirations are 36; and pulse is 92. Bed rest is ordered. This position is ordered for this client primarily to:
    1. Promote thoracic expansion
    2. Prevent the development of atelectasis
    3. Decrease metabolic needs
    4. Prevent infection of others

12. An adult is to have a tracheostomy performed. What is the nursing priority?
    1. Shave the neck
    2. Establish a means of communication
    3. Insert a Foley catheter
    4. Start an IV

13. Which nursing action is essential during tracheal suctioning?
    1. Using a lubricant such as petroleum jelly
    2. Administering 100% oxygen before and after suctioning
    3. Making sure the suction catheter is open or on during insertion

4. Assisting the client to assume a supine position during suctioning

14. An adult has a chest drainage system. Several hours after the chest tube was inserted, the nurse observes that there is no bubbling in the water seal chamber. What is the most likely reason for the absence of bubbling?
    1. His lungs have re-expanded.
    2. There is an obstruction in the tubing coming from the client.
    3. There is a mechanical problem in the pump.
    4. Air is leaking into the drainage apparatus.

15. An adult has a chest drainage system. The client's wife reports to the nurse that her husband is restless. The nurse enters the room just in time to see him pull out his chest tube. The most appropriate initial action for the nurse to take is:
    1. Go get petrolatum gauze and apply over the wound.
    2. Place her hand firmly over the wound.
    3. Apply a sterile 4 × 4 dressing.
    4. Reinsert the chest tube.

16. An adult had a negative PPD test when he was first employed two years ago. A year later, the client had a positive PPD test and a negative chest X-ray. This indicated that at that time the client:
    1. Was less susceptible to a tuberculosis infection than the year before
    2. Had acquired some degree of passive immunity to tuberculosis
    3. Had fought the mycobacterium tuberculosis but had not developed active tuberculosis
    4. Was harboring a mild tuberculosis infection in an organ other than the lung

17. An adult is being treated with Isoniazid (INH) and streptomycin for active tuberculosis. Which of the following symptoms would suggest a toxic effect of Isoniazid?
    1. Paroxysmal tachycardia
    2. Erythema multiforma
    3. Peripheral neuritis
    4. Tinnitus and deafness

18. An adult is being treated with Isoniazid (INH) and streptomycin for active tuberculosis. He is also receiving pyridoxine (vitamin B_6). Why is this medication prescribed for him?
    1. Pyridoxine is bacteriostatic against the mycobacterium tuberculosis.
    2. To enhance his general nutritional status
    3. To prevent side effects of Isoniazid
    4. Pyridoxine acts to increase the effects of streptomycin.

19. The wife of a client with active tuberculosis has a positive skin test for tuberculosis. She is to be started on prophylactic drug therapy. What drug is the drug of choice for prophylaxis of tuberculosis?
    1. Streptomycin
    2. Para-amino-salicylic acid (PAS)

3. Isoniazid (INH)
4. Ethambutol (Myambutol)

20. A farmer who has had a cough for several months has noticed a lack of energy lately. He is being tested for histoplasmosis. Which factor reported by the client would be most related to the diagnosis of histoplasmosis?
1. He drinks raw milk.
2. He cleans chicken houses.
3. He handles fertilizer frequently.
4. He stepped on a rusty nail recently.

21. The nurse is caring for a client who is admitted with histoplasmosis. What drug is most likely to be prescribed for this client?
1. Penicillin
2. Chloromycetin
3. Streptomycin
4. Amphotericin B

22. An adult is to have a thoracentesis performed. What should the nurse do while preparing the client for this procedure?
1. Keep him NPO for 8 hours.
2. Prepare him to go to the operating room.
3. Explain the procedure to him.
4. Administer anticholinergic and analgesic as ordered.

23. The nurse is planning care for a client who has COPD. Which statement is the client most likely to say about activity tolerance?
1. "The most difficult time of the day for me is the first hour after waking up in the morning."
2. "I feel best in the morning after a good night's sleep."
3. "I seem to have more energy after eating a big meal."
4. "I don't know why, but I get my 'second wind' at night and don't want to go to bed."

24. The nurse is caring for a woman who is admitted with pneumonia. On admission, the client is anxious and short of breath but able to respond to questions. One hour later, the client becomes more dyspneic and less responsive, answering only yes and no questions. What is the best action for the nurse to take at this time?
1. Stimulate the client until the client responds.
2. Increase the oxygen from the ordered 6 liters to 10 liters.
3. Assess the client again in 15 minutes.
4. Notify the charge nurse of the change in the client's mental status.

25. A client's PPD test is positive, and a chest X-ray is negative. What is the best interpretation of these data?
1. The client's resistance to tuberculosis is low.
2. The client has been exposed to the organism but has not developed the disease.

3. The client has tuberculosis, but it is not serious.
4. The client has active tuberculosis.

26. An adult with tuberculosis has started taking Rimactane (Rifampin). Which side effect is the client most likely to experience when taking this drug?
1. Reddish-orange color of urine, sputum, and saliva
2. Erythema and urticaria
3. Tinnitus and deafness
4. Peripheral neuritis

27. Which laboratory tests should the client receive before prophylactic drug therapy for tuberculosis is started?
1. Serum creatinine and BUN
2. SGOT (AST) and SGPT
3. CBC and hematocrit
4. WBC and urinalysis

28. A client who had a laryngectomy is nearly ready for discharge. Which instruction is most appropriate for the nurse to give?
1. "Always be sure you have a buddy with you when you go swimming or boating."
2. "You may take a tub bath, but you should not take a shower."
3. "Be sure to have only liquids for another three weeks."
4. "Never cover your stoma with anything."

29. The client asks the nurse why inspiration through the nose is preferable to inspiring through the mouth. What is the best response?
1. It produces greater blood oxygen levels.
2. It is easier to breathe through the nose.
3. The nares humidify, warm, and filter the air.
4. Mouth breathing dilutes the air and reduces the amount of air entering the lungs.

30. While the nurse is suctioning a tracheostomy tube, the client starts to cough. What is the best action for the nurse to take?
1. Suction deeper to pick up secretions.
2. Gently withdraw suction tubing to allow suction or coughing out of mucus.
3. Remove the suction as quickly as possible.
4. Put the suction tube in and out several times to pick up secretions.

Answers and Rationales

1. (1) The sputum has collected during the night. It is most concentrated early in the morning.
2. (1) Hemoptysis is the only abnormal finding. All of the others are within normal range for someone who has undergone an invasive procedure.
3. (1) Postural drainage should be scheduled between meals and close to bedtime.
4. (2) Suctioning should be done under sterile technique for no more than 10 seconds. The

suction should be off as the tube is inserted and applied intermittently as it is withdrawn.

5. (1) Suction should not be applied as the suction tube is inserted, because this will cause the suction tube to appear to attach to the tracheal wall and create a pulling sensation.

6. (1) This position will help to stop bleeding without causing aspiration of any blood dripping down the back of the throat.

7. (2) Cigarette smoking is the greatest risk factor for development of laryngeal cancer.

8. (1) Establishing a means of communication is the highest priority. Teaching the client to use an artificial larynx is a postoperative task. Because the laryngectomy tube will be temporary, the client will not need to learn to suction. That is a nursing function.

9. (3) The stimulus to breathe in a person with COPD is a low O_2 level rather than a CO_2 level, as in normal persons. If high-flow oxygen were given, the O_2 level would increase and the respiratory drive would cease.

10. (2) Distended neck veins and peripheral edema are signs of right-sided heart failure or cor pulmonale—heart failure due to pulmonary causes.

11. (3) Bed rest will reduce metabolic needs in this client who has pneumonia and is having difficulty meeting oxygenation needs. Semi-Fowler's position, not bed rest, will promote thoracic expansion. Isolation prevents infection of others. Deep breathing will help to prevent the development of atelectasis.

12. (2) The nursing priority is to establish a means of communication, because she will not be able to speak after the tracheostomy is performed.

13. (2) 100% oxygen is given before and after suctioning to help prevent hypoxia. Petroleum-based lubricants are not water-soluble and should never be used near an airway. Saline is used as a lubricant. The suction catheter is off during insertion to avoid traumatizing the tissues. She should be in semi-Fowler's position during suctioning. Supine predisposes to aspiration.

14. (2) Cessation of bubbling in the water seal bottle means either an obstruction in the tubing or re-expansion of the lung. This is the night of insertion of the tube. It takes at least 24 hours and often two to three days for the lung to re-expand.

15. (2) The nurse's primary goal has to be to stop air from entering the thoracic cavity and causing the lung to collapse again. Placing a hand firmly over the wound will accomplish this. Number 1 is wrong, because the nurse should not leave the client. Petrolatum gauze would be ideal but the nurse should not leave the client. Number 3 is wrong because a sterile 4 × 4 dressing allows air to enter the thoracic cavity. The nurse should not reinsert the chest tube.

16. (3) A positive PPD test indicates that the client has come in contact with the organism and fought it. A negative chest X-ray says that the client won the fight and does not at that time have active tuberculosis.

17. (3) Peripheral neuritis is a toxic effect of INH. Tinnitus and deafness are side effects of streptomycin.

18. (3) Pyridoxine (Vitamin B_6) prevents the development of peripheral neuritis toxicity of INH.

19. (3) INH is the drug of choice for chemoprophylaxis. All of the other drugs listed can be used in the treatment of tuberculosis.

20. (2) Histoplasmosis is a fungus that grows in chicken and pigeon manure. Drinking raw milk might cause "milk fever." Handling fertilizer could cause "white lung," a COPD illness. Stepping on a nail might cause tetanus.

21. (4) Amphotericin B is the drug of choice to treat histoplasmosis.

22. (3) The nurse should explain the procedure to the client and obtain a permit if one has not already been signed. Thoracentesis is usually done at the bedside. NPO is not necessary. Anticholinergics and analgesics are not ordered.

23. (1) Morning is a difficult time for persons with COPD because secretions have accumulated during the night. They have to do a great deal of hacking and coughing to clear their air passages in the morning. The client with COPD is apt to be short of breath after a big meal because he is an abdominal breather. Most clients with COPD do not get a "second wind" at night. They need a lot of rest.

24. (4) The change in the client's status is significant and indicates hypoxia. The charge nurse or physician must be notified quickly. Stimulating a severely hypoxic client is not appropriate. Increasing the oxygen from 6 liters to 10 liters is not likely to change the client's status. The LPN should notify the charge nurse now, not in 15 minutes.

25. (2) A positive PPD test indicates antibodies against tuberculosis. A positive PPD test and a negative X-ray indicate that the client has been exposed to tuberculosis but has not developed the disease. These findings do not give information regarding the client's resistance. The negative x-ray indicates that the client does not have active tuberculosis.

26. (1) Rimactane (Rifampin) causes body secretions to turn reddish-orange. Erythema and urticaria are not likely to be seen. Tinnitus and deafness is a side effect of streptomycin. Peripheral neuritis is a side effect of isoniazid (INH).

27. (2) SGOT (AST) and SGPT are liver function tests. INH can cause liver toxicity. Serum creatinine and BUN are renal function tests and would test for toxicity to streptomycin or kanamycin. CBC and hematocrit might be indicated if bleeding or bone marrow depression were major expected toxicities. WBC and urinalysis might be indicted for urinary tract infections.

28. (2) Showering is not usually allowed, because water will go into the stoma. The client will never be able to swim. The client does not need a liquid diet for three weeks. The stoma should be covered with a special absorbent scarf to filter and warm the air.

29. (3) The purpose of the nares is to humidify, warm, and filter the air before it enters the lungs. Breathing through the nose does not produce greater blood oxygen levels. It is not easier to breathe through the nose. Mouth breathing does not dilute the air.

30. (2) Allow the client to cough. He will frequently cough out the mucus. If he does not, then the nurse can resuction to pick up secretions. The client's cough is more powerful than the suction catheter.

Chapter 9

The Neurosensory System

ANATOMY AND PHYSIOLOGY

The neurological system receives stimuli from the body and the environment via the sensory system and determines the body's response to stimuli via the motor system. It also maintains human functions of memory and judgment and controls and coordinates movement of all body parts.

STRUCTURES

Neuron (basic element of the nervous system):

A. Dendrites transmit impulses to the cell body.
B. Axons transmit impulses away from the cell body.
C. The myelin sheath is the outer covering for most axons and insulates the nerve fiber

Central Nervous System

A. Brain (Figure 9.1)
   1. Cerebrum:
      a. Divided into right and left hemispheres which make up 80% of total brain weight
      b. Gray matter (cortex) made up of nerve cell bodies
      c. White matter made up of cell processes from cell bodies
   2. External surface of the brain made up of convolutions (gyri) and indentations (fissures or sulci)
   3. The meninges are three layers of fibrous, connective tissues which cover the cerebral hemispheres and spinal cord and provide support and protection, nourishment, and blood supply to underlying structures.
      a. Dura mater is the thick, tough, outermost membrane which provides the most support.
      b. The arachnoid membrane is a delicate layer which helps cushion and protect the brain.
         (1) Separated from the dura mater by the subdural space
         (2) The arachnoid sends tiny finger-like projections (arachnoid villa) through the inner layer of the dura mater to aid in reabsorption of cerebrospinal fluid (CSF) into the blood stream.
         (3) Immediately below the arachnoid is the subarachnoid space in which CSF circulates.
         (4) Large blood vessels lie in the subarachnoid space and provide a major part of the blood supply to the brain.

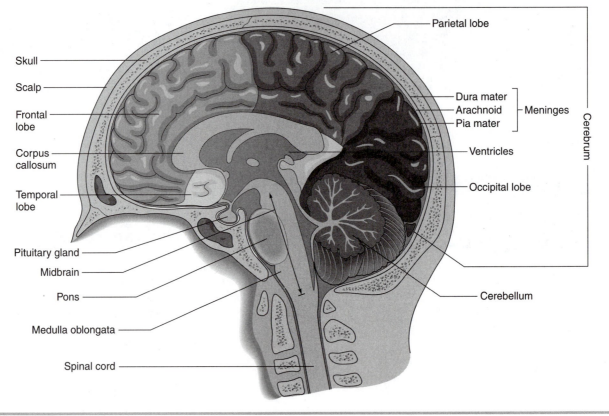

Figure 9.1 Cross section of the brain

c. Pia mater is a thin, delicate membrane which closely adheres to the surfaces of the brain and spinal cord.

4. Lobes:

a. Frontal lobes contain the motor cortex, which controls motor function as well as the motor aspects of speech and the written speech center.

b. Parietal lobes are the principle sensory areas for appreciation and discrimination of sensory impulses (pain, temperature, touch, and so on).

c. Temporal lobes contain the auditory center, auditory speech center, and centers for long and short-term memory.

d. Occipital lobes contain the visual center and the visual speech center.

5. Basal ganglia are areas of gray matter located at the base of each hemisphere that regulate and integrate motor activity in the cerebral cortex.

B. The diencephalon lies deep within the brain and consists of the thalamus and hypothalamus.

1. The thalamus is located on either side of the third ventricle and acts as a relay station for sensory impulses.

2. The hypothalamus makes up the anterior wall of the third ventricle.

a. Controls water balance (manufactures antidiuretic hormone [ADH]), blood pressure, sleep, appetite, and body temperature

b. Control center for pituitary function

c. Affects both divisions of the autonomic nervous system

C. Midbrain (mesencephalon) is a small area between the diencephalon and the pons in which the third and fourth cranial nerves originate. (Figure 9.2)

D. Brain stem:

1. The pons is located between the midbrain and the medulla oblongata and contains ascending sensory tracts and descending motor tracts. The reticular formation (which helps keep us awake) is located deep within the pons and midbrain.

2. The medulla oblongata connects the brain and spinal cord:

a. Motor tracts running from the cortex to the spinal cord cross over at the lower end of the medulla (spinal decussation). This is the reason why the right side of the brain controls the left side of the body and vice-versa.

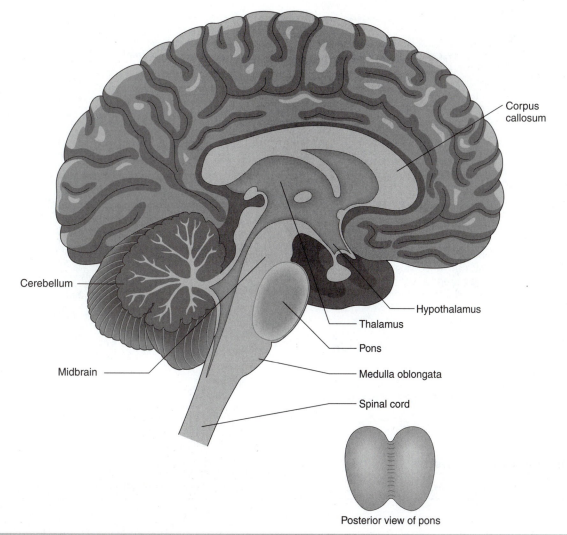

Figure 9.2 Inner structures of the brain

b. Contains vital centers that control respiration, heart rate, vomiting, and hiccoughing

E. The cerebellum is located posteriorly to the pons that interconnects the cerebellum, thalamus, and cerebral cortex to control and coordinate motor movement.

F. Ventricles:
   1. Four irregularly shaped, interrelated spaces within the brain
   2. CSF principally formed by the choroid plexus in the lateral ventricles

G. Spinal cord (Figure 9.3):
   1. Lies within the vertebral canal and extends to the level of the first or second lumbar vertebra
   2. Afferent pathways carry motor impulses via afferent nerves through ascending tracts to the brain.
   3. Efferent pathways carry motor impulses via efferent nerves from the brain through descending tracts to nerves supplying muscles, glands, and other body parts.

   4. The reflex pathway forms a reflex arc within the spinal cord.
      a. A reflex is an involuntary response to a stimulus.
      b. Responses to spinal reflexes are not relayed to and from the brain. Sensory neurons relay impulses from sensory receptors to central neurons located entirely within the cord. Central neurons then send impulses to motor neurons leading to glands and muscles.

Peripheral Nervous System

A. The peripheral nervous system includes cranial and spinal nerves.
   1. Afferent nerves carry impulses toward the central nervous system.
   2. Efferent nerves carry impulses away from the central nervous system.
   3. Mixed contain both types of fibers.

B. Twelve pairs of cranial nerves each having a specific function (Table 9.1)

Table 9.1 Cranial Nerves

Number and Nerve Function

I.	Olfactory	Sensory: carries impulses for smell
II.	Optic	Sensory: carries impulses for vision
III.	Oculomotor	Motor: aids movement of most eye muscles, including pupil constriction
IV.	Trochlear	Motor: innervates eye muscle controlling downward and inward eye movement
V.	Trigeminal	Mixed: sensation to head and face and movement to the muscles of chewing
VI.	Abducens	Motor: muscle for lateral deviation of eye
VII.	Facial	Mixed: movement to most facial muscles and sensation to the tongue
VIII.	Acoustic	Sensory: hearing and balance
IX.	Glossopharyngeal	Mixed: swallowing and sensation to tongue and throat
X.	Vagus	Mixed: impulses for sensation to lower pharynx and larynx; muscles for movement of soft palate, pharynx, and larynx
XI.	Spinal accessory	Motor: provides movement to neck muscles
XII.	Hypoglossal	Motor: movement of tongue

Remember: **O**n **O**ld **O**lympus's **T**owering **T**ops **A** **F**inn **A**nd **G**erman **V**iewed **S**ome **H**ops

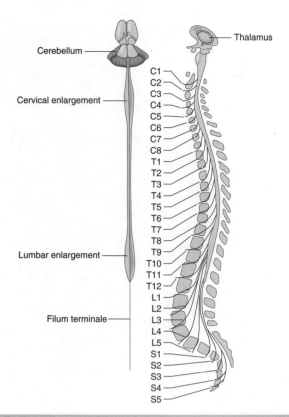

Figure 9.3 Spinal cord and nerves

Table 9.2 Autonomic Nervous System

	Sympathetic (Adrenergic)	Parasympathetic (Cholinergic)
Neurotransmitter	Adrenalin	Acetylcholine
Effects on:		
Eye	Dilates pupil	Constricts pupil
Lacrimal gland	None	Stimulates secretion
Salivary	Thick, scanty, viscous secretions, and dry mouth	Copious, thin, watery secretions
Heart	Increases rate and force of contraction	Decreases rate
Blood vessels	Constricts smooth muscles of skin, abdominal blood vessels, and cutaneous blood vessels	No effect
	Dilates smooth muscle of bronchioles, blood vessels of heart, and skeletal muscles	
Lungs	Dilates bronchi	Constricts bronchi
GI tract	Decreases motility	Increases motility
	Constricts sphincters	Relaxes sphincters
	Inhibits secretions	Stimulates secretion
	Inhibits gallbladder and ducts	Stimulates gallbladder and ducts
	Inhibits glycogenolysis in liver	
Adrenal gland	Stimulates secretion of epinephrine and norepinephrine	No effects
Urinary tract	Relaxes detrusor muscle	Contracts detrusor muscle
	Contracts trigone sphincter (prevents voiding)	Relaxes trigone sphincter (allows voiding)

C. Thirty-one pairs of spinal nerves (Figure 9.3)
   1. 8 cervical
   2. 12 thoracic
   3. 5 lumbar
   4. 5 sacral
   5. 1 coccygeal spinal

Autonomic Nervous System (ANS)

The autonomic nervous system allows the body to maintain homeostasis despite changing environmental conditions and regulates smooth muscles, cardiac muscles, and glands. It is divided into parts that act opposite to each other (Table 9.2).

A. Sympathetic nervous system:
1. Originates from the thoracic and lumbar areas of the spinal cord
2. Speeds up body responses when threatened by real or imagined stressors (fight or flight response)
B. Parasympathetic nervous system:
1. Originates from the cranial and sacral areas of the spinal cord
2. Slows down body processes and promotes protection and restoration of body resources

EYES

A. External Structures of the Eye (Figure 9.4)
1. Eyelids (palpebrae) and eyelashes: protect the eye from foreign particles
2. Conjunctiva:
   a. Palpebral conjunctiva lines inner surface of eyelids; pink in color
   b. Bulbar conjunctiva covers anterior sclera; white with small blood vessels
3. Lacrimal (tear) apparatus:
   a. The lacrimal glands secrete tears that maintain moisture on the anterior surface of the eyeball.
   b. The lacrimal ducts, located in the inner corner of each eye, collect tears and drain them into the nose.
B. Internal Structures of the Eye (Figure 9.5)
1. The eyeball has three layers:
   a. Outer layer:
      (1) Sclera: outer layer made of tough, white connective tissue ("white of the eye"); located anteriorly and posteriorly

(2) Cornea: transparent tissue through which light enters the eye; located anteriorly
b. Middle layer:
   (1) Choroid: contains many blood vessels that provide blood supply for the entire eye
   (2) Ciliary body: anterior to choroid; secretes aqueous humor; muscles change the shape of the lens
   (3) Iris: pigmented membrane behind cornea; gives color to the eye. The pupil is a circular opening in the

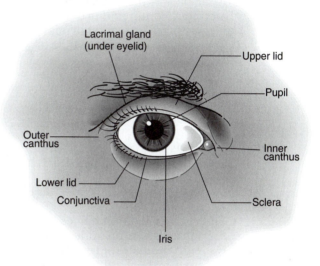

Figure 9.4 Major structures of the eye

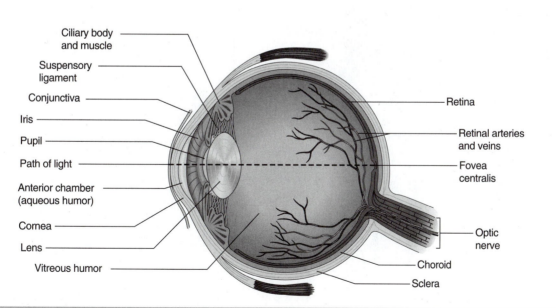
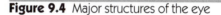

Figure 9.5 Internal structures of the eye

middle of the iris that constricts or dilates to regulate the amount of light entering the eye.
  c. Inner layer: retina
    (1) Light-sensitive layer composed of rods (sensitive to light and aid in peripheral vision) and cones (fine discrimination and color vision)
    (2) Optic disk: area in retina for entrance of optic nerve; has no photoreceptors
  2. Lens: transparent body that focuses image on retina
  3. Fluids of the eye:
    a. Aqueous humor: clear, watery fluid in anterior and posterior chambers in the anterior part of the eye; serves as a refracting medium and provides nutrients to the lens and cornea; contributes to the maintenance of intraocular pressure
    b. Vitreous humor: clear, gelatinous matter that fills the posterior cavity of the eye; maintains the transparency and form of the eye
  4. Visual pathways:
    a. Retina (rods and cones) translates light waves into neural impulses that travel over the optic nerves
    b. Optic nerves for each eye meet at the optic chiasm.
    (1) Fibers from median halves of the retinas cross at the optic chiasm and travel to opposite side of the brain. (Fibers for the right visual field go to the left side of the brain.)

    (2) Fibers from the lateral halves of retinas remain uncrossed.
  c. Optic nerves continue from the optic chiasm as optic tracts and travel to the occipital lobe of the cerebrum, where visual impulses are perceived and interpreted.

EARS: SENSORY ORGANS THAT ENABLE HEARING AND HELP TO MAINTAIN BALANCE (Figure 9.6)

A. External ear:
  1. Auricle (pinna): outer ear composed of cartilage and covered by skin; collects sound waves
  2. External auditory canal: lined with skin; glands secrete cerumen (wax), providing protection; transmits sound waves to tympanic membrane
  3. Tympanic membrane (eardrum): at end of external canal; vibrates in response to sound waves and transmits vibrations to middle ear
B. Middle ear:
  1. Ossicles:
    a. Three small bones; malleus (hammer) attached to tympanic membrane, incus (anvil), and stapes (stirrup)
    b. Ossicles set in motion by sound waves from tympanic membrane
    c. Sound waves conducted by vibration to the footplate of the stapes in the oval

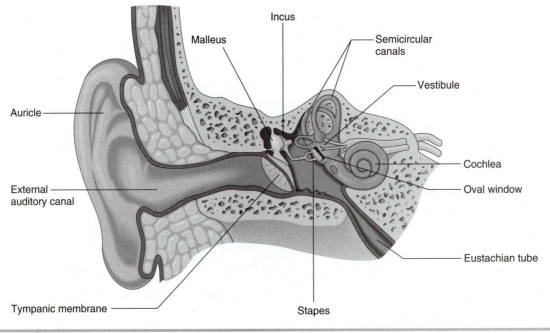

Figure 9.6 Structures of the ear

window (opening between the middle ear and the inner ear)
2. Eustachian tube: connects nasopharynx and middle ear; brings air into middle ear, equalizing pressure on both sides of eardrum.
C. Inner ear
  1. Cochlea:
    a. Contains the organ of Corti, the receptor end organ for hearing

b. Transmits sound waves from the oval window and initiates nerve impulses carried by cranial nerve VIII to the brain
2. Vestibular apparatus:
  a. Organ of balance
  b. Composed of three semicircular canals and the utricle

Diagnostic Procedures

BRAIN SCAN

A. Done to detect tumors, cerebrovascular accidents, abscesses, and other brain lesions
B. Radioisotope injected intravenously and is carried to the brain where it localizes around any lesion that alters the blood-brain barrier

LUMBAR PUNCTURE

A. Hollow needle inserted into the subarachnoid space between the third and fourth lumbar vertebrae
B. Done to obtain a specimen of cerebrospinal fluid or to measure CSF pressure
C. Have client empty bowel and bladder before procedure
D. Position client with back arched during the procedure
E. After procedure, position patient horizontal for 8–12 hours

CEREBRAL ANGIOGRAPHY

A. Dye injected into cerebral circulation via carotid, vertebral, femoral, or brachial artery followed by X-rays to detect tumors, aneurysms, occlusions, hematomas, or abscesses
B. Nursing care before procedure:
  1. Nothing by mouth (NPO) after midnight or a clear liquid breakfast.
  2. Take baseline vital signs and neuro check.
  3. Administer sedation if ordered.
  4. Ask if the client is allergic to shellfish or iodine.
  5. Explain that iodine dye injection may cause a warm, flushed feeling and a salty taste in the mouth.

C. Nursing care after procedure:
  1. Pressure dressing over the site if the femoral or brachial artery is used; ice to decrease swelling
  2. Check for hematoma or bleeding at the puncture site.
  3. Assess for adequacy of circulation; check pulses, color, and temperature of extremity distal to the site used.
  4. Monitor vital signs and perform neuro checks frequently; report any changes immediately.
  5. Keep extremity extended and avoid flexion.

COMPUTERIZED AXIAL TOMOGRAPHY (CAT OR CT SCAN)

A. Noninvasive X-ray technique that produces images of single-tissue planes, and the computer uses the information to construct a picture of the organ scanned
B. Check for allergies to iodine because iodine dye may be used during the procedure.

MAGNETIC RESONANCE IMAGING (MRI)

A. Computer-drawn, detailed pictures of the structures of the body through the use of large magnet, radio waves
B. Nursing care:
  1. Determine that the client has no metal in his or her body, such as pacemaker, internal surgical clips, shrapnel, and so on, because a magnetic force may dislodge or disrupt functioning.
  2. Instruct the client to remove all jewelry and objects containing metal.
  3. Teach the client of the need to remain still while completely enclosed in a narrow

cylinder during the procedure. Report if the client indicates a presence of claustrophobia.

4. Warn the client that thumping and humming sounds will be heard during the test.
5. Have the client void before the test.
6. Sedate the client if ordered.

ELECTROENCEPHALOGRAPHY (EEG)

A. Graphic recording of electrical activity of the brain; several small electrodes placed on the scalp
B. Used to detect the focus of seizure activity and to determine brain death
C. Pretest nursing care: withhold sedatives, tranquilizers, and stimulants for 2–3 days
D. Posttest nursing care: remove electrode paste with acetone and shampoo hair

Nervous System Disorders

INCREASED INTRACRANIAL PRESSURE

A. Increased intracranial pressure occurs when there is an increase in the intracranial bulk due to an increase in any of the major intracranial components: brain tissue, cerebrospinal fluid (CSF), or blood.
B. Causes:
   1. Head injury
   2. Cerebrovascular accident
   3. Brain tumor
C. Assessment findings:
   1. Decrease in level of consciousness (LOC) due to lethargy, drowsiness, or stupor
   2. Headache
   3. Projectile vomiting
   4. Vital sign changes:
      a. Widening pulse pressure (systolic rises while diastolic stays the same)
      b. Pulse slows
      c. Respirations slow
   5. Pupil changes:
      a. Ipsilateral pupil dilation (same side)
      b. Pupils no longer react to light
      c. Fixed, dilated pupils
   6. Contralateral (opposite side) loss of motor function
   7. Papilledema
   8. Glasgow coma scale (Table 9.3):
      a. Standardized system for assessing the degree of neurologic impairment in critically ill clients. Does not replace a complete neurologic check.
      b. Score of 15 indicates that the client is awake and oriented; a score of 7 or below is considered coma; 3 is a deep coma.
   9. Motor function; assess for movement or lack of movement (paralysis) and motor strength
D. Related nursing diagnoses (Table 9.4)

Table 9.3 Glasgow Coma Scale

Subscale	Response	Score
Best eye opening (E)	Spontaneous	4
	To voice	3
	To pain	2
	None	1
Best verbal response (V)	Oriented	5
	Confused conversation	4
	Inappropriate words	3
	Incomprehensible sounds	2
	None	1
Best motor response upper limb (M)	Obeys commands	6
	Localizes to pain	5
	Flexor withdrawal (decorticate posturing)	4
	Abnormal flexion (decorticate posturing)	3
	Extension	2
	Flaccid	1

Table 9.4 Nursing Diagnoses Related to Increased Intracranial Pressure

- Ineffective cerebral tissue perfusion related to an increase in brain tissue, intracranial blood volume, and CSF volume
- Ineffective breathing pattern related to increased ICP and alteration in LOC
- Impaired gas exchange related to increased ICP, and alteration in LOC
- Impaired physical mobility related to alteration in LOC
- Impaired skin integrity related to immobility, and hypothermia therapy
- Risk for injury related to seizure activity, drug therapy (steroids), and decreased level of responsiveness
- Fluid volume excess related to steroid therapy, and syndrome of inappropriate antidiuretic hormone
- Decreased sensory perception (visual, auditory, kinesthetic, and tactile) related to sensory overload/deprivation, sensory deficits, and altered LOC

E. Interventions:
   1. Maintain patent airway and adequate ventilation.
      a. Vital signs and neuro checks
      b. Elevate head of bed 30–45 degrees to reduce cerebral edema
      c. Prevent increase in intracranial pressure (ICP):
         (1) Administer stool softeners as ordered to prevent straining.
         (2) Maintain a calm environment and reduce environmental stimuli.
         (3) Avoid restraints unless absolutely necessary.
         (4) Prevent vomiting and coughing.
      e. Monitor intake and output; limit fluids to 1200–1500 cc/day
      f. Acetaminophen may be ordered; opiates and sedatives are contraindicated because they decrease respirations and alter LOC and pupils; aspirin may cause bleeding.
      g. Osmotic diuretics (Mannitol) and loop diuretics (Lasix) to reduce cerebral edema; hourly outputs
      h. Corticosteroids (Decadron) to reduce cerebral edema
      i. Anticonvulsant (Dilantin) to prevent seizures

HEAD INJURIES

A. Usually caused by trauma such as car accidents, falls, or assaults
B. Types:
   1. Concussion: severe blow to the head that jostles the brain and causes temporary or prolonged alteration in consciousness
   2. Hemorrhage:
      a. Epidural hematoma: accumulation of blood between dura and skull; often due to torn artery; blood accumulates quickly
      b. Subdural hematoma: accumulation of blood between dura and arachnoid; venous bleeding that forms slowly; may be acute or chronic
   3. Fractures
C. Assessment findings:
   1. Concussion: headache, transient loss of consciousness, amnesia, and/or nausea
   2. Hemorrhage:
      a. Epidural hematoma: brief loss of consciousness followed by lucid interval; progressing to severe headache, vomiting, loss of consciousness, seizures, and ipsilateral pupil dilation
      b. Subdural hematoma: headache, changes in LOC, focal neurological deficits, personality changes, and

ipsilateral pupil dilation; chronic may take 4–8 weeks to develop
   3. Fractures: headache, pain over fracture site; leakage of CSF from nose or ears with compound fracture
D. Diagnostic tests:
   1. Skull X-ray to show fracture or intracranial shift
   2. CT scan to show hemorrhage
E. Nursing diagnoses (same as increased intracranial pressure, Table 9.4)
F. Interventions:
   1. Same as care of client with increased intracranial pressure
   2. Observe for cerebrospinal fluid (CSF)
      a. Clear discharge from head wound, ears, or nose
      b. Dextrose positive with Testape or Dextrostix test
      c. Do not clean the ears or nose of a client with a head injury or use nasal suction unless ordered by a physician.
      d. If a CSF leak is present, elevate the head of the bed, instruct the client not to blow his or her nose, and notify physician immediately.
   3. Observe for seizures.
   4. Observe for increased urine output and increased temperature (indicates hypothalamus damage); report immediately.

HYPERTHERMIA

A. Assessment findings:
   1. Body temperature above 105°F
   2. Caused by dysfunction of hypothalamus from cerebral edema, head injury, hemorrhage, CVA, brain tumor, or intracranial seizure
   3. Hyperthermia increases cerebral metabolism, predisposing to seizures and neurologic damage if prolonged.
   4. Interventions (see p. 22)

SEIZURES

A. Manifestation of abnormal and excessive discharge of neurons in the brain
B. Types:
   1. Grand mal; major motor
      a. Tonic phase: limbs contract or stiffen, pupils dilate and eyes roll up and to one side, glottis closes causing noise on exhalation, incontinence, 20–40 seconds
      b. Clonic phase: repetitive movements, increased mucous production
      c. Post ictal (after seizure) period: confusion, drowsiness; person does not remember the seizure

2. Petit mal: Absence seizures; brief loss of consciousness with minor movements
3. Febrile seizure: 5% of children under five get a seizure when temperature is rising
4. Status epilepticus: any type of seizure occurring in rapid succession

C. Assessment findings:
1. Impaired consciousness
2. Disturbances of mental function
3. Excess or loss of muscle tone or movement
4. Disorders of sensation or special senses
5. Disturbances of the autonomic functions of the body
6. Incontinence during grand mal seizure

D. Nursing diagnoses (Table 9.5)
E. Interventions:
1. Administer anticonvulsants as ordered (Table 9.6)
2. Protect from injury
   a. Support head
   b. Do not restrain
   c. Do not use tongue blades
3. Keep airway open:
   a. Side lying position
   b. Suction excess mucous
4. Observe and record seizure:
   a. Events preceding seizure
   b. Order of movements, length of time, and post-ictal state

Table 9.5 Nursing Diagnoses Related to Seizures

- Risk for injury related to uncontrolled tonic/clonic movements during seizure episode
- Risk for ineffective airway clearance related to relaxation of tongue and gag reflexes secondary to disruption in muscle innervation
- Risk for social isolation related to fear of embarrassment secondary to having a seizure in public
- Risk for impaired oral mucus membrane related to effects of drug therapy on oral tissue
- Fear related to unpredictable nature of seizures and embarrassment

CEREBROVASCULAR ACCIDENT

A. Sudden loss of brain function resulting from a disruption of blood supply to part of the brain causing temporary or permanent dysfunction; may be caused by thrombosis, embolism, or hemorrhage
B. Assessment findings:
1. Headache
2. Vomiting
3. Seizures
4. Confusion, decreased LOC
5. Nucchal rigidity (stiff neck)
6. Fever
7. Hypertension, slow bounding pulse, Cheyne Stokes respirations
8. Focal signs related to site of injury:
   a. Hemiparesis and hemiplegia (right-side brain damage causes left-side paralysis)
   b. Aphasia (may be receptive: can't understand speech; expressive: unable to speak)
   c. Homonymous hemianopsia (unable to see one side, right or left of the visual field with both eyes open)
9. CT and brain scan show a lesion.
10. Cerebral arteriography shows an occlusion or malformation of vessels.
C. Nursing diagnoses (Table 9.7)
D. Interventions:
1. Maintain a patent airway
2. Monitor vital signs, neuro checks
3. Administer medications as ordered:
   a. Osmotic diuretic (Mannitol), steroids to decrease cerebral edema
   b. Anticonvulsants to prevent seizures
   c. Anticoagulants for embolic stroke (rule out hemorrhage first)
      (1) Thrombolytic agents such as tissue plasminogen activase (tPA) must be given within 2–3 hours of stroke episode and followed by heparin.
      (2) Heparin
      (3) Wafarin (Coumadin); given following heparin; may be given for a prolonged period of time

Table 9.6 Anticonvulsant Medications

Drug	Action	Side Effects	Serum Levels
Hydantoin (Dilantin)	Inhibits spread of electrical discharge	Gum hyperplasia, hirsutism, ataxia, nystagmus, sedation, gastric distress, red urine	10–20 mcg/ml
Phenobarbital	Elevates the seizure threshold and inhibits spread of electrical discharge	Sedation (in children and elderly may get paradoxical active reaction), habituating	15–40 mcg/ml
Carbamazepine (Tegretol)	Reduces seizure activity	Dizziness, sedation	4–12 mcg/ml

Table 9.7 Nursing Diagnoses Related to Cerebrovascular Accident

- Disturbed sensory perception related to hypoxia and compression or displacement of brain tissue
- Impaired physical mobility related to decreased motor function of (specify) secondary to damage to upper motor neurons
- Risk for constipation related to prolonged periods of immobility, inadequate fluid intake, and inadequate nutritional intake
- Impaired verbal communication related to dysarthria and/or aphasia
- Risk for injury related to visual field deficits, motor deficits, perception deficits, and/or inability to perceive environmental hazards
- Activity intolerance related to deconditioning secondary to fatigue and weakness
- Risk for disuse syndrome related to effects of immobility
- Total incontinence related to loss of bladder tone, lost of sphincter control or mobility to perceived bladder cues
- Self-care deficit related to impaired physical mobility or confusion
- Impaired swallowing related to muscle paralysis or paress secondar to upper motor neuron damage
- Risk for impaired home maintenance related to altered ability to maintain self at home secondary to sensory-motor/cognitive deficits
- Unilateral neglect related to impaired perceptual abilities secondary to effects of cerebral pathology
- Risk for impaired skin integrity related to immobility, incontinence, sensory deficits, and/or motor deficits.
- Risk for disturbed self-concept related to effects of prolonged debilitating condition on achieving developmental tasks and lifestyle.

       (4) Aspirin may be given as an anticoagulant.
   d. Antihypertensives
  4. Keep the client on bed rest.
  5. Maintain fluid and electrolyte balance.
  6. Maintain proper positioning and body alignment.
  7. Promote skin integrity.
  8. Elimination:
   a. Offer bedpan every two hours; catheterize only if necessary.
   b. Stool softeners and suppositories
  9. Communication
   a. Receptive aphasia: inability to decode spoken word
    (1) Give one command at a time.
    (2) Simple instructions
    (3) Nonverbal communication
   b. Expressive aphasia: inability to speak
    (1) Encourage attempts at speech.
    (2) Allow time for the client to answer.
 10. Care of client with homonymous hemianopsia (half blindness)
   a. Loss of half of each visual field resulting in person's inability to see on the paralyzed or affected side
   b. Approach client on the unaffected side.

   c. Place belongings on the unaffected side.
   d. Teach client to scan the environment frequently.

TRANSIENT ISCHEMIC ATTACK (TIA)

A. Temporary episode of neurological dysfunction lasting only a few minutes or seconds caused by decreased blood flow to the brain; most common cause is atherosclerosis of the common carotid artery. Often precedes full-blown stroke or brain attack.
B. Assessment findings:
  1. Sudden loss of motor, sensory, or visual function
  2. Lasts a few seconds to a few minutes
C. Interventions:
  1. Surgical: carotid endartarectomy
   a. Assess temporal pulses after surgery
   b. Assess LOC and orientation after surgery
  2. Medical: anticoagulant therapy
   a. Heparin
   b. Warfarin sodium (Coumadin)
   c. Aspirin or Persantine

SPINAL CORD INJURY
(Figure 9.7)

A. Partial or complete disruption of nerve tracts and neurons resulting in paralysis, sensory loss, altered activity, and autonomic nervous system dysfunction below the level of the lesion
B. Assessment findings:
  1. Cervical injury:
   a. Respiratory paralysis if injury above C-4
   b. Paralysis of all four extremities (quadriplegia)
   c. Loss of bladder and bowel control
  2. Thoracic injury:
   a. Paralysis of lower extremities and major control of body trunk (paraplegia)
   b. Loss of bladder and bowel control
  3. Lumbar injury:
   a. Flaccid paralysis of lower extremities
   b. Loss of bladder and bowel control
  4. Spinal shock:
   a. Loss of all reflex activity below level of cord injury
   b. Lasts a few weeks to a few months after injury
   c. Resolution of spinal shock when reflex activity returns
C. Nursing diagnoses (Table 9.8)
D. Interventions
  1. Immobilize head and spine:
   a. Emergency collar
   b. Halter traction

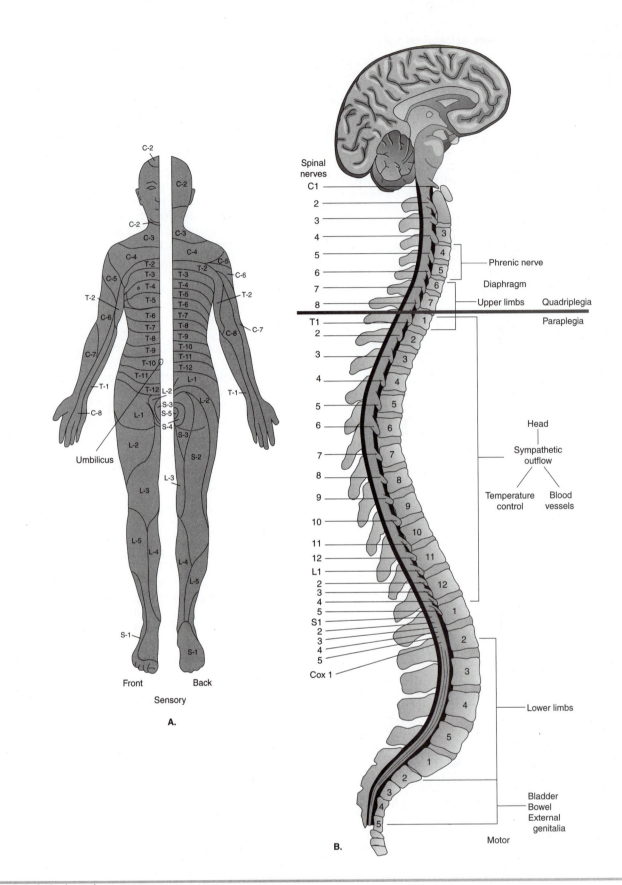

Figure 9.7 Spinal cord

Table 9.8 Nursing Diagnoses Related to Spinal Cord Injury

- Self-care deficit related to sensory-motor deficits secondary to level of spinal cord injury
- Impaired verbal communication related to impaired ability to speak words secondary to tracheostomy
- Interrupted family processes related to adjustment requirements for the situation (time, energy, financial, physical care, and prognosis)
- Risk for aspiration related to inability to cough secondary to injury
- Risk for impaired home maintenance related to inadequate resources, housing, or impaired caregiver(s)
- Grieving related to loss of body function and its effects on lifestyle
- Risk for social isolation related to disability
- Disturbed self-concept related to effects on limitations on achievement or developmental tasks
- Risk for deficient fluid volume related to difficulty obtaining fluids
- Reflex incontinence or urinary retention related to bladder atony secondary to sensory-motor deficits
- Risk for disuse syndrome related to effects of immobility
- Risk for injury related to impaired ability to control movements and sensory-motor deficits
- Risk for infection related to urinary stasis, repeated catheterizations, and invasive procedures (skeletal tongs, tracheostomy, venous lines, and surgical sites)
- Risk for ineffective sexuality patterns related to inability to achieve or sustain an erection for intercourse, limitations on sexual performance, decreased libido, altered self-concept, and/or unwilling/uninformed partner
- Bowel incontinence related to lack of voluntary rectal sphincter control secondary to spinal cord injury above T_{11}
- Bowel incontinence: areflexia related to lack of voluntary sphincter control secondary to spinal cord injury involving sacral reflex arc (S_2–S_4)

  c. Crutchfield tongs
  d. Stryker frame
2. Transport client in position in which found
3. Maintain airway
4. Nasogastric tube to prevent paralytic ileus
5. Steroids to decrease inflammation
6. Skin care
7. Prevent deformities by proper positioning, ROM exercises as indicated
8. Bladder care
   a. During spinal shock, bladder will not empty reflexively; must be catheterized at intervals.
   b. After spinal shock resolves, use Crede maneuver, reflex arc stimulation, and timing for bladder control.
9. Bowel care:
   a. Suppositories, stool softeners
   b. High fiber diet
10. Care for client who develops autonomic dysreflexia
    a. Reflex response to stimulation of the sympathetic nervous system manifested by a sharp rise in blood pressure that may be fatal. Seen in clients with cord lesions above T-6.

b. Stimulus may be over-distended bladder or bowel, decubitus ulcer, chilling
c. Symptoms: severe headache, hypertension, blurred vision, bradycardia, goose bumps, nasal congestion, convulsions
d. Interventions
   (1) Raise client to sitting position to decrease BP
   (2) Check for source of stimulus (full bladder, bowel impaction, or skin ulcer)
   (3) Remove offending stimulus (for example, catheterize client, remove impacted feces, or reposition client)
   (4) Monitor blood pressure
   (5) Administer antihypertensives (hydralazine HCl [Apresoline]) as ordered

MULTIPLE SCLEROSIS

A. Chronic progressive disease of the CNS, characterized by small patches of demyelination in the brain and spinal cord; cause is unknown; may be caused by a virus; may be autoimmune. Affects young adults 20–40 years of age; more women than men. Greater frequency in temperate climates.
B. Assessment findings:
   1. Nystagmus, blind spots, diplopia, blurred vision
   2. Slurred, hesitant, scanning speech
   3. Spastic weakness of extremities
   4. Paresthesias
   5. Mood swings
   6. Intention tremor
   7. Bladder retention or incontinence
   8. Constipation
C. Nursing diagnoses (Table 9.9)

Table 9.9 Nursing Diagnoses Related to Multiple Sclerosis

- Risk for injury related to unsteady gait, visual disturbances, and weakness
- Disturbed self-concept related to prolonged, debilitating condition
- Impaired verbal communication related to dysarthria secondary to nerve damage
- Activity intolerance related to fatigue and difficulty in performing activities of daily living
- Risk for disuse syndrome related to effects of immobility
- Urinary retention related to sensory-motor deficits
- Powerlessness related to inability to control symptoms and the unpredictable nature of the condition (in other words, remissions and exacerbations)
- Impaired physical mobility related to muscle weakness, ataxia, spasticity, or perceptual impairment
- Self-care deficits related to fatigue and muscle weakness
- Sexual dysfunction related to changes in sensation, genitalia, and psychological response to diagnosis

D. Interventions:
    1. No cure or specific treatment
    2. Allow expression of feelings regarding the disease and necessary role changes
    3. Remissions and exacerbations common
    4. Steroids during exacerbations
    5. Baclofen (Lioresal), dantrolene (Dantrum), and diazepam (valium) for spasticity
    6. Prevent injury due to paresthesias and poor ambulation
    7. Assess for bladder incontinence or urinary tract infection
    8. Promote bowel function
    9. Plasmapharesis

MYASTHENIA GRAVIS

A. Progressive neurologic disorder in which there is a disturbance in the transmission of nerve impulses at the myoneural junction, causing extreme muscle weakness
B. Assessment findings:
    1. Diplopia
    2. Dysphagia
    3. Muscle weakness, especially in upper body
    4. Ptosis
    5. Mask-like facial expression
    6. Weak voice, hoarseness
    7. Positive response to Tensilon
C. Nursing diagnoses (Table 9.10)
D. Interventions
    1. Drug therapy:
        a. Anticholinesterase drugs (Cholinergic): ambenonium (Mytelase), neostigmine (Prostigmin), pyridostigmine (Mestinon)
            (1). Block action of cholinesterase and increase levels of acetylcholine at the myoneural junction

Table 9.10 Nursing Diagnoses Related to Myasthenia Gravis

- Risk for injury related to unsteady gait, visual disturbances, and weakness.
- Disturbed self-concept related to prolonged, debilitating condition
- Impaired verbal communication related to dysarthria secondary to nerve damage
- Activity intolerance related to fatigue and difficulty in performing activities of daily living
- Risk for disuse syndrome related to the effects of immobility
- Urinary retention related to sensory-motor deficits
- Powerlessness related to the inability to control symptoms and the unpredictable nature of the condition (in other words, remissions and exacerbations)
- Self-care deficits related to fatigue and muscle weakness
- Risk for ineffective airway clearance related to impaired ability to cough
- Risk for aspiration related to impaired ability to cough, chew, and swallow

(2) Side effects: salivation, sweating, nausea and vomiting, fasiculations
(3) Give medications on time (before meals) with milk and crackers
        b. Corticosteroids (prednisone)
            (1) Used if other drugs are not effective
            (2) Suppress autoimmune response
    2. Thymectomy for some clients who do not respond to drugs
    3. Plasmapharesis for patients who do not respond to other therapy
    4. Avoid fatigue.
    5. Do not give morphine, quinine, curare, neomycin, or streptomycin.
    6. Check gag and swallowing reflexes before feeding.
    7. Mechanical soft diet
    8. Monitor respiratory status
    9. Myasthenic Crisis
        a. Caused by undermedication
        b. Manifested by extreme weakness
        c. Tensilon relieves symptoms
        d. Interventions
            (1) Airway: tracheostomy or endotracheal tube
            (2) Arterial blood gasses
            (3) Increase medications
    10. Cholinergic Crisis
        a. Caused by over-medication
        b. Manifested by weakness and salivation, nausea and vomiting
        c. Symptoms worse with Tensilon
        d. Interventions:
            (1) Atropine as an antidote
            (2) Airway
            (3) Arterial blood gasses

PARKINSON'S DISEASE

A. A progressive neurologic disorder affecting the brain centers that are responsible for control and regulation of movement (extrapyramidal) caused by a deficiency of dopamine; Occurs in the older adult.
B. Assessment findings (Figure 9.8):
    1. Tremors of the upper limbs; "pill rolling"; resting tremor
    2. Rigidity, loss of postural reflexes
    3. Bradykinesia (moves slowly)
    4. Stooped posture
    5. Shuffling, propulsive gait
    6. Monotone speech
    7. Mask-like facial expression
    8. Increased salivation, drooling
    9. Excessive sweating, seborrhea
    10. Lacrimation, constipation
    11. Decreased sexual capacity
C. Nursing Diagnoses (Table 9.11)
D. Interventions
    1. Medications (Table 9.12)

2. Nursing care
   a. Safety when ambulating
   b. Encourage independence as long as possible
   c. Prevent or manage constipation
   d. Psychologic support

GUILLAIN-BARRÉ SYNDROME (INFECTIOUS POLYNEURITIS)

A. Disease affecting the peripheral and cranial nerves; usually follows a viral infection; may be autoimmune
B. Assessment findings:
   1. Ascending paralysis which may progress to respiratory muscles
   2. Paralysis ascends and stays at maximum level for 2–3 weeks and then slowly descends
   3. Abnormal sensations of tingling and numbness
C. Nursing Diagnoses (Table 9.13)
D. Interventions:
   1. No specific therapy
   2. Supportive care of paralyzed, immobilized patient:
      a. Range of motion (ROM) to prevent contractures
      b. Skin care

Table 9.11 Nursing Diagnoses Related to Parkinson's Disease

- Constipation related to excessive salivation, and side effects of medication and inactivity
- Impaired physical mobility due to muscular rigidity
- Risk for injury related to gait disturbances and tremor
- Impaired verbal communication related to muscle impairment
- Ineffective coping related to depression
- Self-care deficit related to immobility, tremors, and bradykinesia
- Impaired swallowing related to neuromuscular impairment

Table 9.12 Drugs Used to Treat Parkinson's Disease

Drug	Action	Side Effects
Levodopa (l-dopa)	Increases the level of dopamine in the brain and relieves tremor, rigidity, and bradykinesia	Anorexia, nausea and vomiting; postural hypotension; confusion, agitation, hallucination; postural hypotension; confusion, agitation, hallucination; cardiac arrhythmias; do not give to patients with narrow angle glaucoma and those taking MAO inhibitors, methyldopa, or antipsychotics; avoid foods and vitamins high in pyridoxine (Vitamin B 6); administer medication with food to decrease GI irritation
Carbidopa—levodopa (Sinemet)	Prevents breakdown of dopamine in the periphery	Causes fewer side effects than l-dopa alone
Bromocriptine (Parlodel)	Stimulates release of dopamine	Used when l-dopa is no longer effective
Anticholinergic drugs: benztropine mesylate (Cogentin), trihexyphenidyl (Artane)	Used in mild cases to relieve tremor and rigidity	Dry mouth, blurred vision, constipation, urinary retention, confusion, hallucinations, tachycardia
Antihistamines: Diphenhydramine (Benadryl)	Decreases tremor and anxiety	Drowsiness

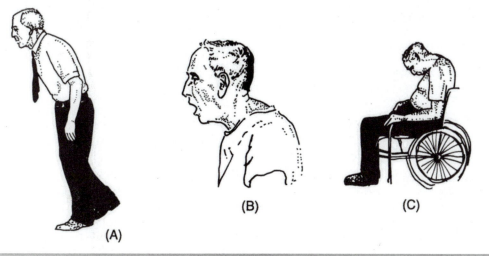

(A)   (B)   (C)

Figure 9.8 The shuffling gait (A), early postural changes (B), and advanced stages (C) of Parkinson's Disease.

Table 9.13 Nursing Diagnoses Related to Guillain-Barré Syndrome

- Risk for aspiration related to impaired ability to cough, chew, and swallow
- Ineffective breathing pattern related to weakness of the respiratory muscles
- Impaired physical mobility related to motor weakness
- Risk for injury related to unsteady gait, visual disturbances, and weakness
- Disturbed self-concept related to prolonged debilitating condition
- Risk for disuse syndrome related to effects of immobility
- Self-care deficits related to fatigue, muscle weakness

    c. Respiratory support
    d. Maintain nutritional status, fluid intake
    e. Allow the client to verbalize fears
    f. Provide diversional activity
E. Full recovery often occurs if good supportive care exists during the illness.

AMYOTROPHIC LATERAL SCLEROSIS (ALS, LOU GEHRIG'S DISEASE)

A. Progressive disease affecting motor neurons in the cortex, medulla, and spinal cord; usually leading to death in 2–6 years; onsets between 40 and 70 years; affects more men than women
B. Assessment findings:
    1. Progressive weakness and atrophy of muscles of hands, forearms, and legs
    2. Dysphagia, drooling
    3. Respiratory difficulties
    4. Difficulty communicating
    5. Emotional lability
C. Nursing diagnoses (Table 9.14)

Table 9.14 Nursing Diagnoses Related to Amyotrophic Lateral Sclerosis

- Impaired physical mobility related to muscle atrophy, weakness, and spasticity
- Imbalanced nutrition, less than body requirements, related to impaired chewing and swallowing
- Impaired verbal communication related to weakness of muscles used for speech
- Ineffective breathing pattern related to weakness of the respiratory muscles
- Powerlessness related to loss of control over life, physical dependence, and presence of fatal disease
- Risk for aspiration related to impaired ability to cough, chew, and swallow
- Risk for injury related to muscle atrophy
- Disturbed self-concept related to prolonged, debilitating condition
- Risk for disuse syndrome related to effects of immobility
- Self-care deficits related to muscle atrophy

D. Interventions:
    1. No known cure
    2. Provide nursing measures for muscle weakness and dysphagia.
    3. Promote adequate respiratory function.
    4. Prevent complications of immobility.
    5. Maintain nutritional status, and fluid intake.
    6. Promote independence as long as possible.

TRIGEMINAL NEURALGIA (TIC DOULOUREUX)

A. Neurologic disorder affecting the fifth cranial nerve; cause unknown
B. Assessment findings:
    1. Excruciating recurrent paroxysms of sharp, stabbing facial pain along the trigeminal nerve
    2. Pain frequently brought on by heat, cold, eating, drinking, and washing the face
C. Nursing diagnosis: alteration in comfort related to nerve damage
D. Interventions:
    1. Assess characteristics of the pain, precipitating factors, and trigger points
    2. Avoid extremes of heat and cold
    3. Antiepileptic drugs (Tegretol and Dilantin), Table 9.6
    4. Alcohol injection of nerve
    5. Surgery
    6. Protect eye if surgery done

BELL'S PALSY

A. Lower motor neuron lesion of the seventh cranial nerve resulting in paralysis of one side of the face; cause unknown; usually self-limiting to a few weeks
B. Assessment findings:
    1. Unilateral paralysis of the facial muscles of expression
    2. Tearing of the eyes
    3. Painful sensations in the face
    4. Sagging of one side of mouth; drooling
    5. Usually occurs between ages of 20 and 40
C. Nursing diagnoses (Table 9.15)
D. Interventions:
    1. Steroids and analgesics
    2. Protect involved eye
    3. Active facial exercises when possible
    4. Moist heat and gentle massage to face
    5. Assist client with eating and mouth care as needed

Table 9.15 Nursing Diagnoses Related to Bell's Palsy

- Acute pain related to nerve damage
- Imbalanced nutrition, less than body requirements, related to difficulty eating secondary to facial paralysis

Eye Conditions

DETACHED RETINA

A. The retina separates from the choroid (vascular layer), and vitreous humor flows between the layers.
B. Assessment findings:
  1. Gaps in vision
  2. Spots before the eyes
  3. Curtain over the field of vision
  4. Blindness if not treated
C. Nursing diagnoses (Table 9.16)
D. Interventions:
  1. Immediate bed rest
  2. Positioning to keep retina next to choroid
  3. Surgical intervention:
    a. Scleral buckling
    b. Scarring by heat, cold, or laser
  4. Postoperative care
    a. Bed rest with both eyes bandaged
    b. Avoid jarring or bumping head
    c. No coughing
    d. Positioning to keep retina next to choroid—may be on operative side
    e. Client teaching

CATARACT

A. Lens of the eye becomes opaque; occurs with aging
B. Assessment findings:
  1. Gradual loss of vision
  2. Distorted, blurred, or hazy vision; loss of visual acuity
  3. Glare in bright lights
  4. Pupils may look milky white
C. Nursing diagnoses (Table 9.16)

D. Interventions:
  1. Surgical removal of the lens under local anesthesia (Figure 9.9)
    a. Surgery done on one eye at a time, usually in same-day surgery unit
    b. Intraocular lens implant often performed
  2. Pre-operative medications as ordered:
    a. Mydriatic eye drops to dilate pupils
    b. Cycloplegic eye drops to dilate pupils and paralyze eye muscles
    c. Topical antibiotics to prevent infection
    d. Acetazolamide (Diamox) and osmotic agents (oral glycerin or IV mannitol) to decrease intraocular pressure to provide a soft eyeball for surgery
  3. Postoperative care
    a. Prevent increase in intraocular pressure and stress on suture line:
      (1) Elevate head of bed 30–45°
      (2) Do not turn on operative side
      (3) No hair washing immediately after surgery
      (4) No bending, stooping, or lifting
      (5) No coughing or vomiting

Table 9.16 Nursing Diagnoses Related to Eye Conditions

- Risk for injury related to impaired vision secondary to condition or eye patches
- Self-care deficit related to impaired vision
- Acute pain: related to retinal tearing (retinal detachment) or increased intraocular pressure after surgery
- Anxiety related to possible loss of vision and/or surgical procedure
- Risk for noncompliance related to side effects of medication, difficulty remembering, and cost of medications (glaucoma)

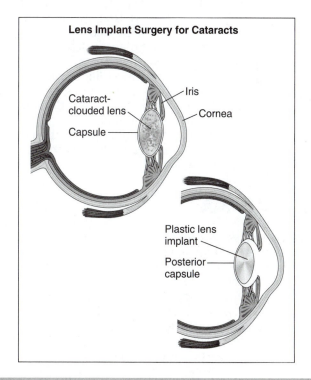

Lens Implant Surgery for Cataracts

Cataract-clouded lens
Capsule
Iris
Cornea
Plastic lens implant
Posterior capsule

Figure 9.9 Lens implant surgery for cataracts

      (6) Give stool softeners as ordered to prevent straining

      (7) Report any signs of increased intraocular pressure: severe eye pain, restlessness, or increased pulse

   b. Protect eye from injury

      (1) Keep eye covered day of surgery; dressings may be removed next day

      (2) Eye shield or glasses during day

      (3) Eye shield at night

   c. Administer medications as ordered

      (1) Topical mydriatics and cycloplegics to decrease spasm of ciliary body and relieve pain

      (2) Topical antibiotics and corticosteroids as ordered

      (3) Mild analgesics as ordered

   d. Provide client teaching concerning:

      (1) The administration of eye drops

      (2) Eye shield at night

      (3) Measures to prevent increase in intraocular pressure: no bending or lifting

      (4) Reporting signs or symptoms of complications immediately: severe eye pain, decreased vision, excessive drainage, or swelling of eyelid

      (5) Cataract glasses or contact lenses

         (a) If lens implant not performed, client needs glasses or contact lenses

         (b) Temporary glasses are worn for 1–4 weeks, then permanent glasses are fitted.

         (c) Cataract glasses distort peripheral vision and magnify objects; have client practice walking, using stairs, and so on, until new spatial relationships become familiar.

         (d) Contact lenses prescribed at one month; cause less distortion of vision

GLAUCOMA

A. Increased intraocular pressure; if not corrected, may lead to atrophy of the optic nerve and eventual blindness

B. Assessment findings:

  1. Acute (closed-angle) glaucoma results from an obstruction to the outflow of aqueous humor; occurs suddenly and is an emergency

   a. Severe pain in and around eye

   b. Rainbows and halos around lights

   c. Cloudy and blurred vision

   d. Pupils dilate

   e. Nausea and vomiting

   f. Within hours may develop GI, sinus, neuro, and dental symptoms

  2. Chronic (open-angle) glaucoma is due to the obstruction of outflow of aqueous humor in the trabecular meshwork or canal of Schlemm; gradual onset; most common form.

   a. Tired feeling in eye

   b. Halos around lights

   c. Slowly decreasing peripheral vision (tunnel vision)

   d. Loss of central vision if untreated

C. Nursing diagnoses (Table 9.16)

D. Intervention:

  1. Medications for chronic glaucoma:

   a. Pilocarpine eye drops (Pilo, Pilocar, e-Pilo): causes pupil to contract, iris is drawn away from cornea, aqueous humor may drain through lymph spaces into Canal of Schlemm

   b. Diamox: decreases production of aqueous humor; do not give when acid base imbalances exist

   c. Mannitol: osmotic diuretic to decrease intraocular pressure for treatment of acute (closed-angle) glaucoma

  2. Surgery:

   a. Iridencleisis, thermosclerectomy, or trabeculectomy for acute glaucoma

   b. Local anesthetic

   c. Safety when ambulating

   d. Liquid or low-residue diet to prevent straining upon defecation

  3. Teach the client:

   a. Glaucoma is controllable, not curable

   b. Avoid emotional upsets

   c. Avoid constricting clothing, extreme exertion, and lifting

   d. Avoid colds

   e. Moderate exercise

   f. Regular bowel habits to prevent straining at stool and increased intraocular pressure

   g. Take daily medications as ordered for life

   h. Medical checkups and Medic Alert bracelet

EYE INJURY

A. Chemical:

  1. Flush immediately for 20 minutes under running water

  2. Take to physician or emergency room

B. Foreign body:

  1. Light dressing only, no pressure dressings as danger of increasing injury to eye

  2. Do not remove glass or metal; take immediately to emergency room

CARE OF THE CLIENT WHO IS BLIND:

A. When approaching the client, knock before entering the room and speak before touching him or her.

B. When ambulating a blind client, the helper should stand slightly ahead of the blind person with the blind person's arm through the helper's.

C. When feeding a blind client, encourage self care when possible. Use the clock approach; have client picture plate as the face of a clock and tell him or her where the food is; for example, the potatoes are at 6 o'clock.

Conditions of the Ear

CARE OF THE CLIENT WITH DIMINISHED HEARING

A. Communication:
1. Attract the client's attention by raising an arm or a hand.
2. Face the client directly when speaking.
3. To make lip reading easier, make sure the client's view of your mouth is not obstructed and you are not standing with your back to a bright light.
4. Speak slowly and distinctly without shouting.
5. Use a low-pitched voice when possible, because the ability to hear high frequencies is usually lost first.
6. Check with the client to be sure instructions are understood.

B. Care of client with hearing aid:
1. If not working, check on-off switch and volume control, battery, and plastic tubing for cracks and loose connections.
2. When not in use, store in a covered container to prevent dust from damaging the mechanism.
3. Wipe clean with soap and water.

MENIERE'S DISEASE

A. Chronic disease of the inner ear characterized by recurrent episodes of vertigo, progressive unilateral nerve deafness, and tinnitus; cause unknown

B. Assessment findings:
1. Sudden attacks of vertigo lasting hours or days
2. Nausea and vomiting
3. Tinnitus, progressive hearing loss
4. Nystagmus

C. Nursing diagnoses (Table 9.17)

D. Interventions:
1. Low-sodium diet and restricted fluid intake to decrease fluid in the inner ear

Table 9.17 Nursing Diagnoses Related to Meniere's Disease

- Risk for injury related to disturbances of balance
- Fear related to possible loss of hearing
- Activity intolerance related to severe vertigo
- Impaired verbal communication related to hearing loss

2. Medications as ordered:
   a. Acute episode: atropine to decrease autonomic nervous system activity; diazepam (Valium)
   b. Chronic: vasodilators; diuretics, mild sedatives, or tranquilizers (diazepam [Valium]); antihistamines (diphenhydramine [Benadryl], Dramamine, Benadryl, or atropine)
3. Encourage the client to stop smoking; smoking aggravates the condition.
4. The patient should move slowly to prevent injury due to dizziness.
5. Side rails to prevent injury due to dizziness
6. Surgery:
   a. Surgical destruction of the labyrinth
   b. Intracranial division of vestibular portion of cranial nerve VIII

OTOSCLEROSIS

A. Fixation of stapes preventing transmission of sound waves to the inner ear; cause unknown, familial tendency

B. Assessment findings:
1. Progressive hearing loss
2. Tinnitus

C. Interventions: stapedectomy
1. Stapedectomy: removal of diseased portion of stapes and replacement with a prosthesis; usually performed under local anesthesia
2. Postoperative care:
   a. Elevate side rails and assist client when out of bed to prevent injury; client may be dizzy

b. Explain to the client that hearing may improve during surgery and then decrease due to edema and packing.

c. Check dressings frequently and report excessive drainage or bleeding.

d. Administer medications as ordered: antibiotics, antiemetics, anti-motion sickness drugs.

e. Assess facial nerve function; ask client to wrinkle forehead, close eyelids, puff out cheeks, smile and show teeth; report if not the same on both sides.

f. Report pain, headache, or vertigo to physician.

g. Teach client not to blow nose or cough and to sneeze with mouth open.

h. Teach client not to shampoo until physician gives approval because ear should be kept dry.

i. Explain to the client that air travel is not allowed for six months.

j. Place cotton ball in meatus after packing is removed; change twice a day.

Sample Questions

1. An adult man fell off a ladder and hit his head and lost consciousness. After regaining consciousness several minutes later, he was drowsy and had trouble staying awake. He is admitted to the hospital for evaluation.
The nursing care plan will most likely include which of the following?
   1. Elevate head of bed 15–30 degrees.
   2. Encourage fluids to 1000 ml q. 8 hrs.
   3. Assist to cough and deep-breathe every two hours.
   4. Chest physical therapy every four hours while awake.

2. A teenager is admitted following a seizure. The next day, the nurse goes into his room and finds him lying on the floor starting to have a seizure. What action should the nurse take at this time?
   1. Carefully observe the seizure and gently restrain him.
   2. Attempt to put an airway in his mouth so he doesn't swallow his tongue and observe the type and duration of the seizure.
   3. Place something soft under his head, carefully observe the seizure, and protect him from injury.
   4. Shout for help so that someone can help you move him away from the furniture.

3. An adult is being treated with phenytoin (Dilantin) for a seizure disorder. Five days after starting the medication, he tells the nurse that his urine is reddish-brown in color. What action should the nurse take?
   1. Inform him that this is a common side effect of phenytoin (Dilantin) therapy.
   2. Test the urine for occult blood.
   3. Report it to the physician because it could indicate a clotting deficiency.
   4. Send a urine specimen to the lab.

4. The nurse is caring for a client who has recently had a CVA. When positioning the client and supporting her extremities, the nurse must remember that when voluntary control of muscles is lost,
   1. The feet will maintain a position of eversion.
   2. The upper extremities will rotate externally.
   3. The hip joint will rotate internally.
   4. Flexor muscles will become stronger than extensors.

5. A stroke victim regains consciousness three days after admission. She has right-sided hemiparesis and hemiplegia and also has expressive aphasia. She becomes upset when she is unable to say simple words. The best approach for the nurse is to:
   1. Stay with her and give her time and encouragement in attempting to speak.
   2. Say, "I'm sure you want a glass of water. I'll get it for you."
   3. Say, "Don't get upset. You rest now and I'll come back later and try to talk to you then."
   4. Encourage her attempts and say, "Don't worry, it will get easier every day."

6. A young man was swimming at the beach when an exceptionally large wave caused him to be drawn under the water. His family members found him in the water and pulled him ashore. He states that he heard something snap in his neck. When a nurse arrives, he is conscious and lying on his back. He states that he has no pain. He is unable to move his legs. How should he be transported?
   1. Position him in a prone position and place on a backboard.
   2. Apply a neck collar and position supine on a backboard.
   3. Log roll him to a rigid backboard.
   4. Position in an upright position with a firm neck collar.

7. A client who is recovering from a spinal cord injury complains of blurred vision and a severe headache. His blood pressure is 210/140. The most appropriate initial action for the nurse to take is:
   1. Check for bladder distention.
   2. Place him in the Trendelenburg position.
   3. Administer prn pain medication.
   4. Position him on his left side.

8. A 27-year-old woman is admitted to the hospital complaining of numbness in both legs, difficulty walking, and double vision of one week duration. Multiple sclerosis is suspected. Orders include: bed rest with bathroom privileges, brain scan, EEG, Lumbar puncture, ACTH 40 Units I.M. bid × 3 days, then 30 Units I.M. bid × 3 days, then 20 Units I.M. bid × 3

days; and passive ROM progressing to active ROM as tolerated. In planning care for this client, which activity is most important to include?
1. Encouraging her to perform all care activities for herself
2. Frequent ambulation to retain joint mobility
3. Scheduling frequent rest periods between physical activity
4. Feeding the client to reduce energy needs

9. The doctor orders a Tensilon test for a woman suspected of having myasthenia gravis. Which statement is true about this test?
1. A positive result will be evident within one minute of injection of Tensilon if she has myasthenia gravis.
2. This is of diagnostic value in only 25% of patients with myasthenia gravis.
3. Administration of Tensilon causes an immediate decrease in muscle strength for about an hour in persons with myasthenia gravis.
4. Tensilon works by blocking the action of acetylcholine at the myoneural junction.

10. When planning care for a woman with myasthenia gravis, the nurse asks her what time of day she feels strongest. The nurse would expect which of the following replies?
1. "I can wash up and comb my hair before breakfast because I feel best in the morning."
2. "I only feel good for about an hour after I take my medication."
3. "I feel strongest in the evening, so I would prefer to take a shower before bedtime."
4. "I feel best after lunch after I've been moving around a little."

11. Which of the following would not be included in the nursing care plan for a client with Parkinson's disease?
1. Restricting his intake of oral fluids
2. Range-of-motion exercises
3. Allowing him to carry out activities of daily living by himself even though he is very slow
4. Providing him with diversionary tasks that require motor coordination of hands

12. The nurse is caring for a client admitted with Guillain-Barré syndrome. On day three of hospitalization, his muscle weakness worsens and he is no longer able to stand with support. He is also having difficulty swallowing and talking. The priority in his nursing care plan should be to prevent:
1. Aspiration pneumonia
2. Decubitus ulcers
3. Bladder distention
4. Hypertensive crisis

13. An adult client is admitted for removal of a cataract from her right eye. Which of the following would the client likely have experienced as a result of the cataracts?

1. Acute eye pain
2. Redness and constant itching of the right eye
3. Gradual blurring of vision
4. Severe headaches and dizziness

14. The client has had a cataract extraction performed. Which statement that the client makes indicates a need for more teaching?
1. "I will take a stool softener daily."
2. "I'm going to start doing calisthenic exercises as soon as I get home."
3. "I'm going to my daughter's for a few weeks until I am recovered."
4. "I am looking forward to watching television during my recovery period."

15. The client is a 50-year-old admitted with the diagnosis of open-angle glaucoma. Which of the following symptoms would the nurse expect the client to have?
1. Severe eye pain
2. Constant blurred vision
3. Severe headaches, nausea, and vomiting
4. Reports of seeing halos around objects

16. The nurse is administering eye drops to a client. Which action is correct?
1. Ask the client to report any blurring of vision and difficulty focusing that occurs after the administration of eye drops.
2. Apply gentle pressure to the naso-lacrimal canal for 1 to 2 minutes after instillation to prevent systemic absorption.
3. Have the client lie down with eyes closed for 45 minutes after giving drops.
4. Gently pull the lower lid down and place medicine in the center of the eye.

17. A 10-year-old boy comes to the school clinic holding his broken pair of glasses. He says that he got hit in the face playing ball and his eye hurts and feels like there's something in it. What should the nurse do before taking him to the emergency room?
1. Thoroughly examine his eyes.
2. Put a pressure dressing on his right eye.
3. Cover both eyes lightly with gauze.
4. Flush his right eye with water for 20 minutes.

18. How should a nurse walk a client who is blind?
1. Stand slightly behind and tell her when to turn.
2. Stand slightly behind and to the side and guide her by holding her hand.
3. Walk slightly ahead with the client's arm inside the nurse's arm.
4. Walk beside the client and gently guide her by grasping her elbow.

19. The client is a 60-year-old man who had a stapedectomy. He is to ambulate for the first time. Which nursing action should be taken?
1. Encourage him to walk as far as he comfortably can.
2. Suggest that he practice bending and stretching exercises.

3. Walk with him, holding his arm.
4. Tell him to take deep breaths while he is ambulating.

20. A client complains of tinnitus and dizziness and has a diagnosis of Meniere's Disease.
She asks the nurse what the cause of Meniere's disease is. What is the nurse's best response?
1. "Meniere's Disease is caused by a virus."
2. "The cause of Meniere's Disease is unknown."
3. "Meniere's Disease frequently follows a streptococcal infection."
4. "It is hereditary. Both of your parents carried the gene for Meniere's Disease."

21. An adult man fell off a ladder and hit his head. His wife rushed to help him and found him unconscious. After regaining consciousness several minutes later, he was drowsy and had trouble staying awake. He is admitted to the hospital for evaluation. When the nurse enters the room, he is sleeping. While caring for the client, the nurse finds that his systolic blood pressure has increased, his pulse has decreased, and his temperature is slightly elevated. What does this suggest?
1. Increased cerebral blood flow
2. Respiratory depression
3. Increased intracranial pressure
4. Hyperoxygenation of the cerebrum

22. The physician has ordered Mannitol IV for a client with a head injury. What should the nurse closely monitor because the client is receiving Mannitol?
1. Deep tendon reflexes
2. Urine output
3. Level of orientation
4. Pulse rate

23. A 17-year-old had one generalized convulsion several hours prior to admission to the medical unit for a neurological workup. Physician's orders include Dilantin 100 mg po tid and Phenobarbital 100 mg po qd. He tells the nurse, "I can't believe I really had a seizure. My mom says she was in the room when it happened, but I don't even remember it." What is the best interpretation of his comments?
1. They indicate an initial denial mechanism, but he will begin to remember the seizure later.
2. Anoxia suffered during the seizure has damaged part of his cerebral cortex.
3. Inability to remember the seizure is a normal response of a person who has had a seizure.
4. They are an indication that he would rather not talk about his seizure at this time.

24. What should the nurse include when teaching the client with Parkinson's disease?
1. He should try to continue working as long as he can remain sitting most of the day.
2. Drooling may be reduced somewhat if he remembers to swallow frequently.

3. He should return monthly for lab tests, which will predict the progression of the disease.
4. Emotional stress has no effect on voluntary muscle control in clients with Parkinson's disease.

25. A 68-year-old woman is brought to the emergency room by ambulance. She was found by her husband slumped in her chair, unresponsive. Tentative diagnosis is cerebrovascular accident (CVA). The physician orders a 15% solution of Mannitol IV. The nurse knows that this drug is given for what purpose?
1. To increase urine output
2. To dissolve clots
3. To reduce blood pressure
4. To decrease muscle spasms

26. An older woman has had a CVA. The nurse notes that she seems to be unaware of objects on her right side (right homonymous hemianopia). Which nursing action is most important in planning to assist her to compensate for this loss?
1. Place frequently used items on the affected side.
2. Position her so that her affected side is toward the activity in the room.
3. Encourage her to turn her head from side to side to scan the environment on the affected side.
4. Stand on the affected side while assisting her in ambulating.

27. A client asks the nurse what causes Parkinson's disease. The nurse's correct reply would be based on which of the following statements? Parkinson's disease is thought to be due to:
1. A deficiency of dopamine in the brain
2. A demyelinating process affecting the central nervous system
3. Atrophy of the basal ganglia
4. Insufficient uptake of acetylcholine in the body

28. The nurse is caring for a client who is very hard of hearing. How should the nurse communicate with this person?
1. Speak loudly and talk in his best ear.
2. Stand in front of him and speak clearly and distinctly.
3. Yell at him using a high-pitched voice.
4. Write all communication on a note pad or magic slate.

29. The day following a stapedectomy, the client tells the nurse that he cannot hear much in the operative ear, and thinks the stapedectomy was a failure. What is the best response for the nurse to make?
1. "There is packing in your ear. You will not hear well for a few days."
2. "The doctors have not yet turned on the stapes replacement. "

3. "You may not have hearing, but you will now be free of pain."
4. "You seem upset that you aren't hearing well."

30. A cataract extraction is performed on the client's right eye. What is the priority nursing care immediately postoperative?
   1. Assist her to turn, cough, and deep-breathe q 2 hrs.
   2. Keep her NPO for four hours.
   3. Assist her in moving her arms and legs in ROM.
   4. Position client on her right side.

Answers and Rationales

1. (1) The head of the bed should be slightly elevated to allow gravity drainage of fluid and reduce cerebral edema. Coughing and forcing fluids are contraindicated because they may raise intracranial pressure. Chest physical therapy would be apt to raise intracranial pressure.

2. (3) Protect his head from injury, and observe the seizure. Never try to restrain a seizing person. Current thinking says do not put an airway in the mouth. Placing something soft under his head will help to protect his head from injury. The question does not indicate that the client is in danger from the furniture.

3. (1) He is receiving Dilantin, which frequently causes the urine to turn reddish-brown in color. There is no indication for testing the urine or notifying the physician. The finding should be recorded on the client's chart.

4. (4) Flexor muscles are stronger than extensors, causing flexion contractures. The hip joint tends to rotate externally.

5. (1) Offering help is always therapeutic. This approach will help her to express herself. The nurse should not routinely anticipate her needs because this does not encourage attempts at speech. Telling her not to get upset is not therapeutic. Encouraging her attempts to speak is therapeutic but telling her not to worry is not therapeutic.

6. (2) He may have a neck or spinal cord injury. The neck and back should be supported and maintained in a rigid position. He should be transported in the position in which he was found. He should not be turned.

7. (1) The symptoms suggest autonomic hyperreflexia, which is usually caused by bladder distention. The patient will need to be catheterized and the physician notified. Autonomic hyperreflexia is a medical emergency. The head is usually elevated to reduce blood pressure.

8. (3) She will need rest periods between activities. She may be too weak to perform all

self activities. Her orders include bed rest, not ambulating ad lib. Feeding her is not necessary and is likely to cause her to be upset.

9. (1) Tensilon works almost immediately to cause an increase in muscle strength by increasing the amount of acetylcholine at the myoneural junction. The test is of value in almost all clients suspected of having myasthenia gravis.

10. (1) Muscle strength is best early in the day. Weakness usually progresses during the day and is at its worst in the evening.

11. (1) Fluids should be encouraged because he has a tendency to drool and lose fluid. Encouraging the client to perform activities of daily living is desirable. He should be encouraged to move frequently to prevent joint contractures. Activities requiring hand coordination will help him to retain function.

12. (1) Because he is having difficulty swallowing and talking, he is at high risk for aspiration pneumonia. He is also at risk for decubitus ulcers, but this is of lesser priority than the airway. Bladder distention is a possibility but not as high a priority as the risk of aspiration pneumonia. There is no evidence that he is at risk for hypertensive crisis.

13. (3) Cataracts are characterized by a gradual blurring of vision. Acute eye pain is characteristic of acute glaucoma or foreign objects in the eye. Redness and itching is more characteristic of an eye infection. Severe headaches and dizziness are not characteristic of cataracts.

14. (2) Bending, stooping, and lifting should be avoided for several weeks following eye surgery. A stool softener is recommended so that the client will not strain at stool. Television and reading are not restricted following cataract extraction. Eye movement is restricted following surgery for detached retina.

15. (4) Chronic glaucoma is characterized by halos around objects. Severe eye pain and severe headaches, nausea, and vomiting are more characteristic of acute glaucoma. Constant blurred vision is characteristic of cataracts.

16. (2) This action will prevent systemic absorption of eye medication and prevent the nose from running. Blurred vision and difficulty focusing is normal immediately after administering eye drops. There is no need to lie down after eye drops are given. Eye drops should be placed in the conjunctival sac, not the center of the eye.

17. (3) Covering both eyes lightly with gauze prevents tracking by the affected eye, which would occur if the unaffected eye was not covered. Examining the eyes should be done only at the emergency room by a physician. A pressure dressing would further damage the eye if broken glass is in the eye. Flushing is appropriate for chemical spills in the eye.

18. (3) Walking slightly ahead of the client allows the nurse to see what is in the way. The client

feels more in control if her arm is through the nurse's rather than the other way around.

19. (3) The client is apt to be dizzy after ear surgery. For safety, the nurse should be with him.

20. (2) The cause of Meniere's Disease is unknown. Glomerulonephritis and rheumatic fever follow a streptococcal infection. As far as is known, Meniere's Disease is not hereditary nor is it caused by a virus.

21. (3) These are classic manifestations of increased intracranial pressure.

22. (2) Mannitol is an osmotic diuretic. Urine output should increase. He must be on intake and output.

23. (3) People seldom remember a seizure; this is a normal response.

24. (2) Swallowing may reduce drooling. Sitting most of the day causes stiffness. There is no lab test to determine disease progression. Emotional stress can aggravate the symptoms.

25. (1) Mannitol is an osmotic diuretic which increases urine output and will decrease intracranial pressure. Streptokinase and tPA dissolve clots and might be ordered for this client. Antihypertensive medications may also be ordered for this client.

26. (3) Encouraging her to turn her head from side to side will do the most to help her learn a skill that will compensate for loss of the visual field. With homonymous hemianopia, the client does not see on the affected or paralyzed side. Choices 1 and 2 will make life more difficult for her. If the nurse stands on the affected side, the client will be unaware of the nurse.

27. (1) A deficiency of dopamine is thought to be the cause of Parkinson's. Multiple Sclerosis is caused by demyelination of the central nervous system. Alzheimer's Disease involves atrophy of the basal ganglia. Myasthenia Gravis is caused by insufficient uptake of acetylcholine in the body.

28. (2) Standing in front of him and speaking clearly and distinctly will allow him to read lips. Speaking loudly is usually not the best approach. Most persons with difficulty hearing hear low-pitched sounds better than high-pitched ones; yelling and speaking loudly tend to raise the pitch of the voice. Written communication might become necessary for some persons. However, that would only be a last resort after all other methods of communication had failed.

29. (1) Packing in the ear will reduce sound wave transmission. Hearing will be muffled until the packing is removed. The stapes replacement does not need to be turned on. The purpose of a stapedectomy is to restore some hearing. Otosclerosis for which the stapedectomy was performed is not a painful condition. It is more appropriate to give the client the information that he needs regarding hearing rather than to focus on the client's feelings.

30. (3) Of these answers, moving arms and legs is the best as it will help to prevent thrombophlebitis. The client should not cough because this will increase intraocular pressure. There is no need to keep her NPO. She should not be positioned on the operative side because this will increase intraocular pressure.

Chapter 10

The Gastrointestinal System

ANATOMY AND PHYSIOLOGY
(Figure 10.1)

A. Overview:
   1. A hollow, muscular tube that extends from the mouth to the anus
   2. Provides the body with fluid, nutrients, and electrolytes
   3. Nutrients are metabolized for energy and tissue building.
B. Major functions:
   1. Secretion of electrolytes, hormones, and enzymes
   2. Movement of ingested products by peristalsis (wave of muscular contraction in the bowel wall that pushes the bolus of food through the gastrointestinal [GI] tract)
   3. Digestion of food and fluids
   4. Absorption of nutrients into the bloodstream

MOUTH

A. Formed by cheeks, hard and soft palate, and tongue
B. Chewing (mastication): teeth break down the food into smaller pieces
C. Saliva:
   1. Lubricates and softens food particles and stimulates the taste buds
   2. Contains the enzyme ptyalin (amylase), which breaks down starches into maltose
D. Swallowing (deglutition): movement down the esophagus requires coordination of peristalsis and relaxation of the lower esophageal sphincter (LES)

ESOPHAGUS

A. A hollow, muscular tube which lies behind the trachea and larynx and extends through the mediastinum and diaphragm and allows food to pass from the mouth to the stomach
B. Composed of the upper esophageal sphincter (UES) and the lower esophageal sphincter (LES). LES is not a distinct sphincter but an area of increased pressure that provides a barrier to protect the esophageal mucosa from the effects of gastric reflux (backward flow of gastric secretions).
   1. Substances such as secretin, cholecystokinin, anticholinergics, cigarettes, fatty foods, and alcohol decrease LES pressure.

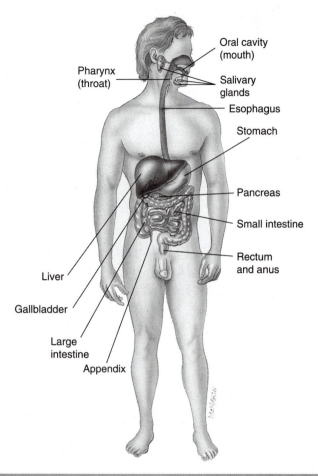

Figure 10.1 Major Structures of the Digestive System

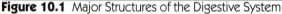

2. Decreased LES pressure can cause problems with gastric reflux and indigestion.

STOMACH

A. Divided into three parts:
   1. The fundus lies above and to the left of the cardiac sphincter.
   2. The body is the central area of the stomach.
   3. The antrum is the lower portion of the stomach (pyloric area).
      a. Cardiac sphincter: located at the proximal end of the stomach; allows inflow of food and prevents backflow
      b. Pyloric sphincter: located between the distal end of the stomach and the duodenum; permits the flow of chyme from the stomach
B. Function:
   1. Storage, mixing, and liquefaction of the bolus of food into chyme
   2. First stage of protein breakdown

3. Digestion of starches (begun in the mouth by ptyalin) continues
   4. Minimal digestion of fats
C. Innervated by the sympathetic and parasympathetic systems. Parasympathetic stimulation (vagus nerve) increases the gastric secretions of acid, gastrin, and pepsin, and increases gastric motility.
D. Secretions:
   1. Secretes 1,500 to 3,000 cc gastric juice per day
   2. Major secretions are hydrochloric acid, pepsin, and mucus
   3. Hydrochloric acid and pepsin provide the corrosive power of gastric secretions.
E. Motor activity:
   1. Stomach empties slowly to accommodate the ability of the duodenum to receive the stomach contents.
   2. The greater the acidity and the greater the caloric density of the stomach contents, the slower the stomach empties.

SMALL INTESTINE

A. Divided into three parts:
   1. Duodenum: begins at the pyloric valve and extends about 10 inches to the jejunum
   2. Jejunum: the middle portion of the small intestine; about 8 feet long and extends to the ileum
   3. Ileum: about 12 feet long and joins the colon at the ileocecal valve, which controls the flow of intestinal contents into the large intestine and prevents backflow into the small intestine
B. Functions:
   1. Completes digestion of the foods
   2. Absorbs the products of digestion
   3. Secretes hormones that control the secretion of bile and pancreatic juices
C. Innervated by sympathetic and parasympathetic fibers
   1. Sympathetic stimulation inhibits the motility of the small intestine.
   2. Parasympathetic stimulation increases intestinal tone and motility.
D. Secretions:
   1. In addition to secretions from the small intestine, the pancreas secretes enzymes, bicarbonate, and water into the duodenum, which act on chyme.
   2. Duodenal hormones (secretin and cholecystokinin [CCK]) regulate pancreas and gallbladder secretions.
E. Absorption:
   1. Carbohydrates are changed to monosaccharides and some disaccharides; CHO digestion takes place primarily in the jejunum.

2. Proteins are changed to amino acids.
3. Fats are changed to fatty acids, monoglycerides, diglycerides, and a few triglycerides.
4. Up to 8 liters of fluid are absorbed daily by the small intestine.
5. Glucose, water-soluble vitamins, protein, and fat are absorbed primarily in the jejunum.
6. Vitamin B_{12} absorption takes place in the ileum provided that the stomach has secreted intrinsic factor and that calcium ions are present.
7. Iron absorption occurs in the duodenum and jejunum.

F. Motor activity:
1. Chyme normally moves forward at a rate of about one to two cm/minute and remains in the small intestine from three to 10 hours.
2. Principal movements of the small intestine are peristalsis and mixing (or segmental) contractions.

LARGE INTESTINE
(Figure 10.2)

A. Extends from the ileocecal valve to the anus and is approximately five to six feet long and is two inches in diameter
B. Divided into three segments:
1. Cecum:
   a. Comprises the first two to three inches of the large intestine; connects with the ileum and the ileocecal valve
   b. The distal end of the cecum forms a blind pouch to which is attached the vermiform appendix located in the right lower quadrant of the abdomen.

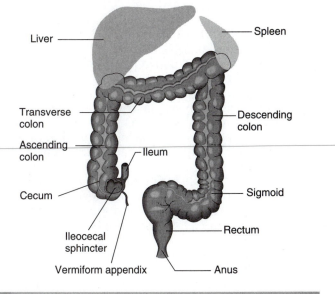

Figure 10.2 Structures of the Colon

2. Colon:
   a. Approximately 4 to 5 feet long and consists of the ascending, transverse, descending, and sigmoid colon
   b. Hepatic flexure is at the juncture of the ascending and transverse colon.
   c. The splenic flexure is at the juncture of the distal portion of the transverse colon and the descending colon.
3. Rectum:
   a. Final segment of the large intestine
   b. Extends from the sigmoid colon to the anal opening
   c. Internal and external sphincters control the opening of the anus

C. Functions:
1. Absorbs the remaining water, urea, and electrolytes (sodium and chloride)
2. Reduces the volume of chyme from 500 cc in the cecum to 100 cc of fluid in the feces
3. Secretes mucus in the proximal half
4. Stores feces in the distal half until defecation

D. Flora:
1. The alkaline environment of the intestines permits the growth of organisms whose function is to break down remaining proteins and indigestible residue.
2. Organisms include E. coli, A aerogenes, Clostridium perfringes, and Lactobacillus.
3. Intestinal bacteria convert urea into ammonium salts and ammonia.

HEPATIC, BILIARY, AND PANCREATIC SYSTEM

Major functions are to produce, detoxify, and store substances that aid in the digestion, absorption, and use of nutrients by the body.

Liver
(Figure 10.3)

A. Largest organ in the body located in the upper-right quadrant of the abdomen just below the diaphragm
B. Blood is circulated through the liver by means of the hepatic portal system.
C. Functions:
1. Production of bile from bilirubin (byproduct of hemoglobin breakdown)
2. Glycogenesis, the conversion of glucose to glycogen
3. Glycogenolysis, the breakdown of glycogen into glucose
4. Gluconeogenesis, the conversion of non-carbohydrate substances into glucose
5. Synthesizes fat from protein and carbohydrates

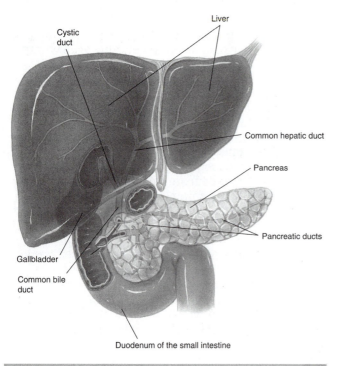

Cystic duct

Liver

Common hepatic duct

Pancreas

Pancreatic ducts

Gallbladder

Common bile duct

Duodenum of the small intestine

Figure 10.3 Liver, Gallbladder, and Pancreas

6. Deamination of amino acids (converts ammonia into urea, which is excreted by the kidneys and intestines)
7. Makes plasma proteins such as albumin, prothrombin, fibrinogen, and clotting proteins
8. Detoxifies hormones, drugs, and other chemicals
9. Serves as a reservoir of blood for use in time of major systemic blood loss
10. Contains Kupffer cells (part of the phagocyte system), which serve as filters to remove bacteria and other debris from the blood as it enters the portal system

Gallbladder
(Figure 10.3)

A. Small pear-shaped sac located just under the right lobe of the liver that serves as a reservoir for bile produced in the liver
B. Bile is transported from the liver by the right and left hepatic ducts; bile is concentrated in the gallbladder and released into the small intestine via the cystic duct and empties into the common bile duct.
C. The presence of fat in the stomach stimulates the secretion of cholecystokinin from the small intestine, causing the gallbladder to contract and the sphincter of Oddi (in the duodenum) to relax, allowing bile to enter the small intestine to aid in fat digestion.

Pancreas
(Figure 10.3)

A. Fish-shaped, grayish-pink gland that stretches horizontally across the posterior abdominal wall in the epigastric and hypochondriac areas of the body
B. Normally produces 1,200 to 3,000 mL of pancreatic juices daily
C. Pancreatic juice is a clear, alkaline solution that includes three major types of digestive enzymes:
  1. Amylase breaks down carbohydrates.
  2. Lipase breaks down fats.
  3. Trypsin breaks down proteins.

DIAGNOSTIC PROCEDURES

A. Upper GI X-rays; Barium Swallow
  1. Radiopaque substance (barium) swallowed at beginning of test
  2. Outlines esophagus and stomach
  3. Client should be NPO for 8 hours before test
B. Lower GI X-rays; Barium Enema
  1. Radiopaque substance (barium) given via enema
  2. Outlines colon
  3. Preparation of client
    a. Laxatives and/or enemas given day before test
    b. Clear liquid or low-residue diet day before test
    c. Encourage client to drink adequate fluids to prevent dehydration
C. Esophagogastroduodenoscopy (EGD)
  1. Visualization of the esophagus, stomach, and duodenum by means of a lighted tube
  2. Client should be NPO for 6–8 hours prior to test
  3. Client will be sedated
D. Sigmoidoscopy
  1. Visualization of the sigmoid colon by means of a lighted tube
  2. Client should take a packaged enema one hour before the procedure.
E. Analysis of Secretions
  1. Gastric analysis; gastric secretions removed via NG tube
  2. Tubeless gastric analysis: ingestion of dye which is displaced by acid and secreted in urine
F. Analysis of stools for culture, fat, and guaiac
G. Cholecystogram (Gallbladder Series)
  1. Check for allergy to seafood or iodine
  2. Telepaque (Diodrast) tablets 12 hours before test
  3. Low-fat diet
  4. NPO after midnight
  5. Dye conjugated in the liver and excreted into the bile, which outlines the gallbladder

6. Poor or no visualization of gallbladder if disease is present
H. Gallbladder sonogram
   1. Sound waves used to visualize abdominal structures
   2. No preparation necessary
I. Cholangiogram
   1. Check for allergy to iodine and seafood
   2. Bile ducts visualized
J. Liver Biopsy
   1. No aspirin or nonsteroidal antiinflammatory drugs (NSAIDs), such as ibuprofen or naproxen sodium, for one week before procedure to prevent excessive bleeding
   2. Clotting studies should be done before the test because the liver makes clotting factors.
   3. Position on left side during biopsy so liver is accessible
   4. Position on right side with bath towel or blanket supporting biopsy site for two hours after biopsy to provide hemostasis and decrease bleeding
   5. Bed rest for 24 hours after biopsy to decrease likelihood of hemorrhage
   6. Observe biopsy site for ecchymosis
K. Paracentesis
   1. Removal of fluid accumulated in the peritoneum; performed diagnostically to examine contents of peritoneal fluid; therapeutic removal of fluid relieves dyspnea
   2. Client should void immediately before test so bladder is not in the abdominal cavity
   3. During procedure, position client sitting up with feet resting on a stool
   4. Maintain client on bed rest following procedure
   5. Apply dry, sterile dressing to the site and observe for drainage.
   6. Monitor vital signs.
L. Liver Function Tests
   1. Bilirubin
      a. 0.1–1.0 mg/dl
      b. Measures bilirubin in the blood. Elevated levels indicate that the liver is not removing bilirubin from the blood as it should.
   2. Total Protein
      a. 6.4–8.3 g/dl
      b. Total measure of albumin and globulin, proteins made by the liver
      c. Instruct client to avoid high-fat foods for 24 hours before the test.
   3. Serum albumin
      a. 3.5–5.0 g/dl
      b. Albumin is a protein made by the liver and is responsible for colloidal osmotic pressure.
   4. Serum globulin
      a. 2.3–3.3 g/dl
      b. Globulin is made by the liver and is important for antibody production.
   5. Alkaline phosphatase
      a. 30-85 InU/ml
      b. Enzyme found in liver tissue, released during liver damage
      c. Fasting may be required.
   6. Prothrombin time
      a. 11–12.5 seconds
      b. Prothrombin, a clotting factor, is made in the liver; elevated levels occur with liver damage.
   7. Blood ammonia
      a. 15–110 µg/dl
      b. The liver normally converts ammonia into urea, which is then secreted by the kidneys; in liver disease the levels will rise.
   8. BUN (blood urea nitrogen)
      a. 10–20 mg/dl
      b. Urea is formed in the liver as the end product of protein metabolism; people with severe primary liver disease will have a decreased BUN.
   9. Serum transaminase studies: SGOT (AST), SGPT (ALT), LDH
      a. Enzymes produced by the liver
      b. Rise in response to liver damage and damage to cardiac muscle and skeletal muscle
   10. Cholesterol
      a. 150–200 mg/dl
      b. Made in the liver
      c. Increased in bile duct obstruction; decreased with severe liver damage
      d. Client should fast for 12–14 hours before test with a low-fat diet before the fast; no alcohol for 24 hours before the test
   11. Gamma-glutamyl Transpeptidase (GGT or GGPT)
      a. Females < 45 years 5–27 U/l; females < 45 years and males 8–38 U/l
      b. Enzyme that detects liver cell dysfunction
      c. Client should fast for 8 hours before test
   12. HB_5AG (Hepatitis B Surface Antigen)
      a. Should be negative
      b. Positive result indicates presence of hepatitis or prior exposure
M. Carcinoembryonic antigen (CEA)
   1. < 5 ng/ml
   2. Protein present in blood stream with some gastrointestinal tract cancers; elevated levels after removal of cancer may indicate a return of cancer.

Related Procedures

ENEMAS

A. Instillation of fluid into the rectum, usually for the purpose of stimulating defecation

B. Types
1. Cleansing enema:
   a. Tap water, normal saline, or soap
   b. Used to treat constipation or fecal impaction, as bowel cleansing before diagnostic procedures or surgery, or to help establish regular bowel functions
2. Retention enema:
   a. Mineral oil, olive oil, cottonseed oil
   b. Used to lubricate or soften a hard fecal mass to facilitate defecation; may be used prior to cleansing enema in persons with fecal impaction

C. Nursing care for a cleansing enema (see Table 10.1)

D. Nursing care for a retention enema; same as cleansing enema except:
1. Oil is used instead of water; usually comes in a prepared kit; administered at body temperature.
2. Administer 150–200 ml of prepared solution
3. Instruct client to retain oil for at least 30 minutes to allow for adequate softening of feces

Table 10.1 Procedure for a Cleansing Enema

1. Explain the procedure.
2. Teach the client to breathe through his or her mouth to help relax the abdominal muscles and prevent cramping.
3. Assemble equipment and prepare solution so temperature is 105–110°F; be sure bedpan, commode, or bathroom is readily available.
4. Place waterproof pad under buttocks.
5. Lubricate tube with water-soluble lubricant and allow solution to fill the tubing, displacing air.
6. With rubber gloves on, insert rectal tube 4–5 inches without using force; have client take several deep breaths during insertion of rectal tube.
7. Administer solution (usually 500–1000 ml) over 5–10 minutes; if cramping occurs, slow the speed of administration of the solution.
8. After administration, have the client retain solution until urge to defecate is very strong (15–30 minutes).
9. Record amount, color, characteristics of stool, and client's response to procedure.
10. Assess for dizziness, light-headedness, abdominal cramps, or nausea.
11. Monitor electrolyte levels if client is receiving repeated enemas.

GASTROINTESTINAL INTUBATION

A. Types
1. Nasogastric tubes
   a. Types
      (1) Levin (single lumen, nonvented stomach tube)
      (2) Salem pump (stomach tube; tube within a tube, vented to provide constant inflow of atmospheric air)
   b. Nursing care:
      (1) Before passing tube, measure tube from tip of nose to tip of ear lobe to tip of xyphoid process and mark
      (2) Lubricate tube with water soluble lubricant
      (3) With client sitting upright, advance tube through nose and nasopharynx
      (4) When passing tube through oropharynx, have client bend forward and sip water through a straw so tube will pass easily into the esophagus
      (5) Test for placement by aspirating gastric contents and checking for acid pH.
2. Nasoenteric tubes
   a. Miller-Abbott: double lumen weighted tubes
   b. Cantor: single lumen weighted tube
   c. Nursing care:
      (1) After tube is passed through pyloric, sphincter tube is advanced 5–7.5 cm (2 to 3 in) every hour
      (2) To facilitate gravity and peristalsis, position the client on his or her right side for two hours, his or her back for two hours, and on the left side for two hours.
      (3) Ambulation, if permitted, helps passage of tube
      (4) Tape tube in place only after placement in small intestine is confirmed by X-ray; usually about 24 hours
3. Sengstaken-Blakemore (triple-lumen tube used to treat bleeding esophageal varices)
4. Nasogastric Tube Feeding/Irrigation
   a. May be given as intermittent bolus feedings or continuous infusion
   b. Assess placement by aspirating contents and assessing for acid pH
   c. Position client in semi-Fowler's position

d. Check for residual before each bolus feeding and every 4–8 hours for continuous feeding; delay feeding if residual is more than 100 ml
e. Nose and mouth care
f. Use correct solution for irrigation, usually normal saline
g. To prevent clogging of tube, administer 50 ml water before and after each dose of medication and each tube feeding, after checking gastric residuals and pH, and every 4–6 hours with continuous feedings
h. Weigh client two or three times/week
i. Monitor intake and output.

GASTROSTOMY TUBE

A. Anterior wall of the stomach is sutured to the abdominal wall and the tube is sutured in place.
B. Initial feedings are small (30–60 ml) feedings of water and 10% glucose; water and milk are instilled after 24 hours; blenderized foods are gradually added to clear liquids until full diet is reached.
C. Plug tube after feeding instilled to prevent leakage; apply dressing.
D. Evaluate skin daily: wash with soap and water, apply zinc oxide or petrolatum ointment; report signs of skin breakdown.
E. Teach client proper technique for gastrostomy feeding:
   1. Assess for residual gastric contents.
   2. Flush with water before and after feeding.
   3. Hold container with feeding no higher than 18 inches above stomach; usually takes 10–15 minutes for bolus feeding of 200 to 500 ml.

TOTAL PARENTERAL NUTRITION

A. Intravenous administration of a hypertonic solution of glucose, nitrogen, and other nutrients to achieve positive nitrogen balance; intravenous catheter is inserted into subclavian vein by physician.
B. Hickman, Broviac, or Groshong central catheters are often used for long-term use.
C. Indications:
   1. Inability of the GI tract to absorb nutrients adequately: malabsorption syndromes, GI obstruction, paralytic ileus, bowel resection, ulcerative colitis
   2. Inability to take food by mouth; coma or anorexia nervosa

Table 10.2 Nursing Diagnoses Related to Total Parenteral Nutrition

- Imbalanced nutrition, less than body requirements, related to inadequate intake of nutrients
- Risk for infection related to contamination of the catheter site or infusion line
- Risk for fluid volume excess or deficit related to altered infusion rate
- Deficient knowledge about home TPN therapy

   3. Excessive nutritional needs that cannot be met by the usual methods: burns, multiple fractures, carcinoma being treated with chemotherapy or radiation, severe infections
D. Nursing diagnoses (see Table 10.2)
E. Nursing care:
   1. Explain procedure to client and tell him that he will be instructed to perform a Valsalva maneuver (have client practice) when catheter is inserted.
   2. Teach client that the area must be kept as clean as possible at all times and that he should not touch the area or pull at the catheter.
   3. If client is ambulatory, tell him that once the catheter is in place, he will be able to continue to ambulate pushing an IV pole.
   4. Prior to procedure, place client in a Trendelenburg position with shoulder hyperextended.
   5. Provide sterile catheter setup tray for the physician; assist with procedure; get client ready for X-ray.
   6. Refrigerate TPN solutions until used.
   7. TPN solutions are always run on a controlled infusion pump at a rate ordered by the physician.
   8. Once infusion is begun, check the infusion rate every 30 minutes; if the client has not received as much as ordered over time, do not try to "catch up" by increasing the rate.
   9. Vital signs every four hours; more often if indicated.
   10. Daily weights, strict I & O, and urines or blood sugar (TPN is a hypertonic glucose solution).
   11. V tubing and filter are changed according to hospital protocol (24 hours).
   12. Dressing changed every 24–48 hours using strict aseptic technique.
   13. Assess insertion site for evidence of infection.
   14. Assess for signs of air embolism.

Disorders of the Gastrointestinal System

NAUSEA AND VOMITING

A. Nausea: a feeling of discomfort in the epigastrum with a conscious desire to vomit
B. Vomiting: forceful ejection of stomach contents from the upper GI tract. Emetic center in medulla is stimulated by things such as local irritation of intestine or stomach or disturbance of equilibrium, causing the vomiting reflex.
C. Nausea and vomiting occur in many conditions: GI problems, central nervous system disorders, metabolic disorders, response to motion, response to pain, and/or side effects of drugs, such as cancer chemotherapy and antibiotics.

Table 10.3 Nursing Diagnoses Related to Nausea and Vomiting

- Impaired comfort related to nausea and vomiting secondary to (specify)
- Risk for imbalanced nutrition: less than body requirements related to nausea and vomiting
- Fluid volume deficit related to nausea and vomiting
- Impaired oral mucous membrane related to dehydration secondary to nausea and vomiting

D. Assessment findings:
   1. Signs of dehydration: dry mucous membrane, poor skin turgor
   2. Electrolyte imbalances; serum sodium, calcium, potassium decreased
   3. Weakness, fatigue, pallor, lethargy
E. Nursing diagnoses (see Table 10.3)
F. Interventions:
   1. Maintain NPO until client is able to tolerate oral fluids
   2. Start oral fluids with clear liquids (ginger ale, warm tea, popsicles) in small amounts; gradually introduce solid foods (toast, crackers) in small amounts.
   3. Administer antiemetics as ordered and monitor effects and side effects (see Table 10.4).
   4. Notify physician or charge nurse if vomiting pattern changes.
   5. Promote fluid and electrolyte balance:
      a. Client may have IV fluids.
      b. Maintain accurate intake and output, including amount and characteristics of vomitus.

DIARRHEA

A. The rapid movement of fecal matter through the intestine, resulting in poor absorption of

Table 10.4 Antiemetics

Drug	Action & Nursing Care	Side Effects
Antihistamines		
Benzquinamide (Emete-Con)	Antiemetic, antihistamine, and anticholinergic	Drowsiness, dizziness, dry mouth, blurred vision
Dimenhydrinate (Dramamine) promethazine (Phenergan) diphenhydramine (Benadryl) cyclizine (Marezine) meclizine (Antivert) hydroxyzine (Atarax, Vistaril)	Used to prevent motion sickness; administer before nausea occurs	
Phenothiazines		
Prochlorperazine (Compazine) chlorpromazine (Thorazine) perphenazine (Trilafon)	Depresses vomiting center in brain	Drowsiness, dizziness, hypotension
trifluoperazine (Stelazine) Metoclopramide HCl (Reglan)	Stimulates motility of the upper GI tract; blocks dopamine receptors at the chemoreceptor trigger zone; administer before cancer chemotherapy	Drowsiness, dizziness, dry mouth, blurred vision
Ondansetron (Zofran)	Used to prevent nausea and vomiting associated with cancer chemotherapy and surgery	Drowsiness, dizziness, dry mouth, blurred vision
Ganisetron (Kytril)	Administer 30 minutes before cancer chemotherapy and radiation therapy to prevent nausea and vomiting	Temporary taste disorder

water and nutrients and producing abnormally frequent evacuation of watery stools
B. Diarrhea is a symptom that may occur with many conditions: chronic bowel disorders, malabsorption conditions, intestinal infections, neoplasms, foods, stress, tube feedings, and medications such as magnesium-based antacids and antibiotics.
C. Assessment findings:
   1. Abdominal cramps, distention
   2. Frequent, foul-smelling, watery stools
   3. Anorexia, thirst, tenesmus (ineffectual and painful straining at stool)
   4. Electrolyte imbalances (decreased sodium and potassium) if severe
D. Interventions:
   1. Have client avoid foods causing diarrhea: milk and milk products
   2. Provide adequate fluids; gradually add bland, high-protein, high-calorie, low-fat, low-bulk foods
   3. Maintain accurate intake and output including amount and characteristics of each stool
   4. Provide good skin care:
     a. Cleanse rectal area with mild soap and water and pat dry after each bowel movement.
     b. Apply A and D ointment or Desitin to promote healing.
     c. Use a local anesthetic as needed.
   5. Administer medications as ordered (see Table 10.5)

CONSTIPATION

A. Infrequent, small, dry, hard stools as a result of decreased motility of the colon or from retention of feces in the colon or rectum
B. May be caused by many things: not enough fiber and fluids in the diet, not enough physical activity, barium retention after X-ray studies, prolonged use of laxatives
C. Assessment findings:
   1. Feeling of abdominal fullness, abdominal distention, pressure in the rectum
   2. Increased flatus
   3. Hardened stool upon digital exam
D. Interventions:
   1. Promote adequate intake of fluids (3,000 ml/day) and fiber-containing foods.
   2. Encourage physical exercise and activity.
   3. Encourage client not to suppress the urge to defecate.
   4. Massage abdomen to promote peristalsis and movement of feces.
   5. Administer medications as ordered (see Table 10.6).
F. Nursing care
   1. Do not give laxatives if abdominal pain, nausea, or vomiting is present or if an intestinal obstruction is suspected.
   2. Avoid over-administration—laxatives should be used for a week or less to prevent the development of dependence.

Table 10.5 Antidiarrheals

Drug	Action & Nursing Care	Side Effects
Bismuth subsalicylate (PeptoBismol)	Has a water-binding capacity and provides a protective coating for intestinal mucosa; contains a high quantity of salicylates; use with caution in persons who are taking other salicylates (aspirin products); may be used in the treatment of helicobacter pylori infection	Bismuth is a heavy metal and should not be used in patients who are receiving radiation therapy; heavy metals may block radiation
Kaolin—Pectate (Kaopectate)	Decreases the water loss in stools; may cause constipation	Kaopectate should not be given if obstructive bowel lesions are suspected.
Loperamide (Imodium)	Loperamide inhibits peristalsis, making intestinal contents take longer to pass through (causing stools to be more firm).	Antidiarrheals should not be used for more than two days without consulting a physician; should not be used in acute diarrhea due to poisons until the toxic material is removed from the GI tract.
Diphenoxylate with atropine (Lomotil)	Lomotil increases smooth muscle tone in the GI tract, inhibits motility, and diminishes gastric secretions; an opium derivative and a controlled substance	Physical dependence may occur, especially when used in large amounts over a period of time; to decrease the risk of physical dependence, atropine is included in the drug; sedation, dizziness, dry mouth, and paralytic ileus
Opium tincture (Paregoric)	Paregoric is a controlled substance because it is opium.	Physical dependence in long-term use, nausea and vomiting, and respiratory depression; monitor respirations

Table 10.6 Laxatives

Drug	Action & Nursing Care	Side Effects
Hyperosmolar or saline cathartics; magnesium citrate; milk of magnesia; potassium citrate; glycerin	Increase the bulk of the stools by attracting and holding large amounts of fluids; give with fluid to prevent dehydration; do not give magnesium to a person in renal failure	Do not give laxatives when the patient has abdominal pain, nausea, vomiting, or other symptoms of appendicitis or intestinal obstruction; avoid over-administration of laxatives
Bowel evacuant; Polyethylene glycol—electrolyte solution (CoLyte, GoLytely, OCL, NuLytely, Colovage)	Induces diarrhea and clean bowel in an electrolyte-sparing manner; used prior to surgery and diagnostic tests; clients must follow directions regarding fluid intake	
Bulk forming; methylcellulose (Cologel); psyllium hydrophilic muciloid (Metamucil)	Increased bulk of the feces stimulating peristalsis by mechanical means; safest of all laxatives	
Emollient—stool softener; docusate salts (Colace, Surfak)	Exerts detergent activity; decreases surface tension of feces and promotes penetration by water and fat; used to prevent constipation, not to treat it; used when straining at stool is contraindicated—MI, rectal surgery, eye surgery, postpartum hemorrhage	
Stimulant; Bisacodyl (Dulcolax); Cascara sagrada; Castor oil; Senna (Senokot)	Acts directly on the smooth muscle of the intestine, stimulating peristalsis	

Table 10.7 Nursing Diagnoses Related to Hiatal Hernia

- Risk for altered health maintenance related to insufficient knowledge of condition, dietary management, hazards of alcohol and tobacco, positioning after meals, pharmacological therapy, and weight reduction (if indicated)
- Pain: heartburn related to regurgitation and eructation
- Risk for altered nutrition: less than body requirements related to anorexia and heartburn

3. Encourage patients to eat a diet high in fiber and to have an adequate fluid intake to promote proper bowel function.
4. Be sure that the client has plenty of fluids.

HIATAL HERNIA

A. Portion of the stomach is herniated through the esophageal hiatus of the diaphragm
B. Assessment findings:
1. Heartburn
2. Dysphagia
C. Nursing diagnoses (see Table 10.7)
D. Interventions:
1. Small, frequent meals
2. High-fiber diet, increased fluids to prevent constipation
3. Upright position during and after meals
4. Head of bed elevated at night
5. Antacids as ordered for heartburn
6. Avoid coughing, bending, straining, smoking, and alcoholic beverages.
7. Wear non-constricting clothing.

8. Avoid anticholinergics such as probanthine, because these make it more difficult for the sphincter to remain closed.
9. Surgery if condition is severe

PEPTIC ULCER DISEASE

Ulcerations of the mucous membrane of the esophagus, stomach, or duodenum caused by the action of the acid gastric juice. There are two kinds of peptic ulcers: gastric and duodenal.

Gastric Ulcers

A. Ulceration of the mucosal lining of the stomach, often in the antrum; caused by Helicobacter pylori. Predisposing factors include smoking, alcohol abuse, emotional tension, and medications such as salicylates, nonsteroidal anti-inflammatory drugs (NSAIDs), and steroids.
B. Assessment findings:
1. Left epigastric pain sometimes radiating to the back 1–2 hours after eating
2. Eating does not relieve pain; weight loss
3. Anemia if bleeding
4. Endoscopy or upper GI series shows ulceration in stomach
5. Blood test positive for Helicobacter pylori
C. Nursing diagnoses (see Table 10.8)
D. Interventions:
1. Stress reduction
2. Teach client about dietary alterations:
   a. Avoid stimulants (caffeine, spices, chocolate, nicotine) and alcohol
   b. Small, frequent meals

Table 10.8 Nursing Diagnoses Related to Peptic Ulcers
- Acute pain related to stomach lesions secondary to increased gastric secretions
- Risk for ineffective health maintenance related to insufficient knowledge of condition, dietary restrictions, contraindications (certain medications, tobacco, caffeine, or alcohol), stress-related factors, and signs and symptoms of complications
- Risk for constipation/diarrhea related to effects of medications on bowel function
- Risk for deficient fluid volume related to hemorrhage
- Fear/anxiety related to change in health status and threat of death

3. Administer ulcer medications as ordered (see Table 10.9):
   a. Antacids
   b. Histamine antagonists
   c. Antisecretory
   d. Anticholinergics
   e. Sucralfate
   f. Antibiotics such as metronidazole (Flagyl) and clarithromycin (Biaxin)

Duodenal Ulcers

A. Ulceration of the mucosal lining of the duodenum, usually in the first 2 cm, caused by Helicobacter pylori. Predisposing factors include smoking, alcohol abuse, emotional tension, and medications such as salicylates, NSAIDs, and steroids.
B. Assessment findings:
   1. Midepigastric pain usually described as burning, cramping, or boring; usually occurs 2–4 hours after eating and is relieved by food
   2. Weight gain may occur as client "feeds the ulcer"
   3. Anemia if bleeding
   4. Endoscopy or upper GI series shows ulceration in duodenum
   5. Blood test positive for Helicobacter pylori
C. Nursing diagnoses (see Table 10.8)
D. Interventions:
   1. Stress reduction
   2. Teach client about dietary alterations:
      a. Avoid stimulants (caffeine, spices, chocolate, nicotine) and alcohol
      b. Frequent meals
   3. Administer ulcer medications as ordered (see Table 10.9):
      a. Antacids
      b. Histamine antagonists
      c. Antisecretory
      d. Anticholinergics
      e. Sucralfate
      f. Antibiotics such as metronidazole (Flagyl) and clarithromycin (Biaxin)

CANCER OF THE STOMACH

A. Cancer usually develops in the distal third of the stomach and may spread through the walls of the stomach into adjacent tissues, lymphatics, regional lymph nodes, other abdominal organs, or through the bloodstream to the lungs and bones; client usually has had helicobacter pylori infections.
B. Assessment findings:
   1. Indigestion, nausea, vomiting
   2. Weight loss
   3. Gastric fullness and later pain
   4. Stool positive for occult blood
   5. Decreased Hgb and Hct
   6. Positive cancer embryonic antigen (CEA)
   7. Histologic changes seen with gastric analysis
C. Nursing diagnoses (see Table 10.10)
D. Interventions:
   1. Allow expression of feelings
   2. Assist the client and family through the grieving process.
   3. Assess dietary pattern and caloric intake.
   4. Provide supplemental feedings as ordered.
   5. Chemotherapy (see p. 55)
   6. Radiation (see p. 57)
   7. Surgery: subtotal or total gastrectomy (see gastric surgery)
   8. Treatment for anemia
   9. Total parenteral nutritional as needed
   10. Monitor electrolyte balance.

GASTRIC SURGERY

A. Surgery performed for peptic ulcer disease that does not respond to treatment or for gastric cancer
B. Procedures:
   1. Gastroduodenostomy (Billroth I): removal of the lower portion of the stomach with anastomosis of the remaining portion of the duodenum
   2. Gastrojejunostomy (Billroth II): removal of the antrum and distal portion of the stomach and duodenum with anastomosis of the remaining portion of the stomach to the jejunum
   3. Gastrectomy: removal of 60%–80% of the stomach
   4. Esophagojejunostomy (total gastrectomy): removal of the entire stomach with a loop of jejunum anastomosed to the esophagus
C. Interventions:
   1. Provide postop care.
   2. Care of nasogastric tube:
      a. Measure drainage accurately; notify charge nurse or physician if no drainage.

Table 10.9 Medications used in the treatment of peptic ulcer

Drug	Action	Side Effects	Nursing Implications
Antacids	Neutralizes gastric acidity; available as tablets and liquid		Chew tablets thoroughly before swallowing and follow with a full glass of water; liquid antacids should be followed by a full glass of water for best action
Magnesium-containing antacids; Milk of Magnesia	Neutralizes gastric acid; provides pain relief	Diarrhea, hypermagnesemia, nausea, and vomiting	Should be taken after meals and h.s.; do not give to persons with renal failure
Aluminum-containing antacids (Amphojel)	Neutralizes gastric acid; provides pain relief	Constipation, fecal impaction, hypophosphatemia, hypercalcemia; interferes with absorption of anticholinergics	Should be taken after meals; observe for constipation
Aluminum-magnesium combination; Magaldrate (Riopan), Maalox, DiGel	Neutralizes gastric acid; provides pain relief	Less diarrhea and constipation	Should be taken after meals
Sodium-containing antacids; Dihydroxy-aluminum sodium carbonate (Rolaids)	Neutralizes gastric acid; provides pain relief	High sodium content may cause sodium and water retention	Do not give to clients on low-sodium diets or pregnant women (may aggravate PIH)
Calcium-containing antacids (Tums)	Neutralizes gastric acid; provides pain relief	Hypercalcemia and hypophosphatemia; can cause rebound hyperacidity	Do not give to persons with severe renal disease; should not be administered with milk or other foods high in Vitamin D
Histamine (H_2) Antagonists	Decreases the acidity of the stomach by blocking the action of histamine; histamine triggers gastric acid secretion		Can be taken for up to two months to treat ulcers
Cimetidine (Tagamet)	As above	Diarrhea, dizziness, confusion, drowsiness, headache, elevated liver function tests, impotence	Monitor liver function tests; antacids decrease absorption of cimetidine; allow at least one hr between cimetidine and antacids; administer with meals
Ranitidine (Zantac)	As above	Vertigo, malaise, blurred vision, jaundice, anaphylaxis; possible interference with action of warfarin	Antacids decrease absorption of ranitidine; allow at least one hr between ranitidine and antacids; incompatible with aluminum; most effective if taken at bedtime; absorption not affected by food
Famotidine (Pepcid)	As above	Headache, dizziness, tinnitus, taste disorder, diarrhea, constipation, anorexia, dry mouth, acne, flushing	Most effective if taken at bedtime; available OTC; limit use to two weeks
Anticholinergics: Atropine, dicyclomine (Bentyl), Belladonna Methaneline bromide (Banthine), Propantheline bromide (Probanthine), glycopyrrolate (Robinul)	Decreases gastric secretions and motility; delays gastric emptying; slows peristalsis	Headache, insomnia, drowsiness, blurred vision, increased pulse, postural blood pressure changes, dry mouth and throat, thirst, constipation, nausea, paralytic ileus, urinary hesitancy and retention, impotence, diaphoresis, urticaria	Take 30 minutes before meals; antacids may interfere with absorption of anticholinergics; client should avoid driving and should change positions slowly; drink plenty of fluids and suck hard candy to relieve dryness of mouth; assess for abdominal distention; have client void before each dose; use cautiously in a hot environment
Sucralfate (Carafate)	Reacts with gastric acid to form a paste that adheres to GI mucosa and allows the ulcer to heal	Constipation, diarrhea, nausea, indigestion, rash, and itching; binds with other medications	Administer one hour before meals and at bedtime; wait two hrs after giving other meds before giving sucralfate
Nizatidine (Axid)	As above	Sleepiness, arrhythmias, diaphoresis	Avoid tomato-based mixed vegetable juices because they decrease the potency of the drug; use with caution in persons with renal disease
Antisecretory Omeprazole (Prilosec)	Blocks formation of gastric acid; it is not a histamine blocker	Headache, dizziness, fatigue, diarrhea, abdominal pain, nausea, skin rash	Instruct patient to swallow capsules whole and not crush or open capsule; take capsules before eating; antacids can be taken with Prilosec

Table 10.10 Nursing Diagnoses Related to Stomach Cancer

- Imbalanced nutrition: less than body requirements related to difficulty swallowing, poor absorption of nutrients, and nausea and vomiting from chemotherapy drugs
- Anticipatory grieving with related feelings of guilt, anger, sadness, and/or denial
- Acute pain related to disease process
- Impaired home maintenance related to debilitation, lack of resources, and/or inadequate support systems
- Fear/anxiety related to situational crises, threat to health/socioeconomic status, role functioning, threat of death, separation from family
- Risk for deficient fluid volume related to vomiting from disease process or chemotherapy drugs
- Impaired oral mucous membrane related to side effects of chemotherapy
- Disturbed body image related to loss of hair from chemotherapy and loss of weight secondary to disease process

    b. Drainage will be bright red for 12–24 hours.
3. Promote respiratory function.
    a. Position the client in mid or high Fowler's position.
    b. Teach the client to splint the upper abdomen before turning, deep-breathing, or coughing.
4. Promote adequate nutrition.
    a. After NG tube removed, provide clear liquids with gradual progression to bland foods
    b. Daily weights
    c. Assess for regurgitation; if present, instruct client to eat smaller amounts of food more slowly
5. Manage "dumping syndrome" (the rapid passage of food from the stomach to small intestine because there is no longer a sphincter).
    a. Assessment findings:
      (1) Dizziness, sweating, nausea, and diarrhea may occur 5–30 min after eating; thought to be due to rapid fluid shifts.
      (2) Symptoms of hypoglycemia (pallor, cool and moist skin) may occur 2–3 hours after eating.
    b. Teach client to avoid salty, high-carbohydrate foods and eat high protein, low carbohydrate, high-fiber foods; avoid liquids with meals; lie down after meals.
    c. Administer antispasmodics as ordered.
6. Provide discharge teaching concerning
    a. Managing dumping syndrome and gradually increasing food intake until able to tolerate three meals a day.
    b. Monitoring weight on a daily basis.
    c. Need to report signs of complications to physician immediately: vomiting, blood in vomitus or stools, diarrhea, pain, weakness, feeling of abdominal fullness
    d. Managing dumping syndrome as described above

HERNIAS

A. Abnormal protrusion of part of an organ or tissue through the structures normally containing it; occurs most frequently in the abdominal cavity
B. Kinds:
    1. Reducible: can be returned by manipulation
    2. Irreducible: cannot be returned by manipulation
    3. Strangulated: irreducible with obstruction to intestinal flow and blood supply
    4. Inguinal: weakness in the abdominal wall where the spermatic cord in men and round ligament in women emerge
    5. Femoral: protrusion through the femoral ring
    6. Incisional: occurs at the site of a previous surgical incision as a result of inadequate healing
    7. Umbilical: protrusion of part of the intestine at the umbilicus, seen most often in infants
C. Assessment findings:
    1. Vomiting
    2. Protrusion of involved area and discomfort at site of protrusion
    3. Abdominal pain and abdominal distention if strangulated, resulting in bowel obstruction
D. Interventions:
    1. Manual reduction; truss or support
    2. Bowel surgery if strangulated
    3. Herniorrhaphy: surgical repair of the hernia by suturing the defect
    4. Post-op nursing care:
      a. Assess for distended bladder
      b. Deep-breathe but no coughing to prevent injury to the site
      c. Splint incision when coughing or sneezing
      d. Ice bags to scrotal area to reduce swelling (inguinal hernia repair)
      e. Scrotal support (inguinal hernia repair)
      f. No strenuous physical activities for six weeks postop

APPENDICITIS

A. Inflammation of the vermiform appendix, usually requiring surgery

B. Assessment findings:
  1. Pain starting in the umbilicus, becoming localized in the right lower quadrant (RLQ) around McBurney's point
  2. Rigid abdomen, guarding, and rebound tenderness
  3. Nausea and vomiting
  4. Low-grade fever
  5. Elevated WBC (14,000–16,000; above 20,000 suggests peritonitis)
  6. Decreased or absent bowel sounds
C. Nursing diagnoses (see Table 10.11)
D. Interventions:
  1. No heat, laxatives, enemas if appendicitis suspected
  2. Appendectomy
  3. Post-op nursing care
     a. Routine postop nursing care
     b. Drains if appendix ruptured
     c. Position in semi-Fowler's to promote drainage and prevent tension on suture line
     d. Promote fluid balance

CHRONIC INFLAMMATORY BOWEL DISORDERS

Regional Enteritis (Crohn's Disease)

A. Chronic inflammatory bowel disease that can affect both the large and small intestines; terminal ileum, cecum, and ascending colon most often involved. Characterized by granulomas that may affect all bowel wall layers, resulting in thickening, narrowing, and scarring of the intestinal wall. Affects both sexes; more common in the Jewish population. Cause is unknown; may be genetic, autoimmune, or infection.
B. Assessment findings:
  1. Right lower quadrant tenderness and pain
  2. Abdominal distention
  3. Nausea and vomiting
  4. Several semisoft stools/day with mucus and pus
  5. Decreased skin turgor, dry mucus membranes
  6. Increased peristalsis
  7. Pallor
  8. Diagnostic tests
     a. Decreased Hgb and Hct if anemia present
     b. Sigmoidoscopy may be normal or show scattered ulcers.
     c. Barium enema or colonoscopy shows narrowing of bowel with areas of strictures separated by segments of normal bowel.
C. Nursing diagnoses (see Table 10.12)

Table 10.11 Nursing Diagnoses Related to Appendectomy

Preoperative

- Acute pain related to inflamed appendix
- Risk for injury related to possibility of rupture
- Risk for deficient fluid volume related to decreased intake secondary to loss of appetite, vomiting, NPO status

Postoperative

- Risk for injury related to surgical procedure, anesthesia
- Anxiety/fear related to surgery
- Acute pain related to surgical incision
- Risk for deficient fluid volume related to NPO prior to and/or after surgery, loss of appetite, vomiting
- Risk for infection related to weakened condition, presence of infective organisms

Table 10.12 Nursing Diagnoses Related to Chronic Inflammatory Bowel Disorders

- Imbalanced nutrition and fluid and electrolyte status related to nausea, vomiting, frequent diarrhea, and GI bleeding
- Altered body image due to disease process
- Risk for impaired skin integrity in perianal area related to frequent diarrhea
- Risk for imbalanced health maintenance related to insufficient knowledge regarding follow-up care

D. Interventions:
  1. Maintain adequate nutrition:
     a. Provide high protein, high calorie, low-residue diet with no milk products if able to tolerate oral intake
     b. TPN feedings or enteral feedings given if client is unable to tolerate oral foods
  2. Record the number and characteristics of stools.
  3. Administer antidiarrheals (see Table 10.5), antispasmodics, anticholinergics (see Table 10.9), azulfidine, or steroids as ordered.
  4. Provide skin care to perianal area as needed.
     a. Wash and dry area after each bowel movement.
     b. Apply analgesic or protective ointment as needed.
     c. Provide sitz baths as needed.
  5. Provide care for a client having bowel surgery.

Ulcerative Colitis

A. Inflammatory disorder of the bowel characterized by inflammation and ulceration that starts in the rectosigmoid area and spreads upward. The mucosa of the bowel becomes edematous and thickened with eventual scar formation. Cause is unknown; may be autoimmune or infection; emotional stress may play a role.

B. Assessment findings:
1. Severe diarrhea: 15–20 liquid stools/day containing blood, mucus, and pus; tenesmus
2. Weight loss, anorexia, weakness
3. Decreased skin turgor, dry mucus membranes
4. Low-grade fever, abdominal tenderness over colon
5. Diagnostic tests
   a. Sigmoidoscopy and colonoscopy reveal mucosa that bleeds easily with ulcer development
   b. Hgb and Hct decreased
C. Nursing diagnoses (see Table 10.12)
D. Interventions same as for Crohn's Disease

Diverticulosis and Diverticulitis

A. A diverticulum is an outpouching of the intestinal mucosa (usually sigmoid colon). Diverticulosis: multiple diverticula of the colon. Diverticulitis: inflammation of the diverticula. Seen most commonly in obese men aged 40–45 who have congenital weakness of intestinal muscle fibers or who have a dietary deficiency of roughage and fiber and chronic constipation.
B. Assessment findings:
1. Intermittent lower-left quadrant pain
2. Constipation alternating with diarrhea containing blood and mucus
3. Barium enema shows diverticula
4. Decreased Hgb and Hct
C. Nursing diagnoses (see Table 10.13)
D. Interventions:
1. High residue, high-fiber diet; may be told to avoid seeds; eight glasses of water
2. Prevent constipation
3. Bulk laxatives or stool softeners
4. Anticholinergics (see Table 10.9), antibiotics

Table 10.13 Nursing Diagnoses Related to Diverticulosis and Diverticulitis

- Acute pain related to intestinal inflammatory process
- Diarrhea related to intestinal inflammatory process
- Constipation related to inadequate dietary intake of fiber
- Risk for impaired skin integrity (perianal) related to diarrhea
- Risk for ineffective individual coping related to the chronicity of the condition and the lack of definitive treatment
- Imbalanced nutrition: less than body requirement related to dietary restrictions
- Risk for ineffective health maintenance related to insufficient knowledge of condition, dietary restrictions, and signs and symptoms of complications

5. Surgery: resection of diseased part of colon with temporary colostomy for severe cases (see bowel surgery)
6. Teach patient to prevent increased intra-abdominal pressure

CANCER OF THE COLON/RECTUM

A. Adenocarcinoma is the most common type of colon cancer; may spread by direct extension through the walls of the intestine or through the lymphatic or circulatory system; metastasis is often to the liver.
B. Assessment findings:
1. Alternating diarrhea and constipation, lower abdominal cramps, abdominal distention
2. Weakness, anorexia, weight loss, pallor, dyspnea
3. Diagnostic tests:
   a. Stool for occult blood positive
   b. Hgb and Hct decreased
   c. CEA positive
   d. Sigmoidoscopy, colonoscopy, barium enema reveal mass/lesion
   e. Digital rectal exam indicates palpable mass
C. Interventions:
1. Care for client receiving chemotherapeutic agents
2. Provide care for client receiving radiation therapy
3. Provide care for client who has had bowel surgery

BOWEL SURGERY

A. May be indicated for Crohn's disease, ulcerative colitis, intestinal obstructions, or colon/rectal cancer
B. Types (see Table 10.14)
C. Nursing diagnoses (see Table 10.15)
D. Interventions:
1. Special preoperative nursing care needs:
   a. Low residue diet for 3–5 days before surgery
   b. Clear liquids only the day before surgery
   c. Bowel prep
      (1) Antibiotics for 3–5 days to decrease bacteria in intestine (Neomycin or other antibiotic poorly absorbed from GI tract)
      (2) Enemas to cleanse bowel
      (3) Give vitamins C and K (decreased by bowel cleansing) to prevent post-op bleeding

Table 10.14 Types of Bowel Surgeries

Type	Procedures
Resection with anastomosis	The diseased part of the bowel is removed and remaining portions are anastomosed, allowing elimination through the rectum.
Abdominoperineal resection	Distal sigmoid colon, rectum, and anus are removed through a perineal incision; permanent colostomy is created; done for cancer of colon and rectum
Permanent colostomy	Consists of a single stoma made when the distal portion of the bowel is removed; most often located in the sigmoid or descending colon
Loop colostomy	A loop of bowel is brought out above the skin surface and held in place by a glass rod. There is one stoma but two openings, a proximal and a distal; often temporary.
Double-barreled colostomy	Colon is resected and both ends are brought through the abdominal wall creating two stomas—a proximal and a distal. Done most often for an obstruction in the descending or transverse colon. May be temporary.
Temporary colostomy	Usually located in the ascending or transverse colon; most often done to rest the bowel
Ileostomy	Opening of the ileum onto the abdominal surface; done for ulcerative colitis and sometimes Crohn's Disease
Continent ileostomy (Kock's pouch)	An intra-abdominal reservoir with a nipple valve is formed from the distal ileum. The pouch acts as a reservoir for fecal material and is cleaned at regular intervals by insertion of a catheter.
Cecostomy	Opening between the cecum and the abdominal base to divert the fecal flow to rest the distal portion of the colon after some types of surgery; temporary

Table 10.15 Nursing Diagnoses Related to Bowel Surgery

1. Risk for ineffective therapeutic regimen management
2. Anxiety and disturbed self-concept related to possible lifestyle changes due to change in normal bowel function
3. Risk for ineffective sexuality patterns related to perceived negative impact of ostomy on sexual functioning
4. Deficient knowledge related to products needed in care of ostomy, irrigations, skin care, and so on
5. Pain related to surgical incision

Table 10.16 Colostomy irrigation

Position the client on the toilet or in high-Fowler's position if possible.
Hang irrigation bag filled with 500–1000 mL normal saline at shoulder height.
Remove air from tubing; lubricate tip of tube or cone with water-soluble lubricant (KY jelly).
With latex gloves on, remove old pouch and clean skin and stoma with water.
Gently dilate stoma and insert irrigation catheter or cone snugly, open tubing, and allow fluid to enter the bowel.
Remove the catheter and allow fecal contents to drain.
Record the amount and character of fecal return.

2. Special postoperative nursing care needs:
   a. Assess for evidence of return of peristalsis: bowel sounds, flatus passed through rectum or stoma
   b. Assess initial stool characteristics
   c. Abdomino-perineal resection postop needs:
      (1) Two wounds, perineal and abdominal
      (2) Warm sitz baths qid for perineal wound
      (3) T binder for perineal wound dressing

3. Colostomy care:
   a. Skin care around stoma with mild soap, water, and pat dry
   b. Skin barrier around stoma to protect skin (Karaya)
   c. No adhesives on irritated skin
   d. Control odor in pouch by frequent changing and use of deodorizers
   e. Teach client to avoid gas-producing foods such as baked beans, broccoli, and cabbage
   f. Stomal drainage will be mucoid-serosanguinous for 24 hours, then liquid.
   g. Irrigate the colostomy as needed (see Table 10.16)
   h. Encourage fluid intake to at least 2,500 ml/day.
   i. Encourage patient to express concerns and feelings about colostomy
   j. Teach patient to care for self
   k. In client who had double-barreled colostomy, irrigate proximal loop if irrigation is needed
4. Ileostomy special post-op needs:
   a. Skin care
   b. Drainage is always liquid, so no irrigations are necessary.

5. Kock's pouch special postop needs:
   a. Teach client how to insert catheter and drain pouch
   b. Eventually client will be able to go several hours between emptying

HEMORRHOIDS

A. Varicose veins of anal canal; internal are above the internal sphincter; external are outside the rectal sphincter
B. Assessment findings:
   1. Bleeding with defecation, hard stools with streaks of blood
   2. Pain with defecation, sitting, or walking
   3. Protrusion of external hemorrhoids visible on inspection
   4. Proctoscopy shows internal hemorrhoids.
   5. Hgb and Hct decreased if excessive bleeding
C. Nursing diagnoses (see Table 10.17)
D. Interventions:
   1. Administer stool softeners, local anesthetics, or anti-inflammatory creams as ordered.
   2. Encourage a high-fiber diet with adequate fluid intake.
   3. Hemorrhoidectomy:
      a. Preoperative care may include laxatives or enemas to promote cleansing of the bowel.
      b. Postoperative nursing care needs:
         (1) Ice packs immediately postop to prevent edema and bleeding
         (2) Inspect rectal area and dressings every 2–3 hours for bleeding; report a significant increase in bloody drainage.
         (3) Sitz baths after each bowel movement after first day to keep area clean
         (4) Spray analgesic to relieve pain.
         (5) Avoid pain medications containing codeine, because they are constipating.
         (6) Prevent urinary infections.

Table 10.17 Nursing Diagnoses Related to Hemorrhoids

- Impaired comfort related to pain upon defecation
- Risk of constipation related to fear of pain upon defecation
- Risk for ineffective health maintenance related to insufficient knowledge of condition, bowel routine, diet instructions, exercise program, and perianal care

Postoperatively:
- Risk for urinary retention related to perineal trauma, edema/swelling, and pain

---

         (7) Use flotation pads or pillows for comfort, not rubber rings.
         (8) Encourage high fluid intake to prevent constipation.
         (9) Administer stool softeners and laxatives daily as ordered.
        (10) Enemas may be ordered on the second day before the first bowel movement.

DISORDERS OF THE LIVER

Hepatitis

A. Inflammation of liver tissue with liver cell damage
B. Types of Hepatitis:
   1. Hepatitis A (infectious hepatitis):
      a. Incubation period 15–45 days
      b. Spread by a virus via the fecal-oral route; poor personal hygiene, contaminated milk, water, shellfish, food
      c. Immunization available for persons at high risk or those traveling to countries where hepatitis A is endemic
   2. Hepatitis B (serum hepatitis):
      a. Incubation period 50–180 days
      b. Spread by blood and body fluids (saliva, semen, vaginal secretions); IV drug abuse, intimate sexual contact
      c. Encourage immunization of health care workers and the general public
   3. Hepatitis C:
      a. Incubation period 7–50 days
      b. Spread by parenteral route, through blood and blood products, needles, syringes
C. Assessment findings
   1. Early (pre-icteric stage–before jaundice):
      a. Nausea, vomiting, fatigue, constipation, diarrhea, weight loss (flu-like)
      b. Right Upper Quadrant (RUQ) discomfort, hepatomegaly, splenomegaly, lymphadenopathy
   2. Later (icteric stage–jaundice)
      a. Fatigue, weight loss
      b. Light-colored stools
      c. Dark urine
      d. Enlarged liver, spleen, lymph nodes
      e. Jaundice, pruritus
   3. Elevated SGPT, SGOT, alkaline phosphatase, bilirubin, ESR
   4. Decreased leukocytes, lymphocytes, neutrophils
   5. Prolonged PT
   6. Serologic tests for antigens for Hepatitis A and B
D. Nursing Diagnoses (see Table 10.18)

Table 10.18 Nursing Diagnoses Related to Liver Disorders

- Activity intolerance related to weakness secondary to reduced energy metabolism of liver
- Risk for infection transmission related to contagious agents (hepatitis)
- Impaired physical mobility related to prolonged bed rest
- Impaired nutrition: less than body requirements related to nausea, anorexia, and impaired utilization and storage of vitamins A, C, K, D, and E
- Risk for injury related to reduced prothrombin synthesis and reduced vitamin K absorption
- Impaired comfort related to pruritus secondary to bile salt accumulation
- Acute pain related to swelling of liver
- Risk for ineffective health maintenance related to insufficient knowledge of condition, rest requirements, precautions to avoid transmission, nutritional requirements, and contraindications (certain medications, alcohol)
- Diarrhea related to excessive secretion of fats in stool secondary to liver dysfunction
- Risk for impaired respiratory function related to pressure on diaphragm secondary to ascites
- Risk for infection related to leukopenia secondary to enlarged, overactive spleen and hypoproteinemia
- Fluid volume excess: peripheral edema related to portal hypertension, lowered plasma colloidal osmotic pressure, and sodium retention
- Potential for complications of liver disease, such as ascites, esophageal varices, and hepatic encephalopathy.

E. Interventions:
  1. Rest
  2. Adequate nutrition: low fat, high CHO, high calorie, high protein diet (low protein diet when liver failure is threatening); no alcohol
  3. Prevent and treat nausea: antiemetics as ordered; avoid temperature extremes in food
  4. Relieve itching:
     a. Do not use soaps and detergents
     b. Bathe in tepid water followed by application of emollient solution
     c. Cut fingernails to avoid skin damage from scratching.
     d. Apply cool, moist compresses to areas that itch.
  5. Prevent spread of hepatitis:
     a. Enteric precautions for hepatitis A
     b. Stool and needle precautions for hepatitis B and C
     c. Administer immune serum globulin to persons exposed to hepatitis A and B.
     d. Teach persons who have had any type of hepatitis that they should not donate blood.
     e. Administer immune serum globulin early to persons exposed to hepatitis A and B as ordered.

  f. Instruct persons with hepatitis B to avoid sexual intercourse while the disease is active.

Cirrhosis of the Liver

A. Chronic, progressive disease in which liver cells are destroyed and replaced by scar tissue; frequently seen in alcoholics but occurs in nonalcoholics
B. Assessment findings:
  1. Fever
  2. Jaundice of skin, sclera, and mucus membranes
  3. Anorexia, nausea, and vomiting
  4. Liver changes: early in the disease, enlarged liver causes right upper quadrant pain; late in disease, liver becomes smaller and nodular
  5. Spleen enlarges
  6. Ascites, distended abdominal veins
  7. Easy bruising and bleeding; prothrombin time prolonged
  8. AST (SGOT), ALT (SGPT), LDH, alkaline phosphatase increased
  9. Serum bilirubin increased
  10. Serum albumin decreased
  11. Hgb and Hct decreased
  12. Muscle atrophy
  13. Wernicke-Korsakoff syndrome:
     a. Central nervous system disorder associated with chronic alcoholism and thiamin (Vitamin B_1) deficiency
     b. Abrupt onset of motor and sensory disturbances and memory problems
     c. Thiamin administration helps visual problems immediately; ataxia and cognitive problems may improve slowly or not at all
  14. Delirium, convulsions, and coma during end stage
C. Nursing diagnoses (see Table 10.18)
D. Interventions:
  1. Rest
  2. Teach client to avoid hepatotoxic drugs
  3. Teach client proper diet, low sodium, high calorie diet with vitamins and minerals, no alcohol
  4. Albumin may be given IV to decrease ascites.
  5. Daily weights as ordered
  6. Measure abdominal girths.
  7. Skin care to relieve itching (see hepatitis)
  8. Monitor intake and output.
  9. Administer diuretics as ordered.
  10. Prevent infection; skin care and reverse isolation if necessary
  11. Neomycin po may be ordered when coma is pending to decrease E. Coli in the bowel (E. Coli makes ammonia, which the liver is supposed to break down).

Bleeding Esophageal Varices

A. Esophageal varices are dilated veins found in the lower esophagus which occur secondary to portal hypertension; bleeding may result from coughing, trauma, or vomiting and is a medical emergency.
B. Assessment findings:
   1. Anorexia, nausea, and vomiting blood
   2. Splenomegaly, ascites, peripheral edema
   3. Decreased serum albumin, RBC, Hct, Hgb
   4. Increased LDH, AST (SGOT), ALT (SGPT), BUN
C. Nursing diagnoses (see Tables 10.18 and 10.19)
D. Interventions:
   1. Maintain a patent airway.
   2. Administer vitamin K as ordered to promote clotting.
   3. Administer Pitressin as ordered to decrease portal pressure by constricting splanchnic vessels.
   4. Assist with insertion of Sengstaken-Blakemore tube
      a. Triple lumen tube that is inserted into the stomach through the nose:
         (1) One lumen inflates an esophageal balloon.
         (2) One lumen inflates the gastric balloon.
         (3) One lumen is for aspirating gastric contents.
         (4) Some tubes have a fourth lumen for aspirating the nasopharyngeal area above the esophageal balloon.
      b. Purposes of tube:
         (1) Inflated balloons exert pressure against esophageal varices.
         (2) Reduced bleeding reduces transfusion requirements.
         (3) Accumulated blood can be removed from the stomach (accumulated blood could precipitate hepatic coma), and iced saline can be infused to further stop bleeding.
      c. Nursing care of client with Sengstaken-Blakemore tube:
         (1) Nurse must be present in the room at all times while the balloon is inflated.
         (2) Assess respiratory status; tube could ride up into oropharynx and block airway.
         (3) Scissors are kept at bedside at all times; in case of respiratory distress, cut across tubing and remove.
         (4) Keep balloon pressure at levels ordered; hemostats are used as clamps.
         (5) Nothing by mouth; no ice chips
         (6) Keep head of bed elevated to avoid gastric regurgitation.
         (7) Take vital signs frequently.
         (8) Assess for chest pain.
         (9) Irrigate suction tube with iced saline as prescribed.
         (10) Esophageal balloon should be deflated for five minutes every 8–12 hours.
         (11) Gastric balloon under traction is not deflated.
         (12) Pressure on tubes and traction is released in 2–4 days.
         (13) Oral hygiene
   5. Surgery may be portosystemic shunts (splenorenal, portacaval) or transesophageal ligation; prognosis poor after surgery; high mortality rates

Cancer of the Liver

A. The liver is a common site for metastasis for cancer of the colon, rectum, stomach, pancreas, esophagus, breast, lung, and melanomas. Primary liver cancer is very rare.
B. Assessment findings:
   1. Weakness
   2. Anorexia, nausea, and vomiting
   3. Right upper quadrant discomfort/tenderness, hepatomegaly, blood-tinged ascites, peripheral edema, ascites, jaundice
   4. Blood tests same as for cirrhosis of the liver plus increased blood sugar and alpha fetoprotein
   5. Liver scan, abdominal X-ray, and liver biopsy all positive
C. Nursing diagnoses (see Table 10.18)
D. Interventions:
   1. Same as for cirrhosis
   2. Provide care for client receiving cancer chemotherapy or radiation therapy
   3. Provide care for client who has had abdominal surgery
   4. Special preoperative care needs for client having liver surgery:
      a. Bowel prep (neomycin p.o.) to decrease ammonia levels
      b. Administer vitamin K to decrease risk of bleeding.
   5. Special postoperative care needs for client having liver surgery:
      a. Monitor for hyper/hypoglycemia.
      b. Assess for bleeding; hemorrhage is the most serious complication.

Table 10.19 Nursing Diagnoses Related to Esophageal Varices

- Deficient fluid volume related to upper-gastrointestinal hemorrhage
- Risk for ineffective health maintenance related to insufficient knowledge of etiology of condition and treatment
- Also see nursing diagnoses related to liver disorders (see Table 10.18)

    c. Assess for signs of hepatic encephalopathy (confusion, slurred speech, tremors, positive Babinski's reflex).

DISORDERS OF THE GALLBLADDER

Cholecystitis and Cholelithiasis

A. Cholecystitis: inflammation of the gallbladder is often associated with cholelithiasis; stones in the gallbladder are usually cholesterol stones
B. Assessment findings:
    1. RUQ or epigastric pain; may radiate to right scapula
    2. Nausea and vomiting
    3. Fat intolerance; pain, belching, nausea, sensation of fullness after eating foods containing fat
    4. Pruritus, easy bruising, jaundice, dark amber urine, steatorrhea (fatty stools)
    5. Liver function tests elevated
    6. Oral cholecystogram (gallbladder series), abdominal sonogram showed gallstones
C. Primary nursing diagnosis is pain related to inflammation and possible infection in biliary tract
D. Interventions:
    1. Relieve pain; never give morphine because it causes spasm of the sphincter of Oddi
    2. Maintain fluid and electrolyte balance.
    3. Instruct the client about a low-fat diet.
    4. Administration of bile acid (chendeoxycholic acid) if ordered
    5. Administer antibiotic if ordered.

Cholecystectomy/Choledochostomy

A. Cholecystectomy (removal of the gallbladder) and choledochostomy (opening of common bile duct, removal of stone, and insertion of T-tube) can be performed via laparoscopy for uncomplicated cases when the client has not had prior abdominal surgery or by abdominal incision.
B. Nursing diagnoses (see Table 10.20)

C. Interventions:
    1. Routine preoperative nursing care
    2. Postoperative nursing care as for abdominal surgery
    3. Monitor functioning of T-tube if present:
        a. Expect 300–500 ml bile-colored drainage during the first 24 hours, then 200 ml/day for the next 3–4 days
        b. Measure and record drainage every shift
        c. Assess skin around T-tube; cleanse frequently and keep dry
    4. Assess for peritonitis.
    5. Teach client a low fat diet
    6. Resumption of ADL in six weeks for abdominal surgery; two weeks for laparoscopy

DISORDERS OF THE PANCREAS

Pancreatitis

A. Inflammation brought about by the digestion of the pancreas by the enzymes it produces; usually caused by alcoholism, biliary tract disease, viral infections, trauma, or medications (steroids, thiazide diuretics, oral contraceptives)
B. Assessment findings:
    1. Extreme upper abdominal pain radiating into the back
    2. Persistent vomiting
    3. Abdominal distention
    4. Weight loss
    5. Steatorrhea (bulky, pale, frothy, foul-smelling stools)
    6. Elevated serum amylase, blood sugar, lipids
    7. CT scan shows enlargement of the pancreas
C. Nursing diagnoses (see Table 10.21)

Table 10.20 Nursing Diagnoses Related to Cholecystectomy

- Risk for impaired respiratory function related to high abdominal incision and splinting secondary to pain
- Risk for infection related to destruction of first line of defense against bacterial invasion
- Acute pain related to surgical incision
- Risk for impaired oral mucus membrane related to NPO state and mouth breathing secondary to nasogastric intubation
- Risk for deficient fluid volume related to vomiting, NG aspiration, or medically restricted intake

Table 10.21 Nursing Diagnoses Related to Pancreas Disorders

- Risk for deficient fluid volume related to decreased intake secondary to nausea and vomiting and fluid loss secondary to nasogastric suction
- Imbalanced nutrition: less than body requirements related to nasogastric suction and NPO status
- Acute pain related to nasogastric suction, distention of pancreatic capsule, and local peritonitis
- Risk for ineffective health maintenance related to insufficient knowledge of disease, contraindications (alcohol, coffee, and large meals), dietary management, and follow-up care
- Risk for infection related to nutritional deficiencies, tissue destruction, and chronic disease

D. Interventions:
1. NPO
2. NG tube to decrease acid stimulation to pancreas
3. Anticholinergics
4. Antacids to decrease acid stimulation to pancreas
5. Pancreatic extracts—give with meals
6. Pain relief; never give morphine because it causes spasm of the sphincter of Oddi
7. Teach client to follow low-fat diet and avoid alcohol and caffeine

Cancer of the Pancreas

A. Head of pancreas is most common site; tumor growth results in common bile duct obstruction with jaundice
B. Assessment findings:
1. Anorexia; rapid, progressive weight loss
2. Dull pain in upper abdomen or left hypochondriacal region with radiation to the back, related to eating
3. Jaundice
4. Serum lipase, bilirubin, and amylase elevated
5. CT scan may show changes
C. Nursing diagnoses (see Table 10.21)
D. Interventions:
1. See pancreatitis.
2. Provide care for client receiving radiation or chemotherapy.
3. Provide pre- and post-operative care for client undergoing Whipple's Procedure (pancreatoduodenectomy).
4. Teach client to follow low-fat, high-calorie diet with vitamin supplements.

Sample Questions

1. A client is admitted to the hospital with a gnawing pain in the mid-epigastric area and black stools for the past week. A diagnosis of chronic duodenal ulcer is made. During the initial nursing assessment, the client makes all of the following statements. Which is most likely related to his admitting diagnosis?
   1. "I am a vegetarian."
   2. "My mother and grandmother have diabetes."
   3. "I take aspirin several times a day for tension headaches."
   4. "I take multivitamin and iron tablets every day."
2. An upper GI series is ordered for a client. Which action is essential for the nurse before the test?
   1. Check to see if the client has an allergy to shellfish.
   2. Instruct the client to have nothing to eat after midnight before the test.

3. Encourage the client to drink plenty of liquids before the test.
   4. Be sure he does not eat fat-containing foods for 18 hours before the test.
3. The client with a duodenal ulcer is ready for discharge. Which statement made by the client indicates a need for more teaching about his diet?
   1. "It's a good thing I gave up drinking alcohol last year."
   2. "I will have to drink lots of milk and cream every day."
   3. "I will stay away from cola drinks after I am discharged."
   4. "Eating three nutritious meals and snacks every day is okay."
4. The client, admitted with appendicitis, overhears the physician say that the pain has reached McBurney's point. She becomes very frightened and asks the nurse to explain what this means. Which is the best response?
   1. "The next time the doctor comes in, we should ask him what he meant by that."
   2. "I've felt that I don't understand the doctor at times either."
   3. "That is the term used to indicate that the pain has traveled to the right lower side."
   4. "McBurney's point refers to severe pain for which surgery is the only treatment."
5. Which blood test results would confirm a diagnosis of appendicitis?
   1. WBC of 13,000
   2. RBC of 4.5 million
   3. Platelet count of 300,000
   4. Positive Heterophil antibody test
6. The nurse is admitting a client with the diagnosis of appendicitis to the surgical unit. Which question is it essential to ask?
   1. "When did you last eat?"
   2. "Have you had surgery before?"
   3. "Have you ever had this type of pain before?"
   4. "What do you usually take to relieve your pain?"
7. The client with appendicitis asks the nurse for a laxative to help relieve her constipation. The nurse explains to her that laxatives are not given to persons with possible appendicitis. What is the primary reason for this?
   1. Laxatives will decrease the spread of infection.
   2. Laxatives are not given prior to any type of surgery.
   3. The patient does not have true constipation. She only has pressure.
   4. Laxatives could cause a rupture of the appendix.
8. A child with appendicitis is scheduled for surgery this evening. The nurse enters the room and sees the child's mother starting to place hot, wet washcloths on her daughter's abdomen so that "she will feel better."

The nurse explains that this action is contraindicated because heat:
1. Can cause the appendix to rupture and cause peritonitis
2. Can mask symptoms of acute appendicitis
3. Will increase peristalsis throughout the abdomen
4. Will arrest progression of the disease

9. A client returns from having had abdominal surgery. Her vital signs are stable. She says she is thirsty. What should the nurse give her initially?
1. Orange juice
2. Milk
3. Ice chips
4. Mouth wash

10. The client who has had an appendectomy and has a penrose drain in place has recovered from anesthesia. The nurse places her in semi-Fowler's position. What is the primary reason for selecting this position?
1. To promote optimal ventilation
2. To promote drainage from the abdominal cavity
3. To prevent pressure sores from developing
4. To reduce tension on the suture line

11. The client is admitted to the hospital complaining of malaise, abdominal discomfort, and severe diarrhea. The diagnosis is possible Crohn's Disease. The client says that he has lost 27 pounds in the last four months even though he has not been dieting. To plan nursing care, which assessment data is most essential for the nurse to obtain?
1. Approximate number and characteristics of stools each day
2. Amount of liquid consumed daily
3. History of previous gastric surgery
4. Bowel sounds in the right lower quadrant

12. The nurse is preparing a client with Crohn's Disease for discharge. Which statement he makes indicates that he needs further teaching?
1. "Stress can make it worse."
2. "Since I have Crohn's Disease I don't have to worry about colon cancer."
3. "I realize I shall always have to monitor my diet."
4. "I understand there is a high incidence of familial occurrence with this disease."

13. A low-residue diet is ordered for a client. Which food would be contraindicated for this person?
1. Roast beef
2. Fresh peas
3. Mashed potatoes
4. Baked chicken

14. The client is to have a sigmoidoscopy in the morning. Which activity will be included in the care of this client?
1. Give him an enema one hour before the examination.

2. Keep him NPO for eight hours before the examination.
3. Order a low-fat, low-residue diet for breakfast.
4. Administer enemas until the returns are clear this evening.

15. The client had a barium enema. Following the barium enema, the nurse should anticipate an order for which of the following?
1. An antacid
2. A laxative
3. A muscle relaxant
4. A sedative

16. The client is found to have colon cancer. An abdomino-perineal resection and colostomy is scheduled. Neomycin is ordered. The nurse explains to the client that the primary purpose for administering this drug is to:
1. Decrease peristalsis in the intestines
2. Decrease the bacterial content in the colon
3. Reduce inflammation of the bowel
4. Help prevent post-operative pneumonia

17. The day after surgery in which a colostomy was performed, the client says "I know the doctor did not really do a colostomy." The nurse understands that the client is in an early stage of adjustment to the diagnosis and surgery. What nursing action is indicated at this time?
1. Agree with the client until the client is ready to accept the colostomy.
2. Say, "It must be difficult to have this kind of surgery."
3. Force the client to look at his colostomy.
4. Ask the surgeon to explain the surgery to the client.

18. The nurse is irrigating the client's colostomy when the client complains of cramping. What is the most appropriate initial action by the nurse?
1. Increase the flow of solution.
2. Ask the client to turn to the other side.
3. Pinch the tubing to interrupt the flow of the solution.
4. Remove the tube from the colostomy.

19. A 32-year-old female is admitted for a hemorrhoidectomy. During the nursing assessment, all of the following factors are elicited. Which one is most likely to have contributed to the development of hemorrhoids? The client:
1. States that she usually cleans herself from back to front after a bowel movement
2. Says her mother and grandmother had hemorrhoids
3. Has had four pregnancies
4. Eats bran every day

20. Following a hemorrhoidectomy, the nurse is instructing the client in self care. Which statement is especially important to include in these instructions?

1. "Wash the anal area with water after defecation and pat it dry."
2. "Gently wipe the anal area after defecation from back to front."
3. "Do not drink more than three glasses of fluid per day until after you have had the first bowel movement."
4. "When you first feel the need to defecate, call me and I will give you the enema the doctor has ordered."

21. The client who has had a hemorrhoidectomy wants to know why she cannot take a sitz bath immediately upon return from the operating room. The nurse's response is based upon which of the following concepts?
    1. Heat can stimulate bowel movement too quickly after surgery.
    2. Patients are generally not awake enough for several hours to safely take sitz baths.
    3. Heat applied immediately postoperatively increases the possibility of hemorrhage.
    4. Sitting in water before the sutures are removed may cause infection.

22. Following a hemorrhoidectomy, the nurse assesses the client's voiding. What is the reason for this concern?
    1. The client has been NPO before and during surgery.
    2. Urinary retention is frequently seen after a hemorrhoidectomy.
    3. The client has a long history of hemorrhoids, making her prone to voiding problems.
    4. The client had several pregnancies, which can make voiding difficult.

23. The client has had a hemorrhoidectomy. Which statement she makes indicates a need for more teaching?
    1. "I'll decrease the amount of fiber in my diet."
    2. "I should drink more liquids at home."
    3. "There seems to be a relationship between bowel regularity and diet."
    4. "Establishing a routine for bowel movements is important."

24. A client with pancreatitis tells the nurse that he fears nighttime. Which of the following statements most likely relates to the client's concerns?
    1. The pain is aggravated in the recumbent position.
    2. The client has fewer distractions at night.
    3. The mattress is uncomfortable.
    4. The pain increases after a day of activity.

25. Warm Aveeno baths are ordered for a client with cancer of the pancreas. What is the chief purpose of this procedure for this client?
    1. Relief of paralytic ileus
    2. Alleviate pruritus associated with jaundice
    3. Relief of bloating and fullness after eating
    4. Reducing the fever associated with the disease

26. A distal pancreatectomy and splenectomy is performed on a client with cancer of the pancreas. He is returned to his room post-operatively. The client is sleepy but can answer simple questions appropriately. His dressing is dry and intact. Vital signs are within normal limits. Which of the following nursing measures must be done before the nurse leaves the room?
    1. Inform his wife that he has returned to his room.
    2. Check to see if the indwelling urinary catheter bag is correctly attached to the bed frame.
    3. Assess to be sure he is not experiencing any discomfort.
    4. Put all four side rails in the high position.

27. The client's temperature rises to 100.4°F (38°C) on the first post-operative day following abdominal surgery. The nurse interprets this to be:
    1. Indicative of a wound infection
    2. A normal physiologic response to the trauma of surgery
    3. Suggestive of a urinary tract infection
    4. An indication of over-hydration

28. The client asks how he contracted hepatitis A. He reports all of the following. Which one is most likely related to hepatitis A?
    1. He ate home-canned corn.
    2. He ate oysters his roommate brought home from a fishing trip.
    3. He stepped on a nail two weeks ago.
    4. He donated blood two weeks before he got sick.

29. The client has had a liver biopsy. The nurse should position him on his right side with a pillow under his rib cage. What is the primary reason for this position?
    1. To immobilize the diaphragm
    2. To facilitate full chest expansion
    3. To minimize the danger of aspiration
    4. To reduce the likelihood of bleeding

30. A client with cirrhosis is about to have a paracentesis for relief of ascites. Which activity is essential prior to the procedure?
    1. Administer thorough mouth care.
    2. Ask the client to empty his bladder.
    3. Be sure his bowels have moved recently.
    4. Have the client bathe with betadine.

31. The client has severe liver disease. Which of the following observations is most indicative of serious problems? The client:
    1. Has generalized urticaria
    2. Is "confused" and can no longer write his name legibly
    3. Is jaundiced
    4. Has ecchymotic areas on his arms

32. An adult has a nasogastric tube in place. Which nursing action will relieve discomfort in the nostril with the NG tube?

1. Remove any tape and loosely pin the NG tube to his gown.
2. Lubricate the NG tube with viscous lidocaine.
3. Loop the NG tube to avoid pressure on the nares.
4. Replace the NG tube with a smaller-diameter tube.

33. An adult is being treated for a peptic ulcer. The physician has prescribed cimetidine (Tagamet) for which reason?
    1. It blocks the secretion of gastric hydrochloric acid.
    2. It coats the gastric mucosa with a protective membrane.
    3. It increases the sensitivity of H_2 receptors.
    4. It neutralizes acid in the stomach.

34. The nurse is assessing a client who may have a hiatal hernia. What symptom is the client most likely to report?
    1. Projectile vomiting
    2. Crampy lower abdominal pain
    3. Burning substernal pain
    4. Bloody diarrhea

35. When an elderly client is receiving cimetidine (Tagamet), it is important that the nurse monitor for which side effect?
    1. Chest pain
    2. Confusion
    3. Dyspnea
    4. Urinary retention

Answers and Rationales

1. (3) Aspirin is very irritating to the gastric mucosa and is known to cause ulcers. Being a vegetarian does not cause ulcers. Ulcers are not known to be inherited. Multivitamins and iron do not cause ulcers.

2. (2) Preparation for an upper GI series is NPO for eight hours. In an upper GI series, the client swallows barium, a radiopaque substance. An iodine dye is not used, so it is not necessary to ask about iodine allergies (shellfish). Fats are restricted before gallbladder X-rays, not for an upper GI series.

3. (2) Milk and cream are now known to cause rebound acidity and are not prescribed for ulcer clients. The other choices all indicate good knowledge. He should not drink alcohol or cola. Three meals and snacks will help keep the stomach from staying empty for long periods.

4. (3) McBurney's point is the area in the right lower quadrant where the appendix is. The client asked for information that the nurse should be able to provide. Answer 4 is not correct. McBurney's point refers to the location of the appendix, not the severity of the pain.

5. (1) An elevated white blood count indicates appendicitis. The RBC and platelet levels given are normal but are not specifically related to appendicitis. A positive Heterophil antibody test indicates infectious mononucleosis.

6. (1) When a person is admitted with possible appendicitis, the nurse should anticipate surgery. It will be important to know when she last ate when considering the type of anesthesia so that the chance of aspiration can be minimized. The other information is "nice to know" but not essential.

7. (4) Laxatives cause increased peristalsis, which may cause the appendix to rupture. Answer 2 is not a true statement. Laxatives may well be given prior to gynecological, rectal, and colon surgery. Answer 3 is true but is not the primary reason why laxatives are not given when a person has appendicitis.

8. (1) Heat can cause drawing of the inflammation and rupture of the appendix, which will cause peritonitis. Heat is not likely to mask the symptoms of appendicitis, increase peristalsis, or arrest progression of the disease.

9. (3) Ice chips can be given to help relieve thirst. Only clear liquids will be given until peristalsis has returned; milk and orange juice are not clear liquids. Mouth wash is not consumed and when used appropriately does not relieve thirst. It may freshen the mouth but does not relieve thirst.

10. (2) The client has a Penrose drain in place. The primary reason for the semi-Fowler's position is to promote drainage. This position may also help reduce tension on the suture line and promote ventilation. Turning will help prevent pressure sores.

11. (1) It is most important for the nurse to know how many stools he has been having each day. Frequent stools are characteristic of Crohn's Disease and may cause dehydration and skin breakdown. The nurse may want to know how much liquid he has been consuming, but that is not the most important. Previous gastric surgery is not usually related to Crohn's Disease. Bowel sounds may be assessed but are not the most important assessment data.

12. (2) Persons with Crohn's Disease are at high risk for the development of colon cancer. The other answers are all correct and therefore do not indicate a need for more instruction.

13. (2) Fresh peas are high in residue. Roast beef, mashed potatoes, and baked chicken are not high in residue. High-residue foods are those that contain skins, seeds, and leaves. Milk products are also to be avoided on a low-residue diet.

14. (1) An enema one hour before the exam will clear the sigmoid colon. A client having an upper GI series will be NPO. A low-fat diet is indicated prior to a gallbladder series. A low-residue diet is part of the preparation for a barium enema. Enemas until clear are sometimes ordered prior to a barium enema or colonoscopy.

15. (2) Barium can be very constipating and may cause blockage of the bowel. Laxatives help to empty the bowel of barium. The other drugs are not appropriate following a barium enema.

16. (2) Neomycin is an antibiotic that is poorly absorbed from the GI tract and will therefore kill the bacteria in the bowel. This must be done before colon surgery to prevent peritonitis. Neomycin is an antibiotic and does not decrease peristalsis or reduce inflammation. Because it is not absorbed from the bowel, it does not kill bacteria outside the GI tract and therefore will not prevent pneumonia.

17. (2) The first stage of adjustment to a major loss is usually denial. The client is denying the colostomy. This empathic response encourages the client to discuss feelings. The nurse should never agree with the client's denial. The denial should not be confronted at this point in time. He needs time to adjust. Notice that the stem of the question focuses on the denial stage.

18. (3) When cramping occurs during a colostomy irrigation or an enema, the nurse should temporarily stop the flow of solution. Having the client take deep breaths may help also. Increasing the flow of solution will increase the cramping. Changing position will not decrease the cramping. It is not necessary to remove the tube; simply stop the flow of the solution briefly.

19. (3) Pregnancy causes increased portal hypertension, which can cause hemorrhoids. Cleaning from back to front after bowel movements may cause cystitis but not hemorrhoids. There may be some familial tendency toward hemorrhoids; however, pregnancies are more directly related. Bran will promote bowel regularity and would help to prevent constipation, which is a risk factor for hemorrhoids.

20. (1) After hemorrhoid surgery, the anal area should be washed with water, no soap, and patted, not rubbed, dry. Wiping should be from front to back to reduce risk of urinary tract infection. Fluids are encouraged because they will promote a soft stool, which will pass more easily. If an enema is used to promote the first bowel movement, it would be given to promote the urge to defecate, not after the client feels the need to defecate.

21. (3) Heat causes vasodilation. In the immediate post-operative period, this could cause hemorrhaging. Ice packs will be applied for the first 24 hours. Sitz baths are ordered after that.

22. (2) The proximity of the anus and the bladder make urinary retention a frequent complication after hemorrhoidectomy. The client was NPO before and during surgery but received IV fluids during and after surgery. The long history of hemorrhoids and the client's previous pregnancies are not the key factors causing bladder retention immediately following surgery.

23. (1) She should increase fiber in her diet. The other actions all indicate a good understanding of her care.

24. (1) The recumbent position aggravates pancreatic pain. The client will be more comfortable on his side with his knees flexed. While the client may have more to distract his mind from pain during the day, this is not the primary reason why pancreatic pain is worse at night.

25. (2) Aveeno baths are used to reduce itching. Jaundice, seen in pancreatic cancer, causes severe itching. Paralytic ileus is not a major feature of pancreatic cancer, and Aveeno baths are not the way to relieve paralytic ileus. Aveeno baths do not relieve bloating and fullness or reduce fever.

26. (4) Side rails are safety devices. When the question asks for an essential action, think of an answer related to safety. It is important to check for correct positioning of the urinary catheter drainage bag and to assess for comfort. However, the side rails are essential. The nurse will notify the client's family after leaving the room.

27. (2) A low-grade temperature on the first post-operative day is a normal response to surgery. It takes at least 72 hours for a wound infection to develop. Urinary tract infections take 48 to 72 hours to develop. Dehydration, not over-hydration, may cause a slight temperature increase in the first few hours after surgery. A temperature elevation the day after surgery could also indicate the development of a respiratory infection, but that was not a choice.

28. (2) Hepatitis A is viral hepatitis and is spread via the fecal-oral route. Shellfish that grow in contaminated waters may have the virus. Home-canned corn might cause food poisoning if it was not properly done. Stepping on a nail might cause tetanus. Donating blood will not cause hepatitis. Receiving blood might cause hepatitis B.

29. (4) The liver is a very vascular organ. It is located on the right side. Lying on the right side will put pressure on it and provide hemostasis and reduce the chance of bleeding. There is no reason to immobilize the diaphragm. Lying on the right side does not immobilize the diaphragm or facilitate chest expansion. Aspiration is not a problem following a liver biopsy.

30. (2) Emptying the bladder is essential prior to a paracentesis so that the bladder will not be punctured during the procedure. Mouth care is not related to a paracentesis. It is not necessary to empty the bowels before a paracentesis. Bathing with betadine is not necessary before a paracentesis.

31. (2) This indicates that the client is going into hepatic coma. He will have urticaria from the jaundice, but this is not the most serious. He will have ecchymotic areas on his body due to the decrease in prothrombin, which is made in the liver. It is not the most serious.

32. (3) Looping the NG tube will prevent pressure on the nares that can cause pain and eventual necrosis. Pinning the tube to the client's gown would cause irritation of the nares each time he moved and might cause dislocation of the tube. Prior to insertion of an NG tube, it is proper to lubricate the tip with viscous xylocaine, but this is not applied to the nostril. A smaller tube might not be large enough to drain the stomach contents; it would still irritate the nose, and it may not be changed without a doctor's order.

33. (1) Cimetidine (Tagamet) is a histamine antagonist that blocks the secretion of hydrochloric acid. Sucralfate (Carafate) coats the gastric mucosa. Cimetidine is an H_2 receptor antagonist; it does not increase the sensitivity, it blocks it. Antacids neutralize acid in the stomach and raise the pH.

34. (3) Heartburn, which is a burning substernal pain, is the most common sign of hiatal hernia in clients who have symptoms. Projectile vomiting is more likely to be associated with pyloric obstruction due to scarring from chronic peptic ulcer disease. Crampy pain in the lower abdomen is commonly associated with lactose intolerance. Bloody diarrhea is more likely to be associated with diverticulitis or ulcerative colitis.

35. (2) Drowsiness, confusion, or mood swings may be side effects of cimetidine. Confusion is particularly common in the elderly. Chest pain is more likely to reflect heartburn, which is a symptom that cimetidine is given to relieve. Dyspnea is a sign of an anaphylactic, allergic reaction to any drug. Allergic reactions to cimetidine are very rare. Urinary retention is associated with anticholinergic drugs. Cimetidine is not anticholinergic.

Chapter 11

The Genitourinary System

ANATOMY AND PHYSIOLOGY

URINARY SYSTEM
(Figure 11.1)

Kidneys

A. Two bean-shaped organs that lie in the retroperitoneal space on either side of the vertebral column
B. Adrenal glands located on top of each kidney
C. Renal parenchyma
   1. Cortex: the outermost layer and the site of glomeruli and proximal and distal tubules of nephron
   2. Medulla: the middle layer formed by collecting ducts and tubules

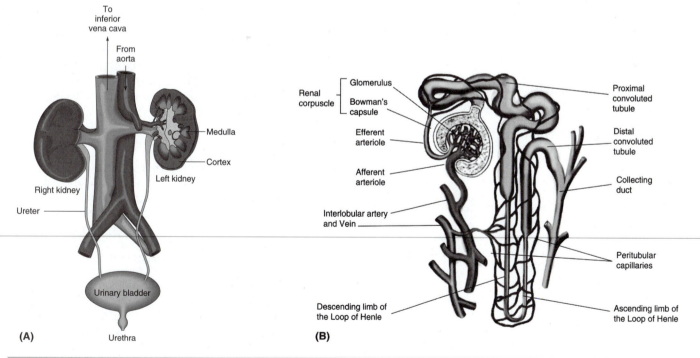

Figure 11.1 Structure and blood flow of the kidneys. (A) The kidneys, ureters, and bladder. (B) A nephron and its associated structures.

D. Renal sinus and pelvis: calyces collect urine from collecting ducts and direct urine from renal sinus to renal pelvis; urine flows from renal pelvis to ureters
E. Nephron: the functional unit of the kidney consists of the following (see Figure 11.1):
   1. Renal corpuscle (vascular system of nephron)
   2. Bowman's capsule: a portion of the proximal tubule that surrounds the glomerulus
   3. Glomerulus: a capillary network permeable to water, electrolytes, nutrients, and wastes, and impermeable to large protein molecules
   4. The renal tubule consists of the proximal convoluted tubule, the descending loop of Henle, the ascending loop of Henle, the distal convoluted tubule, and the collecting duct

Ureters

A. Two tubes approximately 25–35 cm long
B. Extend from the renal pelvis to the pelvic cavity, where they enter the bladder
C. Take urine from the kidneys to the bladder
D. Ureterovesical valve prevents backflow of urine into ureters

Bladder

A. Located behind the symphysis pubis
B. Composed of muscular, elastic tissue that makes it distensible
C. Serves as a reservoir of urine; can hold 1,000 ml–1,800 ml; a moderately full bladder holds about 500 ml
D. Internal and external sphincters control the flow of urine.
E. Urge to void stimulated by passage of urine past the internal sphincter (involuntary) to the upper part of the urethra
F. Relaxation of external sphincter (voluntary) produces emptying of the bladder.

Urethra

A. Small tube that extends from the bladder to the exterior of the body
B. Females:
   1. Located behind the symphysis pubis and anterior to the vagina
   2. 3–5 cm long
C. Males:
   1. Extends entire length of penis
   2. 20 cm long

Regulatory Functions of Kidney:

A. Remove nitrogenous wastes
B. Regulate fluid and electrolyte balance
C. Regulate acid base balance
D. Formation of urine
   1. Glomerular filtration:
      a. Ultrafiltration of blood by the glomerulus; beginning of urine formation
      b. Normally 125 ml/min, is filtered; called glomerular filtration rate (GFR)
   2. Tubular function:
      a. Tubules and collecting ducts carry out the functions of reabsorption of water and electrolytes; secretion; excretion
      b. Functions take place within the proximal convoluted tubule, the Loop of Henle, the distal convoluted tubule, and the collecting ducts
   3. Normal adult produces 1–1 1/2 liters/day of urine
E. Blood pressure control:
   1. Kidneys regulate blood pressure partly through maintenance of volume
   2. Renin-angiotensin system: when blood pressure drops, cells of the glomerulus release renin; renin activates angiotensin to cause vasoconstriction

MALE REPRODUCTIVE SYSTEM (Figure 11.2)

Penis

An external structure that serves as a passageway for urine and sperm; it is capable of distention during sexual excitement. The distal portion, the glans penis, is covered by a prepuce or foreskin that is sometimes removed in a procedure called circumcision.

Scrotum

A saclike structure that hangs from the root of the penis and contains the testes and epididymis; being outside the body helps to maintain a cooler temperature conducive to sperm production.

A. Testes: Small, oval structures suspended in the scrotum that produce sperm (exocrine function) and testosterone (endocrine function)
B. Ductal system:
   1. Epididymis: a soft, cordlike structure that lies along the posterolateral surface of each testis; the head is attached to the top of the testis and the tail is continuous with the vas deferens; stores spermatozoa while they mature

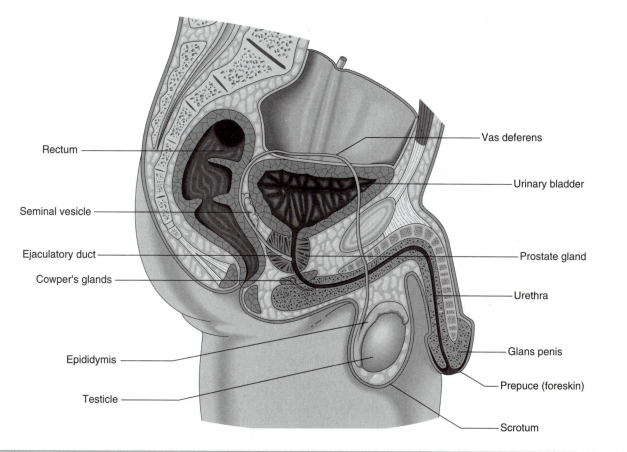

Figure 11.2 Cross section of the male reproductive system.

2. Spermatic cord consists of vas deferens, arteries, veins, nerves, and lymphatic vessels; the vas deferens joins the duct of the seminal vesicles to become the ejaculatory duct.
C. Accessory Glands:
   1. Prostate: a structure about 4–6 cm long located below the bladder and in front of the rectum; enclosed in a firm, fibrous capsule connected to the urethra and ejaculatory ducts secrete a milky fluid that aids in the passage of spermatozoa and helps keep them viable
   2. Cowper's glands lie on each side of the urethra and just below the prostate and secrete a small amount of lubricating fluid.
   3. Seminal vesicles are paired structures parallel to the bladder that secrete a portion of the ejaculate and may contribute to nutrition and activation of sperm.

Diagnostic Tests

A. Urinalysis
B. Clean catch urine
   1. Cleansing
      a. Male: cleanse area around meatus with antiseptic wipe going from meatus outward
      b. Female: client separates labia with one hand and cleanses area with antiseptic wipes; motion is front to back; go down each side with a separate wipe and finally down the center over the meatus with a third wipe
   2. Mid-stream collection: client should void initial urine into the toilet and collect urine midstream
C. Renal Function Tests: several tests over a period of time are necessary
   1. Blood Urea Nitrogen (BUN) 10–20 mg; elevated levels indicate kidneys are not functioning well

2. Serum creatinine: 0–1 mg/dL; elevated levels indicate poor kidney function
3. Uric acid—serum 3.5–7.8 mg/dL; high levels indicate risk of gout and kidney stones

D. Radiologic Tests:
1. Kidney, ureter, bladder (KUB) X-ray—shows size, shape, and position of kidneys
2. Intravenous pyelography (IVP):
   a. Preparation: NPO for 8–10 hrs
   b. Laxative to clear lower bowel
   c. Check for allergies to iodine or shellfish; iodine dye is used to visualize the kidneys.
3. Renal angiography; visualization of renal arterial supply; contrast material injected through a catheter
   a. Nursing care before exam:
      (1) Cathartic or enema
      (2) Shave proposed injection sites (groin or ankle)
      (3) Locate and mark peripheral pulses
   b. Nursing care after exam:
      (1) Vital signs until stable
      (2) Cold to puncture site
      (3) Check for swelling and hematoma
      (4) Palpate peripheral pulses
      (5) CHECK color and temp of extremity

E. Cystoscopy
1. Uses:
   a. Diagnostic to inspect bladder and urethra, insert catheters into ureters, and see configuration and position of ureteral orifices
   b. Treatment uses: remove calculi from urethra, bladder, and ureter; treat lesions of bladder, urethra, prostate
2. Nursing care before procedure: Push fluids if general anesthesia not to be given
3. Nursing care after procedure:
   a. Pink-tinged or tea-colored urine normal
   b. Bright red urine or clots should be reported to the physician.
   c. Back pain and/or abdominal pain may occur; notify the doctor.
   d. Leg cramps from lithotomy position
   e. Warm baths are comforting.

F. Needle Biopsy of Kidney
1. Pre-biopsy care:
   a. Bleeding, clotting, and prothrombin times because kidney is very vascular
   b. X-ray of kidney
   c. Ultrasound to locate kidney
2. Post-biopsy care
   a. Bed rest for 24 hours to decrease chance of bleeding
   b. Vital signs q 5–15 minutes for one hour; then decreased if stable
   c. Check for pain, nausea, or vomiting
   d. Fluids to 3,000 cc

e. Hct and Hgb in eight hrs
f. Avoid strenuous activity for two weeks

G. Catheterization (see Table 11.1)
1. Purposes include:
   a. Empty contents of bladder
   b. Obtain a sterile specimen
   c. Determine residual urine
   d. Irrigate bladder
   e. Bypass an obstruction
2. Sterile procedure
3. Specimen for culture from catheterized client:
   a. Clamp tubing for 15 minutes
   b. Cleanse port (if present) or cleanse catheter distal to bifurcation with antiseptic
   c. Insert sterile needle (with syringe) into port or distal to bifurcation
4. Residual urine:
   a. May be ordered after gynecological or urinary tract surgery or when client

---

Table 11.1 Urinary Catheterization

Insertion of Retention Catheter
1. Using sterile technique, open catheterization tray.
2. Lubricate catheter using sterile water-soluble lubricant provided in tray.
3. Drape client.
4. Cleanse the client's meatus:
   a. For a female: cleanse client's meatus with one downward stroke of the antiseptic-soaked sterile cotton ball or wipe, repeating three or four times; continue to hold client's labia apart until catheter inserted
   b. For a male: hold the penis upright, holding the sides to prevent closing the urethra; cleanse client's meatus with one downward stroke of the antiseptic-soaked sterile cotton ball or wipe, repeating three or four times; continue to hold client's penis until catheter inserted
5. Insert a lubricated catheter 2 to 3 inches beyond the point at which urine begins to flow to ensure it is beyond the neck of the bladder.
6. Instill sterile water into the balloon after the catheter is inserted.
7. Tape the catheter with tape.
   a. Female: tape catheter to the side of the leg
   b. Male: tape catheter to abdomen to prevent pressure on the penoscrotal angle
8. Attach the drainage bag to the bed frame, not side rails, so that it hangs freely.

Removal of Catheter
1. Clamp the catheter.
2. Do not cut the catheter with scissors. The balloon may not totally deflate if it is cut.
3. Withdraw fluid from balloon (usually 5 to 10 ml water in the balloon).
4. Pull gently on the catheter to be sure the balloon is deflated before attempting to remove it in order to prevent damage to urethra from a partially deflated balloon.
5. Record output on I and O record.
6. Wash the perineum with soap and water and dry thoroughly.
7. Instruct client to drink oral fluids as tolerated and observe for signs and symptoms of urinary tract infection.
8. Offer bedpan or urinal every two to four hours after removing catheter until voiding occurs; monitor I and O until voiding well established.

who has been catheterized for a long time has an indwelling catheter removed

b. Catheterize client immediately after client voids. Normal is less than 50 ml.

H. Self Testicular Exam
   1. Hormonally active years (15–35) are tumor-prone years.
   2. Perform exam while showering or bathing.
   3. Use both hands to palpate; carefully examine all scrotal contents.
   4. Locate the epididymis (cordlike structure in the back of the testis).
   5. The spermatic cord (and vas deferens) extends upward from the epididymis.
   6. Feel each testis between the thumb and first two fingers of each hand; testes move freely in the scrotum, are oval-shaped and measure 4–5 cm in length, 3 cm in width, and 2 cm in thickness.
   7. Stand in front of mirror and look for changes in size and shape of scrotum; tumors or cystic masses tend to involve only one side.

SPECIFIC UROLOGIC DISORDERS

Cystitis

A. Inflammation of the urinary bladder caused by an ascending infection after entry via the urinary meatus; more common in females; acute infections usually E. Coli.
B. Assessment findings:
   1. Frequency and urgency to urinate
   2. Burning in the urethra
   3. Suprapubic tenderness, pain in bladder
   4. Pus and blood in urine
C. Nursing diagnoses (see Table 11.2)
D. Interventions:
   1. Urine for culture and sensitivity
   2. Antimicrobial medications:
      a. Bactrim, Septra
      b. Gantrisin
   3. Pyridium: urinary tract anesthetic to kill pain until infection starts to clear
   4. Appropriate urine pH
   5. Force fluids

Urolithiasis

A. Stones in the urinary system
B. Risk factors:
   1. Obstruction and urinary stasis
   2. Proteus infection
   4. Dehydration
   5. Immobilization
   6. Hypercalcemia
   7. Excessive excretion of uric acid
   8. Heredity
C. Characteristics:
   1. More common in men aged 30–50
   2. Tend to recur
D. Assessment findings:
   1. Pain—renal colic
   2. Nausea, vomiting, diarrhea
   3. Hematuria
   4. Symptoms of urinary tract infection
   5. KUB, urinalysis, IVP done to diagnose stone
E. Nursing diagnoses (see Table 11.3)
F. Interventions:
   1. Encourage fluids to a minimum of 3,000 cc/day to flush stones out.
   2. Strain all urine and send to the laboratory for analysis.
   3. Encourage ambulation to help pass the stone.
   4. Allopurinol (Zyloprim) to decrease uric acid production
   5. Pain control
   6. Surgery to remove stone if not passed

Glomerulonephritis

A. An inflammatory disease involving the renal glomeruli of both kidneys caused by antigen-antibody reaction following streptococcal infection causing damage to glomeruli of kidney
B. Assessment findings:
   1. History of pharyngitis or tonsillitis within 7–20 days
   2. Hematuria
   3. Edema
   4. Decreased urine output
   5. Hypertension
   6. Headache
   7. Flank pain
   8. Anemia
   9. Increased BUN

Table 11.2 Nursing Diagnoses Related to Cystitis

- Chronic pain related to inflammation and tissue trauma
- Impaired comfort related to inflammation and infection
- High risk for impaired nutrition: less than body requirements related to anorexia secondary to malaise
- High risk for ineffective health maintenance related to insufficient knowledge of prevention of recurrence (adequate fluid intake, frequent voiding, hygiene measures, and voiding after sexual activity), signs and symptoms of recurrence, and pharmacologic therapy

---

Table 11.3 Nursing Diagnoses Related to Nephrolithiasis

- Acute pain related to inflammation secondary to irritation of stone
- Diarrhea related to renointestinal reflexes
- Risk for ineffective health maintenance related to insufficient knowledge of prevention of recurrence, dietary restrictions, and fluid requirements

C. Nursing diagnoses (see Table 11.2)
D. Interventions:
   1. Rest
   2. Reduce dietary protein if oliguria and elevated BUN
   3. Administer penicillin (for the strep infection) if ordered
   4. Administer antihypertensives if ordered

Pyelonephritis

A. Inflammation of the renal pelvis. Acute pyelonephritis is usually caused by an ascending bladder infection. Chronic pyelonephritis is thought to be a combination of structural abnormalities and infection.
B. Assessment findings:
   1. Acute: fever, chills, nausea, and vomiting
   2. Chronic: client usually unaware of disease; may have bladder irritability, chronic fatigue, or slight, dull ache over kidneys; eventually develops hypertension and atrophy of kidneys
C. Interventions:
   1. Acute:
      a. Administer antibiotics and antispasmodics as ordered
      b. Surgical removal of any obstruction
   2. Chronic:
      a. Antibiotics and urinary antiseptics as ordered
      b. Surgical correction of structural abnormality if possible
   3. Monitor intake and output
   4. Teach client about condition and side effects of drugs

Nephrotic Syndrome

A. A clinical disorder characterized by marked proteinuria, hypoalbuminemia, edema, and hypercholesterolemia
B. Risk factors:
   1. Chronic glomerulonephritis
   2. Diabetes mellitus
   3. Systemic lupus erythematosus
   4. Toxins
   5. Renal vein thrombosis
   6. Primary lipid nephrosis in children
C. Assessment findings:
   1. Insidious onset of pitting edema
   2. Proteinuria
   3. Hypoalbuminemia
   4. Hypercholesterolemia
D. Interventions:
   1. Rest
   2. Low-sodium, high-calorie diet; high protein may be ordered
   3. Protect patient from infection (has hypoalbuminemia and is at risk for infection)

4. Administer diuretics, steroids (Prednisone), and immunosuppressants (Cytoxan) as ordered

Urinary Tract Surgery

A. Interventions:
   1. Monitor vital signs, because hemorrhage and shock are frequent complications.
   2. Pain control
   3. Observe for paralytic ileus.
   4. Intake and output to assure adequate fluid replacement
   5. Daily weights
   6. Deep-breathing, coughing, positioning to prevent respiratory complications
   7. Ambulate early.
   8. Care for drainage tubes that may be present:
      a. Indwelling catheter (dependent position, tape tubing to thigh)
      b. Nephrostomy tube:
         (1) Do not clamp
         (2) Irrigate only with order—3–5 cc normal saline only
         (3) Change dressings as indicated—profuse drainage
B. Kidney Transplant
   1. Donor must match tissue and blood type:
      a. Best donor is a living relative with compatible serum and tissue studies, free from systemic infection, and emotionally stable: identical twin, sibling, parent
      b. Cadavers with serum and tissue cross-matching free from renal disease, cancer, and sepsis and no ischemia or renal trauma
   2. Nursing diagnoses (see Table 11.4)
   3. Interventions:
      a. Routine post-op care
      b. Monitor fluid and electrolyte balance.
         (1) I&O hourly
         (2) May have massive diuresis
      c. Frequent and early ambulation
      d. Vital signs including temperature

Table 11.4 Nursing Diagnoses Related to Renal Transplantation
- Acute pain related to surgical incision
- Risk for infection related to altered immune system secondary to medications
- Risk for impaired oral mucus membrane related to increased susceptibility to infection secondary to immunosuppression
- Fear related to risk of rejection and dying
- Disturbed body image disturbance related to replacement of body part and medication causing changes in appearance
- Risk for noncompliance related to the complexity of treatment regimen and euphoria at receiving the transplant

e. Mouth care (Mycostatin) for candidiasis
f. Administer immunosuppressive agents as ordered:
   (1) Cyclosporine
   (2) Azathioprine (Imuran)
   (3) Cyclophosphamide (Cytoxan)
   (4) Antilymphocytic Globulin (ALG)
   (5) Corticosteroids (prednisone, Solu-Medrol)
g. Teach patient about living with long-term immunosuppressive therapy:
   (1) Avoid crowds, infections.
   (2) Get regular medical care.
h. Assess for signs of acute rejection:
   (1) Occurs most frequently from four days to four months after transplant
   (2) Report any of the following:
      (a) Decreased urine output
      (b) Fever
      (c) Pain, tenderness over transplant site
      (d) Edema, weight gain
      (e) Elevated blood pressure
      (f) Malaise
      (g) Rise in serum creatinine
      (h) Decrease in creatinine clearance

Acute Renal Failure

A. Abrupt cessation of renal function
B. Causes:
   1. Prerenal: event causing decreased blood flow to the kidney
      a. Cardiogenic shock
      b. Hemorrhage
      c. Burns
      d. Septicemia
   2. Intrarenal: damage to nephrons
      a. Diabetes mellitus
      b. Malignant hypertension
      c. Glomerulonephritis
      d. Tumors
      e. Transfusion reactions
      f. Nephrotoxic substances such as medications, chemicals
   3. Postrenal: mechanical obstruction from the tubules to the urethra
      a. Calculi
      b. Benign prostatic hypertrophy
      c. Tumors
C. Assessment findings:
   1. Oliguric phase:
      a. Urine output under 400 cc/24 hrs
      b. Lasts 1–2 weeks
      c. Hyponatremia, hypocalcemia
      d. Hyperkalemia, hyperphosphatemia, hypermagnesemia
      e. Metabolic acidosis
      f. BUN and creatinine elevated

   2. Diuretic phase:
      a. Gradual increase in urine output up to 3–5 liters per day; recovering kidney cannot concentrate urine well, so urine is dilute
      b. Lasts 2–3 weeks
      c. Hyponatremia, hypokalemia, hypovolemia
      d. BUN and creatinine elevated
   3. Recovery phase:
      a. Renal function stabilizes
      b. Improvement for 3–12 months
D. Nursing diagnoses (see Table 11.5)
E. Interventions:
   1. Intake and output
   2. Daily weights
   3. Low-protein, high-CHO diet
   4. TPN sometimes
   5. Fluid and electrolyte balance
   6. Protect from infection
   7. Dialysis

Chronic Renal Failure

A. Progressive, irreversible destruction of the kidneys that continues until nephrons are replaced by scar tissue
B. Risk factors:
   1. Recurrent renal infections
   2. Urinary tract obstructions
   3. Diabetes mellitus
   4. Hypertension
C. Assessment findings:
   1. Stage of diminished renal reserve
      a. Polyuria
      b. Dilute urine with normal chemistries
   2. Stage of renal insufficiency
   3. Stage of renal failure:
      a. Abnormal chemistries
      b. Confusion
   4. Uremia and death
D. Nursing diagnoses (see Table 11.6)
E. Interventions:
   1. Diet that is low in sodium, potassium, and protein and high in carbohydrates
   2. Vitamins and iron (client has low Hct and Hgb)
   3. Aluminum hydroxide gel to buffer high phosphorus levels

Table 11.5 Nursing Diagnoses Related to Acute Renal Failure

- Fluid volume excess related to renal failure
- Risk for injury related to confusion secondary to renal failure
- Imbalanced nutrition: less than body requirements related to anorexia, nausea, vomiting, loss of taste, loss of smell, stomatitis, and unpalatable diet
- Risk for infection related to invasive procedures
- Anxiety related to present status and unknown prognosis

Table 11.6 Nursing Diagnoses Related to Chronic Renal Failure

- Fluid volume excess related to decreased urinary output secondary to disease process
- Risk for injury related to disturbances in thinking process secondary to renal failure
- Imbalanced nutrition: less than body requirements related to anorexia, nausea/vomiting, loss of taste/smell, stomatitis, and/or unpalatable diet
- Ineffective sexuality patterns related to decreased libido, impotence, amenorrhea, sterility
- Disturbed self concept related to effects of limitation on achievement of developmental tasks
- Risk for social isolation related to disability and treatment requirements
- Impaired comfort related to fatigue, headaches, fluid retention, anemia, uremic frost
- Fatigue related to insufficient oxygenation secondary to anemia
- Risk for infection related to invasive procedures
- Powerlessness related to progressively disabling nature of disorder
- High risk for impaired health maintenance related to insufficient knowledge of condition, fluid and sodium restrictions, dietary restrictions (protein, potassium, sodium), daily recording of intake, output, and weights, pharmacological therapy, signs and symptoms of complications, follow-up visits, and community resources

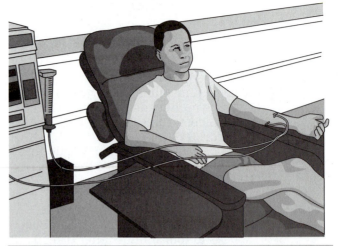

Figure 11.3 Hemodialysis filters waste from the patient's blood. Arterial blood is filtered, then returned into a vein.

concentration; removes fluid that kidneys would normally remove from bloodstream

3. Epogen administered to stimulate hematopoiesis. Dialysis does not substitute for manufacturing role of kidney; in other words, production of erythropoiten to stimulate production of red blood cells

Hemodialysis

A. Shunting of blood from the patient's vascular system through an artificial dialyzing system and return of dialyzed blood to the patient's circulation (see Figure 11.3)
B. Access routes (see Figure 11.4)
   1. A-V fistula:
      a. Internal anastamosis of an artery to an adjacent vein
      b. Takes 4–6 weeks to "mature" before it is ready to use
      c. Fistula accessed by venipuncture
      d. Lasts 3–4 years
   2. Femoral vein and subclavian vein catheterization
      a. Allow immediate access for emergency dialysis
      b. Not for long-term use
C. Nursing diagnoses (see Table 11.7)
D. Nursing care for AV fistula:
   1. Auscultate for a bruit and palpate for a thrill to ensure patency
   2. No I.V.s, I.M.s, or blood pressures on affected arm to prevent damage to fistula
   3. Teach client to avoid restrictive clothing over site
   4. Report bleeding, skin discoloration, drainage, or pain.
E. Nursing care for femoral or subclavian cannulation:
   1. Palpate peripheral pulses in extremity with cannula.

4. Antihypertensives as ordered for hypertension
5. Reduce high potassium levels if needed by the use of Kayexalate enema; insulin and glucose may be given IV to drive potassium into the cells.
6. Calcium and vitamin D may be given because the client has low serum calcium levels.
7. Dialysis
8. Diuretics as ordered
9. Assure safety because client may be confused

Dialysis

A. Purposes:
   1. Remove end products of protein metabolism from blood.
   2. Maintain safe levels of electrolytes.
   3. Correct acidosis.
   4. Remove excess fluid.
B. Principles:
   1. Diffusion: movement of particle from an area of high concentration to an area of low concentration across a semipermeable membrane; removes electrolytes that kidney would normally remove from bloodstream
   2. Osmosis: movement of fluid across a semipermeable membrane from an area of higher concentration to one of lower

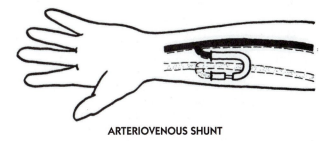

ARTERIOVENOUS SHUNT

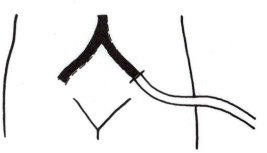

ARTERIOVENOUS FISTULA

FEMORAL VEIN CATHETERIZATION

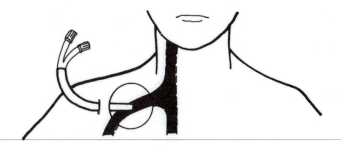

SUBCLAVIAN VEIN CATHETERIZATION

Figure 11.4 Hemodialysis sites.

2. Report bleeding or hematoma formation at site.
3. Observe for bleeding from catheter during dialysis.
F. Nursing care before and during hemodialysis:
   1. Have the client void.

Table 11.7 Nursing Diagnoses Related to Hemodialysis

- Risk for altered health maintenance related to insufficient knowledge of catheter care, precautions, emergency measures, prevention of infection, and activity limitations
- Anxiety related to upcoming shunt insertion
- Risk for injury to vascular access site related to vulnerability
- Risk for infection related to direct access to bloodstream secondary to vascular access
- Powerlessness related to need for treatments to live despite effects on lifestyle
- High risk for ineffective health maintenance related to insufficient knowledge of rationale of treatment, care of site, precautions, emergency treatments (disconnected, bleeding, clotting), pretreatment instructions, and daily assessments (bruit, blood pressure, weights)
- Risk for infection transmission related to frequent contacts with blood and high risk for hepatitis B

2. Weigh the client.
3. Take vital signs before and every 30 minutes during dialysis.
4. Withhold antihypertensives, sedatives, and vasodilators to prevent a hypotensive episode.
5. Observe for bleeding (blood has been heparinized) and report if any is present.
6. Teach the client that headache and nausea are common.
G. Nursing care after dialysis:
   1. Weigh the client.
   2. Observe for hypovolemic shock, which may occur as a result of rapid removal or ultrafiltration of fluid from the intravascular compartment
   3. Assess for dialysis disequilibrium syndrome: nausea, vomiting, elevated blood pressure, disorientation, leg cramps, and peripheral paresthesias

Peritoneal Dialysis

A. Introduction of dialysate solution into the abdominal cavity, where the peritoneum acts as a semipermeable membrane between the dialysate and blood in the abdominal vessels (see Figure 11.5)
B. Nursing diagnoses (see Table 11.8)
C. Nursing care for clients receiving peritoneal dialysis:
   1. Weigh client.
   2. Monitor vital signs before and during procedure.
   3. Have client void before procedure.
   4. Warm dialysate solution to body temperature.
   5. Inflow time 10–20 minutes
   6. Dwell time 30–45 minutes
   7. Drain by gravity.
   8. Continued for 24–72 exchanges

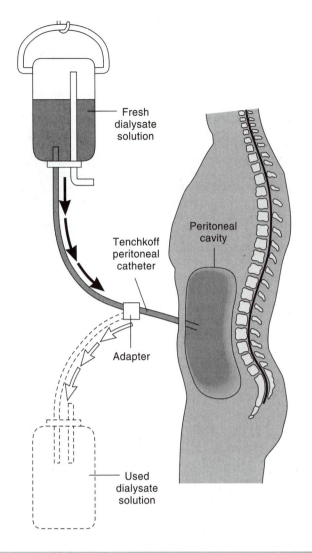

Figure 11.5 Peritoneal dialysis removes wastes through a fluid exchange in the peritoneal cavity.

9. Change the client's position if drainage is not complete.
10. Maintain intake and output.
D. Complications of peritoneal dialysis:
1. Peritonitis: cloudy dialysate suggests peritonitis
2. Respiratory difficulty from pressure of full abdomen
3. Protein loss; most serum proteins pass through the peritoneal membrane and are lost in dialysate fluid; monitor serum protein levels closely

Continuous Ambulatory Peritoneal Dialysis (CAPD)

A. A continuous type of peritoneal dialysis performed at home by the client or others
B. Dialysate is delivered from flexible plastic containers through a permanent peritoneal catheter.

Table 11.8 Nursing Diagnoses Related to Peritoneal Dialysis

- Risk for infection related to direct access to peritoneal cavity, the need to disconnect catheter for treatment, and growth medium potential of the dialysate (high glucose concentration)
- Risk for injury to catheter site related to vulnerability
- Risk for ineffective breathing patterns related to immobility and pressure on diaphragm during dwell time
- Impaired comfort related to rapid instillation, pressure from fluid, excessive suction during outflow, and/or extreme temperature of solution (hot or cold)
- Risk for impaired nutrition: less than body requirements related to anorexia secondary to abdominal distention during dialysis, protein loss in dialysate, or vomiting
- Risk for fluid volume excess related to fluid retention secondary to catheter problems (kinks, blockages) and/or position
- Powerlessness related to need for treatment to live despite effects on lifestyle
- Impaired home maintenance management related to lack of knowledge of treatment procedures
- Risk for impaired health maintenance related to insufficient knowledge of home care, self-care activities, protection of catheter, activity needs, prescribed diet, control of fluid intake/output, medication regimen, signs and symptoms of complications, follow-up visits, and daily recording (intake, output, blood pressure, weights)

C. Following infusion of the dialysate into the peritoneal cavity, the bag is folded and tucked away during the dwell period (usually 4–6 hours)
D. Teach client:
1. Assess the permanent peritoneal catheter for complications such as dialysate leak, exit site infection, obstruction.
2. Follow high protein diet if ordered.
3. Importance of regular blood chemistries
4. Daily weights
5. Cloudy dialysate indicates infection.

DISORDERS OF THE MALE REPRODUCTIVE SYSTEM

Benign Prostatic Hypertrophy

A. Enlargement of the prostate, which accompanies the aging process in the male (seen in men over 50)
B. Assessment findings:
1. Urinary tract infection
2. Hesitancy, difficulty starting urinary stream
3. Elevated PSA (prostate specific antigen), normal is < 4 ng/ml
4. Nocturia, hematuria
5. Dribbling
6. Decrease in size and force of urinary stream

Table 11.9 Nursing Diagnoses Related to Prostate Surgery

- Impaired comfort related to back/leg pains secondary to bladder spasms or clot retention
- Risk for infection related to surgical incision and catheterization
- Risk for urinary retention related to lack of sphincter control secondary to catheterization
- Risk for stress incontinence related to lack of sphincter control and loss of muscle tone secondary to catheterization and prostate
- Risk for impaired sexuality patterns related to fear of impotence resulting from surgical intervention
- Risk for impaired health maintenance related to insufficient knowledge of fluid requirements, activity restrictions, catheter care, urinary control, and follow-up care

7. Urinalysis shows alkaline urine.
8. BUN and creatinine may elevate in time.

C. Interventions:
   1. Cystoscopy for diagnosis
   2. Urinary antiseptics or antibiotics to treat urinary tract infection if present
   3. Medication such as finasteride (Proscar) to shrink the prostate
   4. Prostatectomy
D. Nursing diagnoses (see Table 11.9)

Cancer of the Prostate

A. Second most common cause of cancer deaths in American males over age 55. Highest incidence is in African American men age 60 and older.
B. Assessment findings:
   1. Same as for benign prostatic hypertrophy
   2. Elevated acid phosphatase indicates distant metastasis.
   3. Elevated alkaline phosphatase indicates bone metastasis.
   4. Bone scan to detect bone metastasis
C. Nursing diagnoses (see Table 11.9)
D. Interventions:
   1. Provide care for client receiving chemotherapy.
   2. Provide care for client receiving radiation therapy.
   3. Provide care for client with a prostatectomy.

Prostate Surgery (Prostatectomy)

A. Used for clients with benign prostatic hypertrophy and cancer of the prostate
B. Types of prostatectomies:
   1. Transurethral resection (TUR or TURP):
      a. Insertion of a resectoscope into the urethra to excise prostatic tissue
      b. Most common procedure for BPH
      c. Good for poor surgical risks because it does not involve an incision

   2. Retropubic prostatectomy
      a. Low, midline incision above the pubic bone, below and into the prostatic capsule
      b. Used to remove a large mass high in the pelvic area
   3. Suprapubic prostatectomy
      a. Low abdominal incision into and through the bladder to the anterior aspect of the prostate
      b. Used for large tumors obstructing the urethra
C. Nursing diagnoses (see Table 11.9)
D. Nursing care
   1. Preoperative:
      a. Maintain adequate bladder drainage via a catheter.
      b. Administer antibiotics as ordered.
      c. Monitor vital signs.
      d. Maintain hydration to prevent urinary tract infection or treat existing UTI.
      e. Daily weights
   2. Postoperative:
      a. Observe for shock and hemorrhage, and report signs indicating either.
      b. Monitor bladder drainage from three-way urinary catheter.
         (1) Expect hematuria for 2–3 days.
         (2) Irrigate catheter with normal saline as ordered.
      c. Administer anticholinergics such as propantheline (Probanthine) or antispasmodics for bladder spasms.
      d. Administer stool softeners as ordered.
      e. Restrict caffeinated beverages and teach the client to do so.
      f. Encourage fluids.
      g. Teach the client how to do perineal exercises to help regain bladder control.
      h. Teach the client that he should do no heavy lifting, prolonged travel, or straining during defecation for 8–12 weeks after surgery.

Vasectomy

A. Ligation and transection of a section of the vas deferens. Bilateral vasectomy results in sterility; procedure used as a permanent method of sterilization.
B. No decrease in seminal fluid after vasectomy; seminal fluid is made in the seminal vesicles and prostate, which are not affected by vasectomy.
C. After vasectomy, man is sterile but not impotent.
D. Nursing care:
   1. Ice bags to scrotum to reduce swelling and relieve discomfort
   2. Discoloration of scrotal skin; swelling and edema may occur

3. Client should wear scrotal support for comfort and support
4. Teach client to rest for 48 hours after procedure.
5. Contraceptives should be used until the sperm stored distal to the point of interruption of the vas is evacuated (two negative specimens one month apart).

Sample Questions

1. The nurse is performing a urethral catheterization on a female. After separating the labia, where would the nurse observe the urethral meatus?
   1. Between the vaginal orifice and the anus
   2. Between the clitoris and the vaginal orifice
   3. Just above the clitoris
   4. Within the vaginal cana
2. An adult had an indwelling catheter removed. After she voids for the first time, the nurse catheterizes her as ordered and obtains 200 cc of urine. What is the best interpretation of this finding? The client:
   1. Is voiding normally
   2. Has urinary retention
   3. Has developed renal failure
   4. Needs an indwelling catheter
3. The nurse is preparing to insert an indwelling catheter. What type of technique should the nurse use to perform this procedure?
   1. Clean technique
   2. Medical asepsis
   3. Isolation protocol
   4. Sterile technique
4. After inserting the indwelling catheter, how should the nurse position the drainage container?
   1. With the drainage tubing taut to maintain maximum suction on the urinary bladder
   2. Lower than the bladder to maintain a constant downward flow of urine from the bladder
   3. At the head of the bed for easy and accurate measurement of urine
   4. Beside the patient in his bed to avoid embarrassment
5. The nurse is attempting to pass an indwelling catheter in an adult male and is having difficulty. What is the most appropriate action for the nurse?
   1. Remove the catheter and reinsert it with the client positioned differently.
   2. Try a straight catheter instead.
   3. Try a smaller catheter.
   4. Discontinue the procedure and notify the physician.
6. A client has just had a needle biopsy of the kidney. What should the nurse do immediately following the procedure?
   1. Keep him NPO; take his blood pressure q 5 min for 1 hour and then q 15 min.
   2. Keep him flat for 24 hours; take his blood pressure q 5 min for 1 hour, then q 15 min.
   3. Check his blood pressure q 30 min for 2 hours; monitor I & O ; position in the Sims position.
   4. Check I & O ; send all urine to lab for analysis; ambulate after 8 hours; position in high-Fowler's position.
7. A five-year-old has been wetting his bed since coming into the hospital. The best approach for the nurse to use to help him regain his voluntary bladder control is to:
   1. Put diapers on him until he promises to stay dry.
   2. Leave him in his wet bed so he will learn he should not wet his bed.
   3. Promise him a lollipop if he will call when he needs to void.
   4. Assist him to the bathroom at regular intervals.
8. An adult client has returned to his room following a cystoscopy. When he voids, his urine is pink-tinged. The most appropriate action for the nurse to take is:
   1. Continue to observe him.
   2. Report it immediately to the physician.
   3. Irrigate the catheter with normal saline.
   4. Take his blood pressure every 15 min.
9. An 18-year-old female is seen in the clinic for a bladder infection. Which of the following signs and symptoms would the nurse expect her to manifest?
   1. Burning upon urination
   2. Flank pain
   3. Nausea and vomiting
   4. Elevated potassium
10. The nurse instructs a woman in the proper procedure for obtaining a clean-catch urine specimen. What should the nurse tell her to do?
    1. Clean the perineal area with soap and water and then void into the collection container.
    2. Clean around the urethral opening using antibacterial cleaning pads, wiping from front to back. Urinate and let some of the urine go into the toilet; then collect urine in the sterile container.
    3. Wash the area around the urethra and vagina. Insert the end of the sterile catheter into your urethra and collect the urine that is drained.
    4. Use the special cotton balls and clean your perineal area, wiping in circles from outer labia inward. Collect the urine in the sterile container.
11. A urinalysis reveals white cells and bacteria in the urine of a female client suspected of having a bladder infection. The client is instructed to take the prescribed anti-infective. What else should the nurse include when teaching the client?

1. Limit fluid intake until the pain subsides.
2. Wipe from back to front after voiding.
3. Empty her bladder immediately after having sexual relations.
4. Take the medication until she is pain-free for 48 hours.

12. An adult male is admitted with severe right-flank pain, nausea, and vomiting of four hours duration. The admitting diagnosis is kidney stones. Orders include encourage fluids to 1,000 cc per shift. What is the primary reason for encouraging fluids in this client?
    1. To prevent renal failure
    2. To help the stone pass
    3. To prevent infection
    4. To relieve his dehydration

13. The nurse is straining the urine of a client admitted with possible renal calculi. A small stone is discovered. What should the nurse do?
    1. Send the stone to the laboratory for analysis.
    2. Immediately test for guaiac.
    3. Test the stone for glucose.
    4. Administer pain medication.

14. A client who has kidney stones complains of pain. The nurse finds him pacing the hall. What is the most appropriate action for the nurse to take?
    1. Tell him to get back in bed where he will be more comfortable.
    2. Encourage him to walk if it helps to relieve the pain.
    3. Remind him to walk only when he has someone with him.
    4. Put him back in bed immediately and position him in semi-Fowler's.

15. The nurse is caring for a client who has acute renal failure. His potassium rises to 7.3 mEq/l. A Kayexalate enema is ordered. What is the primary purpose of the Kayexalate enema?
    1. To remove fluid from the extracellular spaces
    2. To exchange potassium ions for sodium ions
    3. To reduce abdominal pressure
    4. To introduce potassium into the bowel

16. The nurse is caring for a client who is in acute renal failure. Which of the following selections would be best to give for a snack?
    1. A slice of watermelon
    2. Orange juice
    3. A turkey sandwich
    4. A dish of applesauce

17. A 67-year-old man is admitted with dysuria that has gotten worse over the past six months. Rectal examination revealed an enlarged prostate. Following urination, he was catheterized and found to have 250 cc of thick, foul-smelling, residual urine. He is admitted with a diagnosis of benign prostatic hypertrophy. Which symptom is least likely to be present in this client?

1. Urinary frequency
2. Pus in the urine
3. Dribbling
4. Decreased force of urinary stream

18. The client who has urinary retention has had an indwelling catheter inserted. Which action is **not appropriate** for the nurse to take?
    1. Limit fluid intake.
    2. Monitor blood pressure frequently.
    3. Weigh the client daily.
    4. Assess renal function.

19. The nurse has inserted an indwelling catheter into an adult male. The nurse tapes the urinary drainage tube laterally to the thigh for which of the following reasons?
    1. To insure patient comfort
    2. To prevent reflux of urine
    3. To maintain tension on the balloon of the Foley
    4. To prevent compression at the penoscrotal junction

20. A client who had a transurethral prostatectomy is returned to the unit with continuous bladder irrigation. The nurse understands that the primary purpose of continuous bladder irrigation for this client is to:
    1. Prevent a urinary tract infection
    2. Maintain bladder tone
    3. Flush blood clots from the bladder
    4. Prevent urethral stricture

21. A 35-year-old man asks the nurse about a vasectomy. In discussing a vasectomy with this man, which information is most important to provide?
    1. A vasectomy involves tubal ligation done by surgery.
    2. This is a permanent method of contraception.
    3. The surgery takes approximately one hour.
    4. A vasectomy may cause intermittent impotence.

22. A client asks the nurse if he can get his wife pregnant after the vasectomy. What is the best response for the nurse to make?
    1. "No. The procedure works immediately and is permanent."
    2. "The first few ejaculations after a vasectomy contain active sperm."
    3. "Yes. You should continue to practice birth control for six months."
    4. "No. The doctor will flush the sperm out after the procedure is completed."

23. A client asks the nurse if he will be able to ejaculate after the vasectomy is done. What is the best response for the nurse to make?
    1. "Yes. This procedure does not affect the ejaculate."
    2. "No. The purpose of a vasectomy is to prevent ejaculation."
    3. "Are you concerned about your sexual identity?"
    4. "My husband had a vasectomy and it doesn't bother us."

24. An adult has been on bed rest for several weeks. A nursing care goal is to prevent the formation of renal calculi. Which of the following liquids is it especially important to include in the client's diet?
    1. Tomato juice
    2. Coffee
    3. Cranberry juice
    4. Milk

25. The physician has prescribed a diuretic for an adult client. Which nursing intervention is most important in relation to diuretic therapy?
    1. Test the urine for sugar and acetone
    2. Measure daily weights
    3. Maintain accurate intake and output
    4. Assess for pedal edema

26. The nurse is caring for an adult who has an indwelling urinary catheter with a continuous bladder irrigation infusing. How should the nurse calculate the urine output when the drainage bag is emptied?
    1. Subtract the total drainage from the amount of irrigation solution used.
    2. Measure the amount of drainage and subtract the amount of solution infused.
    3. Record both the total drainage and the amount of irrigant used on the intake and output record.
    4. Calculate the total fluid intake and subtract this amount from the total drainage.

27. The nurse calculates intake and output for an adult client. His intake for the shift is 1,000 ml. The total amount of drainage emptied from the drainage bag is 2,550 ml. During the shift, 1,825 ml of GU irrigant has infused. What is the client's eight-hour urine output?
    1. 725 ml
    2. 650 ml
    3. 825 ml
    4. 750 ml

28. The nurse is caring for a client admitted for treatment of acute glomerulonephritis. Which question would the nurse ask when obtaining information about the present illness?
    1. "Have you had a sore throat recently?"
    2. "Has anyone in your family had chickenpox recently?"
    3. "Have you had a bladder infection in the last six weeks?"
    4. "Does anyone in your family have a history of kidney disease?"

29. A 78-year-old man is scheduled for a transurethral resection of the prostate (TURP) tomorrow morning for treatment of benign prostatic hypertrophy. What instruction should the nurse give him about the initial post-operative period?
    1. "Void every two hours whether or not you feel the urge to do so."
    2. "Get up and walk to decrease discomfort from bladder spasms."
    3. "Cough and deep-breathe every two hours to prevent clot formation."
    4. "Expect cherry-red urine that will gradually turn pink."

30. A 35-year-old man is admitted with severe renal colic. The nurse should monitor this man for possible complications. Which of the following is a complication of renal colic?
    1. Anemia
    2. Polyuria
    3. Hypertension
    4. Oliguria

31. A woman is being seen in the walk-in clinic for recurrent cystitis. The nurse is teaching her about measures to prevent future episodes of cystitis. What should the nurse include in the teaching?
    1. Drink 1,000 ml of fluid each day, including a serving of cranberry juice at bedtime.
    2. Take a daily bath, and avoid the use of bath oils and soaps.
    3. Take all the medication prescribed, even if you feel better.
    4. Go to the bathroom and void soon after sexual intercourse.

32. A 64-year-old client with late stage chronic renal failure is admitted. What would the nurse expect in the nursing care plan for this client?
    1. Insert a urinary catheter to promote bladder drainage.
    2. Elevate the client's feet when out of bed to promote venous return.
    3. Assess the client's lung sounds each shift to monitor fluid status.
    4. Supplement the client's diet with protein powder shakes to provide essential amino acids to promote healing.

33. The nurse is teaching self-testicular examination to a group of young men on a college campus. Which information should be included in the discussion?
    1. Perform the examination immediately following sexual intercourse.
    2. See your physician for an examination yearly.
    3. A self-testicular exam should be done monthly.
    4. Daily examination of the testicles is recommended.

34. The nurse is caring for an adult who recently received a kidney transplant. Which statement, if made by the client, indicates a lack of understanding of his long-term management?
    1. "I plan to go back to work as soon as I feel strong enough."
    2. "We have started using gloves whenever we are scrubbing things."
    3. "My spouse has helped me work out a schedule for taking all these medications."
    4. "If my face gets puffy or my feet swell, I will stop taking the new medications."

35. An adult is scheduled for an intravenous pyelogram. Which comment by the client is of greatest concern to the nurse?
    1. "I am afraid of needles."
    2. "I get short of breath when I eat crab meat."
    3. "When I had an arteriogram, I felt nauseated when they injected the dye."
    4. "I am allergic to tetanus shots."

Answers and Rationales

1. (2) The urethral meatus is located between the clitoris and the vaginal orifice.
2. (2) After the client has voided, catheterization for retention should yield 50 mL or less. 200 cc indicates a retention of urine.
3. (4) Catheterization is performed by using the sterile technique. Medical asepsis is the clean technique.
4. (2) The drainage bag is positioned below the bladder with tubing angled so that there is a constant downward flow of urine from the bladder. This position helps to prevent ascending infection.
5. (4) Difficulty passing a catheter suggests an obstruction of some nature. The nurse should discontinue the procedure and notify the physician.
6. (2) He should be flat to prevent bleeding from the kidney, a very vascular organ. Blood pressure needs frequent monitoring to determine if he is bleeding. Bleeding is the most common complication following needle biopsy of the kidney.
7. (4) Taking him to the bathroom at regular intervals will help him regain control. Regression is common in children who are hospitalized. Putting diapers on him or leaving him in his wet bed are punitive, which is not therapeutic. Promising him a lollipop is bribing, which is not therapeutic.
8. (1) Pink-tinged urine is normal following a cystoscopy. Bright-red bleeding would need to be reported.
9. (1) Burning upon urination is usually seen in clients with a bladder infection. Flank pain and nausea and vomiting are seen more frequently in persons with kidney infection or stones. Elevated potassium is seen in renal failure.
10. (2) This describes the correct technique for a clean-catch midstream urine collection. Antiseptic wipes, not soap and water, are used. The container must be sterile for urine for culture. A midstream collection is necessary. The initial urine voided may contain organisms from near the urethral opening. The object of the urine culture is to culture urine in the bladder.
11. (3) Failure to empty the bladder after sexual relations is thought to be a cause of bladder infections. Fluids should be encouraged, not restricted. She should wipe from front to back to prevent rectal organisms from entering the bladder, also thought to be a cause of bladder infections. All of the medication should be taken to adequately treat the infection and to prevent the development of resistant organisms.
12. (2) Encouraging fluids will often help the stone to pass. The client in this question has kidney stones; there is no mention of impending renal failure. High fluid intake is advised for clients who have bladder infections. However, that is not the diagnosis for this client. Increasing fluid intake may be indicated for a client who is dehydrated; however, that is not the diagnosis for this client.
13. (1) The stone should be sent to the laboratory for analysis to determine the type of stone. This will help to determine the diet he should follow. Stones do not usually contain blood or glucose. The laboratory needs to do the analysis. Passing the stone may be painful, but the pain is usually relieved after the stone is passed.
14. (2) Walking often helps to relieve the pain and will help the stone to pass. The nurse would instruct the client to have assistance with walking only if he is sedated from pain medication.
15. (2) The client's potassium is dangerously high. The normal level is 3.5–5.0 mEq/l. Kayexalate is a sodium-potassium exchange resin. It removes potassium from the bloodstream. While it will not correct the underlying problem, it will lower the serum potassium to safer levels and perhaps prevent serious or even fatal cardiac dysrhythmias. Kayexalate does not remove fluid or reduce abdominal pressure. Kayexalate does not introduce potassium into the bowel. A client who has hyperkalemia does not need additional potassium.
16. (4) A client in acute renal failure is on a low-sodium, low-protein, low-potassium, high-carbohydrate diet. Applesauce is all of these. Watermelon and orange juice are high in potassium. Turkey contains protein, and the bread contains sodium.
17. (2) Benign prostatic hypertrophy (BPH) causes retention, urinary frequency, dribbling, and decreased force of the urinary stream. It does not cause pus in the urine. If pyuria (pus in the urine) is present, this indicates a secondary infection.
18. (1) Fluid intake should be encouraged to help prevent the development of a urinary tract infection. It is not appropriate to limit fluid intake. Following the removal of urine from a distended bladder, there is a risk of shock. The nurse should monitor the blood pressure. The nurse should weigh the client daily to assess for fluid retention. The nurse would assess renal function by monitoring intake and output.

19. (4) Compression of the penoscrotal junction will cause obstruction of urine flow. Taping the catheter to the thigh straightens out the urethra and prevents compression of the penoscrotal junction. Leaving the penis in a dependent position increases pressure at the penoscrotal junction. Taping the catheter to the thigh does not prevent the reflux of urine. Keeping the tubing gently sloping in a downward direction will help to prevent reflux. There is no need to maintain tension on the balloon of the indwelling catheter. If the balloon is inflated and positioned properly, it will stay in position. The client may or may not be more comfortable with the catheter in this position. However, comfort is not the reason for taping the catheter to the thigh.

20. (3) Continuous bathing of the bladder with the irrigating solution will flush clots from the bladder. The primary purpose of continuous bladder irrigation (CBI) is not to prevent urinary tract infection. CBI does not maintain bladder tone. When a client has CBI, the client has an indwelling catheter. CBI does not prevent urethral stricture formation.

21. (2) A vasectomy is considered a permanent method of contraception even though it is occasionally possible to reverse. A vasectomy is essentially a ligation of the tube (vas Deferens) and is done by surgery, so answer 1 is a true statement. However, the information in answer 2, that this is a permanent method of sterilization, is much more essential. A vasectomy causes sterility but not impotence (inability to maintain an erection); it does not interfere with sexual functioning. The procedure does not take an hour; it takes only a few minutes.

22. (2) The first few ejaculations contain sperm that are already in the tubes. Before he is considered sterile, he should have two ejaculates a month apart that test sperm-free. It is usually at least 6–8 weeks before a man is considered sterile following a vasectomy. The surgeon does not flush the sperm from the man's tubes.

23. (1) A vasectomy does not prevent ejaculation. The ejaculate does not contain sperm. The man's sexual functioning is not affected. The client asks for information. The most appropriate response is to give the information. There is no evidence in the question that the man is concerned about his sexual identity. The nurse should answer the client's question, not interject her own experience in answering this question.

24. (3) Most urinary calculi that form as a result of prolonged immobility are alkaline. Cranberry juice leaves an acid ash, which keeps the urine acidic. The other liquids leave an alkaline ash, which could lead to the development of calculi.

25. (2) A diuretic causes increased urine output. Monitoring daily weights is the best way to assess changes in hydration status. Testing urine for sugar and acetone is not indicated for this client. There is no data stating that the client is a diabetic. Intake and output may be indicated, but daily weights will give a more reliable indication of actual fluid loss. It is not wrong to assess for pedal edema, but daily weights will give a better indicator of fluid loss. Edema can be in places other than the feet.

26. (2) The irrigating solution goes in through the catheter, bathes the bladder, and flows out through the tubing into the collection bag. The nurse should measure the total amount of drainage and subtract the amount of irrigating solution infused, because this is not urine output. Choice number 1 makes no sense because the drainage is larger than the amount of irrigating solution used. The question asked how the nurse calculates total urine output. Answer 3 does not address the issue of calculating the total urine output. Recording total fluid intake will most likely be done for this client, but subtracting it from the drainage does not tell us the client's urine output.

27. (1) Total drainage from the bag is 2,550 ml. The amount of irrigant infused is 1,825 ml. Subtract 1,825 ml from 2,250 ml and the answer is 725 ml of urine.

28. (1) When obtaining a history of the present illness, the nurse questions the client about precipitating factors. Acute glomerulonephritis (AGN) usually occurs 10–14 days after a streptococcal infection. Strep throat or strep-related otitis media is the most common precipitating event. Chicken pox is caused by herpes zoster virus and is not usually associated with AGN. A bladder infection is not usually associated with AGN. AGN follows a streptococcal infection and is not specifically an inherited condition.

29. (4) It is important to tell the client that his urine will be red during the post-surgical period so that he is not frightened. The client will have an indwelling urinary catheter after surgery. He may even have a continuous, normal saline irrigation. There is no need to give instructions regarding voiding until after the catheter has been removed. Walking does not usually relieve bladder spasms. Coughing and deep-breathing are important post-operative interventions, but they do not prevent clot formation.

30. (4) Renal colic is severe pain associated with ureteral spasms when the ureter is irritated by a stone. A stone may occlude the ureter and block urine flow from the kidney. This can also result in hydronephrosis, a complication that can lead to kidney necrosis. Anemia and hypertension are complications of renal failure. Polyuria is not associated with renal colic.

31. (4) Bacteria may enter the urethra during intercourse. Voiding soon after intercourse helps flush organisms from the urinary tract. Daily fluid intake should be at least 2,500 to 3,000 ml to prevent recurring cystitis. Showers, not baths, are recommended. Sitting in a tub may cause a reflux of bacteria into the bladder. Finishing all medication is an appropriate response to a current infection, but does not prevent recurring infections.

32. (3) Lung sounds should be assessed to monitor for pulmonary edema, which is a complication of chronic renal failure. Inserting a catheter does not increase kidney function. The client will be oliguric in late-stage chronic renal failure. Elevating the feet increases fluid flow to the heart, making the heart work harder. This should not be done, because congestive heart failure is associated with chronic renal failure. Protein intake is restricted in chronic renal failure.

33. (3) All males past the age of puberty should perform self-testicular examination every month. The man should do this on the same day every month; such as the 1st or the 15th. The exam should be done in the shower, followed by a visual inspection looking in the mirror. There is no relation to sexual intercourse. Self-testicular examination is performed by the man himself. A physician will examine the testicles when a physical is done. This may not be yearly for young men. Testicular cancer is primarily a disease of young men.

34. (4) A puffy face (moon face) and swollen feet may be side effects of steroid medications. A person who has had an organ transplant will receive immunosuppressant drugs including a steroid for the rest of his/her life. A person who has had a kidney transplant should be able to return to work once strength has been regained. If the client's work involved excessive exposure to infectious agents, the client might have to change jobs. Wearing gloves is an excellent way to reduce the chance of contracting an infection. The client will be taking a number of anti-rejection drugs life-long.

35. (2) Shortness of breath when eating crab meat suggests an allergy to iodine. Iodine dye is used to visualize the kidney during an IVP. This should be reported immediately to the physician. The client will have an intravenous needle, but fear of needles is not the greatest concern. Feeling nauseated or a feeling of warmth along the vein are normal sensations when receiving iodine dye. Tetanus allergy does not indicate an allergy to iodine.

Chapter 12

The Musculoskeletal System

ANATOMY AND PHYSIOLOGY

SKELETAL SYSTEM

A. Consists of joined framework of 206 bones
B. Bone is constantly made and reabsorbed; osteoblasts make and deposit new bone; osteoclasts promote bone reabsorption.
C. Bone marrow:
    1. Red marrow manufactures red blood cells, white blood cells, and platelets.
    2. Yellow marrow is connective tissue composed of fat cells.
D. Classification of bone shapes:
    1. Long bones (for example, humerus, femur)
    2. Short bones; carpals (hand bones), tarsals (foot bones)
    3. Flat bones; ribs, skull, scapula
    4. Irregular bones are of varying shapes (for example, vertebrae, mandible, and ear ossicles).
    5. Sesamoid bones (for example, knee cap)
E. Articulations are places of union between two or more bones.
    1. Joints are categorized by degree of movement; skull sutures have no movement, knees and elbows are freely movable to allow position changes.
    2. Movements allowed by synovial (freely movable) joints include flexion, extension, eversion, inversion, circumduction, abduction, adduction, internal rotation, external rotation, supination, and pronation.

MUSCULAR SYSTEM

A. Types of muscles:
    1. Cardiac muscle is an involuntary, striated muscle that occurs only in the heart (myocardium).
    2. Smooth muscles are involuntary, striated muscles located in hollow structures of the body (for example, digestive tract, blood vessels).
    3. Skeletal muscles are voluntary muscles of the skeletal system.
        a. Muscle fibers are arranged in bundles held together by connective tissue
        b. Entire muscle is encased in a muscle sheath of connective tissue that contains blood and lymph vessels and nerve fibers

B. Nerve fibers carry impulses to muscles at myoneural junctions; a continuous flow of stimuli is necessary to maintain muscle tone.
C. Muscles need a very rich vascular supply to meet the large oxygen demand of the exercising muscle; an "oxygen debt" develops during exercise when oxygen can't be delivered to the muscle fast enough and lactic acid begins to accumulate.

CARTILAGE

A. Dense connective tissue that forms most of the skeleton of an embryo
B. Embryo's cartilage gradually changes into bone by the process of ossification

C. Some cartilage remains in an adult skeleton:
  1. Costal cartilage which connects the ribs to the sternum
  2. Thyroid cartilage
  3. Hyaline cartilage found in the nose septum, the larynx, and the trachea

LIGAMENTS AND TENDONS

A. Dense, fibrous connective tissue containing large numbers of collagen fibers
B. Tendons attach muscles to bone.
C. Ligaments connect bones together at joints and provide stability on movement.

Laboratory / Diagnostic Tests

BLOOD TESTS

A. Erythrocyte sedimentation rate (ESR):
  1. Normal: up to 15–20 mm/hr
  2. Elevated in lupus and arthritis
B. Rheumatoid factor: positive in rheumatoid arthritis and sometimes lupus
C. Lupus erythematosus cells (LE prep): Positive in lupus erythematosus and sometimes rheumatoid arthritis
D. Antinuclear antibodies (ANA): positive in lupus and other autoimmune disorders
E. C-reactive protein: elevated in rheumatoid arthritis
F. Uric acid:
  1. Normal: 2–8.5 mg/dl
  2. Elevated in gout

OTHER TESTS

A. X-rays: used to detect fractures and lesions within the musculoskeletal system
B. Bone scan:
  1. Measures radioactivity in bones two hours after IV injection of a radioisotope; detects bone tumors and osteomyelitis
  2. Nursing care:
    a. Client instructed to drink several glasses of water following injection of radioisotope and then must void immediately before procedure
    b. Client must remain still during scan
C. Arthroscopy:
  1. Insertion of fiberoptic scope into a joint to visualize it, perform biopsies, or remove loose bodies

  2. Performed in operating room under sterile technique
  3. Nursing care after procedure:
    a. Pressure dressing for 24 hours
    b. Client must limit activity for several days.
D. Arthrocentesis: Removal of synovial fluid from a joint for diagnosis or therapy
E. Myelography:
  1. Lumbar puncture used to withdraw a small amount of cerebrospinal fluid (CSF), which is replaced with a radiopaque dye; used to detect tumors or herniated intravertebral discs
  2. Nursing care pretest:
    a. Keep NPO after liquid breakfast
    b. Check for iodine allergy
  3. Nursing care post test:
    a. If dye has been completely removed (oil-based dye), keep client flat for 12 hours
    b. If dye has not been completely removed (water-based dye—Amipaque), keep head of bed elevated (30°–45°) to prevent dye from rising and causing meningeal irritation and even seizures
    c. If water-based dye is used, put client on seizure precautions and do not administer any phenothiazine drugs such as prochlorperazine (Compazine) or hydroxyzine (Vistaril)
F. Electromyography (EMG):
  1. Measures and records activity of contracting muscles in response to electrical stimulation; helps differentiate muscle disease from motor neuron dysfunction
  2. Explain procedure to client and prepare him for discomfort of needle insertion

Related Procedures

RANGE-OF-MOTION (ROM) EXERCISES

A. Movement of joint through its full ROM to prevent contractures and increase or maintain muscle tone
B. Types:
   1. Active: done by client; increases and maintains muscle tone and joint mobility
   2. Passive: done by nurse without help from client; maintains joint mobility only
   3. Active assistive: client moves body part as far as possible and nurse completes exercise
   4. Active resistive: contraction of muscle against an opposing force; increases muscle size and strength
   5. Isometric Exercises:
      a. A form of active exercise that increases muscle tension by applying pressure against a stable resistance; there is no joint movement and the length of muscle does not change
      b. Client presses hands together or pushes against a wall; tension is increased for several seconds and then muscle is relaxed; exercises such as Kegels' or quadriceps setting exercises
      c. Muscle strength and tone are maintained or improved.

ASSISTIVE DEVICES FOR WALKING

A. Cane:
   1. Types: single, tripod cane, quad cane
   2. Client must hold cane in hand opposite affected extremity and advance cane as the affected leg is moved forward
B. Walker: Client holds upper bars of walker at each side and walks toward it
C. Crutches:
   1. Assure proper length:
      a. With client standing, the top of the crutches is two inches below the axilla and the tip of each crutch is six inches in front and to the side of the feet.
      b. Client's elbows should be slightly flexed when hand is on bar.
      c. Weight must be borne by hands, not axillae.
   2. Crutch gaits (see Figure 12.1)
      a. Three point gait:
         (1) Used when weight bearing is permitted on one extremity only
         (2) Advance both crutches and affected extremity, then advance the unaffected leg.
         (3) Stairs:
            (a) When going up stairs, the crutches and affected leg are kept on lower step while the unaffected leg is placed on the upper step, then move the crutches and the affected leg up
            (b) When going down stairs, crutches and affected leg are placed on the lower step, then the unaffected leg is brought down to the lower step
            (c) Remember, "Up with the good, down with the bad."
      b. Four-point gait:
         (1) Used when weight bearing is allowed on both extremities
         (2) Advance right crutch, step forward with left foot, advance left crutch, step forward with right foot (crutch, opposite foot, crutch, opposite foot)
      c. Two-point gait:
         (1) Typical walking pattern; step forward moving right crutch and left leg together; step forward moving left crutch and right leg together
         (2) "Hurry up" four-point gait
      d. Swing to gait:
         (1) Used for clients with paralysis of both lower extremities who are unable to lift feet from floor
         (2) Both crutches are placed forward, client swings forward to the crutches
      e. Swing through gait
         (1) Uses same as swing to gait
         (2) Both crutches are placed forward; client swings body through the crutches

CARE OF THE CLIENT WITH A CAST

A. Cast drying:
   1. Use palms of hands when handling wet cast, finger tips may cause identations in cast and irritate the skin
   2. Support wet cast on pillows until dry (24 hours)
   3. Turn client q two hrs
   4. Do not cover the cast until it is dry.

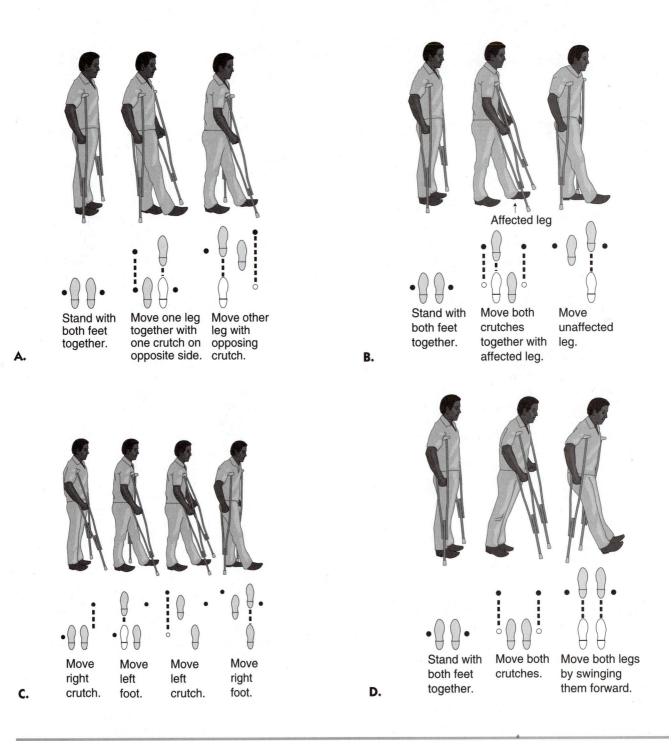

A.
Stand with both feet together.

Move one leg together with one crutch on opposite side.

Move other leg with opposing crutch.

B.
Affected leg

Stand with both feet together.

Move both crutches together with affected leg.

Move unaffected leg.

C.
Move right crutch.

Move left foot.

Move left crutch.

Move right foot.

D.
Stand with both feet together.

Move both crutches.

Move both legs by swinging them forward.

Figure 12.1 Crutch Walking Gaits

5. Do not use heat lamp or hair dryer on plaster cast
6. A fan may be used to circulate air around the cast.
B. Nursing diagnoses for client with a cast (see Table 12.1)
C. Nursing care:
  1. Neurovascular checks:
    a. Check for sensation in movement in fingers or toes of the casted extremity.
    b. Check color, temperature, and capillary refill of casted extremity.
  2. Smell the cast.
  3. Check for bleeding; circle blood spots on cast with a pen to see if bleeding continues.
  4. Check for "hot spots" on cast; may indicate infection.
  5. Petal edges of plaster cast (if rough) with adhesive tape or moleskin (overlap small

Table 12.1 Nursing Diagnoses Related to the Client with a Cast

- Risk for injury related to hazards of crutch walking and impaired mobility secondary to cast
- Risk for impaired skin integrity related to pressure of cast on skin surface
- Self-care deficits related to limitation of movement secondary to cast
- Risk for impaired respiratory function related to imposed immobility or restricted respiratory movement secondary to cast (body)
- Risk for impaired home maintenance management related to the restrictions imposed by cast on performing activities of daily living and role responsibilities
- Risk for ineffective health maintenance related to insufficient knowledge of crutch walking, cast care, exercise program, and signs and symptoms of complications

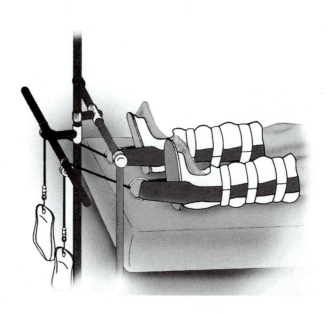

Figure 12.2 Buck's Extension Traction

strips of adhesive tape or moleskin around rough edges).
6. Prevent immobility complications.
7. Give pain medications as ordered.
8. Isometric and ROM exercises as appropriate
9. Keep cast dry; plaster cast will disintegrate if allowed to get very wet

CARE OF THE CLIENT IN TRACTION

A. Traction is the process of putting a limb, bone, or group of muscles under tension by means of weights or pulleys.
B. Purposes of traction:
　1. Align and immobilize a body part
　2. Relieve painful muscle spasms
　3. Correct and prevent deformities
　4. Treat musculoskeletal diseases such as spinal cord compression, dislocations, intervertebral disk disease, painful muscles, and ligaments
C. Types of traction:
　1. Skin traction; weight is borne by the skin; can be applied by fastening traction strips of adhesive tapes to the limbs with woven bandage or by encircling a body part with a halter, corset, or sling; counter-traction is provided by the person's weight
　　a. Buck's extension (see Figure 12.2)
　　　(1) Temporary measure to immobilize the leg in client with a fractured hip
　　　(2) Exerts straight pull on affected extremity
　　　(3) Shock blocks at the foot of the bed produce counter-traction and prevent the client from sliding down in bed
　　b. Russell traction (see Figure 12.3)
　　　(1) Used to treat fracture of the femur

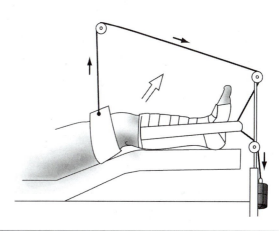

Figure 12.3 Russell's Traction

　　　(2) Knee is suspended in a sling attached to a rope and pulley on a Balkan frame, creating upward pull from the knee; weights are attached to foot of bed creating a horizontal traction
　　　(3) Allows client to move about in bed more freely and permits bending of the knee joint
　　　(4) Hip should be flexed at 20°
　　　(5) Foot of bed usually elevated by shock blocks to provide counter-traction
　　c. Bryant's traction:
　　　(1) Used for children under two years and under 30 pounds to treat fractures of the femur and hip dislocation
　　　(2) Both legs raised at 90° angle to bed

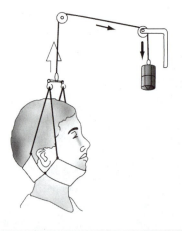

Figure 12.4 Cervical Traction

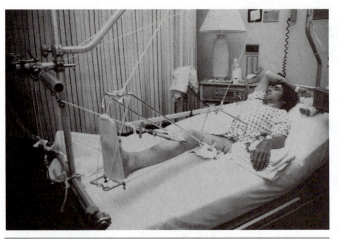

Figure 12.6 Skeletal Traction

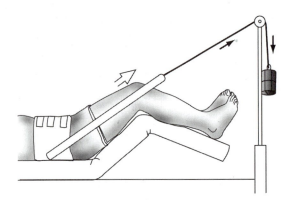

Figure 12.5 Pelvic Traction

Table 12.2 Nursing Diagnoses Related to the Client who Is in Traction

- Risk for impaired skin integrity related to imposed immobility
- Risk for infection related to susceptibility to microorganism secondary to skeletal traction pins
- Risk for colonic constipation related to decreased peristalsis secondary to immobility and analgesics
- Risk for impaired respiratory function related to imposed immobility and pooling of respiratory secretions

(3) Buttocks must be slightly off mattress
(4) Child is own counterweight
  d. Cervical traction (see Figure 12.4)
    (1) Used for soft tissue damage or degenerative disc disease of cervical spine to reduce muscle spasm and maintain alignment
    (2) Cervical head halter attached to weights that hang over head of bed
    (3) Usually intermittent traction
    (4) Elevate head of bed to provide counter-traction
  e. Pelvic traction (see Figure 12.5)
    (1) Used for low back pain to reduce muscle spasm and maintain alignment
    (2) Pelvic girdle with extension straps attached to ropes and weights
    (3) Usually intermittent
    (4) Client in semi-Fowler's position with knee bent
    (5) Secure pelvic girdle around iliac crests

2. Skeletal traction; traction applied directly to the bones using pins, wires, or tongs that are surgically inserted; used for fractured femur, tibia, humerus, cervical spine (see Figure 12.6)
  a. Balanced suspension traction:
    (1) Produced by a counter force other than the client's weight
    (2) Extremity floats or balances in the traction apparatus
    (3) Client may change position without disturbing the line of traction
  b. Thomas splint with Pearson attachment:
    (1) Used with skeletal traction in fractures of the femur
    (2) Hip should be flexed at 20°
    (3) Use foot plate to prevent footdrop
D. Nursing diagnoses related to traction (see Table 12.2)
E. Nursing care of clients in traction:
  1. Check the traction apparatus frequently to assure that ropes are aligned and weights hang freely, that bed is in the proper position, and that the line of traction is with the long axis of the bone.
  2. Maintain client in proper alignment:
    a. Client in center of bed
    b. Do not rest affected limb against foot of bed

3. Neurovascular checks on affected extremity
4. Prevent foot drop:
   a. Use foot plate
   b. Dorsiflexion exercises
5. Prevent thrombophlebitis:
   a. Encourage client to relax and contract muscles of affected extremity.
   b. Have client move unaffected extremity as allowed.
   c. Administer aspirin as ordered.
6. Prevent skin irritation and breakdown.
7. Pin site care for clients in skeletal traction:
   a. Cleanse the pin site with soap and water or peroxide and apply antibiotic ointment as ordered.
   b. Check for redness, drainage, odor

8. Assist with activities of daily living as needed.
9. Encourage ROM and isometric exercises to unaffected extremities.
10. Check carefully for turning orders:
    a. Buck's extension may usually turn to unaffected side.
    b. Russell traction and balanced suspension traction may turn slightly from side to side; may need to make bed from head to foot to limit side to side turning

Disorders of the Musculoskeletal System

FRACTURES

A. A fracture is a break in a bone, usually caused by trauma; a pathologic fracture is a spontaneous bone break found in osteoporosis, osteomyelitis, multiple myeloma, or bone tumors.
B. Types of fractures (see Figure 12.7)
   1. Complete: separation of bone into two parts
   2. Incomplete: fracture does not go all the way through the bone
   3. Comminuted: bone is broken into pieces
   4. Closed or simple: no break in skin
   5. Open or compound: break in skin with or without protrusion of bone

6. Greenstick: one side of the bone is broken, the other is bent (like a green stick when it is bent); seen in children
C. Assessment findings:
   1. Pain, aggravated by motion, tenderness
   2. Loss of motion, edema, crepitus, ecchymosis
   3. Extremity appears shorter
   4. X-ray shows fracture
D. Nursing diagnoses (see Table 12.3):
E. Interventions:
   1. Traction
   2. Reduction:
      a. Closed reduction through manual manipulation followed by application of cast

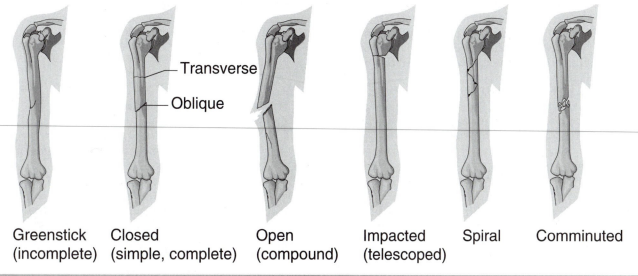

Transverse
Oblique

| Greenstick (incomplete) | Closed (simple, complete) | Open (compound) | Impacted (telescoped) | Spiral | Comminuted |

Figure 12.7 Types of Bone Fractures

Table 12.3 Nursing Diagnoses Related to the Client with a Bone Fracture

- Impaired comfort related to tissue trauma and immobility
- Risk for impaired skin integrity related to mechanical irritants/compression secondary to casts and traction
- Risk for disuse syndrome related to effects of immobility secondary to casts/traction
- Risk for infection related to invasive fixation devices
- Self-care deficits related to impaired ability to use upper/lower limb secondary to immobilization devices
- Risk for ineffective home maintenance management related to fixation device, impaired physical mobility, unavailable support system
- Risk for ineffective health maintenance related to insufficient knowledge of condition, cast care, use of assistive devices, signs and symptoms of complications (numbness, pallor, decreased sensation), and limitations
- Risk for impaired respiratory function related to immobility secondary to traction or their fixation devices

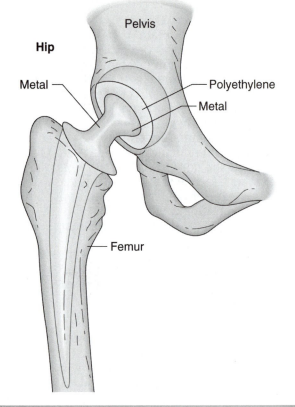

Figure 12.8 Total Hip Replacement

b. Open reduction: the correction of a fracture using surgical intervention
3. Cast (see Care of the Client with a Cast)
4. Monitor for disorientation and confusion in the elderly.
5. Neurovascular checks
6. Prevent complications of immobility.
7. Encourage use of trapeze to facilitate movement.
8. Analgesics as ordered to control pain
9. Care for client with open reduction:
   a. Check dressings.
   b. Empty closed-wound drainage system if present.
   c. Assess LOC.
   d. Turn q 2 h; turn to nonoperative side only; place two pillows between legs while turning, when lying on side.
10. Measures to prevent thrombus formation:
   a. Elastic hose
   b. Dorsiflexion of foot
   c. Anticoagulants such as aspirin; encourage quadriceps setting and gluteal setting exercises
11. Observe for adequate bowel and bladder function.
12. Avoid weight bearing until allowed.
13. Provide care for the client with a hip prosthesis if necessary (similar to care of client with total hip replacement).

TOTAL HIP REPLACEMENT

A. Replacement of both acetabelum and head of femur with prostheses in persons with rheumatoid arthritis or osteoarthritis causing severe disability and intolerable pain and in persons with a fractured hip with nonunion (see Figure 12.8)

Table 12.4 Nursing Diagnoses Related to Fractured Hip

- Impaired physical mobility due to strict post-operative position restrictions
- Risk for infection related to site for bacterial invasion
- Deficient knowledge regarding home care
- Self-care deficit related to prescribed activity restriction
- Disuse syndrome related to surgery and immobility
- Risk for ineffective respiratory function related to postoperative immobility
- Acute pain related to surgical incision
- Risk for ineffective therapeutic regimen management related to insufficient knowledge of home care, incisional care, signs and symptoms of complications, and follow-up care

B. Nursing diagnoses (see Table 12.4)
C. Management:
   1. Cough and deep-breathe every two hours to prevent respiratory complications.
   2. Medicate for pain PRN.
   3. Keep affected leg **abducted** at all times to keep hip in socket.
      a. Place two pillows or an abductor splint between legs when turning or lying on side.
      b. Teach the client not to cross one leg over the other.
   4. Trapeze over bed to assist movement

5. Trochanter rolls to prevent external rotation
6. Raise head of bed 20°–30° for meals if allowed.
7. Turn only to non-operative side.
8. Assist client out of bed in 2–4 days as ordered.
9. No weight bearing until ordered.
10. No adduction or hip flexion.
11. Teach client measures to avoid hip flexion:
    a. Use raised toilet seat.
    b. No bending to put on shoes and socks
    c. Do not sit in low chairs.
12. Assess for indications of hip dislocation, such as sharp hip pain or abnormal position of affected leg (leg shortened and externally rotated).
13. Flex and dorsiflex foot and knee on nonoperative side and operative side when ordered to prevent thrombophlebitis.
14. Teach quadriceps setting and gluteal setting exercises and remind client to do them several times hourly.
15. Assist with exercise to strengthen upper extremities (isometric exercises and use of trapeze).
16. Allow expression of feelings about slow recovery and future activity level.
17. Provide meaningful sensory stimulation.
18. Encourage self care to the extent possible.
19. Before discharge, assure that the client knows the exercise regime ordered and has the phone number of the physical therapist.
20. Contact visiting nurse for ongoing care; home visit to assess needs for railings, ramps, walker, and so on.

KNEE REPLACEMENT

A. Indicated for persons who have severe pain and functional disabilities related to joint surfaces destroyed by arthritis and for persons who have bleeding into the joint such as may occur with hemophilia. Metal and acrylic prostheses are used. Knee replacement may be complete or partial depending on strength of person's ligaments; total replacement needed if ligaments are weakened (see Figure 12.9)
B. Nursing diagnoses (see Table 12.5)
C. Management:
   1. Cough and deep-breathe every two hours to prevent respiratory complications.
   2. Medicate for pain PRN.
   3. Apply ice as ordered to prevent bleeding and edema.
   4. Assess the compression bandage for evidence of bleeding.
   5. Monitor wound suction drainage (200 ml in first eight hours normal; then decreases to less than 25 ml by 48 hours)

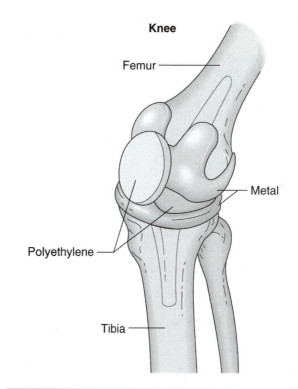

Figure 12.9 Total Knee Replacement

Table 12.5 Nursing Diagnoses Related to Knee Replacement

- Acute pain related to surgery
- Risk for impaired skin integrity related to immobility and surgical incision
- Impaired physical mobility related to surgery
- Risk for injury related to unsteady gait and assistive devices
- Risk for disturbed peripheral tissue perfusion related to surgery and immobility
- Risk for constipation related to activity restriction
- Risk for ineffective management of therapeutic regimen related to insufficient knowledge of activity restrictions, use of supportive devices, rehabilitative program, follow-up care, apparel restrictions, signs of complications, supportive services, and prevention of infection
- Impaired home maintenance management related to post-operative flexion restrictions

6. Maintain continuous passive motion (CPM) device as ordered by physician (see Figure 12.10); CPM promotes healing by increasing circulation and movement of knee joint.
7. Knee immobilizer when out of bed
8. Elevate leg when out of bed in chair.
9. Gradual increase in weight bearing and ambulation
10. Teach client about the use of CPM at home.
11. Assist client in arranging for physical therapy after discharge.

RHEUMATOID ARTHRITIS

A. Rheumatoid arthritis is a chronic, systemic disease characterized by inflammatory changes in connective tissue; it occurs in women more than men (3:1) with peak onset between 35 and 45; may occur in children. The cause remains unknown, although it is usually classified as an autoimmune disease; however, it may be an infectious disease similar to Lyme Disease.

B. Assessment findings:
1. Joint distribution is symmetric; most commonly affects smaller peripheral joints of hands and also commonly involves wrists, elbows, shoulders, knees, hips, ankles, jaw, and cervical spine; joints are painful, warm, and swollen with limited motion; stiff in the morning and after periods of inactivity
2. If not arrested, affected joints progress through four stages of deterioration: synovitis, pannus formation (layer of inflammatory granulation tissue), fibrous ankylosis, and bony ankylosis.
3. Fatigue, anorexia, malaise, weight loss, slight temperature elevation
4. Muscle weakness secondary to inactivity
5. History of remissions and exacerbations
6. Some clients will have subcutaneous nodules, eye, vascular, lung, or cardiac problems

C. Diagnostic tests:
1. X-rays show various stages of joint disease.
2. CBC: anemia is common
3. Erythrocyte sedimentation rate (ESR) elevated
4. Rheumatoid factor and ANA may be positive.
5. C-reactive protein elevated

D. Nursing diagnosis (see Table 12.6)
E. Interventions:
1. Drug therapy:
   a. Aspirin: mainstay of treatment, has both analgesic and anti-inflammatory effect
   b. Nonsteroidal anti-inflammatory drugs (NSAIDs) such as indomethacin (Indocin), phenylbutazone (Butazolidin), ibuprofen (Motrin), fenoprofen (Nalfon), naproxen (Naprosyn), and sulindac (Clinoril)
   c. Gold compounds (chrysotherapy):
      (1) Injectable form: sodium thiomalate (Myochrysine); aurothioglucose (Solganal) is given IM once a week; takes 3–6 months to become effective
      (2) Oral form: auranofin (Ridaura) is effective with smaller doses than injectable; diarrhea is a side effect; blood and urine studies should also be monitored
   d. Corticosteroids:
      (1) Intra-articular injections temporarily suppress inflammation in specific joints; cannot be done indefinitely.
      (2) Systemic administration used only when client does not respond to less potent anti-inflammatory drugs; side effect of system corticosteroids is Cushing's syndrome
2. Physical therapy to minimize joint deformities and maintain function
3. Surgery to remove severely damaged joints (total hip or knee replacement)
4. Bed rest for acute exacerbations:
   a. Resting the joints helps reduce articular inflammation.
   b. Having client lie flat on back with affected joints in a position of extension helps to prevent flexion contractures
   c. Client should lie prone if possible for half hour bid to prevent flexion contractures.
5. Heat or cold treatments as ordered to decrease pain
6. Psychologic support
7. Diversionary activity such as audio tapes of music or books

OSTEOARTHRITIS (HYPERTROPHIC ARTHRITIS)

A. A chronic, nonsystemic disorder of joints characterized by degeneration of articular cartilage; most common form of arthritis; women and men are affected equally; incidence increases with age; also related to obesity, joint trauma, and genetic predisposition

B. Assessment findings:
1. Weight-bearing joints: spine, knees, hips and ends of fingers most affected
2. Pain aggravated by use and relieved by rest, stiffness of joints
3. Heberden's nodes: bony overgrowths at terminal interphalangeal joints
4. Decreased ROM; possible crepitation
5. X-rays show deformity.
6. ESR may be slightly elevated when disease is inflammatory.

C. Nursing diagnosis (see Table 12.6)
D. Interventions:
1. Assess joints for pain and ROM.
2. Relieve strain and prevent further trauma to the joints.
3. Assist with use of cane or walker if needed
4. Assist client with weight-reduction diet as indicated.
5. Help the client to maintain good posture and body mechanics.

Table 12.6 Nursing Diagnoses Related to Arthritis

- Impaired physical mobility related to pain, edema, and joint contractures
- Chronic pain related to swollen, inflamed joints
- Self-care deficit: bathing/grooming/dressing related to joint inflammation or deformity
- Fatigue related to chronic inflammatory process
- Disturbed body image related to joint deformity and side effects of corticosteroid medications
- Risk for infection related to immunosuppressive medications
- Deficient knowledge related to methods to control disease and prevent complications

Table 12.8 Nursing Diagnoses Related to Lupus Erythematosus

- Risk for infection related to immunosuppressive drugs
- Acute pain related to painful swollen joint
- Impaired physical mobility related to pain, edema, and joint contractures
- Deficient knowledge related to methods to control disease and prevent complications
- Self-care deficit: bathing/grooming/dressing related to joint inflammation or deformity
- Fatigue related to chronic inflammatory process
- Disturbed body image related to joint deformity and side effects of corticosteroid medications

Table 12.7 Nursing Diagnoses Related to Gout

- Acute pain related to sudden, intensely painful, swollen joint
- Impaired physical mobility related to pain, edema, and joint contractures
- Deficient knowledge related to methods to control disease and prevent complications

6. Teach client to avoid excessive weight bearing and continuous standing.
7. Physical therapy to maintain joint mobility and muscle strength
8. Promote comfort/relief of pain: analgesics and NSAIDs as ordered; heat or cold as ordered
9. Joint replacement if needed

GOUT

A. Disorder of purine metabolism which causes high levels of uric acid in the blood and the precipitation of urate crystals in the joints, causing irritation and inflammation; occurs most often in males and often is familial
B. Assessment findings:
  1. Joint pain, redness, heat, and swelling often involves the great toe and ankle
  2. Headache, malaise, anorexia
  3. Tachycardia, fever, tophi in outer ear, hands, and feet
  4. Uric acid elevated
C. Nursing diagnosis (see Table 12.7)
D. Interventions:
  1. Drug therapy:
    a. Acute attack: colchicine IV or PO (discontinue if diarrhea or nausea and vomiting occur)
    b. NSAIDs such as indomethacin (Indocin)
    c. Prevention of acute attack: uricosuric agents such as probenecid (Benemid) increase renal excretion of uric acid; allopurinol (Zyloprim) inhibits uric acid formation

    d. Encourage fluids to 2,000 cc to 3,000 ml/day when giving anti-gout drugs to prevent formation of kidney stones.
  2. Low purine diet: avoid protein sources such as meats (especially organ meats), shellfish, fowl (chicken, turkey, goose, and duck), nuts, oats, and beans
  3. Joint rest and protection
  4. Heat or cold therapy
  5. Bed cradle to keep linens off painful joint

SYSTEMIC LUPUS ERYTHEMATOSUS (SLE)

A. Chronic connective tissue disease involving multiple organ systems occurring most frequently in young women; cause unknown; immune, genetic, and viral factors may be involved
B. Pathophysiology:
  1. Defect in body's immunologic mechanisms produces auto antibodies in the serum directed against components of the client's own cell nuclei
  2. Affects cells throughout the body resulting in involvement of many organs, including joints, skin, kidney, CNS, and cardiopulmonary system
C. Assessment findings:
  1. Fatigue, fever, anorexia, weight loss, malaise, remissions, and exacerbations
  2. Joint pain, morning stiffness
  3. Skin lesions: erythematous rash on face, neck or extremities; butterfly rash over bridge of nose and cheeks; photosensitivity
  4. Oral or nasopharyngeal ulcerations
  5. Alopecia
  6. Renal system involvement: proteinuria
  7. Central nervous system involvement; seizures, psychoses
  8. Hematologic disorder; hemolytic anemia, leukopenia, lymphopenia, thrombocytopenia
D. Related nursing diagnosis (see Table 12.8)

E. Diagnostic tests:
1. ESR elevated
2. CBC: anemia; WBC and platelets decreased
3. LE prep positive
4. Anti-DNA positive
5. Chronic false-positive test for syphilis
F. Interventions:
1. Drug therapy (similar to rheumatoid arthritis):
   a. Aspirin and NSAIDs
   b. Corticosteroids
   c. Immunosuppressive agents (Imuran, Cytoxan) when client is unresponsive to other therapy
2. Plasmapharesis
3. Supportive therapy
4. Monitor vital signs, I&O, daily weights
5. Seizure precautions and safety measures if CNS involvement
6. Psychologic support

OSTEOMYELITIS

A. Acute or chronic infection of the bone and surrounding soft tissues, most commonly caused by Staphylococcus Aureus; infection may reach bone through open wound (compound fracture, surgery) through the blood stream, or by direct extension from infected adjacent structures
B. Assessment findings:
1. Malaise, fever, tachycardia
2. Pain and tenderness of bone, redness and swelling over bone
3. Difficulty with weight bearing
4. Drainage from the wound site may be present.
C. Related nursing diagnosis (see Table 12.9)
D. Diagnostic tests:
1. Elevated WBC
2. Elevated ESR
3. Blood cultures may be positive.
4. X-ray may not show evidence of bone infection for some time.
E. Interventions:
1. Analgesics
2. Antibiotics
3. Sterile dressing changes are crucial.
4. Maintain proper body alignment and change position frequently to prevent deformities.
5. Immobilization of affected part
6. Psychologic support
7. Surgery if needed
8. Incision and drainage of bone abscess
9. Sequestrectomy—removal of dead, infected bone, and cartilage
10. Bone grafting after repeated infections

Table 12.9 Nursing Diagnoses Related to Osteomyelitis

- Impaired physical mobility related to pain
- Risk for impaired skin integrity related to immobility
- Deficient knowledge related to home care management
- Acute pain related to inflammation
- Deficient knowledge related to the treatment program

HERNIATED NUCLEUS PULPOSUS (HNP) (Figure 12.10 and 12.11)

A. Protrusion of nucleus pulposus (central part of intervertebral disc) into spinal canal, causing compression of spinal nerve roots and pain in the area innervated by that nerve root; occurs more often in men; 4th and 5th intervertebral spaces in the lumbar region most common; predisposing factors include heavy lifting or pulling and trauma
B. Assessment findings
1. Lumbosacral disc:
   a. Back pain radiating across buttock and down leg (along sciatic nerve)
   b. Weakness of leg and foot on affected side
   c. Numbness and tingling in toes and foot
   d. Positive straight leg raise test: pain on raising leg
   e. Depressed or absent Achilles reflex
   f. Muscle spasm in lumbar region
2. Cervical disc:
   a. Shoulder pain radiating down arm to hand
   b. Weakness of affected upper extremity
   c. Paresthesias (abnormal sensations such as tingling)
C. Diagnostic tests:
1. Myelogram localizes site of herniation
2. CT scan or MRI
D. Related nursing diagnoses (see Table 12.10)
E. Interventions:
1. Conservative:
   a. Bed rest
   b. Traction
   c. Anti-inflammatory agents, muscle relaxants, analgesics
   d. Bed rest on a firm mattress with bed board
   e. Local application of heat and diathermy
   f. Corset for lumbosacral disc
   g. Cervical collar for cervical disc
   h. Epidural injections of corticosteroids
   i. Prevent complications of immobility
   j. Comfort measures to relieve pain
2. Surgery: laminectomy (surgical excision of part of posterior arch of vertebrae and

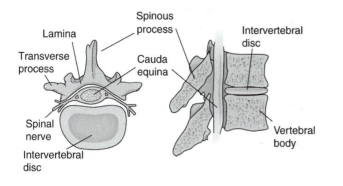

Figure 12.10 Normal intervertebral disc

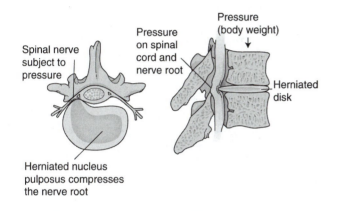

Figure 12.11 Herniated intervertebral disc

Table 12.10 Nursing Diagnoses Related to Herniated Nucleus Pulposus

- Potential alteration in neurological status related to spinal edema or epidural hematoma
- Acute pain related to nerve root compression
- Deficient knowledge regarding correct posture and body mechanics

removal of protruded disc) with or without spinal fusion or diskectomy (excision of an intervertebral disk)
  a. Indications:
    (1) Herniated nucleus pulposus not responsive to conservative therapy
    (2) Spinal decompression as with spinal cord injury
    (3) Remove fragments of broken bone.
    (4) Remove spinal neoplasm or abscess.
    (5) Spinal fusion may be done at the same time if spine is unstable.
  b. Nursing interventions: pre-operative:
    (1) Routine pre-op care
    (2) Teach client log rolling and use of bedpan.
  c. Nursing interventions: post-operative:
    (1) Routine post-op care

(2) Position as ordered: lower spinal surgery—flat; cervical spinal surgery—slight elevation of head of bed
(3) Proper body alignment: cervical spinal surgery, avoid flexion of neck and apply cervical collar
(4) Turn client q 2 h; use log rolling; place pillows between legs while on side
(5) Assess for complications:
  (a) Monitor sensory and motor status q 2–4 h
  (b) With cervical spinal surgery, client may have difficulty swallowing and coughing; check for respiratory distress; suction and tracheostomy set at bedside
(6) Check dressings for hemorrhage, CSF leakage, infection
(7) Administer analgesics as ordered.
(8) Assess for adequate bowel and bladder function; check q 2–4 h for bladder distention; assess bowel sounds; prevent constipation.
(9) Prevent complications of immobility.
(10) Assist with ambulation starting day after surgery using brace or corset if ordered.
(11) If client allowed to sit, use straight back chair and keep feet flat on floor
  f. Client teaching and discharge planning:
    (1) Wound care
    (2) Good posture and proper body mechanics
    (3) Activity level as ordered
    (4) Recognition and reporting of complications such as wound infection or sensory or motor deficits
3. Spinal fusion: fusion of spinous processes with bone graft from iliac crest to provide stabilization of spine; performed in conjunction with laminectomy
  a. Nursing interventions:
    (1) Pre-op care as for laminectomy
    (2) In addition to post-op care for laminectomy, position client correctly:
      (a) Lower spinal fusion: keep bed flat for first 12 hours, then may elevate head of bed (HOB) 20°–30°, keep off back for first 48 hours
      (b) Cervical spinal fusion: elevate HOB slightly; assist with ambulation; apply brace before getting out of bed; apply special cervical collar for cervical fusion
    (3) Promote comfort; may be considerable pain from graft site

(4) In addition to client teaching and discharge planning for laminectomy, teach client:
    (a) Brace will be needed for four months and lighter corset for one year after surgery.
    (b) Takes one year for graft to become stable.
    (c) No bending, stooping, lifting, or sitting for prolonged periods for four months
    (d) Walking without excessive tiring is good.
    (e) Diet modification will help prevent weight gain from decreased activity.

4. Chemonucleolysis:
    a. Used as alternative to laminectomy in selected cases
    b. Chymopapain (papaya derivative) is injected and reduces size of disc, decreasing pressure on affected nerve root
    c. Pre-op care for client receiving chemonucleolysis includes cimetidine (Tagamet) and diphenhydramine HCl (Benadryl) q 6 h to prevent allergic reaction; corticosteroids administered before procedure; not given to persons who are allergic to meat tenderizer or papaya
    d. Post-op care for client receiving chemonucleolysis: observe for anaphylaxis and less serious allergic reactions; monitor for neurologic deficits (numbness or tingling in extremities or inability to void)
    e. Client teaching and discharge planning—teach the client:
        (1) Back strengthening exercises
        (2) Good posture
        (3) Proper body mechanics
        (4) Medications and side effects
        (5) Proper application of corset or cervical collar
        (6) Weight reduction if needed

AMPUTATION OF A LIMB

A. Surgical procedure done for peripheral vascular disease if medical management is ineffective; level of amputation is determined by the extent of the disease process
B. Related nursing diagnosis (see Table 12.11)
C. Nursing interventions
    1. Pre-operative:
        a. Routine pre-op care
        b. Offer support/encouragement and accept client's response of anger/grief, denial

Table 12.11 Nursing Diagnoses Related to Amputation of a Limb

- Risk for disuse syndrome related to impaired movement secondary to pain
- Grieving related to loss of limb
- Altered comfort related to phantom sensations secondary to nerve stimulation secondary to amputation
- Risk for injury related to altered gait and hazards of assistive devices
- Risk for ineffective health maintenance related to insufficient knowledge of adaptations in activities of daily living, stump care, prosthesis care, and gait training
- Risk for body image disturbance related to perceived negative effects of amputation

        c. Discuss:
            (1) Rehabilitation program and use of prosthesis
            (2) Upper-extremity exercises such as pushups in bed, use of overhead trapeze
            (3) Crutch walking
            (4) Amputation dressings/cast
            (5) Phantom limb sensation as a normal occurrence
    2. Post-operative:
        a. Routine post-op care
        b. Prosthesis may be fitted during surgery
        c. Prevent hip/knee contractures.
            (1) Avoid letting client sit in chair with hips flexed for long periods of time.
            (2) Have client assume prone position several times a day and position hip in extension.
            (3) Avoid elevation of stump after 12–24 hours.
        d. Observe stump dressing for signs of hemorrhage, and mark outside of dressing so rate of bleeding can be assessed.
        e. Pain medication as ordered
        f. Ensure that stump bandages fit tightly and are applied properly to enhance prosthesis fitting.
        g. Initiate active ROM of all joints, crutch walking, and arm/shoulder exercises
        h. Provide stump care:
            (1) Inspect daily for signs of skin irritation.
            (2) Wash thoroughly daily with warm water and bacteriostatic soap; rinse and dry thoroughly.
            (3) Avoid the use of irritating substances such as lotions, alcohol, or powders.

Sample Questions

1. A cast has just been applied to a client's left forearm, and he is in 10 lbs Russell traction on his left leg. Which of the following nursing concerns takes priority in the care of this client?
   1. The casted extremity may swell and the cast will become a tourniquet.
   2. Heat conduction from the wet cast can cause burning to the skin below.
   3. Muscle atrophy of the areas involved can lead to decreased muscle tone.
   4. Skin irritation from the cast edges can cause abrasions.

2. The nurse is caring for a client with a newly applied cast. How should the nurse touch and move the wet cast?
   1. Use the palms of the hands.
   2. Use the fingertips only.
   3. Use a towel sling.
   4. Touch the cast only on the petals at the edges.

3. The nurse is caring for a client who has just had a cast applied. Which statement best describes the expected client outcome relative to the circulatory system for a client with a cast?
   1. There will be no increase in pain in the extremity.
   2. The client will have no circulatory impairment.
   3. The integrity of the cast will be maintained.
   4. The client will report any feelings of skin irritation.

4. The nurse gently elevates the client's newly casted arm on a pillow and explains that this is necessary for the first 24–48 hours after casting. What is the chief purpose of this action?
   1. It helps a damp cast to dry more evenly.
   2. It reduces the amount of pain medication needed.
   3. Venous return is enhanced, and edema is decreased.
   4. It is more comfortable than keeping the arm dependent.

5. An adolescent male was in an accident and is hospitalized with multiple fractures. The nurse enters the room and observes that he has his back to the door and is staring at the wall with a sad expression on his face. What is the best response for the nurse to make at this time?
   1. "You seem sad."
   2. "Don't be too down on yourself."
   3. "I know it is hard to be out of school."
   4. "Do you miss your family and friends?"

6. The client is in Russell's traction. Which statement best describes how Russell's traction works?
   1. The legs are suspended vertically with the hip flexed at 90° and knees extended.
   2. A straight pull on the affected leg is assured.
   3. A belt is applied just above and surrounding the iliac crests. The belt is then attached to a pulley system.
   4. Vertical traction is used at the knee at the same time a horizontal force is exerted on the tibia and fibula.

7. The nurse is assessing the leg of a client in Russell's traction. Which area is it essential to assess?
   1. Pedal area
   2. Femoral area
   3. Popliteal area
   4. Inner aspect of the thigh

8. It is necessary to pull the client, who is in Russell's traction, up in bed. Which action should the nurse take?
   1. Leave the weights in place.
   2. Remove the weights completely.
   3. Reduce the weight of the traction by one half.
   4. Have one nurse lift the weights while the others pull the client.

9. The client has been flat in bed in traction for two weeks and she is to be allowed out of bed for the first time today. What must the nurse be particularly alert for when getting the client out of bed?
   1. Renal complications
   2. Depression
   3. Orthostatic hypotension
   4. Skin breakdown

10. The client is a 73-year-old woman who fell in her home and suffered a right hip fracture. She tells the nurse that she was walking across the kitchen and felt something "snap" in her hip and this made her fall. What type of fracture is the client most likely to have had?
    1. Comminuted fracture
    2. Greenstick fracture
    3. Open fracture
    4. Pathological fracture

11. The nurse knows that elderly women have a high incidence of hip fracture for which reason?
    1. Decreased progesterone secretion
    2. Decreased mobility due to arthritic conditions
    3. Increased calcium absorption
    4. Osteoporosis in the skeletal structure

12. The nurse is caring for a person prior to surgery to repair a broken right hip. Which nursing care measure is essential?
    1. Get the client out of bed twice a day to maintain mobility.
    2. Use pillows to maintain the right hip in a state of abduction.

3. Elevate the foot of the bed to 25 degrees.
4. Feed the client to conserve her energy.

13. A femoral head replacement was performed on an elderly client. Post-operatively the nurse positions the client with an abductor pillow between the client's legs. What is the primary reason for this?
    1. This position will promote greater comfort.
    2. Abduction promotes greater circulation to the hip joint.
    3. Abduction will prevent the prosthesis from snapping out of the socket.
    4. This position will help to prevent pressure on the sciatic nerve.

14. The client with rheumatoid arthritis has been taking 15 or 20 extra-strength aspirin a day. Which additional statement she makes would be of greatest concern to the nurse?
    1. "I sometimes have ringing in my ears."
    2. "I have a rash under my arms."
    3. "My fingers are swollen sometimes."
    4. "I don't have very much energy."

15. The physician orders prednisone for a client with rheumatoid arthritis for painful wrists and joints. Which instruction is it essential for the nurse to give the client?
    1. "Take the pills with milk or food."
    2. "Be sure to take the medication between meals."
    3. "Stop the pills at once if your face begins to get puffy."
    4. "Your urine may turn pinkish while taking this."

16. The client is a 64-year-old male admitted to the hospital with severe pain in his right big toe, which is red and swollen. Which nursing care measure is most essential for the nurse to perform at this time?
    1. Use a bed cradle on the bed.
    2. Put a bed board on the bed.
    3. Obtain a heat lamp.
    4. Prepare to catheterize the client.

17. The nurse is to give the client with gout one tablet of colchicine every hour until relief or toxicity occurs. Which of the following is an indication for stopping the colchicine?
    1. Ringing in the ears
    2. Nausea and vomiting
    3. A rash on the client's hips
    4. A temperature of 101°F

18. The nurse is teaching the client with gout about a diet low in purines. Which of the following is lowest in purine?
    1. Roast chicken
    2. Beef liver
    3. Fried shrimp
    4. Scrambled eggs

19. The client is now over an acute episode of gout. He is to be discharged on allopurinol (Zyloprim). What instruction must the nurse give to this client?
    1. "Take your medicine on an empty stomach."

2. "Report any nausea to your physician at once."
3. "Drink two to three quarts of fluids daily."
4. "Do not take over-the-counter cold medicine."

20. The client with arthritis is receiving sodium salicylate and asks the nurse what the drug will do for her. The nurse's reply should include information that the drug is given for which of these effects?
    1. Antipyretic
    2. Antibiotic
    3. Anticoagulant
    4. Anti-inflammatory

21. The client with newly diagnosed rheumatoid arthritis asks what can happen if no treatment is done. The nurse knows that if rheumatoid arthritis is left untreated, which of the following would be most apt to develop?
    1. Bony ankylosis
    2. Chronic osteomyelitis
    3. Pathological fractures
    4. Joint hypermobility

22. The client with rheumatoid arthritis is to receive prednisone 2.5 mg p.m. a.c. and h.s. What is the primary expected action of the drug?
    1. Maintenance of sodium and potassium balance
    2. Improvement of carbohydrate metabolism
    3. Production of androgen-like effects
    4. Interference with inflammatory reactions

23. The client is admitted to the hospital for a diagnostic workup. The client has vague symptoms of malaise, coughing, chest discomfort, low-grade fever, diffuse rashes, and musculoskeletal aches and pains. A diagnosis of probable lupus erythematosus has been made. The night nurse finds the client crying and saying, "I would rather die than suffer with this disease for the rest of my life." Which response by the nurse would be most therapeutic at this time?
    1. Telling the client there are support groups to join after discharge
    2. Offering to stay with the client to discuss concerns and questions
    3. Advising the client to write concerns on paper to discuss with the doctors and nurses tomorrow
    4. Offer the client a back rub and a warm cup of milk

24. The client is an elderly man who has had diabetes and peripheral vascular disease for several years. He now has had a right below-the-knee amputation. Which pre-operative nursing action will do most to help the client adjust to having an amputation?
    1. Encouraging deep-breathing
    2. Asking him if he understands the full effects of the planned surgery

3. Discussing the effects of diabetes on the vascular system
4. Having a recovered amputee visit him

25. The client has returned to the nursing unit following a right below-the-knee amputation. How should the nurse position the client?
    1. Supine with head turned to the side
    2. Place shock blocks under the foot of the bed
    3. Semi-Fowler's position with knees bent
    4. Left lateral with pillows between the knees
26. The day after an amputation, the client begins to hemorrhage from his stump. What action should the nurse take first?
    1. Apply a pressure dressing to the stump.
    2. Place a tourniquet above the stump.
    3. Notify the physician.
    4. Apply an ice pack to the stump.
27. The client continues to recover following a below-the-knee amputation. What nursing action should the nurse employ to help prevent the most common complication following leg amputation?
    1. Clean the wound with hydrogen peroxide three times a day.
    2. Have the client lie prone several times a day.
    3. Ask the client to flex and extend the toes on the remaining leg.
    4. Encourage the client to completely empty his/her bladder.
28. A young adult is discharged to home with crutches. Which exercise should the nurse teach the client in order to strengthen the triceps muscles for crutch-walking?
    1. Pushing the buttocks up off the mattress
    2. Pulling the body up, using an overhead trapeze
    3. Raising the legs straight up and down
    4. Squeezing a rubber ball in each hand
29. The client is ordered to be positioned flat following a myelogram. The nurse understands the primary reason for this is which of the following?
    1. To prevent infection
    2. To prevent spinal headache
    3. To prevent seizures
    4. To promote excretion of dye
30. The client has a fractured right ankle that has just been casted. The nurse is instructing the client in crutch-walking techniques. Which method is most appropriate?
    1. Move the right crutch, then the left foot, then the left crutch, and finally the right foot.
    2. Balance weight on the left foot and move right foot and both crutches forward, then bear weight on both crutches and move the left foot forward.
    3. Move the right crutch and left foot forward together; then the left crutch and right foot.
    4. Move the right crutch and right foot together and then the left crutch and the left foot.

Answers and Rationales

1. (1) The nurse must elevate the extremity to prevent swelling, which could cut off circulation. The wet cast gives a sensation of heat to the client but will not burn the skin. There will be muscle atrophy to both the arm and the leg. However, this is a long-term problem and will best be addressed after the cast and traction are removed. Abrasions are a cause for concern after the cast has dried but not at this time.
2. (1) The nurse should touch the cast using only the palms of the hands to prevent making indentations in a wet cast. Indentations could cause irritation of the skin. Fingertips would cause indentations in the wet cast. A towel sling is not appropriate. The cast is not petalled until it has dried. It would be impossible to move the casted extremity just by touching the petalled area at the edge of the cast.
3. (2) The cast should not be so tight as to cause circulatory impairment, which would be evidenced by swelling and changes in color or temperature. Pain is usually evidence of neurological impairment. The integrity of the cast should be maintained, but that does not describe an outcome relative to the circulatory system. Skin irritation is not an indicator of circulatory impairment.
4. (3) Elevation of the extremity increases venous return and reduces swelling. Elevation does not help a damp cast to dry more evenly. Changing the position of the pillow beneath the cast and not covering the cast will help it dry more evenly. Elevating a casted extremity does not directly reduce the amount of pain medication needed. A casted extremity that is elevated usually is more comfortable than one that is dependent; the chief purpose of elevation is to prevent edema formation. The prevention of edema is what makes the extremity more comfortable.
5. (1) The nurse should open communication. The nurse is sharing with the client the nurse's perception of the client's behavior. This is therapeutic and should open communication. Answer 2 tells him what not to do and will probably block communication. Answers 3 and 4 assume that the nurse knows what is causing his sadness and do not allow him to discuss his feelings.
6. (4) This best describes Russell's traction. Answer 1 describes Bryant's traction. Answer 2 is Buck's extension traction. Answer 3 is pelvic traction.
7. (3) The popliteal area should be assessed for adequacy of circulation. In Russell's traction, there is a vertical pull at the popliteal area that could obstruct circulation. There is no problem site in the pedal or femoral areas or the inner aspect of the thigh.

8. (1) The weights should remain in place at all times. They should not be removed or reduced or lifted up while the client is moved.

9. (3) The client has been flat for two weeks. Orthostatic hypotension is likely. The nurse should let the client dangle on the side of the bed before ambulating. While the client would have an increased possibility of kidney stones after being immobilized, this is not related to getting the client out of bed. Depression and skin breakdown can also occur in clients who have been immobilized. However, they are not apt to cause problems when the client gets out of bed for the first time.

10. (4) The description fits that of a pathological fracture in which the bone fractured first and then she fell. This is usually related to a decrease of calcium in the bone. With a comminuted fracture, the bone is broken into several pieces. A greenstick fracture occurs in children. One side of the bone is broken and the other side is splintered, like breaking a green stick. An open or compound fracture is one in which a wound through the soft tissue communicates with the site of the break.

11. (4) Osteoporosis or the loss of calcium is caused by a number of factors and is often related to the decrease in estrogen following menopause. Osteoporosis is thought to be related to decreased estrogen after menopause, not decreased progesterone. Elderly women do not all have decreased mobility due to arthritis. The cause is usually related to decreased calcium absorption rather than increased calcium absorption.

12. (2) The hip should be maintained in abduction to keep the hip in the best alignment. She cannot get out of bed. The foot is not elevated. There is no data indicating a need to feed the client.

13. (3) Abduction is necessary to keep the hip from coming out of the socket. This position may or may not be most comfortable. Comfort, while important, is not of highest priority. Abduction does not necessarily promote greater circulation to the hip joint. Abduction does not prevent pressure on the sciatic nerve.

14. (1) Tinnitus is a sign of aspirin toxicity. Swollen fingers and decrease in energy are typical of rheumatoid arthritis. A rash under the arms is not likely to be related to aspirin ingestion.

15. (1) Corticosteroids are very irritating to the stomach and are taken with food or milk to reduce the chance of ulcer development. The client will develop a puffy face from the steroid. This is not an indication to discontinue the drug. Steroids should not be stopped abruptly. They should always be tapered. Answer 4 is not true; the urine does not turn pinkish. Dilantin, an anti-seizure drug, may turn the urine pinkish.

16. (1) The pain of gout is very severe. A bed cradle will keep the bed linens off his toe. There is no indication for a bed board. Bed boards are indicated for back problems. A heat lamp is not part of the therapy for gout. There is no indication of a need to catheterize the client.

17. (2) Nausea, vomiting, and diarrhea indicate toxicity to colchicine. Tinnitus indicates aspirin toxicity. Rash and fever are not usual signs of colchicine toxicity.

18. (4) Eggs are lowest in purine. Chicken, organ meats such as liver, and shrimp are high in purines.

19. (3) It is essential to force fluids when taking allopurinol, a uricosuric drug. This will help the uric acid crystals to be excreted in the urine and not collect in the kidneys and form stones. The medicine does not need to be taken on an empty stomach. Nausea can be a side effect of the allopurinol. However, the priority instruction is to drink large amounts of fluid. There is no contraindication with over-the-counter cold medicine.

20. (4) Sodium salicylate has all of the effects except antibiotic. However, it is given to a person with arthritis primarily for its anti-inflammatory effect. The anticoagulant action can be an adverse effect for this client.

21. (1) Bony ankylosis occurs in untreated rheumatoid arthritis. Osteomyelitis is a bone infection and is not related to rheumatoid arthritis. Pathological fractures are usually the result of severe osteoporosis, not arthritis. Joints lose mobility and become ankylosed; they do not have hypermobility.

22. (4) Prednisone is a corticosteroid and has an anti-inflammatory effect. It does affect sodium and potassium balance, carbohydrate metabolism, and causes androgen-like effects; however, these are seen as bothersome side effects when given to a client who has arthritis.

23. (2) Offering help and letting the client express feelings is most therapeutic at this time. Telling the client about support groups may be appropriate later. Advising the client to write her concerns on paper to discuss tomorrow could be appropriate after the nurse had listened to the client's concerns and feelings. At this time, that response closes communication. Giving the client a back rub and a warm cup of milk could be done after listening to the client.

24. (4) Seeing an amputee who is living successfully will do the most to help him adjust to having an amputation. All of the others might be done but do not help him to adjust to an amputation.

25. (2) The foot of the bed should be raised to prevent edema formation in the stump. Shock blocks are the best way to accomplish this. Pillows can be used for the first 24–28 hours only. Note that the client has returned to the

nursing unit. The client will be awake before returning to the nursing unit, and so turning the head to the side is not needed. Positioning the client in semi-Fowler's position with knees bent would cause swelling of the surgical site and is contraindicated. Positioning the client on the side with pillows between the knees is not the most appropriate position.

26. (2) Applying a tourniquet is the best action because the bleeders are usually too large to be controlled by pressure. This is one of the very few times when applying a tourniquet is indicated. An ice pack will be ineffective in controlling hemorrhage from the stump. The nurse should notify the physician but should attempt to stop the bleeding before leaving the client to call the physician.

27. (2) The most common complication is flexion contracture of the hip or knee. Having the client lie prone will help to prevent flexion contractures of the hip and knee. The wound should be kept clean, but not usually with hydrogen peroxide three times a day. Asking the client to flex and extend the toes on the remaining leg will help to prevent thrombophlebitis in the remaining leg and is certainly appropriate. However, thrombophlebitis is not the most common complication following leg amputation. It is appropriate to encourage the client to empty the bladder. However, a bladder infection is not the most common complication following leg amputation.

28. (1) Pushing one's buttocks up off the mattress is a resistive exercise that improves the strength and tone of the triceps muscles. Pull-ups strengthen the biceps muscles. Straight leg raises strengthen the hip flexor and quadriceps. Squeezing a rubber ball strengthens finger flexors.

29. (2) When a client is ordered to be flat following a myelogram, the nurse knows the physician used an oil-based dye. The reason for the flat position is to prevent development of spinal headache. If the client had been ordered to be in a low-Fowler's position, the nurse would know that a water-based dye had been used. The water-based dye is not removed, and the client is in low-Fowler's position to prevent irritation of the meninges and seizures. With a water-based dye, fluids are encouraged to promote excretion of the dye. Positioning does not prevent development of infection.

30. (2) A three-point gait is indicated when the client can bear no weight on one foot. This correctly describes a three-point gait for someone with a right foot problem. Answer 1 describes a four-point gait. The client must be able to bear weight on both feet for this gait. Answer 3 correctly describes a two-point gait. The client must be able to bear weight on both feet for this gait. Answer 4 does not correctly describe any gait.

Chapter 13

The Endocrine System

ANATOMY AND PHYSIOLOGY

Composed of an interrelated complex of ductless glands that secrete hormones into the blood stream and act on distant parts of the body

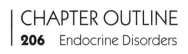
MAJOR FUNCTION IS TO REGULATE BODY FUNCTIONS

A. Negative feedback loop is the major regulatory method:
  1. Decreased concentration of a circulating hormone triggers production of a releasing factor in the hypothalmus.
  2. Releasing factor triggers the production of a stimulating hormone in the anterior pituitary.
  3. Stimulating hormone stimulates its target organ to produce hormones.
  4. Increased concentration of a hormone causes the production of inhibiting factor, resulting in the decreased secretion of the target organ hormone.
B. Some hormones controlled by changing blood levels of specific substances (calcium, glucose)

PITUITARY GLAND (HYPOPHYSIS)
(Figure 13.1 and 13.2)

A. Located in sella turcica at the base of the brain
B. "Master gland" composed of two lobes
  1. Anterior lobe:
    a. Secretes trophic hormones in response to secretions (releasing factors) from hypothalmus
      (1) Thyroid stimulating hormone (TSH)
      (2) Adrenocorticotropic hormone (ACTH)
      (3) Follicle-stimulating hormone (FSH)
      (4) Luteinizing hormone (LH)
    b. Also secretes hormones that have a direct effect on tissues:
      (1) Luteotropic hormone (prolactin)
      (2) Growth hormone (somatotropin)
      (3) Melanocyte-stimulating hormone that relates to pigmentation
  2. Posterior lobe: stores and releases hormones made in the hypothalmus
    a. Antidiuretic hormone regulates fluid balance by causing kidneys to retain sodium and fluid
    b. Oxytocin stimulates uterine contractions

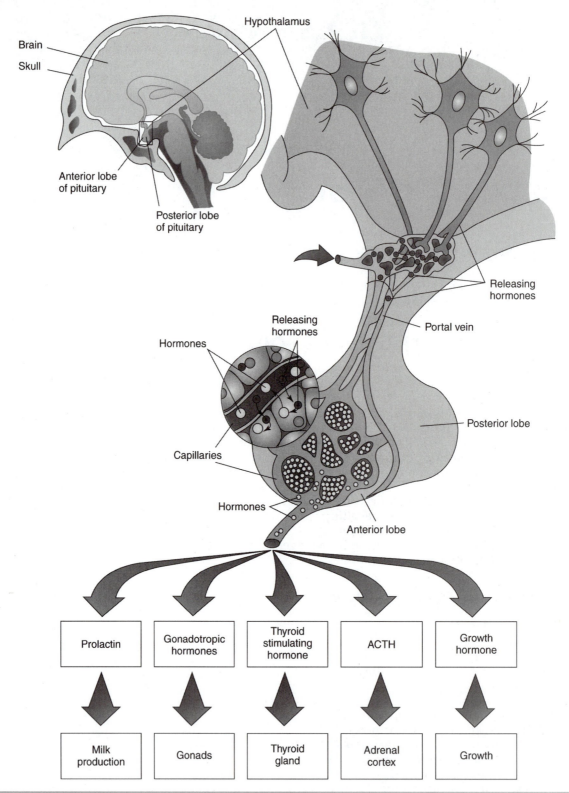

Figure 13.1 The relationship of the hypothalamus with the anterior lobe of the pituitary gland.

ADRENAL GLAND

A. Two small glands, one above each kidney
B. Each gland has two sections:

1. Adrenal cortex secretes three types of hormones:
   a. Glucocorticoids (sugar): Cortisol, cortisone
      (1) Glyconeogenesis

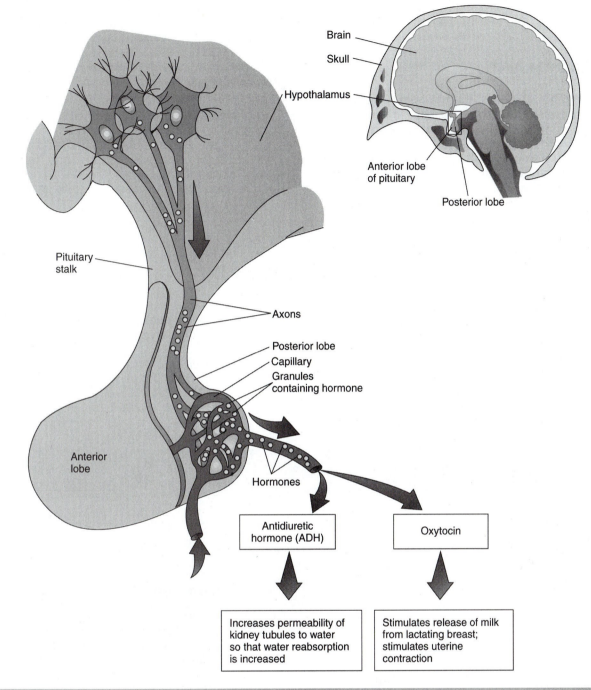

Figure 13.2 The relationship of the hypothalamus with the posterior lobe of the pituitary gland.

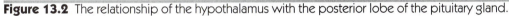

    (2) Protein catabolism
    (3) Mobilization of fatty acids
    (4) Sodium and water retention
    (5) Anti-inflammatory effect
    (6) Stress response
  b. Mineralocorticoids (salt): Aldosterone
    (1) Regulates fluid and electrolyte
        balance
    (2) Promotes sodium, chloride, and
        water reabsorption
    (3) Promotes potassium excretion

  c. Sex hormones:
    (1) Androgens
    (2) Estrogens, progesterone
    (3) Development of secondary sex
        characteristics
2. Adrenal medulla: secretes adrenalin
  (epinephrine), noradrenalin
  (norepinephrine)
  a. Sympathetic nervous system
    response—"fight or flight"
  b. Increases heart rate, blood pressure

    c. Dilates bronchioles
    d. Glycogen to glucose for emergency energy

THYROID GLAND

A. Located in anterior portion of neck; consists of two lobes separated by a narrow isthmus
B. Produces thyroxin (T_4), triiodothyronine (T_3), thyrocalcitonin
C. Thyroid-stimulating hormone produced by the anterior pituitary stimulates the thyroid gland; anterior pituitary is stimulated by thyroid releasing factor produced by the hypothalmus in response to decreased levels of thyroid hormones.
D. Functions:
    1. Controls metabolic rate
    2. Regulates carbohydrate, fat, and protein metabolism
    3. Aids in regulating physical and mental growth and development

PARATHYROID GLANDS

A. Four small glands located in pairs behind the thyroid gland

B. Produce parathormone, which regulates calcium phosphorus balance; parathormone causes increase in serum calcium and decrease in serum phosphorus

PANCREAS

A. Located behind the stomach
B. Endocrine functions: Islets of Langerhans:
    1. Beta cells produce insulin.
    2. Alpha cells produce glucagon (insulin antagonist).
B. Exocrine functions: digestive enzymes:
    1. Amylase
    2. Lipase
    3. Trypsin

GONADS

A. Ovaries:
    1. Located in pelvic cavity
    2. Produce estrogen and progesterone
B. Testes:
    1. Located in scrotum
    2. Produce testosterone

Endocrine Disorders

PITUITARY GLAND

Hyperpituitarism

A. Hyperfunction of the anterior pituitary resulting in over secretion of one or more of the anterior pituitary hormones; frequently caused by a benign pituitary adenoma
B. Assessment findings:
    1. Overproduction of growth hormone resulting in giantism in children and acromegaly (enlarged feet, hands, nose, coarse features, enlarged tongue) in adults
    2. Hyperthyroidism
    3. Reproductive problems
C. Diagnostic tests:
    1. Skull X-ray, CT scan, MRI
    2. Serum and urine hormonal tests
D. Interventions:
    1. Surgical removal or irradiation
    2. Monitor for problems related to hormonal imbalance:
        a. Hyperglycemia

        b. Menstrual
        c. Cardiovascular

Hypopituitarism

A. Hypofunction of anterior pituitary gland causing deficiencies in both the pituitary hormones and the hormones of the target glands; caused by tumor, trauma, surgical removal, or irradiation of the gland
B. Assessment findings:
    1. Hemianopia (half blindness, may occur with a tumor)
    2. Headache (may occur with tumor)
    3. Signs of hormonal disturbances:
        a. Menstrual irregularities
        b. Hypothyroidism
        c. Adrenal insufficiency
        d. Growth retardation before epiphyses closed
C. Diagnostic tests:
    1. Skull X-ray
    2. CT scan
    3. Plasma hormone levels

D. Interventions:
1. Surgical removal of tumor
2. Irradiation of pituitary gland
3. Hormone replacement

Hypophysectomy

A. Partial or complete removal of pituitary gland
B. Indications include pituitary tumors and endocrine-dependent tumors of the breast or prostate
C. Approaches:
1. Craniotomy (usually transfrontal)
2. Transphenoidal: incision made in the inner aspect of the lip and gingiva; sella turcica is entered through the floor of the nose and sphenoid sinuses
3. Cryohypophysectomy: cold used to destroy the pituitary
D. Nursing Care:
1. Nursing care for a craniotomy patient
2. Observe for signs of deficiencies in glands the pituitary regulates—thyroid, adrenal, reproductive.
3. Hourly urines to monitor antidiuretic hormone (ADH)
4. Report outputs above 900 cc in two hours or specific gravity below 1.004, because this indicates diabetes insipidus.
5. Administer hormone replacements as ordered: given immediately and for the remainder of the client's life:
   a. Cortisone replacement
   b. Thyroid replacement
   c. Sex hormone replacement: testosterone for men; estrogen for women
   d. Vasopressin (Lypressin) (ADH) to control diabetes insipidus if posterior pituitary removed
6. Teach client:
   a. No bending in the post-operative period to prevent increased intracranial pressure
   b. Medications must be taken as ordered for life.
   c. Wear identification, such as a Medicalert bracelet.
   d. Transphenoidal approach: special nursing care needs:
      (1) Observe for cerebralspinal fluid leak; test clear drainage for glucose.
      (2) Most leaks resolve within 72 hours with bed rest and head elevation.
      (3) Physician may perform daily spinal taps to decrease CSF pressure
      (4) Elevate head of bed 30° to decrease headache and pressure on the sella turcica
      (5) Administer antibiotics as ordered post-operatively to prevent meningitis.
      (6) Teach client no tooth brushing until sutures removed and incision heals (10 days)

ADRENAL GLAND

Disorders of Adrenal Medulla

A. Pheochromocytoma: functioning tumor that secretes excessive amounts of epinephrine and norepinephrine
1. Assessment findings:
   a. Hypertension, tachycardia, palpitations
   b. Headache
   c. Vomiting
   d. Hyperglycemia
2. Diagnostic tests:
   a. Plasma catecholamines—elevated with pheochromocytoma
   b. Blood and urine tested for sugar—elevated with pheochromocytoma
   c. 24-hour urine for catecholamines and vanillylmandelic acid (VMA)—elevated with pheochromocytoma
   d. X-ray to visualize tumor on adrenal gland
3. Interventions
   a. Surgery—adrenalectomy
   b. Monitor vital signs—especially blood pressure:
      (1) Administer antihypertensives as ordered.
      (2) Promote rest.
      (3) Provide a high-calorie diet and avoid stimulants, such as caffeine.
B. No hypofunction disorders related to the adrenal medulla because epinephrine and norepinephrine are made elsewhere in the body and no replacement is necessary even when gland removed

Disorders of Adrenal Cortex

A. Hyperfunction of the Adrenal Gland (Cushing's Syndrome)
1. Causes:
   a. Primary Cushing's syndrome caused by tumors or hyperplasia of the adrenal cortex
   b. Secondary Cushing's syndrome can be caused by pituitary tumors.
   c. Cushing's syndrome may be caused by prolonged steroid administration.
2. Assessment findings (see Figure 13.3)
   a. Elevated cortisol levels
   b. Obese trunk with thin arms and legs, muscle wasting and purple striae on trunk
   c. Moon face
   d. Buffalo hump
   e. Decreased resistance to infection

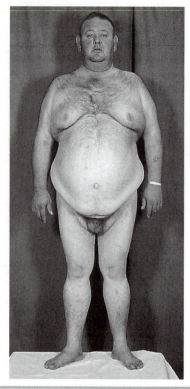

Figure 13.3 Cushing's Syndrome

    e. Maintain skin integrity.
    f. Minimize stress.
    g. Measure I & O and daily weights.
    h. Provide a diet low in calories and sodium and high in protein, potassium, calcium, and Vitamin D.
    i. Monitor the urine or blood for glucose, and give insulin as ordered.
    j. Provide emotional support; inform the client that physical changes will recede after treatment

B. Hypofunction of the Adrenal Gland (Addison's Disease)
  1. Caused by idiopathic atrophy (possibly autoimmune) and destruction of adrenal gland secondary to tuberculosis or fungal infection
  2. Assessment findings:
    a. Fatigue, muscle weakness (caused by hyperkalemia)
    b. Anorexia, nausea, vomiting, weight loss
    c. Hypoglycemia
    d. Hypotension, weak pulse as a result of decreased circulating volume
    e. Bronze pigmentation of skin
    f. Inability to cope with stress
  3. Diagnostic tests:
    a. Low cortisol levels
    b. Serum electrolytes: low sodium and elevated potassium
  4. Nursing diagnoses (see Table 13.2)
  5. Interventions
    a. Hormone replacement therapy:
      (1) Cortisone (Give two thirds of dose in early morning and one third in afternoon)
      (2) Florinef (mineralocorticoid)
    b. Teach that medications must be taken every day for the rest of his life.
    c. Monitor vital signs.
    d. Decrease stress, because the client has little ability to respond to stress (do not even make the client's bed during the crisis until steroids are administered).

    f. Hyperglycemia
    g. Osteoporosis
    h. Hypokalemia resulting in muscle weakness, fatigue
    i. Sodium and fluid retention resulting in hypertension and edema
    j. Mood swings, irritability
    k. Acne
    l. Masculinization in women: menstrual irregularities, decreased libido, hirsutism
  3. Diagnostic tests:
    a. Cortisol levels elevated
    b. Serum electrolytes: potassium decreased and sodium elevated
    c. Blood sugar elevated
  4. Interventions:
    a. Adrenalectomy if condition caused by adrenal tumor or hyperplasia
    b. Hypophysectomy or irradiation of pituitary if caused by a pituitary tumor
    c. Drug dosage adjustment if caused by administration of steroids
  5. Nursing diagnoses (see Table 13.1)
  6. Nursing care:
    a. Monitor vital signs.
    b. Maintain muscle tone.
    c. Prevent injury, because the client is bruised easily and may have osteoporosis.
    d. Prevent exposure to infection, because the client is immunosuppressed.

Table 13.2 Nursing Diagnoses Related to Addisons's Disease

- Risk for deficient fluid volume related to excessive loss of sodium and water secondary to polyuria
- Risk for imbalanced nutrition: less than body requirements related to anorexia and nausea
- Diarrhea related to increased excretion of sodium and water
- Risk for disturbed self-concept related to appearance changes secondary to increased skin pigmentation
- Risk for injury related to postural hypotension secondary to fluid/electrolyte imbalances
- Risk for ineffective health maintenance related to insufficient knowledge of disease, signs and symptoms of complications, risks for crisis (infection, diarrhea, decreased sodium intake, diaphoresis), over-exertion, dietary management, identification card or medallion, emergency kit, and pharmacologic management

e. Prevent exposure to infection, because the client has little ability to respond to stress of any kind.
f. Monitor intake and output; client usually has excessive urine output due to lack of aldosterone.
g. Provide a high protein, CHO, sodium, and low potassium diet.

THYROID GLAND

Diagnostic Tests

A. Serum studies (non-fasting):
   1. Serum T_3 and T_4 levels
   2. Thyroid Stimulating Hormone (TSH): measurement differentiates primary from secondary hypothyroidism
B. Radioactive iodine studies:
   1. Radioactive Iodine Uptake (RAIU): I^{131} given orally; counter measures amount of radioactive iodine taken up by the thyroid after 24 hours; determines thyroid functioning
   2. Thyroid Scan: Radioactive isotope given IV or PO; scanner visualizes the distribution of radioactivity in the gland; determines location, size, shape, and anatomic function of the thyroid gland and can identify areas of increased or decreased uptake; used to evaluate thyroid nodules
   3. Nursing care:
      a. Discontinue thyroid medication for 7–10 days before the test.
      b. Iodine in medications, test dyes (IVP, cardiac catheterization, arteriograms), foods can invalidate test; RAIU should be done before any test using iodine dye

Simple Goiter

A. Enlargement of the thyroid gland not caused by inflammation or neoplasm; low levels of thyroid hormone stimulate production of TRF in the hypothalamus, which causes the anterior pituitary to produce TSH that stimulates the thyroid gland—causing it to enlarge in an attempt to produce more thyroid hormone
B. Types:
   1. Endemic: caused by iodine deficiency
   2. Sporadic
   3. Caused by ingestion of large amounts of goitrogenic foods (foods that decrease thyroxine production—cabbage, soybeans, rutabagas, peanuts, peaches, peas, strawberries, spinach, radishes)
   4. Caused by use of goitrogenic drugs such as propylthiouracil, large amounts of iodine, phenylbutazone, para-amino salicylic acid, cobalt, lithium
B. Assessment findings:
   1. Dysphagia
   2. Enlarged thyroid
   3. Respiratory distress
C. Diagnostic Tests:
   1. Serum T_4 low normal or normal
   2. RAIU uptake normal or increased
D. Interventions:
   1. Drug therapy
      a. Hormone replacement with levothyroxine (Synthroid) (T_4); desiccated thyroid; or liothyronine (Cytomel)
      b. Small doses of iodine (Lugol's or potassium iodide solution) for goiter resulting from iodine deficiency
   2. Teach client about thyroid hormone replacement:
      a. Usually start with small doses and increase to the proper level.
      b. Report any signs of toxicity, such as rapid heart beats, chest pain, severe insomnia, or tremors.
   3. Avoid goitrogenic foods or drugs in sporadic goiter.
   4. Surgery: subtotal thyroidectomy if goiter is large to relieve pressure symptoms and for appearance
   5. Teach the client to use iodized salt to prevent and treat an endemic goiter.

Hypothyroidism (Myxedema)

A. Slowed metabolic processes caused by hypofunction of the thyroid gland with decreased production of thyroid hormone; causes myxedema in adults and cretinism in children; commonly seen in women between 30 and 60.

B. Types:
1. Primary: caused by atrophy of the thyroid gland; thought to be autoimmune
2. Secondary: caused by decreased stimulation from pituitary TSH
3. Iatrogenic: surgical removal of the gland or over treatment of hyperthyroidism with drugs or radioactive iodine
C. Assessment findings:
1. Fatigue, lethargy, and slow, clumsy movements
2. Slowed mental processes, dull look
3. Anorexia, weight gain
4. Constipation
5. Intolerance to cold
6. Dry, scaly skin; dry, sparse hair; brittle nails
7. Menstrual irregularities
8. Generalized interstitial nonpitting edema
9. Bradycardia, atherosclerosis, angina pectoris, MI, CHF
10. Decreased respirations
11. Increased sensitivity to sedatives, narcotics, and anesthetics
12. Myxedemic coma, exaggeration of above manifestations: weakness, lethargy, syncope, bradycardia, hypotension, hypoventilation, subnormal body temperature
D. Nursing diagnoses (see Table 13.3)
E. Interventions:
1. Drug therapy: levothyroxine (Synthroid), thyroglobulin (Proloid), desiccated thyroid, liothyrosine (Cytomel)
2. Myxedemic coma is a medical emergency:
   a. Immediate treatment necessary—high mortality rate
   b. IV thyroid hormones

Table 13.3 Nursing Diagnoses Related to Hypothyroidism

- Imbalanced nutrition: more than body requirements related to intake greater than metabolic needs secondary to slowed metabolic rate
- Activity intolerance related to insufficient oxygenation secondary to slowed metabolic rate
- Constipation related to decreased peristaltic action secondary to decreased metabolic rate and decreased physical activity
- Impaired skin integrity related to edema and dryness secondary to decreased metabolic rate and infiltration into interstitial tissues
- Impaired comfort related to cold intolerance secondary to decreased metabolic rate
- Risk for impaired social interactions related to listlessness and depression
- Impaired verbal communication related to slowed speech secondary to enlarged tongue
- Risk for altered health maintenance related to insufficient knowledge of condition, treatment regimen, dietary management, signs and symptoms of complications, pharmacologic therapy, and sensitivity to narcotics, barbiturates, and anesthetic agents

c. Correction of hypothermia
d. Maintenance of vital functions
e. Treatment of precipitating factors (failure to take medications; infection; trauma; exposure to cold; use of sedatives, narcotics, anesthetics)
F. Nursing care:
1. Monitor vital signs; be especially alert to cardiac complications
2. Daily weights
3. Observe for signs of thyrotoxicosis when administering thyroid medications:
   a. Tachycardia, palpitations, angina
   b. Nausea, vomiting, diarrhea, sweating
   c. Dyspnea
   d. Tremors, agitation
4. Dosage should be increased gradually.
5. Provide a warm, comfortable environment.
6. Low-calorie diet; give increased fluids and roughage
7. Avoid sedatives.
8. Administer stool softeners as ordered.
9. Observe for myxedemic coma.

Hyperthyroidism (Grave's Disease)

A. Hyperfunction of the thyroid gland; thought to be autoimmune; seen in women 30–50 years old
B. Diagnostic tests:
1. Serum T_3 and T_4 levels elevated
2. RAIU increased
C. Assessment findings:
1. Irritability, agitation, restlessness, hyperactivity
2. Increased appetite
3. Weight loss
4. Intolerance to heat
5. Exophthalmos
6. Goiter
7. Warm, smooth skin; soft hair; pliable nails
8. Tachycardia, palpitations, increased systolic pressure
D. Nursing diagnoses (see Table 13.4)
E. Interventions:
1. Drug therapy:
   a. Antithyroid drugs (Propylthiouracil and methimazole [Tapazole]) to block synthesis of thyroid hormone; toxic effects include agranulocytosis
   b. Adrenergic blocking drugs (Propranolol [Inderal]) to decrease sympathetic activity and slow heart rate
2. Radioactive Iodine therapy
   a. I^{131} given to destroy the thyroid gland, thereby decreasing production of thyroid hormone
   b. Hypothyroidism a potential complication
3. Nursing care:
   a. Vital signs
   b. Daily weights

Table 13.4 Nursing Diagnoses Related to Hyperthyroidism

- Imbalanced nutrition: less than body requirements related to intake less than metabolic needs secondary to excessive metabolic rate
- Activity intolerance related to fatigue and exhaustion secondary to excessive metabolic rate
- Diarrhea related to increased peristalsis secondary to excessive metabolic rate
- Impaired comfort related to heat intolerance secondary to excessive metabolic rate
- Risk for impaired tissue integrity: corneal related to inability to close eyelids secondary to exophthalmos
- Risk for injury related to tremors
- Risk for hyperthermia secondary to excessive metabolic rate
- Risk for ineffective health maintenance related to insufficient knowledge of condition, treatment regimen, pharmacologic therapy, eye care, dietary management, and signs and symptoms of complications

   c. Provide for rest
   d. Cool environment
   e. Minimize stress
   f. Diet high in carbohydrates, protein, calories, vitamins, and minerals with supplemental feedings—no stimulants
   g. Protect eyes with dark glasses and artificial tears if exophthalmos is present
   h. Teach patient signs of hyper- and hypothyroidism

F. Thyroid storm:
  1. Uncontrolled and potentially life-threatening hyperthyroidism precipitated by stress, infection, or unprepared thyroid surgery
  2. Assessment findings:
    a. Apprehension, restlessness
    b. Hyperthermia (to 106° F)
    c. Tachycardia
    d. Respiratory distress
    e. Delirium
    f. Coma
  3. Interventions:
    a. Antithyroid drugs, such as propylthiouracil
    b. Corticosteroids, sedatives
    c. Beta adrenergic blockers (Propranolol, Inderal) to slow heart rate
  4. Nursing care:
    a. Maintain a patent airway and adequate ventilation and oxygen
    b. IV therapy as ordered
  5. Thyroidectomy:
    a. Partial or total removal of the thyroid gland
    b. Pre-operative nursing care:
      (1) Administer antithyroid drugs as ordered.

      (2) Propylthiouracil to suppress production of thyroxine and to prevent thyroid storm
      (3) Lugol's solution to reduce the size and vascularity of the thyroid gland and prevent hemorrhage
      (4) Ensure stable cardiac status.
      (5) Ensure that weight and nutritional status are normal.
    c. Post-operative nursing care:
      (1) Monitor vital signs.
      (2) Monitor intake and output.
      (3) Check dressings for signs of hemorrhage; check behind neck for wetness.
      (4) Semi-Fowler's position and support head with pillows
      (5) Tracheostomy set, oxygen, and suction at bedside for 48 hours in case respiratory distress develops
      (6) Observe for signs of tetany (hypocalcemia due to damage or removal of parathyroids).
      (7) Asses for Trousseau's sign—inflating blood pressure cuff on arm causes hand spasm—and Chovstek's sign—gently tapping the facial nerve causes facial grimace
      (8) Calcium gluconate at bedside to give if hypocalcemia develops
      (9) Check for extreme hoarseness.
      (10) Observe for thyroid storm.
      (11) Analgesics and analgesic throat lozenges
      (12) Cool mist humidifier to liquefy secretions
      (13) Encourage fluids
      (14) Cough and deep-breathe every hour.
      (15) Teach client to support neck with hands when turning and moving
      (16) Teach client signs of hypo- and hyperthyroidism
      (17) Teach client about medications if he is receiving thyroid medications
      (18) ROM neck exercises 3–4 times a day after discharge

PARATHYROID GLANDS

Hypoparathyroidism

A. Characterized by hypocalcemia; may be hereditary, idiopathic, or caused by accidental damage to or removal of parathyroid glands during thyroidectomy
B. Assessment
  1. Tetany as evidenced by:
    a. Tingling around lips and of fingers

b. Chovstek's sign—tapping over facial nerve causes twitching of mouth, nose, and eye
c. Trousseau's sign—Blood pressure cuff inflated for three minutes causes carpopedal spasm
d. Painful muscle spasms, fatigue, weakness, muscle cramps, and tremor
2. Dysphagia
3. Laryngospasm
4. Seizures
5. Cardiac dysrhythmias
6. Personality changes, irritability, memory impairment
7. Dry, scaly skin; hair loss; loss of tooth enamel
8. Cataract formation
C. Diagnostic Tests
1. Serum calcium levels decreased (< 8.5 mg/dl); serum phosphorus levels increased
2. Skeletal X-rays reveal increased bone density.
D. Interventions:
1. Calcium gluconate by slow IV drip for acute hypocalcemia
2. Administer medications for chronic hypocalcemia.
a. Oral calcium—calcium gluconate, lactate, carbonate (Os-Cal)
b. Vitamin D (Calciferol) to help absorption of calcium
c. Aluminum hydroxide gel (Amphojel) or aluminum carbonate gel (Basaljel) to decrease phosphate levels
3. Initiate seizure and safety precautions.
4. Reduce environmental stimuli to reduce the likelihood of seizures.
5. Monitor for signs of hoarseness or stridor and Chovstek's and Trousseau's signs.
6. Tracheostomy set, injectable calcium gluconate at bedside
7. Rebreathing bag may be used for tetany or generalized muscle cramps
8. Monitor serum calcium and phosphorus levels.
9. High calcium, low phosphorus diet
10. Teach patient regarding medications and diet and need for follow-up care

Hyperparathyroidism

A. Hyperfunction of the parathyroid glands causing increased secretion of parathormone resulting in hypercalcemia, hypophosphatemia, and altered bone metabolism; seen most frequently in women aged 35–65
B. Primary hyperparathyroidism is caused by tumor or hyperplasia; secondary is caused by Vitamin D deficiency, malabsorption syndromes, or chronic renal failure.

C. Assessment findings:
1. Bone pain (especially in back), bone demineralization, pathologic fractures
2. Renal colic, kidney stones, polyuria, polydipsia
3. Anorexia, nausea, vomiting, gastric ulcers, constipation
4. Muscle weakness, fatigue
5. Irritability, personality changes, depression
6. Cardiac dysrhythmias, hypertension
D. Diagnostic tests:
1. Elevated serum calcium levels (<10.5 mg/dl)
2. Decreased serum phosphate levels
3. Skeletal X-rays show bone demineralization.
E. Interventions:
1. Normal saline given IV
2. Administer diuretics as ordered.
3. Input and Output—observe for fluid overload and electrolyte imbalances
4. Handle client carefully to prevent pathologic fractures.
5. Monitor vital signs.
6. Force fluids, provide acid ash juices; low calcium, high phosphorus diet
7. Strain urine for stones.

PANCREAS DISORDERS

Diabetes Mellitus

A. Hyperglycemia resulting from relative or absolute lack of insulin; chronic, systemic disease characterized by disorders in the metabolism of carbohydrate, fat, and protein; eventually produces structural abnormalities in various tissues and organs
B. Predisposing factors:
1. Heredity
2. Autoimmunity
3. Virus
4. Obesity
5. Stress
C. Types:
1. Type I (Insulin-Dependent Diabetes Mellitus):
a. Secondary to destruction of beta cells in the pancreas resulting in little or no insulin production
b. Usually occurs in children, young adults, or in non-obese adults
2. Type II (Non-Insulin-Dependent Diabetes Mellitus):
a. Secondary to alterations in insulin receptors on cell membrane, causing resistance to insulin
b. Usually occurs in obese adults

D. Pathophysiology:
 1. Lack of insulin causes hyperglycemia (Insulin is necessary for the transport of glucose across the cell membrane.)
 2. Hyperglycemia leads to osmotic diuresis as large amounts of glucose pass through the kidney, resulting in polyuria and glycosuria.
 3. Diuresis leads to cellular dehydration and fluid and electrolyte depletion, causing polydipsia.
 4. Polyphagia results from cellular starvation.
 5. The body breaks down fats for energy; when there is no glucose in the cell, fats cannot be completely metabolized—and ketones (intermediate products of fat metabolism) are produced.
 6. Ketones act as CNS depressants and can cause coma.
 7. Excess loss of fluids and electrolytes leads to hypovolemia, hypotension, renal failure, and decreased blood flow to the brain resulting in coma and death unless treated.
E. Assessment findings:
 1. All types have polyuria, polydipsia, polyphagia, fatigue, blurred vision, and susceptibility to infection.
 2. Type I: anorexia, nausea, vomiting, weight loss
 3. Type II: obesity, eye changes, vulval itching
F. Diagnostic Tests:
 1. Fasting blood sugar elevated (normal 70–110 mg/dl)
 2. Two-hour post-prandial sugar elevated (normal 70–140 mg/dl)
 3. Oral glucose tolerance test elevated (see Table 13.5)
 4. Elevated Hgb A_{1c} levels (normal 2.2%–4.8%)
 5. Clinitest and Testape positive for glucose
 6. Acetest, Ketostix may be positive for acetone.
G. Nursing Diagnoses (see Table 13.6)
H. Interventions
 1. Strict diet
  a. Used with insulin for Type I
  b. Used alone or in combination with oral hypoglycemic agents for Type II
 2. Insulin for Type I
  a. Short acting (regular):
   (1) Used in treating ketoacidosis, during surgery, infection, trauma, management of poorly controlled diabetes, and to supplement longer acting insulin
   (2) See Table 13.7 for onset, peak, and duration.
  b. Intermediate acting (NPH):
   (1) Used for maintenance therapy
   (2) See Table 13.7 for onset, peak, and duration.
  c. Long-acting (Protamine Zinc Insulin)

Table 13.5 Oral Glucose Tolerance Test

Fasting	70–115 mg/dl
30 min	<200 mg/dl
1 hour	<200 mg/dl
2 hours	<140 mg/dl
3 hours	70–115 mg/dl
4 hours	70–115 mg/dl

Urine Test: Negative for glucose

Table 13.6. Nursing Diagnoses Related to Diabetes Mellitus

- Risk for injury related to decreased tactile sensation, diminished visual acuity, and hypoglycemia
- Impaired comfort related to insulin injections, capillary blood glucose testing, and diabetic peripheral neuropathy
- Anxiety/fear related to diagnosis of diabetes, potential complications of diabetes, and self-care regimens
- Risk for ineffective individual/family coping related to chronic disease, complex self-care regimen, and decreased support systems
- Imbalanced nutrition: greater than body requirement related to intake in excess of need, lack of knowledge, and ineffective coping
- Risk for ineffective sexuality patterns (male) related to peripheral neuropathy and/or psychologic problems
- Risk for noncompliance related to the complexity and chronicity of the prescribed regimen
- Risk for ineffective health maintenance related to insufficient knowledge of diabetic exchange diet, weight control, weight maintenance, benefits/risk of exercise, self-monitoring of blood glucose, medications, sick day care, foot care, hypoglycemia, and available resources
- Social isolation related to visual impairment/blindness
- Powerlessness related to complications of diabetes (blindness, amputations, kidney failure, and neuropathy)

Table 13.7 Insulins

Insulin	Onset	Peak	Duration	Solution
Regular	1/2–1 hr	2–4 hrs	6–8 hrs	Clear
NPH	2–4 hrs	6–8 hrs	18–24 hrs	Cloudy
Insulin zinc suspension, extended Ultralente		4–8 hrs	16–20 hrs	Cloudy

   (1) Used for maintenance therapy in patients who experience hyperglycemia during the night with intermediate-acting insulin
   (2) See Table 13.7 for onset, peak, and duration.
  d. Administration of insulin:
   (1) Open bottle may be stored at room temperature (store extras in refrigerator).
   (2) Gently roll between palms; do not shake.

(3) Use sterile technique.
(4) When mixing insulins, draw up clear before cloudy.
(5) Rotate sites to prevent lipodystrophy; arm, abdomen, and thigh sites may be used; rotate within same area, preferably abdomena; do not go from arm to abdomen to thigh because absorption rate is different in different areas.
(6) Insert needle at 90° angle unless the client is emaciated.

e. Insulin pumps:
(1) Insulin pumps are small, externally worn devices that closely mimic normal pancreatic functioning.
(2) Contain a 3 ml syringe attached to a long (42 inch), narrow lumen tube with a needle or Teflon catheter at the end; the needle or Teflon catheter is inserted into the subcutaneous tissue (usually on the abdomen) and secured with a tape or a transparent dressing
(3) Needle or catheter changed at least every three days
(4) Pump is worn either on a belt or in a pocket.
(5) Pump uses only regular insulin.
(6) Insulin can be administered via the basal rate (usually 0.5–2.0 units/hr) and by a bolus dose (which is activated by a series of button pushes) prior to each meal.

f. Drug interactions:
(1) Advise patient not to smoke within 30 minutes after insulin injection because cigarette smoking decreases absorption of subcutaneously administered insulin.
(2) Marijuana use may increase insulin requirements.
(3) Advise the patient not to drink alcohol. Excessive alcohol intake may require reduction in insulin dosage because alcohol potentiates the hypoglycemic effect of insulin.

3. Oral hypoglycemic agents:
a. Used for Type II diabetics who are not controlled by diet and exercise
b. Increase the ability of islet cells to secrete insulin
c. Reduce glucose output by the liver
d. Enhance peripheral sensitivity to insulin
e. Hypoglycemic agents (see Table 13.8)
f. Glucophage (Metformin):
(1) May decrease dosage of other hypoglycemic agents
(2) Do not give to clients with severe liver or renal disease.

Table 13.8 Oral Antidiabetic Agents

Drug	Onset	Duration
Glucotrol	1–1 1/2 hrs	16–24 hrs
Micronase (Diabeta)	15 min.–1 hr	10–24 hrs
Metformin (Glucophage)	2–2 1/2 hrs	10–16 hrs

g. Acarbose (Precose) and Miglitol (Glyset):
(1) Delay glucose absorption and digestion of carbohydrates, resulting in smaller rise in blood glucose concentration after meals, lowering post-prandial hyperglyclemia
(2) Do not enhance insulin secretion.

h. Troglitazone (Rezulin):
(1) Reduces plasma glucose and insulin; exact mechanism unknown
(2) Potentiates action of insulin in skeletal muscle and decreases glucose production in liver
(3) Rezulin has been associated with an increased incidence of infection, headache, and liver damage.

4. Exercise:
a. Decreases the body's need for insulin
b. Best performed after meals when the blood sugar is rising
c. Regular exercise is desirable; avoid sporadic exercise.
d. Food intake may need to be increased before exercising. Take a snack.

I. Interventions:
1. Administer insulin as ordered; monitor for hypoglycemia.
2. Special diet; may count carbohydrates or low fat, high fiber
3. Do finger sticks to check blood glucose levels.
4. Meticulous skin and foot care
a. Wash the feet with mild soap and water and pat dry.
b. Apply lanolin to feet to prevent drying.
c. Cut toenails straight across.
d. Avoid constricting garments.
e. Wear clean, absorbent socks (cotton, white).
f. Wear properly fitting shoes.
g. Never go barefoot.
h. Inspect feet daily.
i. Prevent injury.
5. Provide emotional support.
6. Observe for chronic complications:
a. Atherosclerosis
b. Microangiopathy (eyes and kidneys)
c. Kidney disease (recurrent pyelonephritis and diabetic nephropathy)
d. Premature cataracts

e. Diabetic retinopathy

f. Peripheral neuropathy:

(1) Affects peripheral and autonomic nervous systems

(2) Causes diarrhea, constipation, neurogenic bladder, impotence, and decreased sweating

(3) Teach client to avoid application of very hot and very cold substances to extremeties because of potential damage from lack of sensation.

7. Nutrition therapy

a. Goals:

(1) Maintain a near-normal blood glucose level.

(2) Achieve optimal serum lipid levels.

(3) Provide adequate calories to maintain or attain a reasonable weight.

(4) Prevent and treat acute complications of insulin-treated diabetes.

(5) Improve overall health through optimal nutrition.

b. Protein intake should make up 10 to 20 percent of daily calorie intake.

c. Total fat intake varies: if lipids normal, 30% or less of calories should come from fat; if weight loss is desired or client has elevated lipid levels, fat intake should be reduced.

J. Ketoacidosis (DKA):

1. Acute complication of diabetes mellitus characterized by hyperglycemia and ketones in the body, often causing metabolic acidosis

2. Occurs in insulin-dependent diabetics

3. Precipitating factors: undiagnosed diabetes, noncompliance to treatment, infection, cardiovascular disorders, physical or emotional stress

4. Assessment findings:

a. Slow onset: hours to days

b. Polydipsia, polyphagia, polyuria

c. Nausea, vomiting, abdominal pain

d. Warm, dry, flushed

e. Dry mucus membranes; soft eyeballs

f. Kussmaul respirations or tachypnea, acetone breath

g. Changes in LOC

h. Hypotension, tachycardia

5. Diagnostic tests

a. Serum glucose and ketones are elevated.

b. BUN, creatinine, Hct elevated (dehydration)

c. Serum sodium decreased; potassium may be normal or elevated at first; will decrease after insulin administration

d. ABGs show metabolic acidosis with compensatory respiratory alkalosis.

6. Interventions:

a. Maintain a patent airway.

b. IV fluids:

(1) Normal saline, then hypotonic NaCl

(2) When blood sugar drops to 250 mg/dL, may add 5% dextrose to IV

(3) Potassium added when urine output is adequate

(4) Observe for fluid overload, hypo- and hyperkalemia.

c. Insulin as ordered

d. Monitor blood sugar levels frequently.

e. Monitor urine for sugar and acetone frequently.

f. Hourly outputs

g. Vital signs

h. Discuss reasons for ketosis and teach the client.

K. Insulin Reaction/Hypoglycemia:

1. Abnormally low blood sugar (below 50 mg/dL)

2. Usually caused by too much insulin, too little food, or nutritional and fluid imbalances from nausea and vomiting or excessive exercise

3. Rapid onset—minutes to hours

4. Assessment findings

a. Headache, dizziness, difficulty with problem solving

b. Restlessness, hunger, visual disturbances

c. Slurred speech

d. Alterations in gait

e. Decreasing LOC

f. Cold, clammy, pale skin

g. Diaphoresis

5. Diagnostic test—serum glucose below 50–60 mg/dl

6. Interventions:

a. Administer oral sugar in the form of candy or sweetened orange juice if the client is alert.

b. If client unconscious, 1 mg glucagon IM, IV, or SC as ordered or 20–50 cc 50% dextrose may be given IV push

c. Explore with client the reasons for hypoglycemia and provide additional teaching as needed.

L. Hyperglycemic Hyperosmolar Nonketotic Coma (HHNK):

1. Occurs in non-insulin dependent diabetics or nondiabetic persons

2. Precipitating factors: undiagnosed diabetes, infections or other stress, medications (Dilantin, thiazide diuretics), dialysis, hyperalimentation, major burns, pancreatic disease

3. Assessment—similar to ketoacidosis but without Kussmaul respirations and acetone breath

4. Diagnostic tests:
   a. Very high blood glucose
   b. BUN, creatinine, Hct Elevated (dehydration)
   c. Urine positive for glucose
5. Nursing care similar to client in DKA, not including measures to treat ketosis and metabolic acidosis

Sample Questions

1. What should be included in the nursing care plan for a client with diabetes insipidus?
   1. Blood pressure every hour
   2. Strict intake and output
   3. Urine for ketone bodies
   4. Glucose monitoring qid
2. What must the nurse do when preparing a client for a CT scan?
   1. Administer a laxative prep.
   2. Encourage fluids.
   3. Explain the procedure.
   4. Administer a radioisotope.
3. Antibiotics are ordered for a client who has had a transphenoidal hypophysectomy. He asks why he is receiving an antibiotic when he does not have an infection. The nurse's response is based on the knowledge that:
   1. Antibiotics will help to prevent respiratory complications following surgery.
   2. Meningitis is a complication following transphenoidal hypophysectomy.
   3. Fluid retention can cause dangerously high cerebral spinal fluid pressure.
   4. Hormone replacement is essential after hypophysectomy.
4. Twelve hours after a transphenoidal hypophysectomy, the client keeps clearing his throat and complains of a drip in his mouth. In order to accurately assess this, the nurse should test the fluid for:
   1. Sugar
   2. Protein
   3. Bacteria
   4. Blood
5. The client is ready for discharge following an adrenalectomy. Which statement that the client makes indicates the *best* understanding of the client's condition?
   1. "I will continue on a low-sodium, low-potassium diet."
   2. "My husband has arranged for a marriage counselor because of our fights."
   3. "I will stay out of the sun so I will not turn splotchy brown."
   4. "I will take all of those pills every day."
6. What is the nursing priority when administering care to a client with severe hyperthyroidism?
   1. Assess for recent emotional trauma.
   2. Provide a calm, non-stimulating environment.
   3. Provide diversionary activity.
   4. Encourage range-of-motion exercises.
7. Which problem is most likely to develop if hyperthyroidism remains untreated?
   1. Pulmonary embolism
   2. Respiratory acidosis
   3. Cerebral vascular accident
   4. Heart failure
8. Which nursing care measure is essential in a client with exophthalmos?
   1. Administer artificial tears.
   2. Encourage the client to wear her glasses.
   3. Promote bed rest.
   4. Monitor her pulse rate every four hours.
9. A client who has just had a thyroidectomy returns to the unit in stable condition. What equipment is it essential for the nurse to have at the bedside?
   1. Tracheostomy set
   2. Thoracotomy tray
   3. Dressing set
   4. Ice collar
10. What is the best way to assess for hemorrhage in a client who has had a thyroidectomy?
    1. Check the pulse and blood pressure hourly.
    2. Roll the client to the side and check for evidence of bleeding.
    3. Ask the client if he/she feels blood trickling down the back of the throat.
    4. Place a hand under the client's neck and shoulders to feel bed linens.
11. Which finding would be the greatest cause for concern to the nurse during the early post-operative period following a thyroidectomy?
    1. Temperature of 100°F
    2. A sore throat
    3. Carpal spasm when the blood pressure is taken
    4. Complaints of pain in the area of the surgical incision
12. An adult is admitted to the hospital with a diagnosis of hypothyroidism. Which findings would the nurse most likely elicit during the nursing assessment?
    1. Elevated blood pressure and temperature
    2. Tachycardia and weight gain
    3. Hypothermia and constipation
    4. Moist skin and coarse hair
13. Which diet would most likely be ordered for the client with hypothyroidism?
    1. High protein, high calorie
    2. Restricted fluids, low protein
    3. High roughage, low calorie
    4. High carbohydrate, low roughage
14. An adult with myxedema is started on thyroid replacement therapy and is discharged. The client returns to the doctor's office one week later. Which statement that the client makes is most indicative of an adverse reaction to the medication?

1. "My chest hurt when I was sweeping the floor this morning."
2. "I had severe cramps last night."
3. "I am losing weight."
4. "My pulse rate has been more rapid lately."

15. The nurse's next door neighbor calls. He says he cannot awaken his 21-year-old wife. The nurse notes that the client is unconscious and is having deep respirations. Her breath has a fruity smell to it. The husband says that his wife has been eating and drinking a lot recently and that last night she vomited before lying down. What is the most appropriate action for the nurse to take?
    1. Start cardiopulmonary resuscitation.
    2. Get her to a hospital immediately.
    3. Try to rouse her by giving her coffee.
    4. Give her sweetened orange juice.

16. The client is diagnosed as having insulin-dependent diabetes mellitus (IDDM). She received regular insulin at 7:30 a.m. When is she most apt to develop a hypoglycemic reaction?
    1. Mid-morning
    2. Mid-afternoon
    3. Early evening
    4. During the night

17. The nurse is teaching a client to administer insulin. The instructions should include teaching the client to
    1. Inject the needle at a 90-degree angle into the muscle.
    2. Vigorously massage the area after injecting the insulin.
    3. Rotate injection sites.
    4. Keep the open bottle of insulin in the refrigerator.

18. An adolescent with IDDM is learning about a diabetic diet. He asks the nurse if he will ever be able to go out to eat with his friends again.
    1. "You can go out with them, but you should take your own snack with you."
    2. "Yes. You will learn what foods are allowed so you can eat with your friends."
    3. "When you get food out in a restaurant, be sure to order diet soft drinks."
    4. "Eating out will not be possible on a diabetic diet. Why don't you plan to invite your friends to your house?"

19. At 10 a.m., a client with IDDM becomes very irritable and starts to yell at the nurse. Which initial nursing assessment should take priority?
    1. Blood pressure and pulse
    2. Color and temperature of skin
    3. Reflexes and muscle tone
    4. Serum electrolytes and glucose

20. An elderly woman has been recently diagnosed as having non-insulin-dependent diabetes mellitus (NIDDM). Which of the following complaints she has is most likely to be related to the diagnosis of diabetes mellitus?
    1. Pruritus vulvae

2. Cough
3. Eructation
4. Singultus

21. A client has a transphenoidal hypophysectomy to remove a pituitary tumor. When the client returns to the nursing unit following surgery, the head of the bed is elevated 30°. What is the primary purpose for placing the client in this position?
    1. To promote respiratory effort
    2. To reduce pressure on the sella turcica
    3. To prevent acidosis
    4. To promote oxygenation

22. The nurse is discussing discharge plans with a client who had a transphenoidal hypophysectomy. Which statement made by the client indicates a need for more teaching?
    1. "I won't brush my teeth until the doctor removes the stitches."
    2. "I will wear loafers instead of tie shoes."
    3. "Where can I get a Medic Alert bracelet?"
    4. "I will take all these new medicines until I feel better."

23. A woman with a tumor of the adrenal cortex says to the nurse, "Will I always look this ugly? I hate having a beard." What is the best response for the nurse to make?
    1. "After surgery you will not develop any more symptoms, but the changes you now have will linger."
    2. "That varies from person to person. You should ask your physician."
    3. "After surgery, your appearance should gradually return to normal."
    4. "Electrolysis and plastic surgery should make your appearance normal."

24. The client develops hypoparathyroidism after a total thyroidectomy. What treatment should the nurse anticipate?
    1. Emergency tracheostomy
    2. Administration of calcium
    3. Oxygen administration
    4. Administration of potassium

25. A woman with newly diagnosed IDDM says she wants to have children. She asks if she will be able to have children and if they will be normal. What is the best answer for the nurse to give?
    1. "Women with diabetes should not get pregnant because it is very difficult to control diabetes during pregnancy."
    2. "Babies born to diabetic mothers are very apt to have severe and non-correctable birth defects."
    3. "You should be able to safely have a baby if you go to your doctor regularly during pregnancy."
    4. "You should consult carefully with a geneticist before getting pregnant to determine how to prevent your baby from developing diabetes."

26. A client is admitted to the hospital with recently diagnosed diabetes mellitus and is to have fasting blood work drawn this morning. At 7:00 a.m., the lab has not arrived to draw the blood. The client's dose of regular insulin is scheduled for 7:30 a.m. What is the best action for the nurse to take?
    1. Give the insulin as ordered.
    2. Withhold the insulin until the lab comes and the client will be eating within 15–30 minutes.
    3. Withhold the insulin until the blood has been drawn and the client has eaten.
    4. Do not administer insulin until the blood work has been drawn and the results have been called back to the unit.

27. An adolescent with newly diagnosed IDDM asks the nurse if he can continue to play football. What is the best answer for the nurse to give?
    1. "Now that you have diabetes, you should not play football because you may get a cut that will not heal."
    2. "If you work with your physician to regulate the insulin dosage and your diet, you should be able to play football."
    3. "It would be better for you to work as equipment manager so you will not be under as much stress."
    4. "You can probably continue to play football if you can regulate it so that you have the same amount of exercise each day."

28. The client is a 62-year-old woman who is 30 pounds overweight. She comes to the doctor's office complaining of headaches, frequent hunger, excessive thirst, and urination. The presenting complaints suggest that the nurse should assess for other signs of which condition?
    1. Hypothyroidism
    2. Acute pyelonephritis
    3. Addison's disease
    4. Diabetes mellitus

29. An elderly client with NIDDM develops an ingrown toenail. What is the best action for the nurse?
    1. Put cotton under the nail and clip the nail straight across.
    2. Elevate the foot immediately.
    3. Apply warm, moist soaks.
    4. Notify the physician.

30. A woman with hypothyroidism asks the nurse why the doctor told her she cannot have a sedative. The nurse's response is based on which of the following facts?
    1. Sedatives potentiate thyroid replacement medication.
    2. Clients with hypothyroidism have increased susceptibility to all sedative drugs.
    3. Sedatives will have a paradoxical affect on clients with hypothyroidism.
    4. Sedatives would cause fluid retention and hypernatremia.

Answers and Rationales

1. (2) Diabetes insipidus is excessive urine output due to decreased amounts of antidiuretic hormone. Because of the excessive urine output, it is necessary to monitor intake and output.

2. (3) Explanation is all that is necessary. The client is not given a radioisotope. Fluids are not pushed prior to the procedure. The client frequently is given an iodine dye, so the nurse should ask about allergies to shellfish.

3. (2) A transphenoidal approach goes through the roof of the mouth, which has many organisms. Meningitis can occur. Answer 1 is a true statement but not the primary reason in this case. Antibiotics do not lower spinal fluid pressure. Answer 4 is a true statement, but antibiotics are not hormones.

4. (1) Dripping in the back of the throat after a transphenoidal hypophysectomy may be cerebrospinal fluid (CSF). CSF contains glucose. Saliva and mucus do not.

5. (4) The client must take steroid replacements every day for the rest of his/her life. Answer 1 is not an appropriate diet. The fights should decrease as mood swings decrease after surgery.

6. (2) A calm environment is important to reduce activity. Hyperthyroidism makes a person hyperactive and easily distractible. There is no reason to assess for emotional trauma. The hyperthyroid client is usually hyperactive, so there would be no need for range of motion exercises.

7. (4) Hyperthyroidism causes tachycardia, which can be severe enough to cause heart failure. Pulse rates can be 100 to 150/minute.

8. (1) Exophthalmos (protrusion of the eyes) may be so severe that the eyelids cannot close. Artificial tears will keep the eyes moist so that abrasions do not occur.

9. (1) Swelling in the operative site could cause airway obstruction. The nurse should have a tracheostomy set and oxygen at the bedside for 48 hours after thyroidectomy. A thoracotomy tray is not indicated. This client is not likely to need intervention in the thoracic cavity. A dressing set is unlikely to be needed. An ice collar might be indicated, but is not critical to have at the bedside.

10. (4) Following a thyroidectomy, the client is in semi-Fowler's position so drainage would go to the back of the neck. Because of the neck incision, the client should not be rolled to the side. The bleeding is unlikely to be inside the throat. Blood trickling down the throat might be seen in a client who has had a tonsillectomy.

11. (3) Carpal spasm is a sign of tetany and is known as Chovstek's sign. Tetany may occur if the parathyroids have been inadvertently removed. The parathyroids regulate calcium phosphorus balance. Hypocalcemia causes tetany. Most clients who have been intubated during surgery have a sore throat. Pain in the incision area is normal in the immediate post-operative period.

12. (3) Hypothyroidism causes decreased metabolic rate, which will cause lowered body temperature and pulse and decreased digestion of food. The skin is dry and the hair thins.

13. (3) Hypothyroidism causes constipation and obesity. A diet high in roughage and low in calories is appropriate. The client should not be given a high-calorie diet. There is no need for fluid restriction or alteration in protein.

14. (1) Chest pain on exertion suggests angina. In addition to a slow heart rate, the client with hypothyroidism frequently has atherosclerosis. Thyroxin will increase the heart rate, and the heart will require more oxygen. Angina is a likely and serious complication that can occur. She will also probably lose weight and have an increased pulse. These are expected when taking thyroxin. Cramps are not likely to be related to taking thyroxin.

15. (2) Her symptoms suggest ketoacidosis. She must receive medical treatment at once. Coffee will not help her. She is unresponsive. Sweetened orange juice is not indicated for ketoacidosis. It would be appropriate for hypoglycemia. There is no indication for CPR.

16. (1) Hypoglycemic reactions occur at peak action time. Peak action time for regular insulin is two to four hours after injection.

17. (3) Injection sites should be rotated to prevent tissue damage. Insulin is injected at a 90-degree angle into the deep subcutaneous tissue, not the muscle. Insulin does not need to be refrigerated. The open vial should be kept in the box to protect it from light. Insulin should not be kept at temperature extremes, such as the glove compartment of the car on a hot day.

18. (2) Eating out with friends is very important to an adolescent. Snacks will be allowed on his diet. He should be taught how to use the exchange lists in managing his diet.

19. (2) The nurse should immediately assess the skin. Behavior change and irritability suggest hypoglycemia. If the client is hypoglycemic, the client will have pale, cold, clammy skin, and needs treatment (ingestion of a rapid acting carbohydrate) at once.

20. (1) Pruritus vulvae (itching of the vulva) frequently accompanies diabetes. Monilial infections are common due to the change in pH. Eructation is belching or burping, and singultus is hiccups. Neither of these is particularly related to diabetes.

21. (2) Slight head elevation will reduce pressure on the sella turcica, where the pituitary gland is located, and edema formation in the area. This position may help promote respiratory effort. However, that is not the primary reason in this client. This position does not prevent acidosis or promote oxygenation.

22. (4) Because the pituitary or master gland was removed, the client will need to take life-long medications, not just until the client feels better. All of the other actions are appropriate. The client should not bend over to tie shoes, because this increases intracranial pressure. Answer 1 is correct. Remember, the client had a transphenoidal procedure in which the incision is in the mouth above the gum line. The client must take medications daily for the rest of his/her life so a Medic Alert bracelet is appropriate.

23. (3) A gradual return to normal will occur after adrenalectomy, when there are no longer abnormal amounts of steroids being produced.

24. (2) Hypoparathyroidism causes a decrease in calcium, which is manifested by tetany.

25. (3) Most diabetic women can safely have babies if they receive good medical supervision during pregnancy. There is a slightly higher incidence of fetal loss and malformations in babies of diabetic mothers, but not enough to preclude the chance of a normal baby. There is no way to prevent the child from later developing diabetes. Diabetes is an inherited condition.

26. (2) Regular insulin onsets within 30 minutes. It should not be given until he can eat within 15–30 minutes so that he will not develop hypoglycemia.

27. (2) Diabetes is not a contraindication for sports. Changes in activity level will alter the utilization of glucose, so he will need to work closely with his physician to regulate exercise, insulin, and diet control.

28. (4) The symptoms are the cardinal symptoms of diabetes mellitus: polydipsia, polyphagia, and polyuria. The client with hypothyroidism would have fatigue, weight gain, and complain of being cold all the time. The person with acute pyelonephritis would probably complain of frequent urination and flank pain and might have a fever. The person with Addison's disease would have polyuria, low blood sugar, and might go into hypovolemic shock.

29. (4) An ingrown toenail may cause infection, which can be very serious for the diabetic client. The physician should be notified. It is not appropriate for the practical nurse to initiate treatment.

30. (2) In hypothyroidism, the metabolic rate is decreased. This causes an increased susceptibility to sedative drugs.

Chapter 14

The Integumentary System

ANATOMY AND PHYSIOLOGY

The integumentary system consists of the skin, hair, nails, and various glands. The skin is the largest organ of the body. It forms a barrier between the internal organs and the external environment and participates in many vital functions of the body.

SKIN

A. Functions:
 1. Protection: serves as a barrier to chemicals and microorganisms and to loss of water and electrolytes
 2. Regulates temperature through evaporation and radiant cooling
 3. Serves as sensory perception organ for touch, temperature, pressure, and pain
 4. Plays a role in metabolism by excreting water and sodium and producing vitamins
B. Layers of the Skin (see Figure 14.1)
 1. Epidermis:
     a. The avascular, outermost layer of the skin
     b. Keratinocytes produce keratin, which is responsible for the formation of hair and nails.
     c. Melanocytes produce melanin, the pigment that gives color to the skin and hair.
 2. Dermis:
     a. The layer below the epidermis
     b. Made up of blood and lymph vessels, nerve fibers, and the accessory organs of the skin
     c. Elasticity of skin results from the presence of collagen, elastin, and reticular fibers in the dermis.
 3. Subcutaneous Layer:
     a. A connective tissue layer that stores fat
     b. Important in temperature regulation

HAIR

A. Covers most of the body except the palms of the hands, the soles of the feet, lips, nipples, and parts of the external genitalia
B. Hair functions as protection from external elements.

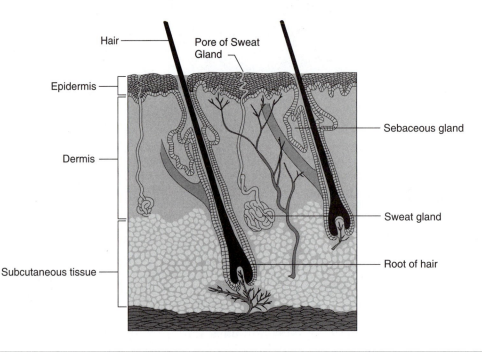

Figure 14.1 Layers of the Skin

C. Hair growth is controlled by hormones and by blood supply.
D. Loss of body hair is called alopecia.

NAILS

A. Hard, transparent plate of keratin on the dorsal surface of the fingers and toes
B. Grows from its root, which lies under a thin fold of skin called the cuticle
C. Nail growth is continuous throughout life (0.1 mm/day); fingernails grow faster than toenails
D. Systemic illness may be reflected by changes in nails
   1. Clubbing:
     a. Enlargement of fingers and toes
     b. Nail becomes convex
     c. Caused by chronic hypoxia (chronic pulmonary or cardiovascular disease)

   2. Beau's line:
     a. Transverse groove
     b. Caused by temporary stop in nail growth due to local trauma or severe illness

GLANDS

A. Eccrine sweat glands:
   1. Located all over the body
   2. Help with heat regulation
B. Apocrine sweat glands:
   1. Odiferous glands
   2. Found primarily in axillary, nipple, anal, and pubic areas
   3. Bacterial decomposition of excretions causes body odor.
C. Sebaceous glands:
   1. Oil glands that produce sebum
   2. Located all over the body except for palms of hands and soles of feet

Laboratory and Diagnostic Studies

A. Serum electrolytes including calcium, chloride, sodium, magnesium, and potassium
B. Hematologic studies: Hgb, Hct, RBC, WBC
C. Biopsy:
   1. Removal of a small piece of skin for examination

   2. Instruct the client to keep the area dry until healing occurs.
D. Skin testing:
   1. Administration of allergens or antigens on the surface of the dermis or into the dermis to determine hypersensitivity

2. Patch test:
   a. Small samples of test material are applied to a disc and the disc is taped to the upper back; may be 20 or 30 discs.
   b. Instruct client to keep the test area dry while the tape is in place.
   c. Return in 48–72 hrs as directed to have discs removed and the test site examined and evaluated
3. Skin scrapings: tissue samples scraped from suspected fungal lesions

LESIONS OF THE SKIN

A. Surface lesions:
   1. Contusion: an injury that does not break the skin and is characterized by swelling, discoloration, and pain
   2. Papule: a small, solid, raised skin lesion that is less than 0.5 cm in diameter
   3. Plaque: a solid, raised lesion that is greater than 0.5 cm in diameter
   4. Macule: a discolored, flat skin lesion such as a freckle or flat mole that is less than 1 cm in diameter
   5. Patch: a localized change in skin color greater than 1 cm in diameter
   6. Scale: flaking or a dry patch made up of an excess of dead epidermal cells
   7. Crust: a collection of dried serum and cellular debris
   8. Wheal: a smooth, slightly elevated, swollen area that is redder or paler than the surrounding skin that is usually accompanied by itching; an insect bite or a reaction to an allergy skin test
   9. Ecchymosis: purplish patch caused by bleeding into the skin; a bruise
   10. Petechiae: a small pinpoint hemorrhage
   11. Verucae: skin lesions caused by the human papilloma virus; warts
B. Fluid-filled lesions:
   1. Cyst: a closed sack or pouch containing fluid or semisolid material
   2. Pustule: a small, circumscribed elevation of the skin containing pus
   3. Vesicle: a circumscribed elevation of skin containing fluid that is less than 0.5 cm in diameter; a blister
   4. Bulla: a large vesicle or blister that is more than 0.5 cm in diameter
   5. Abscess: a localized collection of pus within a circumscribed area and associated with tissue destruction
C. Lesions through the skin:
   1. Laceration: a torn or jagged wound or an accidental cut wound
   2. Ulcer: an open sore or erosion of the skin or mucous membrane resulting in tissue loss; usually with inflammation
   3. Fissure: a groove or crack-like sore
   4. Fistula: an abnormal passage from an internal organ to the body surface or between two internal organs

CONTACT DERMATITIS

A. A skin rash caused by direct contact between the skin and a substance to which the person is allergic or sensitive, such as poison ivy, poison oak, deodorants, cleaning agents, or latex
B. Assessment findings:
   1. Itching, swelling, blistering, oozing, and scaling
   2. History of exposure to an allergen
   3. Skin testing can determine sensitivity to the allergen.
C. Nursing diagnoses (see Table 14.1)
D. Interventions:
   1. Burrow's solution dressings for 20 minutes four times a day to help clear oozing lesions
   2. Help provide relief from itching:
      a. Avoid soaps and detergents.
      b. Use tepid water for bathing followed by an application of emollient lotion.

Table 14.1 Nursing Diagnoses Related to Skin Disorders

- Impaired skin integrity related to lesions and inflammatory response
- Impaired comfort; pruritus related to dermal eruptions
- Risk for social isolation related to fear of embarrassment and negative reactions of others
- Risk for disturbed self-concept related to appearance and response of others
- Risk for ineffective management of therapeutic regimen related to insufficient knowledge of condition, topical agents, and contraindications
- Risk for infection related to broken skin and tissue trauma

c. Provide cool, light, nonrestrictive clothing; avoid wool, nylon, and fur.
d. Keep nails short to avoid skin damage from scratching.
e. Apply cool, moist compresses to pruritic areas.
3. Topical steroids and antibiotics may be ordered.
4. Teach the client to allow crusts and scales to drop off skin naturally as healing occurs.
5. Teach the client to avoid identified irritants.

PSORIASIS

A. A chronic type of dermatitis that involves a turnover rate of the epidermal cells that is seven times the normal rate; often familial; not contagious.
B. Assessment findings:
  1. Mild pruritus
  2. Sharply circumscribed bright red macules, papules, or patches covered with silvery scales
  3. Seen mostly on scalp, elbows, and knees
  4. Thick yellow toenails
C. Nursing diagnoses (see Table 14.1)
D. Interventions:
  1. Topical corticosteroids; apply occlusive wraps over topical steroids
  2. Coal tar preparations; protect areas from direct sunlight for 24 hours
  3. Ultraviolet light
  4. Antimetabolites (methotrexate) to slow cell growth
  5. Provide emotional support and allow clients to discuss their feelings about lesions.
  6. Instruct client to cover affected areas with clothing if sensitive about appearance

SKIN CANCER

A. Types of skin cancers
  1. Basal cell:
    a. Most common
    b. Locally invasive; rarely metastasizes
    c. Often located on the face between the hairline and upper lip
    d. Easily treated with removal in physician's office
  2. Squamous cell:
    a. Grows more rapidly than basal cell
    b. Can metastasize
    c. Frequently seen on mucous membranes, lower lip, neck, and dorsum of hands
  3. Malignant melanoma:
    a. Least-frequent skin cancer but most serious

Table 14.2 Nursing Diagnoses Related to Skin Cancer
- Acute pain related to surgical excision and grafting
- Anxiety related to possible life-threatening condition (melanoma) and disfigurement
- Deficient knowledge about early signs of melanoma

    b. Capable of invasion and metastasis to other organs
B. Precancerous skin lesions:
  1. Leukoplakia: shiny white patches in the mouth and on the lip
  2. Nevi (moles):
    a. Some types can become malignant.
    b. Change in color to black, bleeding, and irritation may signal change to malignant
  3. Senile keratoses: brown, scale-like spots on older persons
C. Assessment findings:
  1. Most often seen in light-skinned Caucasians
  2. History of exposure to ultraviolet light; works outdoors, excessive use of tanning booths
  3. Skin lesions with irregular borders and multiple colors
  4. Biopsy reveals malignant cells
D. Nursing diagnoses (see Table 14.2)
E. Interventions:
  1. Surgical excision: type and depth varies with type of skin cancer
  2. Radiation therapy:
    a. Used for cancer of the eyelid, the tip of the nose, and areas in or near vital structures
    b. Used mostly in older people because radiation therapy itself may cause cancer 15 or 20 years later
  3. Teach client to limit contact with chemical irritants to reduce recurrence.
  4. Teach client to protect self against ultraviolet radiation from sun:
    a. Avoid exposing skin to sun
    b. Use a sun block containing para-amino benzoic acid (PABA)
  5. Teach client to report any lesions that change in size or appearance and any lesions that do not heal.

HERPES ZOSTER (SHINGLES)

A. Acute viral infection of the nervous system caused by the chicken pox virus (varicella)
B. Assessment findings:
  1. Pain that follows nerve root; does not cross midline of front or back
  2. Itching, burning along affected nerve root

3. Cluster of skin vesicles along affected nerve root, usually on trunk, thorax, or face
4. Seen often in persons who are immunocompromised

C. Nursing diagnoses (see Table 14.1)
D. Interventions:
   1. Antiviral agents such an acyclovir (Zovirax) or famciclovir (Famvir) reduce severity significantly when given early.
   2. Analgesics
   3. Corticosteroids
   4. Acetic acid compresses or white petrolatum to lesions
   5. Teach client that condition is contagious to anyone who has not had varicella (chicken pox) or who is immunocompromised.

HERPES SIMPLEX VIRUS, TYPE I

A. This common virus causes cold sores, fever blisters, canker sores, and herpetic whitlow.
B. Assessment findings:
   1. Cluster of vesicles that may ulcerate or crust
   2. Tingling, itching, burning
C. Nursing diagnoses (see Table 14.1)
D. Interventions:
   1. Antiviral agents such an acyclovir (Zovirax) or famciclovir (Famvir) reduce length and severity of outbreak; used when client has recurring episodes
   2. Keep lesions dry.
   3. Instruct client to avoid direct contact when lesions present because virus can be communicable

BURNS

A. Types of burns
   1. Thermal:
      a. Most common type of burn
      b. Caused by flames, scalding, and contact with hot metal and grease
   2. Smoke inhalation: occurs when smoke causes respiratory tissue damage
   3. Chemical: caused by tissue contact, ingestion, or inhalation of acids, alkalis, or vesicants
   4. Electrical:
      a. Occurs from direct damage to nerves and vessels when an electric current passes through the body
      b. Causes include contact with electric wires and lightning
B. Classification of burns (see Figure 14.2)
   1. Partial thickness
      a. Superficial (first degree):
         (1) Affects epidermis only

      (2) Examples: sunburn, hot liquid splash
      (3) Painful
      (4) Erythema, blanching on pressure, no vesicles
      (5) Will heal without grafting
   b. Deep (second degree):
      (1) Involves epidermis and dermis
      (2) Examples: flame burn, scalding
      (3) Very painful
      (4) Fluid-filled vesicles; red, shiny, wet after vesicles rupture
      (5) Can heal without grafting
   2. Full thickness (third and fourth degree)
      a. Involves epidermis, dermis, and subcutaneous layers
      b. Nerve endings and hair follicles damaged
      c. May involve muscle or bone (fourth degree)
      d. Examples: flame, chemicals, scalding, electric current
      e. Wound is dry, white, leathery, or hard; may have black appearance
      f. Will not heal without grafting
C. Assessment findings:
   1. Assess extent of burns using Rule of Nines (see Figure 14.3)
      a. Appropriate for adults only; for children, use the Lund and Browder method, which considers child's age in proportion to relative body part size
      b. Body is divided into 11 areas of 9%
      c. Head neck 9%; each arm 9%; anterior trunk 18%; posterior trunk 18%; each leg 18%; and genitalia 1%
   2. Findings according to depth of burn as discussed above
   3. Severity of burn:
      a. Major: partial thickness greater than 15%; full thickness greater than or equal to 10%
      b. Moderate; partial thickness 15%–25%; full thickness less than 10%
      c. Minor: partial thickness less than 15%; full thickness less than 2%
   4. Assess for airway and pulmonary involvement, especially if the burn involved chemicals, severe smoke, or took place in a small space such as a closet.
   5. Assess for concomitant injuries such as fractures and lacerations.
   6. Assess pre-existing physical and psychological status.
D. Nursing diagnoses (see Table 14.3)
E. Interventions:
   1. Emergent phase:
      a. Stop the burning process:
         (1) Thermal: stop, drop, and roll or smother flames with a blanket

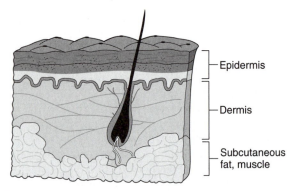

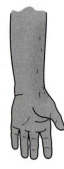

Epidermis

Dermis

Subcutaneous
fat, muscle

Skin red, dry

First degree, superficial

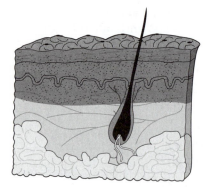

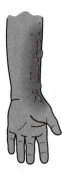

Blistered, skin moist, pink or red

Second degree,
partial thickness

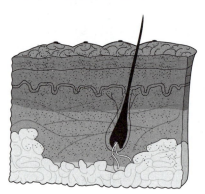

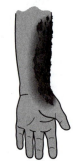

Charring, skin black, brown, red

Third degree, full thickness

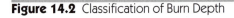

Figure 14.2 Classification of Burn Depth

    (2) Chemical: remove any clothing that contains the chemical and flush area with large amounts of water
    (3) Electrical: turn off the power
  b. For electrical burn, note position of victim, identify entry/exit routes, maintain an airway, and perform an ECG to detect dysrhythmias.
  c. For smoke inhalation, establish a patent airway.
  d. Wrap in dry, clean sheet or blanket to prevent further wound contamination and provide warmth.

  e. Assess how and when the burn occurred.
  f. Transport immediately.
  g. Insert an indwelling catheter.
  h. Assess tetanus immunization status; will need tetanus toxoid if previously immunized, immune globulin if no previous tetanus immunization
2. Shock phase (first 24–48 hours post-burn):
  a. Fluid shifts from plasma to interstitial space
  b. Hematocrit rises (fluid loss is plasma)
  c. Metabolic acidosis

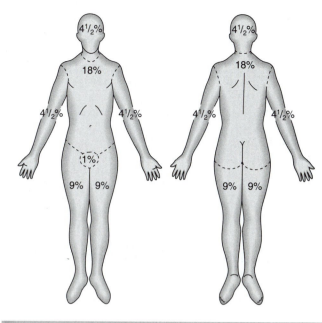

Figure 14.3 Rule of Nines

Table 14.3 Nursing Diagnoses Related to Burns

- Acute pain related to trauma to tissue and nerves, edema formation, and manipulation of impaired tissue
- Risk for deficient fluid volume related to loss of fluids through wounds (first 24–48 hours)
- Risk for fluid volume excess related to fluid shifts secondary to burns (48–72 hours post-burn)
- Risk for impaired respiratory function related to inadequate oxygen exchange secondary to smoke inhalation, edema of respiratory passages
- Risk for infection related to loss of protective layer secondary to thermal injury
- Impaired nutrition: less than body requirements related to increased caloric requirements secondary to thermal injury and inability to ingest sufficient quantities to meet increased requirements
- Impaired physical mobility related to acute pain secondary to thermal injury and treatments
- Fear related to painful procedures and possibility of death
- Post-trauma response related to life-threatening event
- Self-care deficit related to impaired range of motion ability secondary to pain and contractures
- Risk for social isolation related to infection control measures and separation from family and support systems
- Risk for disuse syndrome related to effects of pain and immobility
- Disturbed sleep pattern related to position restrictions, pain, and treatment interruptions
- Risk for disturbed perceptions related to excessive environmental stimuli, stress, imposed immobility, sleep deprivation, and protective isolation
- Grieving related to actual or perceived impact of injury on life (appearance, relationships, occupation)
- Anxiety related to pain secondary to thermal injury treatments and immobility
- Anxiety related to sudden injury, treatments, uncertainty of outcome, and pain

   d. Serum K⁺ rises (cell damage)
   e. Protein loss from plasma loss
   f. Monitor vital signs
   g. Monitor urine output hourly; maintain 50 to 100 ml/hr
   h. Give half of first day's fluid in first eight hours after burn
   i. Formulas for fluid replacement based on body surface area of client and amount of body surface area burned

3. Diuretic phase: post-shock phase starts 48–72 hours after burn
   a. Capillary permeability stabilizes and fluid shifts from interstitial spaces to plasma
   b. Observe for pulmonary edema and circulatory overload.
   c. Check vital signs; CVP rises.
   d. Hct decreases.
   e. Monitor output (increases).
   f. Check lab values; Potassium (K⁺) decreases.

4. Convalescent phase:
   a. Starts when diuretic phase completed and wound healing and coverage begin
   b. Dry, waxy-white appearance of full-thickness burn changing to dark brown; wet, shiny, and serous exudate in partial thickness burn
   c. Hyponatremia

5. Pain control:
   a. Medication: small frequent doses; may receive morphine sulfate IV
   b. Positioning to prevent pain and contractures
   c. Administer analgesics 30 minutes before wound care.
   d. Monitor vital signs following analgesic administration.

6. Nutritional needs:
   a. NPO until bowel sounds heard
   b. Nasogastric tube may be inserted to prevent stress (Curling's) ulcers.
   c. High calorie, high protein diet
   d. Tube feedings may be initiated.
   e. Sometimes TPN needed because client cannot ingest enough calories to meet nutritional needs
   f. Prevent stress ulcers by giving Maalox every two hours and/or cimetidine (Tagamet) as ordered.

7. Prevent wound infection:
   a. Provide asepsis (reverse isolation).
   b. Wound care (debridement, hydrotherapy)
   c. Antimicrobial therapy:
     (1) Silver nitrate 0.5% solution
       (a) Apply to moist dressings bid.
       (b) Discolors everything it touches
       (c) Poor penetration
       (d) Causes hypokalemia, hyponatremia, hypochloremia

(2) Sulfamylon:
  (a) Broad spectrum
  (b) Penetrates tissue well
  (c) Never use a dressing; apply with a sterile, gloved hand.
  (d) Medicate for pain prior to applying Sulfamylon.
  (e) Breakdown of drug causes acidosis; Kussmaul respirations
(3) Silver sulfadiazine:
  (a) Broad spectrum includes yeast
  (b) Can be washed off with water
(4) Gentamicin 0.1%:
  (a) Cream penetrates well.
  (b) Nephrotoxic; check creatinine levels
(5) Povidone-iodine (Betadine) solution:
  (a) Administer analgesics before administration.
  (b) Assess for metabolic acidosis.
  (c) Assess renal function studies.

8. Biologic dressings (skin grafts):
  a. Types
    (1) Allograft: from the same species; usually cadaver
    (2) Xenograft, heterograft: from an animal (pig or dog)
    (3) Human amniotic membrane
    (4) Autograft (self): only permanent graft
  b. Pre-operative nursing care:
    (1) Donor site: cleanse with antiseptic soap the night before and the morning of surgery as ordered
    (2) Recipient site: apply warm compresses and topical antibiotics as ordered
  c. Post-operative nursing care:
    (1) Donor site:
      (a) Keep area covered for 24–48 hours
      (b) Use a bed cradle to prevent pressure and provide air circulation.
      (c) Outer dressing may be removed 24–72 hours after surgery, maintain fine mesh gauze (innermost dressing) until it falls off spontaneously
      (d) Trim the loose edges of gauze because it loosens with healing.
      (e) Administer analgesics as ordered (donor site more painful than recipient site).
    (2) Recipient site:
      (a) Elevate when possible to reduce edema.
      (b) Protect from pressure by using a bed cradle.
      (c) Apply warm compresses as ordered.

  (d) Assess for hematoma and fluid accumulation under graft.
  (e) Monitor circulation distal to graft.
  (3) Provide emotional support.
9. Prevent contractures and deformities:
  a. ROM first post-burn day
  b. Position carefully to promote good alignment.
10. Provide client teaching and discharge planning concerning:
  a. Applying lubricating lotion to maintain moisture on surfaces of healed graft for at least 6–12 months
  b. Protecting grafted skin from direct sunlight for at least six months
  c. Protecting graft from physical injury
  d. Reporting changes in graft (fluid accumulation, pain, hematoma)
  e. Hair may not grow in graft site; pigmentation may not be normal; most grafts do not sweat.
  f. Sensation may not return in the graft site.
  g. Maintain sterility if changing wound dressings.
  h. Prevent injury to wound site by avoiding trauma and constrictive clothing over the site.
  i. Adhere to a prescribed diet.
  j. Report any signs of infection, such as foul-smelling drainage.
  k. Support sources in the community

Sample Questions

1. Burns of what part of the body have the highest mortality rate?
   1. Lower torso
   2. Upper part of the body
   3. Hands and feet
   4. Perineum
2. Which of the following persons with burns has the poorest prognosis?
   1. A 20-year-old with second- and third-degree burns over 60% of the body
   2. An 80-year-old with second- and third-degree burns over 50% of the body
   3. A 35- year-old with second- and third-degree burns over 60% of the body
   4. A 2-year-old with second- and third-degree burns over 30% of the body
3. Which of these clients should have his clothing removed immediately?
   1. A 32-year-old man who was burned while working on high tension wires
   2. A 14-year-old who suffered severe smoke inhalation during a fire at school
   3. A 78-year-old who was burned during a fire that started when the client fell asleep while smoking

4. A 19-year-old who spilled chemicals on himself in the chemistry lab at school

4. A 28-year-old man received severe burns of the chest, abdomen, back, legs, and hands when the house caught fire. In the emergency room, a nasogastric tube was inserted and the client was ordered NPO. What is the primary reason for maintaining NPO on this client?
   1. To prevent the deadly complication of aspiration
   2. To make the client more comfortable
   3. To help prevent paralytic ileus
   4. To help prevent excessive fluid loss

5. An indwelling catheter was inserted in a severely burned client for which reason?
   1. To prevent contamination of burned areas
   2. To measure hourly urine output
   3. To prevent urinary tract infection
   4. To detect internal injuries quickly

6. A severely burned man had his last tetanus shot when he started work at his job two years ago. What should the nurse expect to administer now?
   1. Tetanus toxoid booster
   2. Tetanus antitoxin
   3. Hyperimmune human tetanus globulin
   4. DPT booster

7. A severely burned client is to be admitted from the emergency department. What type of room should the nurse prepare for the client?
   1. A semi-private room with a non-infectious client
   2. A room with a post-operative client
   3. An isolation room
   4. A private room with a private bath

8. The nurse is planning care for a newly burned client. What is the priority nursing observation to be made during the first 48 hours after the burn?
   1. Hourly blood pressure
   2. Assessment of skin color and capillary refill
   3. Hourly urine measurement
   4. Frequent assessment for pain

9. Cimetidine (Tagamet) is ordered IV every six hours for a person with severe burns. What is the primary reason for administering Tagamet?
   1. To prevent infection
   2. To restore electrolyte balance
   3. To promote renal function
   4. To prevent Curling's ulcers

10. A client who was severely burned goes to the Hubbard tank daily. Tanking sessions are limited to a half hour for which reason?
    1. A longer period of time is too tiring.
    2. Eschar becomes difficult to remove with longer soaking.
    3. Prolonged soaking causes electrolyte dilution.
    4. The water becomes too cool and may cause chilling.

11. Silver nitrate dressings are applied to burns on an adult. What should be included in the nursing care plan?
    1. Change the dressings every two hours.
    2. Keep the dressings wet.
    3. Carefully monitor fluid intake.
    4. Observe for black discoloration.

12. Which assessment is essential when the client is having silver nitrate dressings applied?
    1. BUN
    2. Blood gases
    3. CBC
    4. Serum electrolytes

13. A young man has extensive burns on the front and back of the chest. His treatment includes the use of sulfamylon to the burned areas. What is the best method for applying topical antimicrobials?
    1. With the sterile, gloved hand
    2. With a sterile applicator
    3. With sterile 4 × 4's
    4. By aerosol spray

14. An electrician was wearing a glove that had a hole in it when he grabbed a "hot" wire. His coworkers came to him immediately and called the rescue squad. When the industrial nurse reached him, the electric current had been shut off. What action should the nurse take initially?
    1. Dress the entrance and exit wounds.
    2. Check respirations and pulse rate.
    3. Remove clothing from the burned area.
    4. Roll him in a blanket.

15. A client who has just been diagnosed with psoriasis asks the nurse what should be done to prevent family members from getting the condition. What should the nurse include when responding to this question?
    1. Showering daily with antiseptic soap should be sufficient.
    2. Wearing clothing over the affected part and washing clothes separately from the rest of the family is all that is necessary.
    3. Psoriasis is not contagious, so no special precautions are necessary.
    4. Psoriasis is transmitted primarily by direct contact with the skin.

16. The nurse is teaching a class on the prevention of cancer. Which information should be included regarding how to reduce the risk of skin cancer?
    1. Avoid prolonged exposure to the sun.
    2. Shower immediately after being out-of-doors.
    3. Avoid strong perfumes, hand creams, and body lotions.
    4. After being in the woods or in tall grass, check for ticks.

17. The client mentions all of the following to the nurse. Which should the client be encouraged to report to the physician immediately?

1. A small mole on the right thigh that has looked the same ever since the client can remember
2. A pigmented area that is pink-red in color and has been present since birth
3. Three small warts on the right hand that have been present for some time
4. A black and purple mole that is growing larger and has a funny shape

18. The nurse is caring for an adult who has herpes zoster. What medication is most likely to be administered to this client?
   1. Penicillin
   2. Acyclovir
   3. Tetracycline
   4. Benadryl

19. The nurse is caring for a person who has severe poison ivy. Soaks with Burrow's solution are ordered. What is the primary reason for using Burrow's solution soaks?
   1. To disinfect the wound
   2. To prevent pain from the lesions
   3. To stop the pruritus associated with the condition
   4. To help dry the oozing lesions

20. A woman who has herpes simplex I around the mouth and nose asks the nurse if she can give the sores to her husband. What should the nurse include when answering this client?
   1. Herpes simplex I is a fever blister and is not contagious.
   2. She should not kiss her husband or anyone else because it can be transmitted to susceptible persons.
   3. Fever blisters are seen only in persons who have fevers.
   4. The virus is transmitted through coughing and sneezing.

Answers and Rationales

1. (2) Persons with burns of the upper part of the body frequently have respiratory involvement. Airway problems increase the mortality rate.
2. (2) The very old and the very young are at the highest risk and have the highest mortality rate. The very old are half-dehydrated before the burn occurred and have greater difficulty with the fluid shifts. The very young have a greater percent of their body weight that is supposed to be water. They have more difficulty with the fluid shifts that occur following a burn.
3. (4) Clothing should be removed from persons with chemical burns so that they will not be further contaminated. A flame burn should be smothered, and if necessary soak the area with water but do not remove the clothing until the person is in the emergency room. A person who suffered from smoke inhalation does not have an immediate need to remove clothing. A person who received an electrical burn does not have an immediate need to have his clothes removed.
4. (3) Burn victims are very prone to paralytic ileus. The client will remain NPO until bowel sounds have returned.
5. (2) Measurement of urine output is a high priority. Fluid replacement is based on output. The goal is to prevent the client from going into shock by maintaining a urine output of 50–100 ml/hr.
6. (1) Tetanus toxoid is given when the client has had prior tetanus inoculations. Hyperimmune tetanus globulin is given when the person has not had prior tetanus immunization. DTP is not given past the age of six years. Tetanus antitoxin is given when a person has not been immunized and considerable time has elapsed from the time of the injury. Tetanus antitoxin helps to fight a tetanus infection that is developing. Tetanus toxoid and immune globulin help to prevent tetanus infection from developing.
7. (3) Burn victims should be placed in isolation because they are very susceptible to infection.
8. (3) Fluid replacement is based on hourly measurement of urine output. The other observations are important and should be done, but they are not the highest priority.
9. (4) Curling's (stress) ulcers occur frequently in burn victims. Tagamet is a histamine blocker that reduces gastric acid and helps to prevent the development of ulcers.
10. (3) The water in the Hubbard tank is hypotonic, and sodium loss occurs through the open wounds. The bath may be painful and fatiguing for the patient. The primary reason is the physiologic problem of sodium loss.
11. (2) Silver nitrate dressings must always be kept wet or the silver nitrate is not effective. Silver nitrate does cause black discoloration, but this is incidental and not a major nursing consideration.
12. (4) Silver nitrate can cause depletion of potassium, sodium, and chloride; therefore, serum electrolytes are essential.
13. (1) The sterile, gloved hand is the preferred way to apply topical antimicrobials.
14. (2) Electric burns cause cardiac arrhythmias. Checking respiration and the pulse rate is highest priority. There is no need to remove clothing or roll a victim of an electric burn in a blanket because there are no flames. Dressing wounds is of lesser priority than assessing cardiac and respiratory functioning.
15. (3) Psoriasis is not contagious.
16. (1) Prolonged exposure to ultraviolet rays is the major risk factor for skin cancer. Showering immediately after being outdoors will not reduce the risk of skin cancer. Skin cancer is not caused by perfumes, hand creams, or body lotions. Checking for ticks after being outdoors

is helpful in preventing Rocky Mountain Spotted Fever and Lyme Disease but will not prevent skin cancer.

17. (4) A mole that changes shape and has multiple colors and irregular borders is suggestive of malignant melanoma. This should be reported immediately. A mole that has not changed in appearance is of no particular concern. The pigmented area that has been present since birth sounds like a nevus or a birthmark and is not of particular concern. The client may want to report the three small warts and have them removed for cosmetic reasons. They are not an immediate threat to her health and do not need to be reported immediately.

18. (2) Acyclovir, an antiviral agent, is most likely to be given to the person who has herpes zoster, a infection with the chicken pox virus that affects the nerves. Penicillin and tetracycline are given for bacterial infections. Benadryl is an antihistamine and will help with itching. The person who has herpes zoster or shingles is likely to need pain medication, not antihistamines.

19. (4) Burrow's solution is used to help dry up oozing lesions such as poison ivy. It does not disinfect, prevent pain, or stop itching.

20. (2) Herpes simplex I can be transmitted through direct contact if the other person has any breaks in the skin or mucous membrane. She should not kiss anyone until after the lesions have disappeared. While blisters do sometimes occur when a person has a fever, a fever is not necessary for a herpes simplex infection. Herpes simplex virus is transmitted by direct contact, not coughing and sneezing.

Chapter 15

The Female Reproductive System, Maternity, and Newborns

ANATOMY AND PHYSIOLOGY OF THE FEMALE REPRODUCTIVE SYSTEM

ANATOMY

External Structures (See Figure 15.1):

A. Mons veneris: the rounded, fleshy prominence over the symphysis pubis; site of pubic hair
B. Labia majora: lengthwise folds of skin extending from the mons to the perineum that protect the labia minora, the urinary meatus, and the vaginal introitus
C. Labia minora: thinner, lengthwise, hairless folds of skin, extending from the clitoris to the fourchette
   1. Labia minora have a rich nerve supply and are very sensitive.

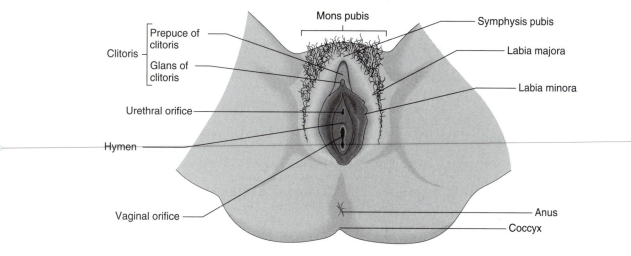

Figure 15.1 External structures of the female reproductive system.

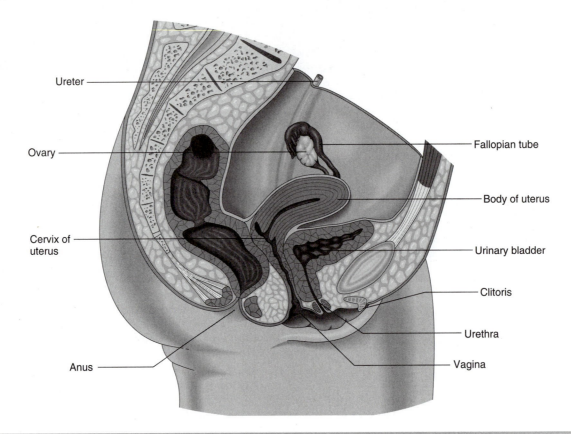

Ureter

Ovary

Cervix of
uterus

Anus

Fallopian tube

Body of uterus

Urinary bladder

Clitoris

Urethra

Vagina

Figure 15.2 Internal structures of the female reproductive system.

2. Glands in the labia minora lubricate the vulva (external genital organs in the female).
D. Clitoris: small, erectile organ located beneath the pubic arch containing many nerve endings and very sensitive to touch; source of female sexual pleasure; secretes a fatty substance called smegma
E. Vestibule: space between the labia minora into which the urethra and vagina open; also contains lubricating glands
   1. Urethra: tubular passage from which urine is discharged from the body; located between the clitoris and the vagina
   2. Skene's glands (also called paraurethral glands): secrete a small amount of mucus; susceptible to infections
   3. Bartholin's glands: small glands located on either side of the vaginal orifice; secrete clear mucus during sexual arousal; susceptible to infection, cysts, and abscesses
F. Fourchette: posterior junction of the labia minora
G. Perineum: skin-covered opening between the vaginal opening and the anus
   1. Paired muscle groups underlie the perineum and form a supportive "sling" for the pelvic organs.
   2. Distends greatly during the birth process

Internal Structures (See Figure 15.2):

A. Uterus: hollow, pear-shaped muscular organ in the pelvic cavity in which the fertilized ovum becomes embedded and in which the developing embryo and fetus is nourished; comprised of fundus, corpus, isthmus, and cervix. The cervix has internal and external os, separated by the cervical canal. The wall of the uterus has layers.
   1. Endometrium: inner, highly vascular layer shed during menstruation and after delivery
   2. Myometrium: muscular layer comprised of smooth muscle fibers running in three directions; expels fetus during birth process, then contracts around blood vessels to prevent hemorrhage
   3. Perimetrium: membranous outer layer
B. Ovaries: oval, almond-sized organs on either side of the uterus that produce ova and hormones
C. Fallopian tubes: tubes that extend from the ovaries to the uterus that serve as the passageway for the ova

The Pelvis

The bony passage through which the baby passes during birth; composed of sacrum, coccyx, and the ilium, pubis, and ischium; relationship between size and shape of pelvis and baby affects labor and delivery

A. Pelvic measurements:
 1. True conjugate: from the upper margin of symphysis pubis to the sacral promontory, should be at least 11 cm as determined by ultrasound or X-ray
 2. Diagonal conjugate: from the lower border of the symphysis pubis to the sacral promontory; should be 12.5–13 cm; obtained by vaginal examination
 3. Obstetric conjugate: from the inner surface of the symphysis pubis, slightly below the upper border to the sacral promontory; the most important pelvic measurement; can be estimated by subtracting 1.5–2 cm from diagonal conjugate
 4. Inter tuberous diameter: measures the outlet between the inner borders of the ischial tuberosities; should be at least 8 cm
B. Pelvic shapes:
 1. Gynecoid: classic female pelvis; wide and well rounded in all directions; ideal for delivery of infant
 2. Platypelloid: wide but flat; may still have vaginal delivery
 3. Android: narrow, heart-shaped; male-type pelvis; not well-suited for delivery of infant
 4. Anthropoid: narrow, oval-shaped; resembles ape pelvis; not well-suited for delivery of infant

The Breasts

A. Paired mammary glands on the anterior chest wall between the second and sixth ribs, comprised of glandular tissue, fat, and connective tissue
B. The nipple and areola are darker in color than the breasts.
C. Responsible for lactation after delivery

PHYSIOLOGY

Menstrual Cycle (See Figure 15.3)

A. The regularly occurring physiologic changes in the endometrium that result in its shedding:
 1. Involves pituitary, ovarian, and uterine interaction
 2. Controls regular ripening and release of an ovum, preparation for its fertilization, and implantation in a thickened endometrium
 3. When fertilization/implantation do not occur, the endometrium is shed (menstruation), and the cycle begins again.
B. Stages of cycle:
 1. Menstruation: first days of cycle when endometrium is shed
 2. Proliferative phase (follicular phase): estrogen causes a build-up of the endometrium
 3. Ovulation: release of ovum, usually 14 days (plus or minus two) before end of cycle
 4. Secretory phase (luteal phase): progesterone secreted by corpus luteum, causing buildup of endometrial tissue with an enriched blood supply to nourish the embryo
 5. If conception does not take place, estrogen levels drop and the endometrium thins and is shed during menstruation. Follicle-stimulating hormone (FSH) and luteinizing hormone (LH) from the anterior pituitary cause the ovum to ripen, and the cycle starts over again.

Menopause (Climacteric)

A. Decline in ovarian function and hormone production
B. Characterized by irregular menses and sometimes vasomotor instability (hot flashes) and loss of bone density
C. See also Menopause

Conditions of the Female Reproductive System

BREAST CONDITIONS

Fibrocystic Breast Disease

A. Mammary dysplasia or chronic cystic mastitis; most common benign breast lesion; true cystic disease poses increased risk for breast cancer
B. Assessment findings:
 1. Presence of one or more lumps in the breast and a feeling of fullness and tenderness in the premenstrual period; cysts may be solid or fluid-filled; can be palpated and are mobile, round, and tender
 2. Diagnosis confirmed by mammogram, fine needle aspiration, or surgical biopsy
C. Interventions:
 1. Surgical removal of cysts
 2. Decreasing or removing caffeine from diet may decrease cyst formation; takes at least two months to show results

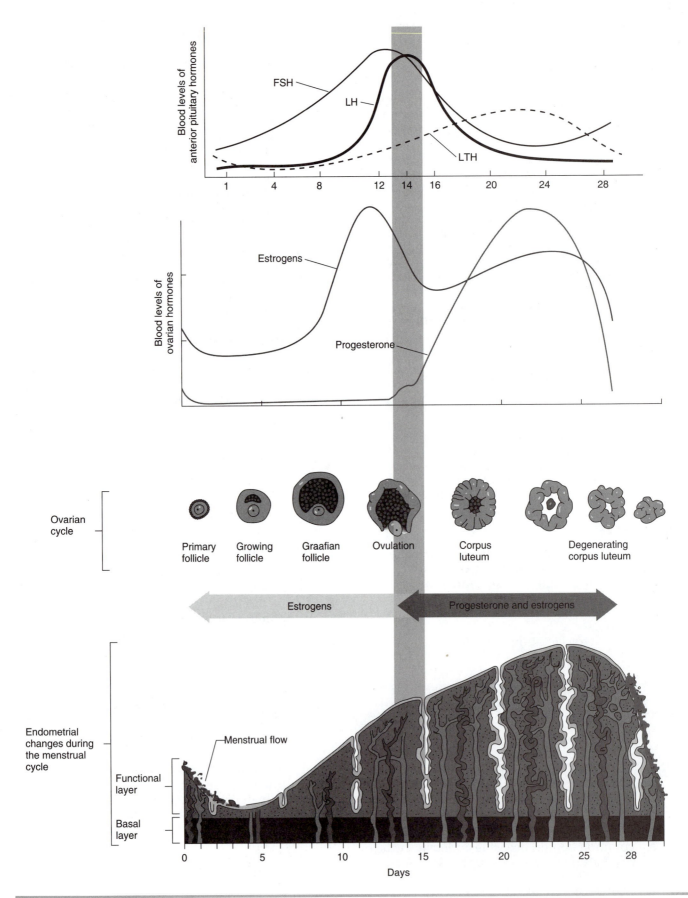

Figure 15.3 Menstrual cycle.

3. Decreasing sodium intake and the prescription of a mild diuretic the week before menses may help decrease discomfort.
4. Danazol (Danocrine) may be prescribed to suppress menses; gives "false menopause."
5. Teach the client that cysts usually decrease or disappear after menopause.

Breast Cancer

A. Common neoplasm in women; leading cause of death in women age 40–44
B. Assessment findings:
  1. Lump that can be palpated is usually the first symptom (upper outer quadrant most frequent)
  2. Breast skin dimpled
  3. Discharge from nipple
  4. Breasts do not appear symmetrical.
  5. Surgical biopsy provides a definitive diagnosis.
  6. Early detection essential:
    a. Annual exam by M.D. or nurse practitioner
    b. Mammograms: baseline at ages 35–40; every other year ages 40–50; every year age 50 and up
    c. Breast self-examination: done monthly after menstrual period when breasts are soft (if woman no longer has periods, have client choose a date such as the first or her birthday to help remember); see Table 15.1 for Procedure for Self Examination of Breasts

C. Nursing diagnoses related to breast cancer (see Table 15.2)
D. Interventions:
  1. Surgery (see Mastectomy)
  2. Chemotherapy
  3. Radiation therapy
  4. Hormonal therapy: Tamoxifen (anti-estrogen drug) to prevent recurrence

Mastectomy

A. Several types of procedures are available. Five-year survival rates are similar when Tamoxifen is used following any type of surgery.
  1. Lumpectomy: removal of lump and surrounding tissue
  2. Simple mastectomy: removal of breast only, no lymph nodes removed
  3. Radical mastectomy: removal of breast, muscle layer down to chest wall and axillary lymph nodes (rarely done)
  4. Modified radical mastectomy: removal of breast and lymph nodes
B. Nursing diagnoses related to mastectomy (see Table 15.3)
C. Nursing care:
  1. Routine pre- and post-op care
  2. Elevate client's arm on operative side on pillows to minimize lymphedema.
  3. Do not use the arm on the affected side to take blood pressure or give injections; should not be used for intravenous lines or obtaining blood samples.
  4. Turn only to the back and unaffected side.
  5. Check the client for bleeding; check under client (remember gravity).

Table 15.1 Procedure for Self Examination of Breasts

- In the shower: With fingers flat, move them gently over every part of each breast. Use the right hand for the left breast and the left hand for the right breast. Check for lumps, hard knots, or thickening.
- In front of a mirror: Inspect breasts with arms at side and raised; look for changes in contour, swelling, dimpling of the skin, or changes in nipple.
- Lying down: To examine the right breast, put a pillow under your right shoulder and your right hand behind your head; with the left hand, fingers flat, press gently in small circular motions around an imaginary clock. A ridge of firm tissue in the lower curve of each breast is normal; move in an inch toward the nipple and keep circling to examine every part of the breast, including the nipple; squeeze the nipple and report any discharge unless lactating or pregnant.

  To examine the left breast, repeat as above except putting the pillow under the left shoulder and putting your left hand behind your head and examining with the right hand.

  Instead of examining the breast in a full circle as described above, the woman may use an up-and-down approach or a wedge approach. The examination should be conducted in the same way each time.

Table 15.2 Nursing Diagnoses Related to Breast Cancer

- Disturbed body image relating to mutilation
- Anxiety related to surgery, unknown prognosis, and changes in functioning
- Impaired comfort related to surgery
- Ineffective sexuality patterns related to perceived loss of attractiveness
- Anticipatory grieving related to loss of breast; threatened loss of life

---

Table 15.3 Nursing Diagnoses Related to Mastectomy

- Risk for impaired physical mobility (shoulder, arm) related to lymphedema, nerve/muscle damage, and pain
- Risk for injury related to compromised lymph, motor, and sensory function in arm on affected side
- Grieving related to loss of breast and change in appearance
- Risk for ineffective therapeutic regimen related to insufficient knowledge of wound care, exercises, breast prosthesis, signs and symptoms of complications, hand/arm precautions, community resources, and follow-up care

6. Start ROM exercises immediately on the unaffected side.
7. On affected side: day of surgery, start movement with fingers and hands, then wrist and elbow; progress to shoulder movements and abduction (out to the side); encourage client to continue hair brushing and wall-climbing exercises after discharge
8. Teach client how to reduce risk of injury on affected side: not to carry heavy packages on affected side; be aware of possible altered sensation on affected side; avoid excessive exposure to the sun; do not cut cuticles on affected side
9. Teach client monthly self breast exam on remaining breast; breast cancer in one breast increases the risk of breast cancer in remaining breast
10. Teach the client that prosthesis and breast reconstruction procedures are available.
11. Encourage the client to utilize the Reach to Recovery support group as indicated.
12. Be aware of emotional concerns: grief at loss of body part, change in body image

CONDITIONS OF THE UTERUS

Fibroid Tumors (Myomas)

A. Benign tumors of the uterine muscle; usually occurring after age 30
B. Assessment findings:
   1. Low abdominal and back pain
   2. Menorrhagia
C. Interventions:
   1. Surgical removal; may include removal of uterus
   2. Shrink with progesterone
   3. Fibroids usually disappear after menopause.

Uterine Prolapse

A. Uterus descends so that cervix is in vagina (first degree), cervix outside of vagina (second degree), or entire uterus outside of body (third degree); occurs most often in women who have given birth to several children
B. Often associated with cystocele (herniation of bladder into vagina) and rectocele (herniation of part of rectum into vagina)
C. Assessment findings:
   1. Pelvic pressure, backache
   2. Urinary retention, incontinence
D. Interventions:
   1. Surgery usually the preferred treatment: anterior and posterior repair of vagina with possible hysterectomy
   2. Nonsurgical options include pessary and Kegel exercises

Endometriosis

A. Endometrial tissue (tissue that normally lines the uterus) found outside the uterus in the pelvic cavity, on the ovary, tubes, or elsewhere
B. Assessment findings:
   1. Pelvic area pain, severe dysmenorrhea
   2. May cause infertility
C. Interventions:
   1. Hormone therapy (Danazol, oral contraceptives) to stop ovulation
   2. Surgery to remove endometrial implants

Cancer of the Cervix

A. Believed to be caused by human papilloma virus infection (genital warts); good prognosis when detected and treated early
B. Assessment findings:
   1. Detected by pap smear (class IV or V) followed by tissue biopsy
   2. No symptoms in early stages
C. Interventions:
   1. Preinvasive: may treat with laser or cryosurgery, cervical conization, or hysterectomy
   2. Invasive: treated with internal radiation and radical hysterectomy

Cancer of the Endometrium

A. Fourth most common cancer in women; most common is pelvic cancer
B. Assessment findings:
   1. Abnormal uterine bleeding pre- or post-menopause
   2. Risk factors include women who receive unopposed estrogen (no progesterone), nulliparity, and late menopause (after age 52)
   3. Diagnosis is confirmed by endometrial biopsy or D&C.
C. Interventions:
   1. Cancer in situ: total abdominal hysterectomy, bilateral salpingectomy, and oophorectomy
   2. Metastasis: surgery and radiation or chemotherapy

Ovarian Cancer

A. Early detection is difficult, usually metastasized by the time the mass is palpated.
B. Risk factors:
   1. High-fat diet
   2. Smoking and alcohol intake
   3. Using talcum powder in the perineal area
   4. History of breast, colon, or endometrial cancer
   5. Family history of breast or ovarian cancer
   6. Nulliparity, infertility, and anovulation

C. Assessment findings:
1. Few early symptoms
2. Irregular menses, menorrhagia, and breast tenderness
3. Early menopause
4. Abdominal discomfort, pelvic pressure
5. Urinary frequency
6. A combination of a long history of ovarian dysfunction and vague, undiagnosed, persistent gastrointestinal symptoms suggest early ovarian malignancy.
7. Blood test may reveal the Ca-125 antigen.

D. Interventions:
1. Total abdominal hysterectomy, bilateral salpingectomy, and oophorectomy
2. Chemotherapy
3. Radiation
4. Prognosis poor if not detected early; 75% of cases have metastasis at diagnosis

Hysterectomy

A. Removal of uterus either through the vagina or through an abdominal incision
B. Types:
1. Total: removal of uterine body and cervix
2. Subtotal: removal of uterine body, leaving cervix in place (rare in this country)
3. Salpingo-oophorectomy: removal of tubes and ovaries; requires abdominal route
4. Radical hysterectomy: removal of uterine body, cervix, connective tissue, part of vagina, and pelvic lymph nodes
C. Nursing Diagnoses (see Table 15.4)
D. Interventions
1. Pre-operative:
   a. Routine pre-operative care
   b. Clearly explain loss of menses and surgical menopause if ovaries removed; no loss of sexual functioning following hysterectomy
   c. Allow the client to express feelings and possible grief.
2. Post-operative care:
   a. Routine post-operative care

Table 15.4 Nursing Diagnoses Related to Hysterectomy

- Interrupted family processes
- Anxiety related to fear of cancer, surgery
- Grieving related to loss of childbearing capability
- Ineffective sexuality patterns related to loss of organs
- Risk for infection related to surgical intervention and presence of urinary catheter
- Risk for disturbed self-concept related to significance of loss
- Risk of ineffective therapeutic regimen management related to insufficient knowledge of perineal/incisional care, signs of complications, activity restrictions, loss of menses, hormone therapy, and follow-up care
- Disturbed body image related to loss of uterus and childbearing capability

b. Check bleeding, vaginal, as well as abdominal, if total abdominal hysterectomy
c. Monitor urine output, catheter at first and then the ability to void after catheter removed
d. Encourage the expression of feelings: grief, change in body image, and end of childbearing years
e. Discuss estrogen replacement if ovaries are removed.

SEXUALLY TRANSMITTED DISEASES

Infections occurring predominantly in the genital area and spread by sexual contact

Herpes

A. Caused by herpes simplex virus type 2; transmitted sexually but can be transmitted in other ways, such as by touching a cold sore on the lips and then touching the genital area; may be transmitted to fetus during delivery and can cause death of the newborn
B. Assessment findings:
1. Painful blisters on internal and external genitalia that later develop crusts
2. Flu-like symptoms may occur three or four days after the lesions appear: headache, myalgia, low-grade fever
3. Inguinal lymphadenopathy
4. Dysuria
5. Lesions subside in two weeks unless a secondary infection develops.
6. Recurrent infections are less painful than the initial outbreak; usually heralded by a tingling, burning sensation.
7. Virus ascends the peripheral sensory nerves and remains inactive in the nerve ganglia and may recur, especially when the person is under stress.
C. Nursing diagnoses (see Table 15.5)
D. Interventions:
1. No cure
2. Acyclovir (Zovirax); famciclovir (Famvir) used to treat infections and reduce recurrence
3. Cesarean section if active lesions at time of delivery, because there is a high risk of

Table 15.5 Nursing Diagnoses for Sexually Transmitted Diseases

- Risk for infection transmission
- Impaired skin/tissue integrity
- Deficient knowledge regarding condition, prognosis, complications, therapy needs, and transmission
- Ineffective sexuality patterns
- Acute pain (in some conditions)

transfer to fetus during birth and a significant risk of death to the newborn if infection is acquired

4. Teach client that she is communicable when lesions are present and during prodromal period; teach client to have no sexual activity when lesions are active.

Chlamydia

A. Most frequent sexually transmitted disease; can be transmitted to fetus during birth process if mother has disease
B. Assessment findings:
   1. Symptoms occur 1–5 weeks after exposure; in some cases, client may be asymptomatic
   2. Females:
      a. Itching and burning
      b. Odorless, thick, yellow-white vaginal discharge
      c. Dull abdominal pain and metrorrhagia
   3. Males:
      a. Painful urination
      b. Watery discharge from penis
C. Nursing diagnoses (see Table 15.5)
D. Interventions:
   1. Tetracycline or erythromycin for both partners
   2. Use a condom for three to six months after treatment.

Gonorrhea

A. Caused by the bacteria Neisseria gonorrhea; can be passed to fetus during birth process and cause ophthalmia neonatorum (blindness) in the newborn; incubation period is only 3–5 days
B. Assessment findings:
   1. May be asymptomatic
   2. Female: heavy, purulent discharge
   3. Male: pain and burning upon urination and white discharge from penis
   4. Increased risk of premature rupture of membranes in pregnant woman
C. Nursing diagnoses (see Table 15.5)
D. Interventions:
   1. Must be reported to public health nurse (required by law)
   2. Penicillin therapy or erythromycin if allergic to penicillin
   3. All sexual contacts must be treated.
   4. All newborns should receive eye prophylaxis with erythromycin ointment, even if the mother is not known to have gonorrhea.

Syphilis

A. Caused by treponema pallidum (a spirochete); spirochete crosses placenta after 16–18th week of pregnancy and infects fetus, causing congenital syphilis
B. Assessment findings:
   1. Primary syphilis: chancre on genitalia and lymphadenopathy
   2. Latent period: symptoms disappear without treatment in 4–6 weeks; organism still in body
   3. Secondary syphilis: rash (on soles of feet and palms of hands as well as body), malaise, alopecia; symptoms may disappear without treatment
   4. Tertiary syphilis: occurs later in life and can affect any organ system, especially cardiovascular and neurologic systems
   5. Diagnosis is made by dark field examination and serology (VDRL).
C. Nursing diagnoses (see Table 15.5)
D. Interventions:
   1. Must be reported:
      a. Penicillin
      b. Treatment of contacts
E. Nursing diagnoses (see Table 15.5)

Trichomonas Vaginalis

A. Caused by protozoan
B. Assessment findings:
   1. Women have profuse, foamy-white, green, or yellow discharge and itching, burning, and dysuria.
   2. Men may have no symptoms or may develop urethritis, an enlarged prostate, or epididymitis.
C. Nursing diagnoses (see Table 15.5)
D. Interventions:
   1. Metronidazole (Flagyl) for woman and partners
   2. Treatment for seven days; use a condom during treatment
   3. Teach client not to drink alcohol when taking Flagyl; alcohol taken with Flagyl causes severe GI upset.
   4. Flagyl causes a metallic taste in the mouth.

Candida Albicans

A. Caused by yeast normally found in the vagina; overgrowth may occur in diabetes, pregnancy, and when taking antibiotics or steroids
B. Assessment findings:
   1. Thick, white, cheesy patches on vaginal walls or oral mucosa (thrush)
   2. Itching
   3. Cheesy patches may occur in the mouth of the newborn (thrush) as a result of infection during birth.
C. Nursing diagnoses (see Table 15.5)
D. Interventions include topical nystatin (Mycostatin), chlotrimazole (Gyne-Lotrimin), or miconazole (Monistat)

Condyloma Acuminata (Genital Warts)

A. Caused by human papilloma virus; cancer of the cervix thought to be caused by infection with human papilloma virus
B. Assessment findings include flesh-colored to pink-colored papillary growth anywhere in the vulvar area or glans penis.
C. Nursing diagnoses (see Table 15.5)
D. Interventions include cautery, cryotherapy, and weekly applications of podophyllin.

Acquired Immunodeficiency Syndrome (AIDS)

Suppression of the cellular immune response, acquired by exposure to the human immunodeficiency virus, leading to opportunistic infections and malignancies. The virus is transmitted through sexual contact and blood; crosses the placenta and can infect the fetus in utero.

Pelvic Inflammatory Disease (PID)

A. Caused by ascending infection from vagina through uterus, tubes, and into pelvic cavity
B. Assessment findings:
   1. Abdominal pain, dysmennorhea, dyspareunia (painful intercourse)
   2. Nausea and vomiting
   3. Fever, malaise
   4. Foul-smelling vaginal discharge
   5. Increased incidence of sterility following PID
   6. Untreated can progress to peritonitis
C. Nursing diagnoses (see Table 15.5)
D. Interventions:
   1. Antibiotics; may be given orally or intravenously depending on the extent of infection
   2. Hysterectomy in extreme cases
   3. Semi-Fowler's position to facilitate drainage of the pelvis
   4. Analgesics

FERTILITY MANAGEMENT

Infertility

A. Inability to conceive after at least one year of unprotected sexual relations or the inability to deliver a live infant after three consecutive pregnancies; in the male, inability to impregnate a female after at least one year of unprotected sexual relations; affects at least 10 to 15% of all couples
B. Diagnostic tests for infertility:
   1. Sperm analysis to identify number and motility
   2. Basal body temperature and cervical mucous identification of ovulation
   3. Plasma progesterone level
   4. Endometrial biopsy
   5. Postcoital test
   6. Hysterosalpingography: X-ray of uterus and tubes following dye insertion
   7. Pelvic ultrasound
   8. Laparoscopy
C. Interventions
   1. Clomisphere (Clomid) and Pergonal induce ovulation; may cause multiple births, may cause hyperstimulation of ovary, given with caution, requires close follow-up
   2. Antibiotics or surgery for blocked tubes
   3. Uterine factors: antibiotics, surgery
   4. Low sperm count: no good therapy
   5. Alternatives for infertile couples:
      a. Artificial insemination by husband or donor
      b. In vitro fertilization, GIFT
      c. Adoption
      d. Surrogate parenting
      e. Embryo transfers

Contraception (See Tables 15.6–15.11)

A. Assessment:
   1. Knowledge about or previous experience with family planning

Table 15.6 Fertility Awareness Methods of Contraception

Method	Basal body temperature method (BBT)	Ovulation method (Billings method)	Sympto-thermal method combines BBT and ovulation method
Mode of Action	Abstinence during fertile period		
Effectiveness	Very low	Theoretically high; requires strong motivation	
Client Responsibilities	Take temperature each morning before rising and record on chart; avoid intercourse when temperature drops and for next three days	Check cervical mucus; avoid intercourse on "wet" days when mucus has spinnbarkeit pattern; may use other symptoms such as mittleschmerz to help determine time for abstinence	
Advantages	Increased awareness of one's body; avoidance of artificial substances; couple cooperation; acceptable to most religions; no side effects		
Disadvantages and Side Effects	No side effects; many couples find periods of abstinence unacceptable	Low effectiveness if used alone because sperm can live approximately 72 hours in fertile cervical mucus	

Table 15.7 Hormonal Methods of Contraception

Method	"mini pill" progesterone 0.35 mg daily
Mode of Action	Suppresses ovulation by suppressing FSH & LH (fools body into thinking it's pregnant); makes cervical mucus impervious to sperm; alters endometrium
Effectiveness	99.7%
Client Responsibilities	Take pill same time each day; take one full cycle before dependence for contraception
Advantages	Easy to take for those motivated; not related to time of intercourse; most effective means; may decrease dysmenorrhea, irregular periods
Disadvantages and Side Effects	Discomforts simulating pregnancy: breast tenderness, water retention, nausea, chloasma, fatigue, decreased libido, headaches; also: breakthrough bleeding, depression; increases susceptibility to monilia, no withdrawal bleeding. Hazards: thrombus formation, pulmonary embolus, hypertension. Contraindicated: obesity, hypertension, sickle cell disease, smokers, diabetes, migraine headaches, age above 35–40, menstrual irregularity, cystic breast changes, liver disease, cancer, clotting problems.

Table 15.8 Mechanical Contraceptives/Chemical Barrier

	Condoms	Diaphragm	Cervical cup	Spermicides
Method				
Mode of Action	Barrier: holds sperm away from cervical mucus and ovum	Physical and chemical barrier: blocks sperm from reaching ovum	"Cup" held over cervix by suction	Forms chemical barrier that holds and kills sperm and decreases motility
Effectiveness	75% to 95% if used properly	65 to 97%	85%	65% when used alone; up to 100% if used with a condom
Client Responsibilities	Condom applied to erect penis before any penile insertion; small space must be left at end; must be removed before erection is lost	Must be fitted by practitioner, refitted after birth or gain or loss of 10–20 lbs.; insert up to one hour before intercourse with 1 tsp. spermicidal jelly in dome and around rim; check placement after insertion by touching cervix through diaphragm; leave in place and avoid douching for six hours after intercourse; repeat intercourse within six hours requires repeat application of spermicide	Insert cup	Insert in supine position just before intercourse; no douching for six hours after; repeat application with repeated intercourse
Advantages	Small, lightweight, disposable, inexpensive; available; no side effects; requires no medical exam or supervision; protects against STDs	Safe, effective; no side effects	May be left in place 1–2 days	Increases effectiveness of mechanical barriers; easy to use; adds vaginal lubrication; no medical exam required; available OTC; some protection against STDs
Disadvantages and Side Effects	Breakage; displacement; possible vaginal irritation; dulled sensation; timing may interfere with arousal	Some object to manipulation of genitals; some feel it interferes with spontaneity; initial exam and fitting may be expensive; may cause vaginal irritation	Cup must be custom made; increased risk for infection	Messiness; can be allergic response; some feel that it lessens sensation; not very effective when used alone

    2. Need for genetic counseling
    3. Problems with fertility
    4. Religious or ethical concerns
B. Types (see Tables 15.6 through 15.10)
C. Nursing diagnoses related to infertility (see Table 15.11)

Table 15.9 Intrauterine Device

Method	Unmedicated I.U.D., Lippes loop, SAF-T, coil	Medicated I.U.D., copper-7	Progestasert
Mode of Action	Alters rate of egg's passage through tubes; discourages implantation because of altered endometrium	Alters endometrium to discourage implantation	Releases progesterone; discourages implantation
Effectiveness	97–99%	95–97%	97%
Client Responsibilities	Check for string monthly after menses; medicated units must be removed and changed q. 1–3 years	Same	Same
Advantages	No direct relationship to coitus; no need to remember to take or use something (good for unmotivated people)	Same	Same
Disadvantages and Side Effects	Must be inserted and removed by practitioner	Hazards: undetected expulsion; uterine perforations; infection	Side effects: heavy flow; spotting between periods, cramping (especially in early months); allergy to copper—must be removed; higher incidence of infertility secondary to infection; not for women who want more children

Table 15.10 Sterilization: Permanent Termination of Fertility

Method	Female: tubal ligation	Male: vasectomy
Mode of Action	Prevents union of sperm and egg	Vas deferens ligated and severed to prevent passage of sperm
Effectiveness	Approaches 100% if ligatures don't slip	100% after ejaculate is free of sperm for three months
Client Responsibilities	None	Use other contraception until ejaculate is free of sperm for three months.
Advantages	Permanent; normal hormones and menstruation continue	Relatively simple surgical procedure; permanent
Disadvantages and Side Effects	Psychologic trauma in some women; slight risk of tubal or abdominal pregnancy if ligature slips; reversals may not be possible	Psychologic impotence; reversal may not be successful

Table 15.11 Nursing Diagnoses Related to Infertility

- Deficient knowledge
- Disturbed self-esteem
- Ineffective sexuality patterns
- Grieving related to loss of anticipated pregnancy

Sample Questions

1. A 45-year-old woman has been having menorrhagia and metrorrhagia for several months. She is also feeling very tired and run down. Which is the most likely explanation for her fatigue?
   1. Hormonal changes related to menopause
   2. Psychological exhaustion produced by continuous worry about her illness
   3. Interference with digestion due to pressure on the small bowel
   4. Decreased oxygen-carrying capacity of the blood due to chronic loss of iron stores

2. A 45-year-old woman was found to have several large fibroid tumors. She is to have an abdominal panhysterectomy. She asks what a panhysterectomy includes. The nurse knows that a panhysterectomy consists of the removal of:
   1. Uterine fundus and body
   2. Uterine fundus and body and uterine cervix
   3. Uterine fundus and body, uterine cervix, fallopian tubes, and ovaries
   4. Uterine fundus and body, uterine cervix, fallopian tubes, ovaries, and vagina

3. The nurse is caring for a woman who had a hysterectomy. Which vascular complication should the nurse be especially alert for because of the location of the surgery?
   1. Thrombophlebitis
   2. Varicose veins
   3. Cerebral embolism
   4. Aortic aneurysm

4. The nurse is caring for an adult woman who had a vaginal hysterectomy today. The client is now returned to the nursing care unit following an uneventful stay in the post-anesthesia care unit. What is the priority nursing action for this client?
    1. Offer her the bedpan.
    2. Encourage coughing and deep breathing.
    3. Immediately administer pain medication.
    4. Assess chest tubes for patency.

5. A young woman has been having lower abdominal pain and amenorrhea. She is diagnosed as having an ovarian cyst. She asks the nurse what the usual treatment is for an ovarian cyst. What is the best response for the nurse to make?
    1. "Most women with your condition are placed on estrogen therapy for six to 12 months until the symptoms disappear."
    2. "The most effective treatment for ovarian cysts is to shrink the cyst with radiation therapy."
    3. "Ovarian cysts are usually surgically removed."
    4. "Steroid therapy is often given. The cyst usually resolves in three months."

6. A 39-year-old woman is seen in the gynecology clinic and asks the nurse about menopause. What is the best explanation for the nurse to give her?
    1. "It usually occurs about the age of 40. You can expect severe hot flashes."
    2. "It usually occurs after the age of 45 and frequently marks the end of a woman's sex life."
    3. "You can expect to have symptoms for about three years while your body adjusts to additional hormones."
    4. "No more ovarian hormones are produced, so you will stop menstruating."

7. A 42-year-old woman sees her physician because of painless spotting between periods that is worse after intercourse. A pap smear is done. The results come back as Stage III. The client is admitted to the hospital for further testing and treatment. She asks the nurse what a Stage III pap smear means. The nurse's response is based on the knowledge that a Stage III pap smear indicates that
    1. Only normal cells are present.
    2. Atypical cells are present.
    3. Cells suggestive but not diagnostic of malignancy are present.
    4. Many malignant cells are present.

8. A woman is to have internal radiation as part of her treatment for cancer of the cervix. In teaching her about the pre-operative preparation for this procedure, the nurse should include which information?
    1. A high-residue diet will be ordered.
    2. An indwelling catheter will be inserted.
    3. A nasogastric tube will be inserted.
    4. Several units of blood will be ready for transfusion if needed.

9. The nurse is caring for a woman after insertion of radium rods for treatment of cancer of the cervix. The nurse positions her in a supine position with legs extended for which reason?
    1. To keep the rods in the correct position
    2. To prevent the urinary bladder from becoming over-distended
    3. To reduce pressure on the pelvic and back areas
    4. To limit the amount of radiation exposure

10. The nurse is caring for a woman after the insertion of radium rods for treatment of cancer of the cervix. Which discomfort should the nurse anticipate that the client may have while the rods are in place?
    1. Headache
    2. Urinary retention
    3. Constipation
    4. Uterine cramps

11. The nurse is caring for a woman the day after the insertion of radium rods for treatment of cancer of the cervix. The woman calls the nurse and says, "There is something between my legs. It fell out of me." What is the most appropriate initial action for the nurse to take?
    1. Call the radiation safety officer.
    2. Put on rubber gloves and put the radiation rod in the bathroom until help arrives.
    3. Using long forceps, place the radium needle in a lead-lined container.
    4. Calmly reinsert the rod in the vagina.

12. A 14-year-old female comes to the clinic for contraceptive advice. She says she wants to take the pill. Vital signs are within normal limits. She tells the nurse she has been having intercourse for the past year without protection. What question is it most important for the nurse to ask her?
    1. How much exercise do you get each day?
    2. What do you usually eat each day?
    3. How many cigarettes do you smoke each day?
    4. Are you under stress?

13. A young woman asks the nurse if oral contraceptives have any side effects. What is the best response for the nurse to make?
    1. "Nausea, fluid retention, and weight gain."
    2. "Why do you ask? Look at the benefits."
    3. "Are you concerned about something?"
    4. "Increased libido, decreased breast size, and diarrhea."

14. A client asks the nurse the difference between an IUD (intrauterine device) and the diaphragm. The nurse's response should be based on which information?
    1. The diaphragm is inserted into the uterine cavity, and the IUD covers the cervix.
    2. The IUD is 97% effective, and the diaphragm is 50% effective.
    3. The IUD is placed into the uterine cavity by the doctor, and the diaphragm is placed into the vagina each time by the user.

4. The IUD must be used with contraceptive jelly, and the diaphragm does not require contraceptive jelly.

15. A young woman tells the nurse that her boyfriend used a "rubber" once. What is the most important information about condoms for the nurse to provide the client?
   1. Always use Vaseline as a lubricant.
   2. Apply the condom to the penis right before ejaculation.
   3. You don't need a medical prescription.
   4. It must be applied before any penile-vaginal contact.

16. A woman is to have a routine gynecological examination tomorrow. What instructions should the nurse give this client?
   1. "Bring a urine sample with you."
   2 "Be sure to drink plenty of fluids in the morning before you come so that your bladder will be full."
   3. "Be sure not to douche today or tomorrow."
   4. "Don't eat breakfast. You will be able to eat right after the exam."

17. A 46-year-old woman visits her gynecologist because she has been spotting. She is to be evaluated for carcinoma of the cervix. If she has cancer of the cervix, she is most likely to report that vaginal spotting occurred at what time?
   1. On arising
   2. While sitting
   3. After intercourse
   4. On stair climbing

18. The nurse is discussing self breast examination with a group of women in a clinic. One woman asks, "When should I do this examination?" What is the best response for the nurse?
   1. "You should perform self breast examination early in the morning for most accurate results."
   2. "Self breast examination should be done a few days after your period every month."
   3. "Self breast examination should be done by women after the age of 40 on the first of every month."
   4. "Self breast examination is best done just before you expect your menstrual period."

19. The physician prescribes clomiphene (Clomid) for a woman who has been having difficulty getting pregnant. When discussing this drug with the woman, the nurse should know that which of the following is known to be a side effect of clomiphene?
   1. Infertility
   2. Multiple births
   3. Vaginal bleeding
   4. Painful intercourse

20. A newly married couple asks the nurse which method of contraception is the best and the one that they should use. Which response is most helpful to the couple?
   1. "The pill is the best because it is 100% effective with few side effects."
   2. "The best method is the one that you both agree upon and will use consistently."
   3. "The condom is the best because it prevents diseases as well as pregnancy."
   4. "No method is completely effective; you should practice abstinence until you are ready to have children."

21. A woman is being treated for trichomonas vaginalis with metronidazole (Flagyl). Which statement the woman makes indicates a need for further teaching?
   1. "My husband is also taking the medication."
   2. "I will take Flagyl with meals."
   3. "The doctor said I might get a metallic taste in my mouth while I am taking Flagyl."
   4. "I will drink only one glass of wine per meal while I am taking Flagyl."

22. A client who is being treated for syphilis says to the nurse, "Why does the doctor want to know who I have had sex with?" What should the nurse include when responding to this question?
   1. It really is not any of the physician's concern.
   2. The physician wants to help her make better decisions about her lifestyle.
   3. Reporting of sexual contacts is mandatory so that the contacts can receive testing and treatment.
   4. Studies need to be done on sexual activities to learn how to reduce the spread of the disease.

23. During the early period following a right modified radical mastectomy, which nursing action would be appropriate to include in the client's plan of care?
   1. Position the patient in the right lateral position.
   2. Encourage a high fluid intake.
   3. Ambulate as soon as sensation and motion have returned.
   4. Elevate the right arm on pillows.

24. The nurse is caring for a client who has had a right modified radical mastectomy this morning. Which exercise should the nurse encourage the client to perform this evening?
   1. Hair combing exercises with the right arm
   2. Wall climbing exercises with the right arm
   3. Movement of the fingers and wrists of the right arm
   4. Exercises of the left arm only

25. The client is being discharged following a left simple mastectomy. Which statement the client makes indicates an understanding of discharge teaching?
   1. "I won't let anyone take blood pressures on my left arm."
   2. "I understand that I should not have sexual relations for at least three months."
   3. "I won't move my arm any more than necessary."
   4. "I will not lift my arm above my head for the next two weeks."

Answers and Rationales

1. (4) Menorrhagia means heavy menstrual flow, and metrorrhagia means bleeding between periods. Such increased loss of blood results in fatigue due to the chronic loss of blood (iron stores). Hormonal changes may cause fatigue, but the data in this question do not support that reason. Excessive worry can cause fatigue, but the data in this question do not support that. There is no data to support interference with digestion due to pressure on the small bowel. If the woman has fibroid tumors, there may be pressure on the bowel—but that would not cause interference with digestion and fatigue.

2. (3) A panhysterectomy consists of the removal of the entire uterus, including the cervix and the tubes and ovaries. The vagina is left intact.

3. (1) Persons who have had surgery in the pelvic area are apt to develop thrombophlebitis. Varicose veins are a complication of pregnancy.

4. (2) Coughing and deep-breathing are very important in the immediate post-operative period. She will have an indwelling catheter after a vaginal hysterectomy. Pain medication is given for pain. There is no indication of pain. She will not have chest tubes after pelvic surgery.

5. (3) Large ovarian cysts are usually surgically removed. Women who have small ovarian cysts may be given birth control pills (progesterone) to suppress ovarian activity and resolve the cyst. Radiation therapy, estrogen, and steroids are not appropriate for persons with ovarian cysts.

6. (4) Menopause is the cessation of production of ovarian hormones. Amenorrhea will occur. Not all women have hot flashes. It is not the end of a woman's sex life. It is the end of her capacity to reproduce. It occurs when a woman is in her 40s or 50s.

7. (3) Stage III is characterized by cells suggestive but not diagnostic of malignancy. Stage I contains normal cells. Stage II contains atypical cells. Stage IV contains malignant cells.

8. (2) During the time the radium rods are in place, the client should have as little movement as possible to prevent dislodgment of the radium. She will have an indwelling catheter in place so her bladder will not become full and also to prevent damage to the bladder from the radiation. She will have an enema before the procedure and a low-residue or clear liquid diet before surgery and while the rods are in place. There is no need for a nasogastric tube or blood transfusions.

9. (1) The client is kept flat to prevent the rods from becoming dislodged. She will have an indwelling catheter in place. Positioning does not reduce radiation exposure.

10. (4) Uterine cramping occurs frequently. She will be on a clear liquid or low-residue diet so that she is not likely to be constipated. She will have a catheter in place so she will not have urinary retention.

11. (3) There should always be long forceps and a lead-lined container readily available whenever a person has radium inserted. The nurse should pick up the rod with the long forceps and immediately place it in a lead-lined container. The radiation safety officer should then be notified. Leaving the rod between the client's legs exposes her and others to unnecessary radiation. Rubber gloves offer no protection from radiation. The nurse does not reinsert the radium.

12. (3) Cigarette smoking is a contraindication for the use of the pill. There is a higher incidence of thromboembolic problems when a person smokes.

13. (1) These are side effects of the pill. Answer 2 and answer 3 do not answer the question asked. Answer 4 is not correct.

14. (3) The IUD must be inserted into the uterus by the physician. The woman inserts the diaphragm before each act of intercourse. Both types are very effective when used as directed. The diaphragm requires contraceptive jelly; the IUD does not.

15. (4) Pre-ejaculatory secretions may contain sperm. It must be applied before there is any penile-vaginal contact. Vaseline should never be used as a lubricant. Lubricants should always be water soluble, such as K-Y jelly or Surgilube. Answer 3 is a true statement but not the most important information to give the client.

16. (3) There is no special preparation for a gynecological exam. The patient should not douche, however. There is no need to bring a urine specimen. The client may be asked to give a specimen prior to the examination. Drinking plenty of fluids would be appropriate prior to a pelvic ultrasound examination. There is no need to fast before a gynecological exam.

17. (3) Post-coital (after intercourse) spotting is often seen with cancer of the cervix. The other responses are not correct.

18. (2) The best time to perform self breast examination is a few days after your period begins because the breasts are least tender at this time. It should be done every month. Answer 1 is incorrect. It does not matter what time of day the exam is performed. Self breast examination should be done monthly, starting right after puberty. The incidence of breast cancer does increase in age, but it can occur in teenagers. The breasts are most tender just before the period starts; this is the least desirable time to do a self breast examination.

19. (2) One of the major side effects of fertility drugs such as clomiphene, which increases

ovulation, is multiple births. Clomiphene is used to treat infertility; it does not cause infertility. Clomiphene does not cause vaginal bleeding or painful intercourse.

20. (2) The best method for any couple is one they will use consistently. The only 100% effective method is abstinence, which is not a realistic choice for most couples. To be effective, contraception must be used consistently and correctly. Answer 1 is not correct. If the pill is not taken exactly as directed, pregnancies can and do occur. The pill has several side effects, including nausea, weight gain, and enlarged breasts. Answer 3 contains correct information in that the condom does help to prevent disease transmission. However, with a married couple this is not likely to be an issue. Answer 4 is an unrealistic answer for a married couple and therefore is not very helpful.

21. (4) Alcohol taken with Flagyl causes an Antabuse-like reaction, nausea, and vomiting. The client should drink no alcoholic beverages. The husband (partner) should also be treated, even if he has no symptoms, to prevent reinfection. Flagyl, unless it is extended release, should be taken with food to decrease GI side effects. People commonly get a metallic taste when taking Flagyl.

22. (3) Sexual contacts must be reported so that they can be contacted, tested, and treated to avoid the serious complications of untreated syphilis. Answer 1 is not correct. It is possible that there might be some truth to answer 2. However, the information regarding contacts is usually obtained in a nonjudgmental manner for the reasons described above. Answer 4 is not correct.

23. (4) The arm on the affected side should be elevated on pillows to help prevent the development of lymphedema. The client should not be positioned on the affected side. Once the client is awake following anesthesia, the head of the bed will be elevated. The client may have liquids following surgery, but there is no particular need to encourage a high fluid intake. The client will begin to ambulate fairly quickly. However, the client will not have had an epidural anesthetic for a mastectomy, so the return of sensation and motion is not an issue. A mastectomy is too high for an epidural. Epidurals are not given for surgery above the waist.

24. (3) The day of surgery, the client should be encouraged to move the fingers and wrists of the affected arm. Hair combing and wall climbing exercises will be performed later, not the day of surgery. The client should be encouraged to exercise the fingers and wrists of the affected extremity the day of surgery as well as exercising the unaffected arm.

25. (1) The person who has had a mastectomy should not have blood drawn or blood pressures taken on that arm. There is no reason why she should not have sexual relations for three months. As soon as she feels well enough, sexual relations can resume. She should use a position that does not put pressure on her left side. Answer 3 and answer 4 are incorrect. A woman who has had a mastectomy will need to perform arm exercises regularly. These will include lifting the arm above the head in exercises like hair combing and wall climbing.

The Antepartal Client

ONSET OF PREGNANCY/FETAL DEVELOPMENT

Fertilization

A. Takes place in the outer third of the fallopian tube
B. Gametes (mature germ cell—egg or sperm): carry 23 chromosomes (22 autosomes and one sex chromosome)
C. Zygote: fertilized ovum rapidly divides as it travels through tube

Implantation

A. Takes place in upper uterine wall 7–9 days after fertilization

B. Endometrium is now called decidua
C. Progesterone is produced by the corpus luteum to maintain the lining of the uterus.

Placenta

A. Forms after third week; takes over pregnancy hormone production completely by third month
B. Acts as an endocrine organ; produces high level of estrogen and progesterone HCG, HPL
C. Maternal and fetal blood do not mix; the exchange of nutrients, waste, and gases is by diffusion.
D. Placenta is a barrier to large molecules only; drugs and viruses pass through.

Developmental Stages

A. Fertilized ovum: from conception through first two weeks of pregnancy
B. Embryo: from end of second week through end of eighth week; organs laid down during this time
C. Fetus: from end of eighth week to termination of pregnancy; continued development of organs

Fetal Circulation/Umbilical Cord

A. Two arteries that carry blood back to the mother (unoxygenated blood)
B. One vein that carries blood to the fetus (oxygenated blood)
C. Wharton's jelly
D. Cord with two vessels instead of the normal three is often associated with fetal anomalies

Fetal Growth and Development

A. Organ systems develop from three primary germ layers:
   1. Ectoderm: outer layer; produces skin, nails, nervous system, and tooth enamel
   2. Mesoderm: middle layer; produces connective tissue, muscles, blood, and circulatory system
   3. Endoderm: inner layer; produces linings of gastrointestinal and respiratory tracts, endocrine glands, and auditory canal
B. Timetable for fetal development (see Figure 15.4):
   1. Four weeks: all systems in rudimentary form; heart beating; length 0.4 cm; weight 0.4 gm
   2. Eight weeks: head large in proportion to rest of body, some movement; length 2.5 cm; weight 2 gm
   3. 12 weeks: sex distinguishable; kidneys secrete urine; can suck and swallow; length 6–8 cm; weight 19 gm
   4. 16 weeks: more human appearance; earliest movement felt by mother; meconium in bowel; scalp hair develops; length 11.5–13.5 cm; weight 100 gm
   5. 20 weeks: vernix caseosa and lanugo appear; movement usually felt by mother; heart rate audible with fetoscope; length 16–18.5 cm; weight 300 gm

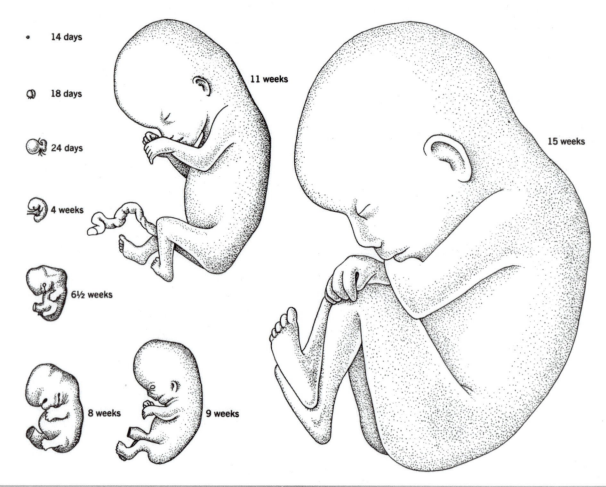

Figure 15.4 Changes in body size of embryo and fetus during development in the uterus

6. 24 weeks: body well proportioned; skin red and wrinkled; can hear; length 23 cm; weight 600 gm
7. 28 weeks: infant viable but immature if born; body less wrinkled; nails present; length 27 cm; weight 1,100 gm
8. 32 weeks: subcutaneous fat depositing; L/S ratio in lungs 1.2:1; skin smooth and pink; length 31 cm; weight 1,800–2,100 gm
9. 36 weeks: lanugo disappearing; body plump; L/S ratio in lungs 2:1; sleep/wake cycle; length 35 cm; weight 2,200–2,900 gm
10. 40 weeks: full-term pregnancy; baby active with good muscle tone; strong suck reflex; male has testes in scrotum; little lanugo; length 40 cm; weight 3,200 gm or more

Effects on Fetal Development

A. Teratogen: "Monster Maker" (nongenetic factor that can produce malformations of the fetus; affects those cells undergoing rapid growth; worst effects in first trimester; weeks 3–8 are highest peak for damage to the developing embryo)
B. Types of teratogens:
   1. Chemicals
   2. Radiation
   3. Drugs: all drugs except insulin and heparin should be considered teratogenic
      a. Alcohol, one of the worst, can cause fetal alcohol syndrome.
      b. Hydantoin (Dilantin) is an example of a known teratogen.
   4. Bacteria and viruses
      a. Syphilis:
         (1) Spirochete causing syphilis does not cross placenta until 16th–18th week of pregnancy when the placenta is developed; treatment with penicillin before this time assures that the baby will not have congenital syphilis
         (2) Causes late abortions, stillbirths, and congenital syphilis
      b. Gonorrhea can cause ophthalmia neonatorum when the infant comes in contact with the bacteria during the birth process
      c. TORCH infections:
         (1) Toxoplasmosis: protozoan contracted by ingesting raw meat or kitten feces
         (2) Other viral infections
         (3) Rubella (German measles): when contracted in the first trimester, causes congenital heart disorders such as cataracts, blindness, deafness, and mental retardation
         (4) Cytomegalovirus (member of the Herpes family): causes congenital and acquired infection that affects liver, brain, and blood
         (5) Herpes virus Type II: transmitted to infant during vaginal delivery; cesarean section usually done if the woman has active lesions
            (a) Herpes affects blood, brain, liver, lungs, CNS, eyes, and skin.
            (b) 96% of babies who get herpes will die, and half the survivors have neurological or visual abnormalities.

PREGNANCY

Signs of Pregnancy

A. Presumptive (subjective):
   1. Amenorrhea
   2. Nausea and vomiting (first three months)
   3. Fatigue (first three months)
   4. Urinary frequency (first three months)
   5. Breast changes
   6. Quickening (16–18 weeks)
   7. Leukorrhea
B. Probable (objective):
   1. Uterine enlargement
   2. Chadwick's sign (bluish coloration or mucous membranes of cervix, vagina, and vulva—eight weeks)
   3. Goodell's sign (softening of cervix—six weeks)
   4. Hegar's sign (softening of the isthmus of the cervix–10 weeks)
   5. Braxton-Hicks contractions (felt after 28 weeks)
   6. Positive human chorionic gonadotropin (HCG) pregnancy test
   7. Ballottement—rebounding of the fetus against the nurse's fingers on palpation
   8. Pigmentation changes: chloasma, linea nigra, striae gravidarum
   9. Uterine souffle: soft blowing sound (blood flow to placenta) same rate as maternal pulse
C. Positive:
   1. Fetal heartbeat: Doppler at 8—10 weeks; fetoscope at 20 weeks
   2. Fetal movements felt by examiner
   3. Fetal outline—by X-ray or sonogram
D. Estimated Date of Delivery:
   1. Human pregnancies last 40 weeks or 10 lunar months.
   2. Naegele's rule—first day of last menstrual period (LMP) minus three months plus seven days
   3. Other landmarks used include fundal height, quickening, and sonogram.

Physical Adaptations to Pregnancy

A. Uterus:
   1. Early growth is influenced by estrogen.
   2. 500—1,000 fold increase in capacity (2 oz. prepregancy to 2 lbs. at term)
B. Vagina:
   1. The epithelium undergoes hypertrophy and hyperplasia.
   2. Increased vascularity
   3. pH (3.5–6) good environment for Monilia, which causes thrush in newborn
   4. Increase in discharge
C. Breasts:
   1. Increase in size and nodularity, straiae
   2. Superficial veins prominent
   3. Hypertrophy of Montgomery's tubercles
   4. Darkening of areola
   5. Colostrum—nipple stimulation may cause contractions
D. Skin:
   1. Areola darkens
   2. Abdominal striae, linea nigra
   3. Diaphoresis
   4. Chloasma
   5. Pruritis due to estrogen and progesterone
   6. Vascular spider nevi, chest, neck, arms, and legs
E. Cervix:
   1. Shorter, larger, and more elastic
   2. Increased vaginal discharge due to increased secretions
   3. Forms mucous plug which is discharged early in labor
F. Perineum:
   1. Increased vascularity
   2. Kegel exercises help to promote circulation and prevent stasis of blood.

G. Respiratory:
   1. Increase in volume of up to 40–50 % between 16th–34th week
   2. Diaphragm is pushed upward and rib cage flares out; breathing changes from abdominal to chest.
   3. Oxygen consumption is increased 15%.
   4. Estrogen can cause stuffiness, epistaxis, and changes in voice.
H. Cardiovascular:
   1. Cardiac output increased by 30%
   2. Blood volume increased; peaks at 30–40 weeks 50% above prepregnant state
   3. Plasma volume increases greater than RBC and hemoglobin, causing "pseudo anemia."
   4. Pulse rate increases by 10–15 beats.
   5. BP remains same or often drops in second trimester.
I. Gastrointestinal Tract:
   1. Nausea and vomiting–first trimester
   2. Constipation, flatulence, heartburn
   3. Gums may bleed
J. Urinary Tract:
   1. Frequency during first and third trimesters due to pressure on bladder
   2. Glomerular filtration rate increases, causing glycosuria.
   3. Increase in urinary infections
K. Metabolism/Nutrition:
   1. Increase in basal metabolic rate by 20%
   2. Water retention; dependent edema
   3. Weight gain:
      a. 20–30 lbs with average of 25 lbs for average woman with single pregnancy
      b. First trimester: 2–3 lbs; second and third trimesters: 12 oz./week
   4. Increase in need for calories, protein, iron, calcium, vitamins, and minerals (see Table 15.12)

Table 15.12 Nutrient Needs During Pregnancy

Nutrient	Daily Requirement	Sources
Calories	Usually 300 kcal over nonpregnant needs; may be modified if over-/underweight	Prefer sources containing other nutrients, not "empty" calories
Protein	30 g over normal to total of 74–76 g; more needed if adolescent or carrying twins	Milk, meats, eggs, cheeses, legumes, tofu, whole grains, nuts
Iron	18 mg	Liver, kidney, dried beans, red meat, dried fruits, dark green leafy vegetables; usually given supplement after first trimester; give iron sources with vitamin C to increase absorption
Calcium	1,200 mg	Dairy products; broccoli, salmon (with bones), dark leafy vegetables fair source; if not eating dairy products, acceptable supplement recommended
Sodium	0.5 gram	Table salt, meat, eggs, dairy products, carrots; no difficulty getting enough sodium; do not restrict without physician order
Vitamins	Fat- and water-soluble needed	Well-balanced diet with fruits and vegetables, whole grains; vitamin supplement often given but not mega vitamins because these can be associated with birth defects
Folic acid	4.0 mg	Dark green and leafy vegetables; should start increasing folic acid before getting pregnant to prevent neural tube defects

L. Endocrine:
 1. Increase in size and activity of thyroid
 2. Increase in size and activity of anterior lobe of pituitary
 3. Increase in size and activity of adrenal cortex

Emotional Adaptations to Pregnancy

A. Body image:
 1. Ambivalence about body changes
 2. Partner's attitudes may affect woman's reactions
B. Mood Swings:
 1. Emotional lability caused by hormone changes
 2. Ambivalence, anxiety or fear, ambivalence normal first trimester
 3. Acceptance of pregnancy comes at about 20 weeks or by quickening (when mother feels baby move)
C. Intimacy:
 1. Increased need for love and esteem
 2. Heightened sexual desire often occurs during second trimester.
 3. Sexual desire less during first trimester (nausea and fatigue) and third trimester (size)
 4. Husband may fear harming infant; alternate positions may help.

Developmental Tasks of Pregnancy

A. Maternal role:
 1. "I am pregnant." (Accepts biological fact)
 2. "I am going to have a baby." (Accepts fetus as distinct from self)
 3. "I am going to be a mother." (Prepares for birth and parenting)
B. Paternal role:
 1. "She is pregnant, and I am the father." (Accepts biological fact)
 2. "We are going to have a baby." (Accepts reality of pregnancy)
 3. "I am going to be a father. I know my role during the birth process." (Prepares for birth and parenting)
C. Sibling preparation, depends on age of child; should be prepared for new arrival and assured of parents' continuing love for him or her

Prenatal Care

A. Assessment; initial visit:
 1. Complete medical and obstetric history; includes gravida (number of pregnancies) and para (number of deliveries of viable-age fetuses)
 2. Lab work: CBC, blood type, Rh, serology, rubella titer
 3. Vital signs, weight, urine for protein and sugar

 4. Physical exam: fundal height, fetal heart rate, fetal activity
 5. Internal exam:
  a. Adequate pelvis
  b. Signs of pregnancy (first visit)
  c. Vaginal cultures for sexually transmitted diseases, pap test
 6. Psychosocial assessment
B. Ongoing assessments:
 1. Vital signs, weight, urine for protein and sugar
 2. Physical exam; fundal height, fetal heart rate, fetal activity
 3. Internal exam for cervical changes (signs of "ripe" cervix) during last few weeks
C. Nursing diagnoses (see Table 15.13)

Table 15.13 Nursing Diagnoses Related to Pregnancy

- Disturbed body image
- Deficient knowledge
- Anxiety related to fears
- Interrupted family processes
- Risk for impaired parenting
- Imbalanced nutrition, less than or more than body requirements
- Ineffective sexuality patterns

D. Teaching during pregnancy:
 1. Importance and frequency of checkups:
  a. Every month through month seven
  b. Every two weeks for month eight
  c. Then, every week
 2. Nutrition and weight gain:
  a. Recommend gain of 20–30 lbs.
   (1) 11 lb.: fetus, placenta, amniotic fluid
   (2) 2 lb.: uterus and breasts
   (3) 4 lb.: increased blood volume
   (4) 3 lb.: tissue fluid
   (5) 5 lb.: maternal stores
  b. Nutritional needs (see Table 15.12)
 3. Discomforts (see Table 15.14)
 4. Danger signs: to be reported to caregiver immediately:
  a. Bleeding
  b. Rupture of membranes
  c. Regular contractions occurring before due date
  d. Signs of pregnancy-induced hypertension:
   (1) Severe headaches
   (2) Visual disturbances
   (3) Swelling in face, hands
   (4) Epigastric pain
   (5) Decrease in urine output
  e. Burning upon urination
  f. Fever
  g. Severe, persistent vomiting
  h. Decrease in fetal activity
 5. Hygiene: important, increased leukorrhea; showers rather than tub baths late in pregnancy

Table 15.14 Discomforts of Pregnancy

Problem	Trimester	Nursing Care
Nausea and vomiting (due to increased HCG)	1	Offer small frequent meals and snacks; crackers and dry toast; avoid fatty, odorous foods
Urinary frequency (due to pressure on the bladder)	1, 3	Kegel exercises (alternately tightening and relaxing perineal muscles); wear sanitary pad PRN
Breast tenderness (due to increased levels of estrogen and progesterone)	1, 3	Wear a well-fitting support bra; don't use soap on nipples; teach nipple rolling exercises.
Leukorrhea (due to increased secretions)	1, 3	Wear cotton underwear, bathe often; avoid pantyhose, avoid douching; observe for signs of infection.
Heartburn (due to esophageal reflux)	2, 3	Small, frequent meals; avoid spicy, fried, fatty foods
Constipation (due to sluggish bowel and iron supplements)	2, 3	Increase fluid and fiber intake; exercise as tolerated; stool softener
Flatulence (due to sluggish intestine)	2, 3	Avoid gas forming foods; maintain normal bowel patterns
Hemorrhoids (due to constipation or increased venous pressure)	3	Avoid constipation; use ointments and creams, sitz baths; avoid tight-fitting underwear.
Backache (due to enlarged uterus causing an exaggerated lumbosacral curve)	3	Good alignment; wear comfortable shoes; pelvic rock exercises; sit upright
Shortness of breath (due to pressure on the diaphragm)	3	Elevate hands above head when supine.
Varicose veins (due to weight gain and venous stasis)	3	Avoid standing or sitting in one position for a long time; elevate hips when lying down or sitting; support hose
Edema of legs and feet (due to venous stasis)	3	Elevate feet when possible; avoid sitting or standing.
Fainting (due to postural hypotension)	3	Change position to left side to relieve pressure; change positions slowly.
Leg cramps (due to nerve pressure and decreased calcium)	3	Extend affected leg and flex ankle pushing upward; increase calcium.

6. Rest and exercise:
   a. Employment usually allowed unless teratogens involved or client has complications or is at risk for complications
   b. Exercise: usually good; no new sports or difficult routines
7. Drugs, smoking, alcohol:
   a. Nothing without permission of physician
   b. Smoking related to increased prematurity and small for gestational age (SGA) babies
   c. Alcohol: high blood alcohol levels related to fetal alcohol syndrome
8. Sexuality during pregnancy: need for adaptation with regard to positions; beware of "danger signs"
9. Preparation for childbirth and baby care:
   a. Childbirth classes: Lamaze, Bradley, and so on; purpose is to decrease fear, increase knowledge, conditioning, breathing, and relaxation exercises
   b. Parenting classes: includes specific how-to's, attitudes, introduce support groups

Assessment of Fetal Well-Being

A. Fetal growth:
   1. Maternal weight gain—20 to 30 lbs.
   2. Fundal height: McDonald's method 20–31 weeks correlates with 20–31 cm.

B. Antepartal testing:
   1. Fetal movement count by mother; kick counts
   2. Sonogram: sound and echo patterns used to identify structures within the body; can tell size of fetus, fetal anomalies, sex, growth patterns; very safe procedure
   3. Non-stress test:
      a. Reactive: three periods of movement with increased heart rate at least 10 BPM
      b. Non-reactive: no movement or no acceleration; indicates problems
   4. Nipple stimulation or contraction stress test (oxytocin challenge test): oxytocin given until three good uterine contractions within a 10-minute period; monitor observed for deceleration (decrease in fetal heart rate) pattern
      a. Negative: adequate placental functioning
      b. Positive: late decelerations; poor placental functioning; fetus at risk
   5. Biophysical profile: collection of data on fetal breathing movements, body movements, muscle tone, reactive heart rate, and amniotic fluid volume; used to identify fetuses at risk for asphyxia
   6. L/S ratio: uses amniotic fluid to determine fetal lung maturity by measuring amounts of lecithin and sphingomyelin; ratio of 2:1 indicates less chance of developing

respiratory distress syndrome; 2:1 level usually reached by 35–36 weeks
7. Amniocentesis: location and aspiration of amniotic fluid for examination; can be done after forth week; identifies chromosomal aberrations, sex, levels of alphafetoprotein, and other chemicals indicative of neural tube defects and inborn errors of metabolism, gestational age, Rh factor

ANTEPARTAL COMPLICATIONS

Risk Factors for Antepartal Complications

The antepartal client should be assessed for factors known to increase maternal or fetal risk during pregnancy.

A. Age:
   1. Younger than 18 and older than 35 years
   2. Prone to complications of pregnancy such as PIH and to fetal problems; increase in Down's syndrome in babies born to older women
B. Multiparity (over 4):
   1. Prone to pregnancy complications
   2. At risk for labor and delivery complications
C. Over- or underweight
D. Drug and alcohol abuse increase the risk of fetal developmental problems.
F. Smoking increases the risk for low birth weight babies and babies with developmental difficulties, such as attention deficit hyperactivity disorder.
G. Previous blood transfusions increase the risk of HIV and hepatitis infections.
H. Lack of prenatal care increases the risk of both maternal and fetal complications.
   1. Poverty increases risk of complications due to poor nutritional status and lack of prenatal care.
   2. Women who are uneducated, unmarried, and/or have an unwanted pregnancy are at risk because they often lack adequate prenatal care.
I. Difficulty conceiving may increase the risk for difficulty carrying the pregnancy to term.
J. Pre-existing maternal medical problems increase the risk to mother and possibly the fetus during pregnancy.

Cardiac Problems

A. May be the result of congenital heart defects or a result of rheumatic fever resulting in heart disease

B. Classification of cardiac problems:
   1. Class I: known cardiac disease with no limitation in activity
   2. Class II: slight limitation in activity
   3. Class III: considerable limitation of activity; even ordinary activity produces symptoms
   4. Class IV: symptoms of cardiac insufficiency even at rest
C. Major dangers:
   1. Increased cardiac workload during pregnancy can cause congestive heart failure (CHF)
   2. Greatest maternal danger from CHF
      a. Blood volume peaks at end of second trimester
      b. During labor: 20% increase in blood volume due to milking effect of contractions
      c. During delivery: sudden increase in blood volume when uterus contracts fully at birth and after placenta
D. Prenatal care
   1. Assessment findings:
      a. Signs of cardiac decompensation, particularly when blood volume peaks at weeks 28–32
      b. Shortness of breath
      c. Cough and dyspnea
      d. Edema
      e. Heart murmurs
      f. Palpitations
      g. Rales
   2. Nursing diagnoses (see Table 15.15)
   3. Nursing care: prenatal:
      a. Prevent infection; teach client to report signs of infection.
      b. Provide high-protein diet; restrict weight gain.
      c. Check for anemia.
      d. Anticoagulant therapy must be heparin (coumadin is teratogen).
      e. Promote adequate rest.
      f. Monitor vital signs.
   4. Nursing care: labor and delivery:
      a. Avoid frequent changes of position; keep head of bed in low semi-Fowler's position.
      b. Avoid pain; epidural anesthesia used for vaginal delivery.

Table 15.15 Nursing Diagnoses Related to Cardiac Conditions During Pregnancy

- Decreased cardiac output
- Fluid volume excess
- Risk for impaired gas exchange
- Risk for impaired fetal gas exchange
- Activity intolerance
- Deficient knowledge
- Fear

c. Avoid cesarean section (more stress); forceps may be used to shorten second stage.
   d. Monitor vital signs q 15 min. or more frequently if needed.
   e. Administer oxygen and pain medication as ordered.
   f. ECG, fetal monitor, oxygen
   g. Monitor the IV carefully.
5. Nursing care: postpartum:
   a. Critical time first 48 hours after delivery; CHF may develop during diuresis period
   b. At greater risk for hemorrhage because pitocin not usually used
   c. Intake and output
   d. Antiembolism stockings to prevent clot formation
   e. Prophylactic antibiotics may be given to prevent infections.
   f. Breastfeeding allowed, will need help with baby and home after discharge

Diabetes Mellitus

A. Types:
   1. Type 1 (insulin dependent); pre-existing diabetes
   2. Type 3: (gestational); onset during pregnancy, reversal at termination of pregnancy
B. Pathophysiology:
   1. Maternal insulin does not cross placenta; by 12 weeks, fetus makes insulin; does not affect maternal blood sugar level
   2. Interaction of estrogen, progesterone, HCS/human placental lactogen (HPL) (one hormone with two names), and cortisol raise maternal resistance to insulin (ability to use glucose at the cellular level)
   3. If pancreas cannot respond by producing additional insulin, excess glucose moves across placenta to fetus, where fetal insulin metabolizes it and acts as growth hormone, producing a large baby
   4. First trimester fetus draws large amounts of glucose for growth; maternal insulin needs decrease
   5. Second and third trimesters: anti-insulin effect of hormones may increase insulin needs to 100–200 units/day
C. Nursing diagnoses (see Table 15.16)
D. Nursing care: prenatal:
   1. Monitor closely; seen by obstetrician every 1–2 weeks
   2. Home glucose monitoring; often long-acting and sliding-scale insulin
E. Nursing care: labor and delivery:
   1. Assess infant for maturity and well being by amniocentesis, stress and non-stress testing, and estriol levels.

Table 15.16 Nursing Diagnoses Related to Diabetes in Pregnancy

- Deficient knowledge
- Imbalanced nutrition
- Risk for impaired adjustment
- Risk for infection
- Risk for fetal injury

   2. Cesarean section after 38 weeks if any changes in above
   3. May go to term if all prenatal tests within acceptable limits
F. Nursing care: postpartum:
   1. Regulate insulin.
   2. Assess the infant for hypoglycemia.
   3. Assess for infection.
   4. May breastfeed
G. Complications:
   1. Polyhydramnios
   2. Greater incidence of fetal anomaly
   3. Pregnancy-induced hypertension
   4. Hypo- and hyperglycemia; acidosis dangerous to fetus

Hyperemesis Gravidarum

A. Cause is probably hormonal; occurs frequently with hydatidiform mole, multiple pregnancy
B. Nursing diagnoses (see Table 15.17)

Table 15.17 Nursing Diagnoses Related to Hyperemesis Gravidarum

- Deficient fluid volume related to excessive gastric losses and reduced intake
- Imbalanced nutrition, less than body requirements related to inability to ingest/digest/absorb nutrients (prolonged vomiting)
- Risk for ineffective individual coping

C. Interventions:
   1. Maintain fluid and electrolyte balance; intake and output
   2. NPO, I.V., slowly resume foods on anti-nausea regime
   3. Decrease stress; provide emotional support.

Polyhydramnios (Excessive Amniotic Fluid)

A. Causes:
   1. Maternal diseases: pregnancy-induced hypertension, diabetes
   2. Fetal anomaly (esophageal atresia)
   3. Erythroblastosis
   4. Multiple pregnancies
B. Interventions:
   1. Relieve pressure by amniocentesis or delivery.

2. Check the baby carefully for anomalies.
3. Post partum: monitor closely because there is a greater risk of hemorrhage relating to the uterus having been over-distended

Abortion (Expulsion of Fetus Before Age of Viability; Spontaneous or Induced)

A. Causes:
1. Abnormality of fetus or placenta (most common cause)
2. Infection
3. Abnormality of reproductive tract
4. Injury
B. Types:
1. Threatened: slight bleeding, cramping, intervention may prevent abortion
2. Inevitable: bleeding, rupture of membranes, cervical dilation, contractions, abortion cannot be avoided
3. Complete: when abortion occurs, all products of conceptions are expelled
4. Incomplete: when abortion occurs, parts are retained; may need oxytocic or D&C
5. Missed: fetal death, but products are retained; may develop infection or DIC
6. Habitual: aborts three or more pregnancies in succession
7. Therapeutic: termination of a pregnancy by medical intervention
8. Criminal: abortion done outside medical facilities, against the law (abortion under medical supervision in first trimester is legal in the U.S.; under certain circumstances in some states, second trimester abortions are legal if done in a hospital)
C. Assessment findings:
1. First trimester bleeding
2. Cramping
D. Nursing diagnoses (see Table 15.18)
E. Interventions:
1. Bed rest with increased fluids to decrease uterine activity
2. Save all pads and any tissue passed.
3. Observe for shock, infection, DIC, or thrombophlebitis.
4. RhoGam if Rh negative
5. Emotional support; do not give false encouragement

Table 15.18 Nursing Diagnoses Related to Abortion
- Deficient fluid volume related to excessive blood loss
- Anxiety related to changes in health status of fetus/self, threat of death
- Deficient knowledge
- Grieving related to perinatal loss
- Risk for ineffective sexuality patterns

Ectopic Pregnancy

Pregnancy that occurs outside the uterus, usually in the tube

A. Causes:
1. Malformation of tubes
2. Narrowing or blockage of tubes; often from infection or PID
3. Tumors
4. Adhesions
B. Assessment findings:
1. Spotting
2. Low HCG levels
3. Sharp abdominal pain/rupture of tube
4. Unilateral pelvic mass
5. Shock
6. Sonogram shows empty uterus, may show mass
C. Nursing diagnoses (see Table 15.19)

Table 15.19 Nursing Diagnoses Related to Ectopic Pregnancy
(In addition to diagnoses related to abortion)
- Acute pain related to distention/rupture of fallopian tube

D. Interventions:
1. Surgery: salpingectomy (removal of tube)
2. Prevent shock; transfusion
3. Routine post-op care
4. Emotional support (can get pregnant with one tube removed; at greater risk for a second tubal pregnancy)

Hydatidiform Mole

The fertilized ovum degenerates and the chorionic villi change into a mass of clear, fluid-filled, grape-like vesicles.

A. Cause is unknown; more common in the orient; most common in women over 40
B. Assessment findings:
1. Uterus larger than expected for gestational age
2. High HCG levels increase symptoms of early pregnancy, such as nausea and vomiting
3. Bleeding; spotting to profuse after twelfth week
4. Passing grapelike clusters through the vagina
5. Symptoms of preeclampsia earlier than usual (before 24th week)
6. No fetal heart sounds or palpation of fetal parts
7. No fetal skeleton on ultrasound
C. Nursing diagnoses (see Tables 15.17 and 15.18)
D. Interventions:
1. Surgical removal: D&C or hysterotomy, hysterectomy often in women over 40

2. Usual post-op care
3. Contraception for at least one year following so that HCG levels can be monitored
4. Close medical follow-up for HCG levels; choriocarcinoma may occur after molar pregnancy
5. Emotional support for loss

Pregnancy-Induced Hypertension

Vasospastic hypertension occurring during pregnancy; usually onsets between 20th and 24th weeks and disappears after pregnancy completed; occurs in 5%–7% of all pregnant women

A. Risk factors:
  1. Incidence higher in primigravidas
  2. Multiple pregnancies
  3. Diabetes
  4. Hydatidiform mole
  5. Poor nutrition
  6. Essential hypertension
  7. Familial tendency
  8. Very young and very old obstetrically
B. Mild Preeclampsia
  1. Assessment findings:
    a. Three cardinal symptoms: proteinuria, hypertension, edema; must have two of three
    b. Proteinuria: 300 mg/liter in a 24-hour specimen (+1)
    c. Hypertension: over 140/90 or increase of 30 systolic/15 diastolic over base on two consecutive occasions at least six hours apart
    d. Oliguria
    e. Edema in upper part of body, hands, and face
    f. Excessive weight gain in short period of time (+3 lb/month in second trimester; +1 lb/week in third trimester; or +4.5 lb/week at any time)
  2. Nursing diagnoses (see Table 15.20)
  3. Interventions:
    a. Promote bed rest as long as signs of edema or proteinuria are minimal; left side usually recommended

Table 15.20 Nursing Diagnoses Related to Pregnancy-Induced Hypertension

- Deficient fluid volume (isotonic) related to plasma protein loss
- Ineffective renal tissue perfusion related to decreased blood flow (vasoconstriction) to kidney and relative hypovolemia
- Impaired fetal gas exchange related to vasospasm and relative hypovolemia
- Imbalanced fetal nutrition related to perfusion and relative hypovolemia
- Deficient knowledge
- Risk for injury may be related to loss of consciousness during seizure

b. Well-balanced diet with adequate protein and roughage
c. Frequent physician visits; once or twice a week
d. Monitor blood pressure
e. Symptoms may appear up to 48 hours postpartum
C. Severe preeclampsia:
  1. Assessment findings:
    a. Headaches, visual disturbances
    b. Epigastric pain (impending convulsion)
    c. Blood pressure of 150–160/100–110 mm Hg
  2. Nursing diagnoses (see Table 15.20)
  3. Interventions:
    a. Goal is to prevent seizures and to deliver as mature an infant as possible
    b. Monitor vitals, daily weight, edema, protein in urine, and fetal vital signs.
    c. Diet: high in protein, adequate fluid intake, no sodium restriction unless ordered
    d. Bed rest; lie on left side to increase placental perfusion
    e. Input and Output
    f. Seizure precautions:
      (1) Restrict visitors.
      (2) Minimize all stimuli.
      (3) Monitor for hyperreflexia.
      (4) Administer sedatives as ordered.
    g. Suction and O_2 at bedside
    h. Magnesium sulfate ($MgSO_4$) given IM or IV
      (1) $MgSO_4$ is a CNS depressant given to prevent seizures and lower blood pressure.
      (2) Before giving or hourly if continuous drip:
        (a) Check respirations; do not give if less than 14
        (b) Monitor urine output; should be at least 30 cc/hr
        (c) Check reflexes before giving and at intervals after (loss of knee jerk reflex indicates toxicity)
        (d) Calcium gluconate (antidote for $MgSO_4$ toxicity) at bedside
      (3) $MgSO_4$ may slow contractions; client may need pitocin.
      (4) Watch for precipitous delivery and abruptio placenta.

Placenta Previa

A. Placenta attaches low in the uterus, either near or covering the cervical os
B. Causes uncertain but occurs more often in older mothers (over 35) and multiparity
C. Types:
  1. Complete: completely covers os

2. Partial: partial covering of os; cesarean delivery usually recommended if 30% or more of cervical os is covered
3. Low lying: near cervical os
D. Assessment findings:
   1. Painless, bright red bleeding after the seventh month
   2. Bleeding sometimes intermittent
   3. Sonogram shows placental placement
E. Nursing diagnoses (see Table 15.21)

Table 15.21 Nursing Diagnoses Related to Placenta Previa

- Risk for deficient fluid volume
- Impaired fetal gas exchange related to altered placental blood flow
- Fear related to threat of death to self or fetus
- Risk for deficient diversional activity related to activity restrictions

F. Interventions:
   1. Bed rest if partial or low lying
   2. Immediate C-section if heavy bleeding and complete
   3. Transfusion if severe bleeding
   4. Observe for hemorrhage; count pads, check vitals, and FHR.
   5. Emotional support
   6. No vaginal exams; can result in severe bleeding

Abruptio Placenta

A. Premature separation of the placenta from part or all of the normal implantation site; usually occurs after 20th week of pregnancy
B. Cause is essentially unknown but seen more frequently in women with hypertension, previous abruptio placentas, late pregnancies, and multigravidas
C. Assessment findings:
   1. Bleeding: either concealed or apparent; signs of shock
   2. Board-like abdomen, severe pain, tenderness, lack of contractions
   3. Bradycardia or absence of fetal heart rate (utero-placental insufficiency)
   4. Late decelerations
D. Nursing diagnoses (see Table 15.22)

Table 15.22 Nursing Diagnoses Related to Abruptio Placenta

- Deficient fluid volume related to excessive blood loss
- Impaired fetal gas exchange related to altered placental blood flow
- Fear related to threat of death to self or fetus
- Acute pain related to collection of blood between uterine wall and placenta

E. Interventions:
   1. Immediate cesarean section

2. Treat for blood loss and shock; monitor urine output.
3. Assess for DIC, infection, and anemia.
4. Provide support for the parents; outlook for the baby is poor.

Adolescent Pregnancy

A. Increased risk of complications due to immaturity of maternal system (especially under age 15)
   1. Prematurity
   2. Low birth weight
   3. Pregnancy-induced hypertension
   4. Cesarean section
   5. Poor socioeconomic adjustment
B. Nursing diagnoses (see Table 15.23)

Table 15.23 Nursing Diagnoses Related to Adolescent Pregnancy

- Interrupted family processes related to situational/developmental transition
- Social isolation related to alterations in physical appearance
- Disturbed body image/self esteem related to situational/maturational crisis, and biophysical changes
- Also see Table 15.12 Nursing Diagnoses Related to Pregnancy.

C. Interventions:
   1. Emphasis on developmental needs of adolescent
   2. Nutrition
   3. Decision making: adoption, keeping infant

Stillbirth/Neonatal Loss

A. Important for parents to be involved in decisions such as whether to be on O.B. or GYN floor
B. Better to see and hold infant; helps bring closure
C. Need to grieve for this baby; no reassurances like "there will be others"

Sample Questions

1. A 21-year-old married woman thinks she may be pregnant. She goes to her physician and tells the nurse that the drugstore test was positive for pregnancy. She asks the nurse if the test is reliable. What is the best response for the nurse to make?
   1. "The tests are quite reliable. In order to be sure you are pregnant, I need to get some more information from you."
   2. "The tests are less reliable than the one the doctor does. We will have to repeat it."
   3. "Those kits are not very reliable. Your doctor should make the diagnosis."
   4. "They are very reliable. You can be sure you are pregnant."

2. The nurse is assessing a woman who thinks she may be pregnant. Which information from the client is most significant in confirming the diagnosis of pregnancy?
   1. She is experiencing nausea before bedtime and after meals.
   2. The client says she has gained six pounds and her slacks are tight.
   3. She has noticed it is difficult to sleep on her "stomach" because her breasts are tender.
   4. The client has a history of regular menstrual periods since age 13, and she has missed her second period.

3. After her examination by the physician, the antepartal client tells the nurse the doctor said she had positive Chadwick's and Goodell's signs. She asks the nurse what this means. What is the best response for the nurse to make?
   1. "Chadwick's sign is a dark blue coloring of the vagina and cervix. Goodell's sign is softening of the cervix of the uterus."
   2. "These help to confirm pregnancy. They refer to color changes and changes in the uterus caused by increased hormones of pregnancy."
   3. "Those are medical terms. You don't need to be concerned about them."
   4. "It refers to changes that occasionally happen in pregnancy but are unlikely to cause problems."

4. An antepartal client asks when her baby is due. Her last menstrual period was August 28. Using Naegele's rule, calculate the EDC (estimated date of confinement).
   1. May 21
   2. May 28
   3. June 4
   4. June 28

5. In establishing a teaching plan for a client who is in the first trimester of pregnancy, the nurse identifies a long list of topics to discuss. Which is most appropriate for the first visit?
   1. Preparation for labor and delivery
   2. Asking the woman what questions and concerns she has about parenting
   3. Nutrition and activity during pregnancy
   4. Dealing with heartburn and abdominal discomfort

6. When a woman in early pregnancy is leaving the clinic, she blushes and asks the nurse if it is true that sex during pregnancy is bad for the baby. What is the best response for the nurse to make?
   1. "The baby is protected by his sac. Sex is perfectly alright."
   2. "It is unlikely to harm the baby. What you do with your personal life is your concern."
   3. "In a normal pregnancy, intercourse will not harm the baby. However, many women experience a change in desire. How are you feeling?"

4. "Intercourse during pregnancy is usually alright, but you need to ask the doctor if it is acceptable for you."

7. The doctor told a pregnant woman to eat a well-balanced diet and increase her iron intake. She says, "I hate liver. How can I increase my iron?" What is the best response for the nurse to make?
   1. "Although liver is a good source of iron, beets, poultry, and milk are also good sources."
   2. "Many people dislike liver. Red meats, dark green vegetables, and dried fruits are also good sources of iron."
   3. "You should eat liver as it is the best source of iron. There are lots of ways to disguise the taste."
   4. "You can eat almost anything you like because your prenatal vitamins have all the vitamins and minerals needed for a healthy pregnancy."

8. The nurse is teaching a prenatal class. A woman in the class who is eight months pregnant asks why her feet swell. The nurse includes which of the following information in the answer?
   1. Swollen feet during pregnancy can indicate a serious problem.
   2. The enlarging baby reduces venous return, causing retention of fluid in the feet and ankles.
   3. Swelling of the feet during pregnancy is usually related to pregnancy-induced hypertension.
   4. Swelling of the feet during pregnancy is due to the increased blood volume and will disappear after delivery.

9. A woman who is at about six weeks gestation asks if she can listen to the baby's heart beat today. What should be included in the nurse's reply?
   1. The heart is not beating at six weeks.
   2. The heart is formed and beating but is too weak to be heard with a stethoscope.
   3. The heart beat can be heard with an electronic fetoscope.
   4. The heart does not start beating until 20 weeks gestation.

10. A woman who is in early pregnancy asks the nurse what to do about her "morning sickness." What should the nurse include in the reply?
   1. Eating a heavy bedtime snack containing fat helps to keep nausea from developing in the morning.
   2. Eating dry crackers before getting out of bed may help.
   3. Drinking liquids before getting up in the morning helps relieve nausea.
   4. The doctor can prescribe an antiemetic if she has had three or more vomiting episodes.

11. A woman who is 38 weeks gestation tells the nurse that she sometimes gets dizzy when she lies down. Which information is it important for the nurse to give the client?
    1. This is a sign of a serious complication and should be reported to the physician whenever it occurs.
    2. Try to sleep in an upright position on your back to prevent the dizziness.
    3. Try lying on your left side rather than on your back.
    4. Sleeping on your back with several pillows should help.

12. The nurse asks the newly pregnant woman if she has a cat for which of the following reasons?
    1. Cats may suffocate new babies and should not be in the home when a baby arrives.
    2. Cat feces may cause toxoplasmosis, which can lead to blindness, brain defects, and stillbirth.
    3. If the mother gets scratched by a cat, the baby may develop heart defects.
    4. Cats are jealous of babies and may try to kill them during infancy.

13. The nurse is caring for a woman who is 30 weeks gestation and has gained 17 pounds during the pregnancy, has a blood pressure of 110/70, and she states that she feels warmer than everyone around her. Which interpretation of these findings is most correct?
    1. All of these findings are normal.
    2. Her weight gain is excessive for this point in pregnancy.
    3. The blood pressure is abnormal.
    4. She should be evaluated for a serious infection, because pregnant women are usually cooler than other people.

14. What should the nurse do to assess for a positive sign of pregnancy?
    1. Perform a pregnancy test on the woman's urine.
    2. Auscultate for fetal heart sounds.
    3. Ask the woman when she had her last menstrual period.
    4. Ask the woman if her breasts are tender.

15. An oxytocin challenge test is ordered for a woman who is 42 weeks pregnant. What should the nurse plan for in the care of this client?
    1. Place her in the supine position during the test.
    2. Keep her NPO before the test.
    3. Have her empty her bladder before the test.
    4. Prepare the client for the insertion of internal monitors.

16. A woman comes to the doctor's office for her routine checkup. She is 34 weeks gestation. The nurse notes all of the following. Which would be of greatest concern to the nurse?
    1. Weight gain of two pounds in two weeks
    2. Small amount of dependent edema
    3. Fetal heart rate of 155/minute
    4. Blood pressure of 150/94

17. A pregnant woman is admitted to the hospital. Her initial admitting vital signs are blood pressure 160/94; pulse 88; respirations 24; and temperature 98°F. She complains of epigastric pain and headache. What should the nurse do initially?
    1. Insert an indwelling catheter.
    2. Give Maalox 30 cc now.
    3. Contact the doctor stat with findings.
    4. Supportive care for impending convulsion

18. Magnesium sulfate is ordered for a client who is hospitalized for PIH. What effects would the nurse expect to see as a result of this medication?
    1. Central Nervous System depression
    2. Decreased gastric acidity
    3. Onset of contractions
    4. Decrease in number of bowel movements

19. A client with PIH asks the nurse, "When will I get over this?" What is the best response for the nurse to make?
    1. "Your disease can be controlled with medication."
    2. "After your baby is born."
    3. "After delivery, you will need further testing."
    4. "You could have this condition for years."

20. A 40-year-old who is 28 weeks gestation comes to the emergency room with painless, bright-red bleeding of 1 1/2 hours duration. What condition does the nurse suspect this client has?
    1. Abruptio placenta
    2. Placenta previa
    3. Hydatidiform mole
    4. Prolapsed cord

21. A woman who is 28 weeks gestation comes to the emergency room with painless, bright-red bleeding of 1 1/2 hours duration. Which of the following would the nurse expect during assessment of this woman?
    1. Alterations in fetal heart rate
    2. Board-like uterus
    3. Severe abdominal pain
    4. Elevated temperature

22. A woman is admitted with suspected placenta previa. What test will be done to confirm the diagnosis?
    1. Internal exam
    2. Non-stress test
    3. Oxytocin challenge test
    4. Ultrasound

23. A pregnant 16-year-old asks the nurse if she should have an abortion. How should the nurse respond initially?
    1. "You should ask your parents for advice."
    2. "Abortion is the deliberate killing of a human being."
    3. "An abortion would let you finish growing up before you have children."
    4. "What are your feelings about abortion?"

24. A 25-year-old is four months pregnant. She had rheumatic fever at age 15 and developed a systolic murmur. She reports exertional dyspnea. What instruction should the nurse give her?
    1. "Try to keep as active as possible, but eliminate any activity which you find tiring."
    2. "Carry on all your usual activities, but learn to work at a slower pace."
    3. "Avoid heavy housework, shopping, stair climbing, and all unnecessary physical effort."
    4. "Get someone to do your housework, and stay in bed or in a wheelchair."

25. A pregnant woman comes for her sixth-month checkup and mentions to the nurse that she is gaining so much weight that even her shoes and rings are getting tight. What should the nurse plan to include in her care?
    1. Teaching about the food pyramid and the importance of a well-balanced diet
    2. Further assessment of her weight, blood pressure, and urine
    3. Encouraging the use of a comfortable walking shoe with a medium heel
    4. Reassurance that weight gain is normal as long as it does not exceed 25 pounds

Answers and Rationales

1. (1) The tests are quite reliable. They are based on the presence of HCG (human chorionic gonadotropin), which is secreted during pregnancy. Physician tests use the same principle. The nurse should take a history to confirm the results of the tests. The physician will examine the woman to help confirm the test results.

2. (4) Amenorrhea in an otherwise healthy woman of childbearing age is strongly suggestive of pregnancy. Nausea, weight gain, and tender breasts are all presumptive signs but are not as significant as amenorrhea.

3. (2) This answer is most appropriate to give the client. Answer 1 is a true statement but uses vocabulary that is inappropriate for the client. These changes are normal changes and occur in most pregnancies. Answer 3 is a real put-down to the client. Answer 4 is not correct. These are normal findings that help to confirm the diagnosis of pregnancy.

4. (3) Add nine months or take away three months and then add seven days. August 28 minus three months is May 28. Adding seven days would make it May 35. Since there are only 31 days in May, the days are carried into June—making June 4 the EDC. Answer 1 subtracts seven days instead of adding seven days. Answer 2 does not add seven days. Answers 3

and 4 subtract only 2 months instead of 3 months and do not add seven days.

5. (3) Nutrition and activity are important concerns from the first trimester onward. Labor and delivery is a third trimester concern, and parenting is of most concern in either the third trimester or post delivery. Heartburn and abdominal discomfort do not usually occur until the third trimester.

6. (3) Intercourse is not harmful during a normal pregnancy. This response recognizes the changes in libido which may occur during pregnancy and allows for the expression of feelings. Answer 1 is factual information but answer 3 allows the woman to express her feelings. The questions says "she blushes." This may indicate that the woman has concerns about sex. Answer 2 gives factual information but does not allow the woman to express her concerns. Answer 4 again does not give the woman a chance to discuss this with the nurse. The nurse should be able to answer this question.

7. (2) This answer recognizes that a dislike of liver is common and suggests good sources of iron. Answer 1 includes information that is not correct; milk contains no iron. Answer 3 has some correct information; liver is high in iron. It is also high in cholesterol. There are many other sources of iron. It is not necessary to eat liver to get iron in the diet. At one time, eating liver regularly was thought to be the best way to get iron. Answers 3 and 4 are not the best answers. Prenatal vitamins do contain iron. However, they should not be considered a substitute for a proper diet.

8. (2) The enlarging fetus presses on the veins returning fluid from the lower extremities, causing fluid retention. Swelling of the upper extremities or face may indicate pregnancy-induced hypertension. There is an increased blood volume during pregnancy, but this does not by itself cause swelling in the lower extremities.

9. (2) The heart chambers are formed and the heart is beating by four weeks gestation. However, it can not be heard even with a fetoscope. Answer 1 is incorrect. The heart is beating by four weeks. Answer 3 is not correct. It cannot be heard at this time. Answer 4 is incorrect. The heart rate will be audible with a standard fetoscope by 20 weeks, but it has been beating since about four weeks.

10. (2) Eating dry carbohydrates in the morning before rising often helps. The woman should avoid fatty foods and those with strong odors. Drinking liquids in the morning usually makes morning sickness worse, not better. Antiemetics are not prescribed because of the possible teratogenic effect on the developing embryo.

11. (3) Dizziness when lying on the back suggests that she may have vena caval syndrome—pressure on the vena cava from the enlarged uterus and fetus that decreases venous return and causes the blood pressure to drop. Lying on the left side usually reduces pressure on the vena cava and prevents the drop in blood pressure and dizziness. Sleeping in an upright position on her back will cause vena caval syndrome. Sleeping on the back with several pillows is similar to answer 2, which was incorrect.

12. (2) Cats may become infected with toxoplasmosis, which if ingested by the mother can cause toxoplasmosis and can lead to neurological lesions causing blindness, brain defects, and death. Parents should be alert for safety with any pet, but cats do not suffocate new babies or try to kill them. It is not being scratched by a cat that is the biggest danger during pregnancy; it is the possibility of developing toxoplasmosis from the feces. Raw meat can also carry toxoplasmosis.

13. (1) All of these findings are within normal limits. Weight gain during the first trimester is usually 3–5 pounds. After that, the normal weight gain is around 12 ounces (3/4 of a pound) a week. Using these guidelines, her weight gain should be 16–18 lbs. Her blood pressure is well within normal limits, even though we are not given a baseline. Pregnant women have a high metabolic rate and usually feel warmer than everyone else.

14. (2) Fetal heart sounds, sonograms, and X-rays are positive signs of pregnancy. A positive pregnancy test is a probable sign of pregnancy. Amenorrhea and breast tenderness are presumptive signs of pregnancy.

15. (3) The mother should empty her bladder before oxytocin is given and contractions begin. It is not necessary to be supine; the head will be elevated. NPO is not essential. The monitor with an oxytocin challenge test is external, not internal.

16. (4) A B.P. of 150/94 is indicative of pregnancy-induced hypertension. Weight gain of a pound a week, slight dependent edema, and a fetal heart beat of 155 are all normal.

17. (4) Epigastric pain and headache suggest that a seizure is imminent. Supportive care to protect the client from injury is essential. An indwelling catheter may be inserted but only after the nurse assures that the client is safe should a seizure occur. The epigastric pain is most likely related to preeclampsia, not gastritis. The doctor should be notified, but the client should be made safe first.

18. (1) Magnesium sulfate is a central nervous system depressant. It is given to prevent seizures. Magnesium hydroxide gel is an antacid. Oxytocin is given to initiate contractions. Magnesium sulfate may decrease contractions. Magnesium sulfate does not cause constipation. Some laxatives contain magnesium.

19. (2) Preeclampsia is pregnancy-induced hypertension and disappears shortly after the birth of the baby.

20. (2) Placenta previa is characterized by painless bleeding in the third trimester. Abruptio is characterized by abdominal pain and a rigid abdomen with or without obvious bleeding. Shock develops rapidly in placenta abruptio. Hydatidiform mole is characterized by severe nausea and vomiting and the passage of grapelike vesicles. Prolapsed cord often occurs when the membranes rupture and is not characterized by bleeding.

21. (1) The history suggests placenta previa. The baby may well develop fetal distress. A boardlike abdomen and severe pain are characteristic of abruptio placenta. Elevated temperature is not characteristic of placenta previa.

22. (4) A sonogram will show the position of the placenta in the uterus. An internal exam will probably not be done because it can cause severe bleeding when there is a placenta previa. The non-stress test and the oxytocin challenge test are done to see how the fetus responds to contractions.

23. (4) The nurse should initially encourage the client to formulate and express her thoughts and concerns. The nurse should not try to impose her/his values on the client as answers 2 and 3 do. Answer 1 tells the client what to do and is not appropriate for an initial response, although discussing the issue with her parents should be encouraged.

24. (3) The client reports exertional dyspnea. The answer relates to avoiding exertion or things requiring extra effort. The data do not suggest that it is necessary at this point to stay in bed or in a wheelchair. Answers 1 and 2 do not relate to the data, which includes exertional dyspnea.

25. (2) Her symptoms suggest pregnancy-induced hypertension; particularly significant is the fact that her rings are getting tight. Upper body edema is highly suggestive of PIH. The nurse should record her weight and note how much weight has been gained in the last month. Monitoring blood pressure for elevation and checking urine for protein will help to determine if this woman has PIH. Dietary teaching as described in answer 1 is important, but the action relating to the data in the question is assessment for PIH. The advice in answer 3 regarding a comfortable walking shoe is also appropriate for a pregnant woman but does not relate to the data in this question. More important than total weight gain is the pattern of weight gain. A sudden increase in weight gain may indicate fluid retention accompanying PIH, even if the total is not yet 25 or 30 lbs.

The Intrapartal Client

OVERVIEW OF NORMAL LABOR

Rhythmic contraction and relaxation of the uterine muscles with progressive effacement and dilation of the cervix, leading to expulsion of the products of conception

Passenger

A. Fetal head:
   1. Usually the largest part of the baby
   2. Bones of the head are joined by membranous sutures which allow for overlapping or molding during the birth process
   3. Biparietal diameter measures approximately 9.25 cm and is the part of the head that goes through the smallest diameter of the pelvis during normal delivery; molding decreases diameter
   4. Anterior and posterior fontanels are the intersection points of the sutures and are important landmarks during labor to determine the position of the fetus
      a. The anterior fontanel is larger, diamond-shaped, and closes at about 18 months of age.
      b. The posterior fontanel is smaller, triangular, and usually closes at about 2–3 months of age.
B. Fetal shoulders:
   1. Can be manipulated during labor to allow the passage of one shoulder at a time
   2. Shoulder dystocia may occur in large, post-date infants
C. Fetal lie: head to feet axis of baby in relation to mother:
   1. Longitudinal lie can be either cephalic (head first) or breech (bottom first) presentation
   2. Transverse lie: shoulder or arm presentation
D. Presentation: body part of passenger that enters pelvic passageway first:
   1. Cephalic: head is presenting part, usually vertex (occiput); most favorable for birth
   2. Breech: buttocks or lower extremities present first. Types are:
      a. Frank: thighs flexed with legs extending straight up; buttocks present
      b. Full or complete: thighs and legs flexed (baby in a squatting position); buttocks and feet present
      c. Footling: one or both feet present

   3. Shoulder: scapula is presenting part; baby in a horizontal or transverse lie; cesarean birth indicated
   4. Face presentation may be full face, brow, or chin (mentum); difficult to deliver vaginally; may need a cesarean delivery.
E. Attitude: relationship of fetal parts to one another:
   1. Flexion: normal fetal position and allows uncomplicated delivery
   2. Extension: neck extension causes chin, face, or brow to enter pelvis and complicates delivery
F. Position: part of baby in the pelvis and relationship to the left or right and anterior posterior axes of the mother
   1. Cephalic positions:
      a. Left occiput anterior (LOA): most common, occiput is in left anterior segment of mother's pelvis; face is down; favorable for delivery
      b. Left occiput transverse (LOT): occiput is turned directly toward mother's left side
      c. Left occiput posterior (LOP): occiput in left posterior segment of pelvis; face is up; mother has back discomfort during labor; rotation to anterior position usually occurs before delivery
      d. Right occiput anterior (ROA): occiput in right anterior segment of mother's pelvis; face is down; favorable for delivery
      e. Right occiput transverse (ROT): occiput is turned directly toward mother's right side
      f. Right occiput posterior (ROP): occiput in right posterior segment of pelvis; face is up; mother has back discomfort during labor; rotation to anterior position usually occurs before delivery
   2. Breech positions:
      a. Left sacral anterior
      b. Left sacral transverse
      c. Left sacral posterior
      d. Right sacral anterior
      e. Right sacral transverse
      f. Right sacral posterior
   3. Methods of assessing fetal position:
      a. Leopold's maneuvers: external palpation of maternal abdomen to determine baby's outline and thus the presentation and position
      b. Auscultation of fetal heart tones and determination of quadrant of maternal abdomen where FHT is best heard

c. Vaginal examination: determine location of sutures and fontanels and determine the relationship of the fetus to the maternal bony pelvis

Passage

Shape and measurement of maternal pelvis and distensibility of birth canal

A. Pelvis:
   1. False: helps support gravid uterus; true: bony canal composed of inlet, mid pelvis, and outlet
   2. Gyneroid shape most favorable for childbirth
   3. Station: relationship of presenting part to ischial spines:
      a. O station (engagement): presenting part at the level of the ischial spines; may occur two weeks before labor in primipara; usually occurs at beginning of labor in multipara
      b. When the presenting part is above ischial spines, station is written as a negative number; –1 through –5 with –5 being very high; an unengaged presenting part may be described as "high" or "floating"
      c. When presenting part is below the ischial spines, station is written as a positive number; + 1 through + 5 with + 5 being on the perineal floor
   4. Soft tissues: cervix, vagina, perineal floor stretches and dilates with force of contractions to accommodate passage of the fetus

Powers

Forces of labor acting together to expel the fetus and placenta

A. Uterine contractions (involuntary):
   1. Frequency: measured from beginning of one contraction to beginning of next contraction
   2. Duration: length of the contraction measured from the beginning to the end of the same contraction
   3. Intensity: strength of contraction; measured with fingertips lightly on fundus measuring the depressability of the uterus; described as mild (tense fundus but can be indented with fingertips), moderate (firm fundus, difficult to indent with fingertips), or strong (very firm fundus, cannot indent with fingertips)
   4. Regularity: discernible pattern of contractions; becomes better established as labor progresses

B. Voluntary bearing-down efforts:
   1. After full dilatation of the cervix, mother uses abdominal muscles to push and help expel the fetus; similar to bearing down for defecation
   2. Contraction of levator ani muscles

Psychologic Response

A woman who is relaxed and participating in the birth process usually has a shorter, less intense labor; maternal anxiety slows labor. Preparation for childbirth usually includes relaxation methods.

Mechanisms of Labor (Vertex Presentation)

A. Engagement: presenting part at ischial spines; head is fixed in the pelvis
B. Descent: constant; head keeps getting lower as it passes through the pelvis
C. Flexion: "attitude" of fetus, chin on chest, curled up in fetal position
D. Internal rotation: fetal skull rotates from transverse to anterior posterior at pelvic outlet and passes the midpelvis
E. Extension: fetal head extends and passes under symphysis pubis and is delivered occiput first, followed by face and chin
F. External rotation (restitution): head rotates back to full alignment on the same side as before for shoulder delivery
G. Expulsion: entire body delivered; this time is recorded as the time of birth

Onset of Labor

A. It is unknown how labor begins. Possibilities include hormonal changes, size, weight, and maturity of the infant, volume of uterus, competency of the cervix, and aging of the placenta.
B. Prodromal (False) versus True Labor (see Table 15.24)

Stages of Labor

A. First stage: from the onset of labor through complete dilatation of the cervix:
   1. Latent phase: from 0–4 cm
   2. Active phase: from 4–8 cm
   3. Transition phase: from 8–10 cm
B. Second stage: from complete dilatation of the cervix through delivery of the infant
C. Third stage: from the delivery of the infant through the delivery of the placenta
D. Fourth stage: from the delivery of the placenta until the mother is stable, usually 1–2 hours after delivery; this is an arbitrary time during which the vital signs should stabilize and any

Table 15.24 Prodromal (False) versus True Labor

Characteristic	Prodromal (False) Labor	True or Advancing Labor
Contractions	Irregular intervals; constant or irregular duration; constant or irregular intensity	Increasing frequency; increasing duration; increasing intensity Tending to become more regular in pattern
Cervix	Lack of cervical dilation or effacement (although many believe that Braxton Hicks contractions do efface)	Cervical effacement and dilatation
Presenting part	Fails to descend	Descends
Show	Absent	Present
Walking	Produces relief from contractions	Intensifies contractions
Other		Membranes frequently rupture

tendency for immediate hemorrhage should be controlled; a critical period for every mother

E. Cervical changes in first stage of labor:
 1. Effacement: shortening and thinning of the cervix
 2. Dilation: enlargement or widening of the cervical canal to 10 cm or complete dilation
 3. In primigravida, effacement usually well underway before dilation begins; in a multipara, effacement and dilation progress together

Duration of Labor

A. Average length of labor for primigravida:
 1. Stage one: 12–13 hours
 2. Stage two: 1 hour
 3. Stage three: 3–4 minutes
 4. Stage four: 1–2 hours
B. Average length of labor for multipara:
 1. Stage one: 8 hours
 2. Stage two: 20 minutes
 3. Stage three: 4–5 minutes
 4. Stage four: 1–2 hours

NURSING CARE DURING LABOR

Fetal Assessment

Auscultation

A. Auscultate fetal heart rate (FHR) every 15–30 minutes during first stage labor and 5–15 minutes during second stage labor.
B. Normal rate 120–160 with some variability
C. Best recorded during the 30 seconds immediately following a contraction

Electronic Fetal Monitoring

A. Continuous monitoring during labor of the FHR and uterine contractions (UC):
 1. External monitor is applied to the mother's abdomen; information is less precise; easier to apply; can be applied before membranes have ruptured; very little danger associated with use
 2. Internal monitor is applied by physician directly to the fetal presenting part; cervix must be dilated and membranes must be ruptured; precise information collected; sterile technique essential to reduce risk of intrauterine infection
B. Types of patterns:
 1. Variability: normal
 2. Early deceleration:
  a. Deceleration (slowing) of FHR begins early in contraction, stays within normal range, and returns to baseline by end of contraction.
  b. Thought to be caused by fetal head compressing against cervix
  c. Normal pattern
 3. Late deceleration:
  a. Deceleration of FHR begins late in contraction; exceeds 20 beats/minute; does not return to baseline by end of contraction
  b. Thought to be caused by uteroplacental insufficiency
  c. Ominous sign of fetal distress
  d. Change maternal position, administer oxygen, discontinue any oxytocin infusion, prepare for immediate delivery if pattern continues
 4. Variable deceleration:
  a. Onset of deceleration not related to uterine contraction with abrupt swings in FHR, usually with rapid return to baseline
  b. Thought to be caused by compression of the umbilical cord
  c. Change maternal position to relieve pressure on cord, administer oxygen if no improvement, discontinue oxytocin if infusing, prepare client for vaginal exam to assess for prolapsed cord
  d. If cord prolapsed, cesarean delivery is necessary

Maternal Care During Labor

Nursing Management of the First Stage of Labor (See Table 15.25)

Table 15.25 Phases of First Stage of Labor

Latent Phase	Active Phase	Transition Phase
Early labor Effacement phase 0–4 cm dilation Mother excited, anxious	Active labor Dilating phase 5–7 cm dilation Hard work; utilize breathing and relaxing techniques	8–10 cm dilation Most difficult time for mothers to cope
<u>Contractions</u> Mild, q 10–20 min. × 20–30 sec.	<u>Contractions</u> Mod., q 3–5 min. × 30–60 sec.	<u>Contractions</u> Intense, q 2–3 min. × 60-90 sec.; may have dual peak; increase in bloody show; irritable, nausea and vomiting; amnesia between contractions
<u>Time</u> 8–9 hrs nullipara 5–6 hrs multipara	<u>Time</u> nullipara dilates 1.2 cm/hr multipara dilates 2.5 cm/hr	<u>Time</u> nullipara 2 hrs multipara 1 hr

A. Admission:
1. Baseline data for vital signs, fetal heart rate
2. Onset and nature of contractions
3. Membranes; intact or ruptured, color of fluid
4. Cervical changes
5. When the woman last ate
6. Client's understanding of labor process
7. How client is responding to labor

B. Assessing progress in labor
1. Effacement: thinning and shortening of cervix:
   a. Expressed as 0 to 100%
   b. Primipara usually effaces first, then begins to dilate.
   c. Multipara effaces and dilates simultaneously.
2. Dilation: opening of cervix from 0–10 centimeters
3. Station
   a. –5 to –1 as head lowers
   b. 0 presenting part engaged
   c. +1 to +5 down to perineum
4. Membranes: ruptured or intact:
   a. Litmus test: acid-base; urine is acid (red color on litmus paper); amniotic fluid is alkaline (blue color on litmus paper)
   b. Fern test; dried amniotic fluid shows a fern-like pattern when viewed under the microscope
   c. If woman does not deliver within 24 hours of rupture of membranes, there is an increased risk of infection; baby needs to be isolated; mother watched for infection
   d. Meconium-stained amniotic fluid may be normal if baby is breech; otherwise, it indicates fetal distress.

5. Maternal vital signs:
   a. Temperature every four hours until membranes rupture, then every two hours
   b. Pulse and respirations every four hours and prn
   c. Blood pressure every half hour and prn
6. Fetal heart rate every 15 minutes; immediately after rupture of membranes

C. Nursing diagnoses (see Table 15.26)

Table 15.26 Nursing Diagnoses Related to Normal Labor

Stage	Nursing Diagnoses
1, 2	Deficient knowledge
1, 2	Impaired comfort related to uterine contractions
1, 2	Risk for ineffective coping, individual/couple
1	Deficient fluid volume related to NPO status during labor
1	Powerlessness
1, 2	Urinary retention related to decreased intake, mechanical compression of bladder, or effects of regional anesthesia
1, 2	Risk for impaired gas exchange for fetus
1, 2	Ineffective breathing pattern
1, 2	Impaired oral mucus membranes related to dehydration and mouth breathing
2	Increased cardiac output related to repeated, prolonged bearing down efforts
2	Risk for impaired skin/tissue integrity
2	Risk for fatigue

D. Nursing interventions
1. Positioning:
   a. Change frequently.
   b. Left lateral often encouraged to promote increased blood flow to uterus and kidneys
   c. Avoid supine position as it may cause hypotension (vena caval syndrome).
2. Touch/presence usually increases relaxation and decreases fear.

3. Hygiene: client has increased perspiration, bloody show, often loss of urine and feces
4. Keep bladder empty; full bladder slows descent of fetus
   a. Encourage client to void every 1–2 hours.
   b. Catheterize if bladder full and client unable to void
5. Breathing:
   a. Encourage client/couple to use breathing techniques learned in prepared childbirth classes.
   b. Help mother who has not taken childbirth classes breathe with contractions.
6. Pain management:
   a. Apply pressure to back prn; encourage breathing and visualization techniques learned in prenatal classes.
   b. Assist in the administration of agents for analgesia if ordered (see Table 15.27).
      (1) Central nervous system depressants such as sedatives and narcotics usually not given when delivery is expected within two hours because infant may have depressed respiratory effort at birth; remember: "if Mom is sleepy; baby will be sleepy"
      (2) Medications may be given IV and sometimes IM.
      (3) Monitor vital signs carefully after the administration of analgesic agents.
      (4) Mother must remain in bed with side rails up following administration of analgesic agents.
   c. Care for woman who has had anesthesia for labor and delivery (see Table 15.28):

      (1) Assess vital signs closely for maternal hypotension/fetal bradycardia.
      (2) Elevate head of bed if epidural used
      (3) Assess for pain relief.
      (4) Assess contractions regularly.

Nursing Management of Second Stage of Labor

A. During second stage labor, mother has intense, strong contractions every 2–3 minutes lasting 60 to 90 seconds; second stage should not last longer than one to two hours.
B. Assessment:
   1. Progress of descent
   2. Maternal and fetal vital signs
   3. Maternal pushing efforts
   4. Signs of imminent delivery:
      a. Vaginal distention
      b. Bulging of perineum
      c. Crowning
   5. Birth of baby
C. Nursing diagnoses (see Table 15.25)
D. Interventions:
   1. Encourage the father's participation in the delivery area.

Table 15.27 Analgesia Used in Labor

Drug	Purpose

Sedatives
  secobarbital (Seconal)
  pentobarbital (Nembutal)
  phenobarbital (Luminal)
	Relieve anxiety

Narcotics
  morphine
  meperidine (Demerol)
  Pentazocine (Talwin)
  nalbuphine HCl (Nubain)
	Pain relief

Narcotic antagonists naloxone (Narcan)	Reverse narcotic respiratory depression in mother or neonate

Analgesic potentiating drugs
  promethazine (Phenergan)
  promazine (Sparine)
  propiomazine (Largon)
  hydroxyzine (Vistaril)
	Raise analgesic effect without increasing amount of analgesic agent

Table 15.28 Anesthesia Used for Labor and Delivery

Type of Anesthesia	Comments

Inhalation
  methoxyflurane (Penthrane)
  nitrous oxide
	Administered by trained personnel only; observe mother for nausea and vomiting, uterine relaxation, and hemorrhage after delivery

Regional
  tetracaine (Pontocaine)
  lidocaine
  bupivacaine (Marcaine)
  mepivacaine (Carbocaine)
	Medication introduced to specific area to block pain impulses; always administered by trained personnel

Lumbar epidural Caudal	May be continuous or intermittent during labor or delivery; epidural very commonly used; usually given after 4 cm dilation to prevent slowing labor; no post-spinal headache
Saddle block, low spinal	Given when delivery is imminent; mother at risk for spinal headache; keep flat for 6–8 hours after delivery and encourage oral fluids to reduce headache
Peripheral nerve blocks paracervical	Used only in first stage of labor; causes fetal bradycardia; rarely used
pudendal	Medication administered transvaginally to block pudendal nerve; useful for delivery and episiotomy
perineal (local)	Injected into perineum during delivery for episiotomy

2. Prepare mother for delivery in birthing room, delivery chair, or by transferring to delivery room if needed.
3. Encourage pushing effort to promote descent of the infant.
   a. Position mother as directed: may be side lying, upright, on hands and knees, in delivery chair, in delivery bed, or on delivery table
   b. Encourage mother to work with natural urge to push by performing several sustained pushes (5–7 seconds) with each contraction
4. Clean the vulva and perineum in preparation for delivery.
5. Maintain fetal monitoring or monitor every five minutes when close to delivery.
6. Record the time of delivery.

Third Stage of Labor

A. Watch for signs of placental separation.
   1. Cord lengthening
   2. Increased bleeding
   3. Uterus contracts
B. Palpate fundus immediately after delivery of placenta; gently massage if not firm
C. Immediate care of neonate:
   1. A-B-C: airway, breathing, cardiac functioning
   2. Maintain clear airway with suctioning; position head down to promote drainage
   3. Clamp cord: plastic clamp to replace Kelly clamp; cut cord to stump or slightly longer if infant is high risk
   4. Provide warmth: overhead warmer, dry quickly to decrease heat loss by evaporation; place newborn on warm surfaces (mother) and cover cold surfaces such as the scale
   5. Resuscitate if needed.
   6. Apgar scoring at one minute and at five minutes (see Table 15.29):
      a. 7–10: good prognosis
      b. 4–6: depressed infant, fair prognosis
      c. 0–3: severely depressed, poor prognosis; requires intense resuscitation
   7. Identification, weight, measurement (foot prints, arm bands)

8. Promote bonding through early nursing if mother desires and infant is stable; have parents hold the newborn.
9. Eye prophylaxis: erythromycin or tetracycline to treat possible chlamydia or gonorrhea to prevent eye damage to newborn
10. Gross examination to detect obvious congenital anomalies
11. Aquamephyton (vitamin K) to prevent hemorrhagic disease of the newborn

Fourth Stage Management

A. Nursing diagnoses (see Table 15.30)
B. Assessment of fundus every 15 minutes:
   1. Fundus must remain firm; should be at or slightly above umbilicus

Table 15.30 Nursing Diagnoses Related to the Postpartal Period

- Acute pain related to tissue trauma, edema, muscular contractions
- Risk for deficient fluid volume
- Impaired urinary elimination related to physiological return to nonpregnant state
- Constipation related to decreased muscle tone associated with diastasis recti, dehydration, analgesia, anesthesia, pain
- Disturbed sleep pattern related to pain, intense excitement, anxiety
- Risk for interrupted family processes
- Disturbed body image
- Risk for impaired parenting
- Deficient knowledge
- Ineffective role performance

   2. If not firm, massage it.
   3. Methergine or pitocin may be ordered if fundus is not firm.
C. Assess lochia, perineum, blood pressure, and pulse every 15 minutes.
   1. Turn mother to side to assess lochia as pooling under buttocks may occur.
   2. Report if bleeding is excessive or if there is no bleeding (may be a clot in the uterus).
   3. Assess perineum, episiotomy for bleeding; apply ice as ordered.
   4. Report changes in blood pressure and pulse.

Table 15.29 Apgar Scoring

Category	0 points	1 point	2 points
Heart Rate	none	< 100	> 100
Respiratory Effort	none	slow, irregular	good cry
Muscle Tone	absent, limp	some flexion	active motion
Reflex Irritability	no response	grimace	active cry
Color	blue	body pink, extremities blue	all pink

D. Encourage mother to void; if unable to void, ask for catheterization order; measure first voiding.
E. Encourage attachment/bonding with infant; mother may breastfeed if desired.

COMPLICATIONS OF LABOR AND DELIVERY

Emergency Childbirth

A. Stay with mother.
B. Do not prevent birth of the baby.
C. Maintain sterile environment if possible; if not, as clean as possible.
D. Rupture membranes if not ruptured.
E. Have mother pant.
F. Support perineum and baby's head to prevent tearing of perineum and too rapid delivery of the head.
G. Feel for cord around neck; slip over the head if present.
H. Clear mucous from baby's nose and mouth.
I. Hold baby in head down position to promote drainage of secretions.
J. Keep baby warm and dry.
K. Place the baby on the mother's abdomen.
L. Do not cut the cord until sterile implements available.
M. Deliver placenta: signs of separation include gush of blood, lengthening of cord, and change in shape of uterus
N. Inspect the placenta for completeness; save the placenta.
O. Massage the uterus to prevent bleeding.
P. Put the baby to mother's breast to promote uterine contractions and facilitate bonding.
Q. Check the mother for fundal firmness and bleeding.

Dystocia

Prolonged or difficult labor

A. Causes:
1. Cephalo Pelvic Disproportion (C.P.D.) due to large baby, poor presentation such as shoulder, face, breech; small or unfavorably shaped pelvis; may require cesarean delivery
2. Full bladder may prevent descent of fetus; encourage mother to empty bladder; obtain catheterization order if needed.
3. Dysfunctional uterine contractions
   a. Hypertonic:
      (1) Strong contractions that have no effect on cervix; cervix does not dilate; mother becomes exhausted

(2) Sedate mother; try to "knock out" poor labor pattern.
(3) Never use pitocin.
b. Hypotonic, primary, or secondary:
   (1) Seen after prolonged labor, epidural, with over-distended uterus
   (2) Treated with oxytocin stimulation
      (a) Close monitoring of fetal heart tone
      (b) Infusion given piggyback by pump
      (c) If tetanic contraction, stop flow immediately

Breech Presentation

A. Usually delivered by cesarean section
B. Vaginal delivery of breech associated with increased risk of prolapsed cord and high fetal morbidity/mortality

Multiple Pregnancy

A. Increased risk especially for second and third babies
B. Increased likelihood of premature labor due to over-distended uterus
C. Uterine dystocia common due to over-distended uterus
D. Postpartum hemorrhage due to over-distended uterus

Premature Labor

A. Labor that occurs before 37 weeks:
1. Assessment of labor: distinguish false labor from true labor
2. Pharmacologic control:
   a. Ritodrine hydrochloride (Yutopar), terbutaline I.V. initially, then P.O.
   b. Observe for maternal hypotension, pulmonary edema, and tachycardia.
   c. Antidote is propranolol (Inderal).
   d. Magnesium sulfate may be used.
3. Betamethasone given to promote fetal lung maturity if delivery can be delayed 24 hours
4. Irreversible labor :
   a. Prepare for delivery of high risk infant.
   b. Need neonatologist and neonatal intensive care unit (NICU) to properly care for infant; mother may be transferred if the hospital is not equipped with NICU.

Induction of Labor

A. Indications include both maternal disease and fetal conditions such as fetal distress.

B. Methods include the artificial rupture of membranes (AROM) and administration of I.V. pitocin to stimulate uterine contractions.
C. Nursing management:
1. Close monitoring of fetal heart rate
2. Stop pitocin if contractions longer than 90 seconds or if fetal distress; potential for uterine rupture

Fetal Distress

A. Causes
1. Acute uteroplacental insufficiency:
   a. Excessive uterine activity associated with pitocin
   b. Maternal hypotension caused by epidural, vena caval compression, supine position, or internal hemorrhage
   c. Placental separation: abruptio, previa
2. Chronic uteroplacental insufficiency:
   a. Hypertensive diseases
   b. Diabetes
   c. Post maturity
3. Umbilical cord compression
B. Interventions:
1. Electronic fetal monitoring usually done
2. Report any abnormalities.
3. Labor may be induced or cesarean section may be performed if the baby's condition is not satisfactory.

Premature Rupture of Membranes (PROM)

A. Loss of amniotic fluid, prior to term, unconnected with labor
B. Dangers associated with this are a prolapsed cord, infection, and possible premature delivery.
C. Causes:
1. Chronic pyelonephritis
2. Incompetent cervix
3. Multiple pregnancy
4. History of premature births
5. Sepsis
6. Placental disorders
D. Interventions:
1. Bed rest
2. Maternal and fetal vital signs
3. Assess for signs of infection: q 2h temperatures; antibiotics and delivery indicated if infection present
4. Check for a prolapsed cord.
5. Ritodrine might be given to slow/prevent contractions.
6. Betamethasone (Celestone) is given to promote fetal lung development.
7. Emotional support
8. Delivery if near term or other complications present

Prolapsed Cord

A. Cord is in the vagina, ahead of the presenting part
B. Occurs when membranes rupture or with contractions that follow rupture of membranes
C. Associated with breech presentations and rupture of membranes before engagement
D. Emergency situation: if compression of the cord occurs, fetal hypoxia may result in central nervous system damage or death
E. Interventions:
1. Check FHT immediately after membranes rupture and again in five minutes.
2. Vaginal exam by RN or physician after membranes rupture to check for prolapsed cord; if cord prolapsed into vagina, push upward against presenting part to lift it off cord; do not remove hand from vagina
3. Trendelenburg or knee chest position for mother to keep fetal head away from cord
4. Oxygen
5. Prepare the mother for an immediate cesarean section.
6. If cord protrudes from vagina, cover with sterile gauze soaked in sterile normal saline; do not replace cord

Surgical Obstetrics

A. Episiotomy: incision into perineum, enlarges vaginal opening, speeds up second stage; prevents tearing
1. Types:
   a. Midline or median: most common, straight back toward rectum, least discomfort
   b. Mediolateral: 45 degrees to left or right, more painful, complication of dyspareunia; cuts through muscle
2. Degrees: episiotomy or lacerations:
   a. First degree: involves vaginal mucosa and skin perineum
   b. Second degree: into perineal body, involves levator ani muscle
   c. Third degree: entire perineum and into rectal sphincter
   d. Fourth degree: all the way through rectal mucosa
3. Interventions:
   a. Day of delivery, apply ice pack to perineum
   b. Sitz baths may be ordered after 24 hours.
B. Forceps delivery, vacuum extraction used when mother unable to push or need to speed up delivery
C. Cesarean delivery: delivery through abdominal incision
1. Maternal and fetal indications:
   a. CPD
   b. Previous c-section; vaginal birth after cesarean (VBAC) quite common

c. Fetal distress
d. Malpresentation such as breech, shoulder, face, brow
e. Maternal illness
f. Multiple births

2. Types (see Figure 15.5):
   a. Classical: vertical incision

Skin incision

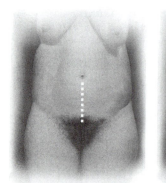

Vertical through skin

Uterine incision

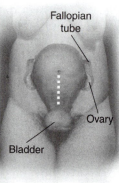

Fallopian tube

Ovary

Bladder

Vertical through uterus

A.

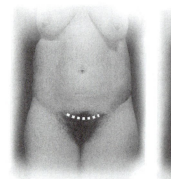

Horizontal through skin
(first skin crease under hairline)

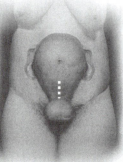

Vertical through lower
uterine segment

B.

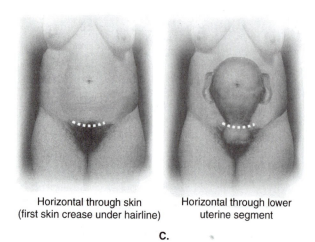

Horizontal through skin
(first skin crease under hairline)

Horizontal through lower
uterine segment

C.

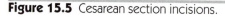

Figure 15.5 Cesarean section incisions.

b. Low transverse: fewer complications, less discomfort

3. Interventions:
   a. Cesarean section is abdominal surgery; care for woman is care of person with abdominal surgery plus postpartal care: lochia checks, fundal checks.
   b. Emotional support
   c. Vaginal birth after cesarean (VBAC) often successful if uterine incision was low transverse and reasons for initial cesarean are not still present (such as small maternal pelvis)

Sample Questions

1. A 23-year-old woman, G1 P0, is admitted to the labor room with contractions every five minutes lasting 45 seconds. Upon vaginal exam, she is noted to be completely effaced and 5 cm. dilated. Station is 0. She asks the nurse for pain medication. What is the best response for the nurse to make?
   1. "I'll ask your doctor for medication."
   2. "Can you hold out for a few more minutes? It's too soon for you to have medication."
   3. "Pain medication will hurt your baby. We would rather not give you any unless absolutely necessary."
   4. "Can your husband help you with your breathing techniques?"

2. After several hours of active labor, a woman says to the nurse, "I have to push. I have to push." What is the best initial response for the nurse to make?
   1. "Pull your knees up to your chest and hold on to them. Take a deep breath and push down as though you are having a bowel movement."
   2. "Let me have the RN examine you before you start to push."
   3. "That means the baby is coming. I'll take you into the delivery room now."
   4. "Women often feel that way during labor. Turn on your left side and you will be more comfortable."

3. A laboring woman is to be transferred to the delivery room. The nurse is positioning her on the table when she has a very strong contraction and starts to bear down. What should the nurse tell her to do?
   1. Pant
   2. Bear down strongly
   3. Put her legs up in the stirrups
   4. Ignore the contraction

4. A 32-year-old, G 2 P1 is admitted to the labor room. Her previous delivery was a normal, spontaneous vaginal delivery without complications. She has been having contractions for four hours at home. The registered nurse examines her and determines

that she is 4 cm. dilated and 70% effaced. The fetus is in the breech position. She calls for the nurse saying, "My water just broke!" What should the practical nurse do initially?
1. Notify the physician.
2. Do a vaginal exam.
3. Check the fetal heart rate.
4. Prepare for delivery.

5. The fetus is in the breech position. Inspection of the amniotic fluid after the membranes rupture shows a greenish-black cast to the fluid. What is the best interpretation of this finding?
   1. The baby is in acute distress.
   2. The fluid is contaminated with feces from the mother.
   3. The mother has diabetes mellitus.
   4. It may be normal since the baby is presenting breech.

6. A woman in labor does not continue to dilate. The physician decides to perform a cesarean section. A healthy 7 lb, 12 oz baby boy is delivered. What is the most essential nursing intervention in the immediate postpartum period?
   1. Check the fundus for firmness.
   2. Assess the episiotomy for bleeding.
   3. Assist the woman with accepting the necessity of having had a c-section.
   4. Encourage fluid intake.

7. A woman, G2 P2, who has just had an unexpected cesarean delivery asks the nurse if having a cesarean means that she can not have any more children. What is the best response for the nurse to give this mother?
   1. "Most women are able to have another child after having had a cesarean delivery."
   2. "Since you have two healthy children, it would be better not to attempt another delivery."
   3. "Is it important for you to have more children?"
   4. "That is a question you will have to discuss with your physician."

8. A 26-year-old, gravida 3, para 0, in early labor is admitted to labor and delivery. She is not sure if her membranes have ruptured. She has had some leakage of fluid. How should the nurse begin the assessment?
   1. "Tell me about your other labor experiences."
   2. "How old are your other children?"
   3. "Did you bring an example of the fluid that was leaking with you?"
   4. "Describe your contractions to me."

9. A woman, 38 weeks pregnant, arrives in the labor and delivery suite and tells the nurse that she thinks her membranes have ruptured. The nurse uses phenaphthazine (Nitrazine) paper to test the leaking fluid. The nurse expects the Nitrazine paper to turn which color if amniotic fluid is present?

1. Red
2. Orange
3. Blue
4. Purple

10. A 29-year-old gravida 1, para 0 woman is admitted to labor and delivery. She is three centimeters dilated, 80% effaced, and head at 0 station. She and her husband have been to prepared childbirth classes and are eager to give birth naturally. During her first contraction in the hospital, which lasts 30 seconds, the nurse observes the client using rapid pant-blow breathing. What is the most appropriate response for the nurse to make at this time?
    1. "Don't pant. It's too early in labor for panting."
    2. "Continue using pant-blow breathing until the RN checks to see if you are fully dilated."
    3. "Good. You are using your breathing from class. Keep it up."
    4. "What kinds of breathing techniques did you learn in childbirth class?"

11. The physician is performing an amniotomy on a woman in labor. What is the most important nursing action during this procedure?
    1. Assist the physician.
    2. Keep the mother informed.
    3. Monitor fetal heart tones.
    4. Encourage slow chest breathing.

12. The nurse is caring for a woman in labor who is having contractions every five to seven minutes that last 45–50 seconds. Her husband asks if this is transition because his wife is getting restless and irritable and feels pressure. What is the best response for the nurse to make?
    1. "Transition is still a long way off. Don't you remember this from your classes?"
    2. "Her contractions are not typical of transition, but I'll have the RN check her."
    3. "The contractions are typical of transition. You are very observant."
    4. "It's impossible to tell where she is without doing an exam."

13. As labor progresses, a client becomes increasingly irritable with her husband, complaining of lower back pain and fatigue. What is the most appropriate response for the nurse to make?
    1. Have the client turn on her side and give her a back rub.
    2. Ask the client if she would like the doctor to give her something for the discomfort.
    3. Reassure the husband that irritability is normal now and teach him to apply pressure to his wife's lower back.
    4. Encourage the client to try and get some rest and ask her husband if he would like to take a coffee break.

14. An epidural block is ordered for a woman in labor. Which nursing action is essential because the client has epidural anesthesia?
    1. Monitoring the uterus for uterine tetany
    2. Giving oxytocin to counteract the effect of the epidural in slowing contractions
    3. Having the woman lie flat in bed to avoid post-anesthesia headache
    4. Monitoring blood pressure for possible hypotension

15. The nurse is positioning a laboring woman who has not reached the transition phase. The nurse should avoid placing her in the supine position because the supine position has which effect?
    1. It increases gravitational forces and prolongs labor.
    2. It causes decreased perfusion of the placenta.
    3. It may impede free movement of the symphysis pubis.
    4. It frequently leads to transient episodes of hypertension.

16. A woman in labor is experiencing very strong contractions every two to three minutes, lasting 60–75 seconds. She complains of a severe backache and is irritable. The best interpretation of these data is that the woman is in which stage/phase of labor?
    1. Early first stage of labor
    2. Transition phase of labor
    3. Late second stage of labor
    4. Early third stage of labor

17. A woman who is completely dilated is pushing with contractions. After 30 minutes of pushing, the baby is still at 0 station. What is the most appropriate nursing action at this time?
    1. Assess for a full bladder.
    2. Prepare for a cesarean delivery.
    3. Monitor fetal heart tones.
    4. Turn the mother to her left side.

18. Which nursing action has the highest priority for a client in the second stage of labor?
    1. Help the mother push effectively.
    2. Prepare the mother to breastfeed on the delivery table.
    3. Check the fetal position.
    4. Administer medication for pain.

19. A woman, gravida 5 para 4, is unable to get to the hospital since labor has progressed very rapidly. The nurse, who lives upstairs, comes down to assist her with the emergency home delivery. The nurse examines the woman and assesses that the perineum is bulging. What is the priority nursing measure at this time?
    1. Encourage the woman to pant during the contraction.
    2. Place a clean sheet under the perineal area.
    3. Accurately time the contractions.
    4. Contact the physician by phone for instructions.

20. During an emergency home delivery, the head is beginning to crown. What is the most appropriate action for the nurse to take at this time?
    1. Instruct the mother to push down vigorously.
    2. Press down on the fundus to expel the baby.
    3. Apply gentle perineal pressure to prevent rapid expulsion of the head.
    4. Direct the mother to take prolonged deep breaths to improve fetal oxygenation.

21. What is the most common complication associated with too rapid delivery in precipitate labor?
    1. Pitting edema of the baby's scalp
    2. Dural or subdural tears in fetal brain tissue
    3. Premature separation of the placenta
    4. Prolonged retention of the placenta

22. The nurse has just completed emergency delivery of a term infant. What is the priority nursing concern at this time?
    1. Controlling hemorrhage in the mother
    2. Removing the afterbirth
    3. Keeping the infant warm
    4. Cutting the umbilical cord

23. What should the nurse do to stimulate the separation of the placenta after home delivery of a baby?
    1. Ask the mother to push down vigorously.
    2. Push the fundus down vigorously.
    3. Encourage the baby to breastfeed.
    4. Place gentle tension on the umbilical cord.

24. A woman delivered a baby in the car on the way to the hospital. In the emergency room, the physician examined the mother. What is the priority action for the nurse at this time?
    1. Gently tug on the cord and massage the uterus to see if the placenta is ready to be delivered.
    2. Clamp and cut the cord with sterile scissors.
    3. Note and record the Apgar score.
    4. Clear the mucus from the baby's mouth and nose.

25. A woman who is giving birth at home wonders if her baby will need drops in the eyes because she knows that neither she nor her husband have gonorrhea. The best answer for the nurse to give should include which of the following?
    1. It is desirable for the baby to receive the eye drops, but it is not essential.
    2. If you do not want your baby to have the eye drops, you must sign a waiver stating that you refuse them.
    3. The baby needs the drops but does not have to receive them for up to two hours after birth.
    4. The drops are needed to prevent the eye condition known as retrolental fibroplasia.

26. The nurse is caring for a laboring woman who has a history of rheumatic heart disease. How should the nurse position her during labor?

1. Supine
2. Semirecumbent
3. Side-lying
4. Sitting

27. The nurse is caring for a laboring woman who has a history of rheumatic heart disease. Which instruction should the nurse give to her during the second stage of labor?
    1. Avoid prolonged bearing down.
    2. Breathe shallowly and rapidly.
    3. Sit on the side of the bed.
    4. Sleep between contractions.

28. A woman spontaneously delivers a baby girl who is immediately handed to the nurse. Which action is of highest priority for the nurse?
    1. Do an Apgar assessment.
    2. Check neonatal heart rate.
    3. Apply identification bracelets.
    4. Clean the nasopharynx.

29. At one minute after birth, an infant is crying, has a heart rate of 140, has acrocyanosis, resists the suction catheter, and keeps his arms extended and his legs flexed. What is the Apgar score?
    1. 4
    2. 6
    3. 8
    4. 10

30. The delivery room nurse is explaining Apgar scoring to new parents. Which information pertaining to the purpose of a five-minute Apgar score should be included in the explanation?
    1. It evaluates the effectiveness of the labor and delivery.
    2. It measures the adequacy of transition to extrauterine life.
    3. It assesses the possibility of respiratory distress syndrome.
    4. It gives an estimate of the gestational age of the infant.

31. The nurse is caring for a woman who has had a spinal anesthetic. Which of the following would be most likely to occur after spinal anesthesia?
    1. The client states that she is dizzy and light-headed.
    2. The temperature is 101°F.
    3. The nurse observes the client shivering.
    . The client develops a red, itchy rash on her back and chest.

32. What action is essential for the nurse during the fourth stage of labor?
    1. Firmly massage the fundus every 15 minutes.
    2. Take the vital signs q 1 h.
    3. Turn the client on her side during a lochia check.
    4. Assist the client to the bathroom to void.

33. Which of the following is the most important nursing assessment during the fourth stage of labor?
    1. Bonding behaviors
    2. Distention of the bladder
    3. Ability to relax
    4. Knowledge of newborn behavior

34. A woman who is 32 weeks gestation is admitted with contractions every four minutes. Ritodrine is given for which of the following purposes?
    1. To suppress uterine activity
    2. To make her more comfortable
    3. To enhance contractions
    4. To increase fetal oxygenation

35. The nursing care plan for a woman who has placenta abruptio should include careful assessment for signs and symptoms of:
    1. Jaundice
    2. Hypovolemic shock
    3. Impending convulsions
    4. Hypertension

Answers and Rationales

1. (1) Analgesia can usually be safely given after 5 cm of dilation and until one to two hours before delivery. Answer 2 is not appropriate, because according to the data given, the mother is a good candidate for some type of analgesia. Answer 3 is not true. Pain medication too early may slow labor, and pain medication too late may depress the baby's respirations and heart beat. Pain medication given appropriately is often very helpful during labor. Answer 4 is not appropriate. It does not address the question that the client asked about pain medication.

2. (2) Before encouraging the mother to push, the nurse should determine that the mother has completed transition and is fully dilated. She should not push before she is fully dilated. Answer 1 is a good description of pushing. However, the woman should not push until she is fully dilated. Most women need to push for a while before the baby is born. Answer 4 is a true statement; however, it is not the best response for the nurse to make.

3. (1) When it is not desirable for a woman to push, such as when moving from bed to table, she should be instructed to pant. It is not possible for a woman to pant and push at the same time. The mother will probably be unable to put her legs up in stirrups during a contraction. At this stage of labor, she will be unable to ignore contractions.

4. (3) The practical nurse should initially check the fetal heart rate, and then the registered nurse should perform a vaginal exam. A breech fetus is at high risk for a prolapsed cord when the membranes rupture. Following assessment of

the fetal heart rate, the RN will perform a vaginal exam. A woman with a breech presentation may need a cesarean delivery. After the initial assessments, the physician will be notified because this baby is in a breech position. The physician is not automatically notified when the membranes rupture.

5. (4) Breech presentations frequently have amniotic-stained fluid. Amniotic-stained fluid in a vertex presentation is a sign of fetal distress. Maternal diabetes does not cause amniotic-stained fluid unless the fetus happens to be in distress.

6. (1) Checking the fundus for hemorrhage is of highest priority. The placenta has separated from the uterus in a woman who has had a cesarean delivery just as it does in a vaginal delivery. Both types of deliveries have a risk of postpartum hemorrhage. It is essential to keep the fundus firm for both types of deliveries. The woman who had a cesarean delivery has no episiotomy. Assisting with emotional adjustment will be a part of nursing care but is not the highest priority. Encouraging fluid intake is important but is not the highest priority.

7. (1) A cesarean delivery is not in itself a contraindication for another pregnancy. Many women can have a vaginal delivery after a cesarean. The old rule of only two cesarean deliveries is no longer true. Remember this client had one vaginal delivery and one cesarean. Answer 2 does not give accurate information. Choice #3 does not answer the question. Answer 4 contains some truth, but the nurse should be able to give general information to this mother.

8. (4) This is the appropriate assessment in early labor. Because she is para 0, the nurse knows that she has not carried a pregnancy at least 20 weeks. She has not had labor and has not given birth, so answers 1 and 2 are not appropriate. It is not reasonable to expect the woman to bring a sample of the fluid with her.

9. (3) Amniotic fluid is alkaline and turns Nitrazine paper blue. Urine is acidic and turns Nitrazine paper red.

10. (4) Panting is not the appropriate breathing pattern at this time. Panting is important when the woman has the desire to push but she should not push. Further assessment is needed to help her alter her breathing to a more appropriate pace. If she continues panting at this time, she will be at risk for developing respiratory alkalosis and exhausting herself. Answer 1 is a true statement but is a put-down to the client. Answer 2 is not correct. Her contractions are not compatible with late first stage labor (transition), when the pant-blow breathing pattern is appropriate. Answer 3 is not correct. She is using an inappropriate breathing technique.

11. (3) Amniotomy can be stressful for the fetus. Assessing the fetal heart rate is the priority nursing measure during amniotomy. Keeping the mother informed is not as important as fetal safety. The procedure is painless, so breathing techniques are not necessary.

12. (2) Contractions during transition usually occur every 2–3 minutes and last 60–90 seconds. Her contractions are not typical of transition, but the only way to be sure is to have the RN do a vaginal exam. Answer 1 ignores the symptoms and puts the client down. Answer 3 is incorrect information; her contractions are not typical of transition. Irritability and restlessness can be signs of transition. Answer 4 is not a useful response. It is not completely true, and it is certainly not a therapeutic response.

13. (3) Rubbing the lower back usually helps the husband deal with his feelings of helplessness and fosters the couple's sense of mutual experience. Answer 1 is not appropriate, because it is better for the mate to give the back rub if he is able and willing than for the nurse to do it. Answer 2 is not appropriate because she has said that she wants to have a natural childbirth. Answer 4 is not realistic. It is not realistic to encourage a woman in active labor to rest. Sending the husband away is not appropriate.

14. (4) Hypotension is a frequent side effect of regional anesthesia. Maternal hypotension causes fetal bradycardia and hypoxia. Answer 1 is not correct, because epidural anesthesia does not cause uterine tetany. Answer 2 is not correct. Even though contractions are sometimes slowed after administering an epidural, oxytocin is not routinely administered. Answer 4 is not correct. The woman who has had an epidural anesthesia will have her head elevated to prevent respiratory depression. Post-anesthesia headache occurs after spinal or saddle block anesthesia, not after epidural anesthesia.

15. (2) Pressure of the uterus against major blood vessels reduces circulation, causing decreased perfusion of the placenta. Answer 1 is not correct; the supine position does not prolong labor. Choice #3 is not correct; the supine position does not impede free movement of the symphysis pubis. Answer 4 is not correct; the supine position does not cause transient episodes of hypertension in the laboring woman.

16. (2) Contractions during the transition phase typically occur every 2–3 minutes and last 60–90 seconds. The woman is often irritable and has a backache. Answer 1 is not correct. Early first stage labor contractions are usually several minutes apart, lasting only a few seconds. Backache and irritability are not common in early first stage labor. Answer 3 is not correct. Late second stage labor is the

"pushing stage" just before delivery. Early third stage labor is after delivery of the baby, just before the placenta is expelled. Third stage labor is usually only a few minutes.

17. (1) Lack of descent is often related to a full bladder. Answer 2 is not correct. Until a full bladder has been ruled out as a cause of failure to descend, cesarean delivery would not be considered. Answer 3 is not correct. Routine fetal assessment will of course be done. However, there is no specific data suggesting a fetal problem and no need for additional fetal monitoring. Answer 4 is not correct. Position is not the most likely cause for failure to descend. Turning the mother to the left side would be an appropriate intervention for a sudden drop in blood pressure resulting from vena caval syndrome.

18. (1) The second stage of labor is the pushing stage. The nurse should help the mother push effectively. Answer 2 is not correct. The mother cannot breastfeed the infant until it is born. Breastfeeding on the delivery table might be an appropriate action in the third stage of labor. Answer 3 is not correct. Checking the fetal position is not the highest priority action during second stage labor. Answer 4 is not correct. Pain medication should not be administered in the second stage because it will cause a sleepy baby.

19. (2) The woman is a G5 P4, and the perineum is bulging. Delivery is imminent. Contamination will be minimized by catching the infant on a clean surface. Answer 1 is not correct. The woman will not need to be encouraged to push; she will be doing it on her own. Secondly, it will be more appropriate to have her pant so that the delivery can be controlled. Answer 3 is not correct. Delivery is imminent. There is no time or need to time the contractions. Answer 4 is not correct. Delivery is imminent. There is no time to contact the physician for instructions. The nurse should be able to handle this emergency delivery.

20. (3) Applying gentle counter pressure to the perineum prevents too rapid expulsion of the head, which can lead to increased intracranial pressure in the infant and laceration in the mother. Answer 1 is not correct. The mother will be encouraged to pant so that the delivery can be controlled. Answer 2 is not correct. The nurse does not press down on the fundus to expel the baby. Answer 4 is not correct. There is no need to tell the mother to take prolonged deep breaths. Applying gentle perineal pressure is by far the most appropriate action for the nurse at this time.

21. (2) The sudden change of pressure tends to tear away dural linings. The mother can also get perineal tears. Answer 1 is not correct. Edema of the scalp is not a complication with precipitate labor. Sometimes prolonged labor

can cause caput succadaneum, where the baby has bleeding under the scalp. Answers 3 and 4 are not correct. Rapid delivery is not particularly associated with placental problems.

22. (3) Newborns have immature temperature regulating mechanisms. The nurse should dry the infant and place it in a blanket or towel on the mother's abdomen. Answer 1 is not correct. The first concern is clearing the infant's airway and keeping the infant warm. The mother is not likely to hemorrhage at this time. Maternal hemorrhage would be more likely after delivery of the placenta. Answer 2 is not correct. The afterbirth or placenta should separate and deliver itself within five to 15 minutes after the baby is born. The nurse should care for the baby until this happens. Answer 4 is not correct. There is no hurry to cut the cord. The cord should never be cut with anything that is not sterile because the baby could develop a fatal infection.

23. (3) Breastfeeding stimulates uterine contractions, which will help the placenta to separate. Answer 1 is not correct. Having the mother push down vigorously will not stimulate the placenta to separate. Answer 2 is not correct. The nurse should not push down on the fundus. This is not necessary for the placenta to separate. Answer 4 is not correct. The nurse should never pull on the cord. This could cause inversion of the uterus.

24. (4) A clear airway for the infant is first priority. Answer 1 is not correct. Tugging on the cord before the placenta is expelled could cause inversion of the uterus. Answer 2 is not correct. The cord does not need to be cut immediately. Clearing the infant's airway is a much higher priority. Answer 3 is not correct. The nurse may assess the infant and get an Apgar score. However, the airway is a much higher priority than the Apgar.

25. (3) Antibiotic eye drops have to be instilled into the neonate's conjunctival sacs to prevent infection, not just from gonorrhea and chlamydia but also from pathogens in the birth canal such as pneumococcus and streptococcus. It is safe to wait up to two hours to instill the drops. This allows time for maternal-child eye contact and interaction, which facilitates attachment. Answers 1 and 2 are not correct. There is a legal requirement to give the baby eye prophylaxis. Answer 4 is not correct. Retrolental fibroplasia results from too much oxygen concentration in immature retinal vessels during oxygen therapy for the compromised neonate.

26. (2) Semirecumbent or semi-Fowler's position would be the most appropriate position to reduce the cardiac work load and ease breathing. The laboring woman who has a history of rheumatic heart disease is at risk for

congestive heart failure. The supine and side-lying positions would increase the cardiac work load. Sitting upright is not the best choice.

27. (1) The woman with cardiac disease should not bear down excessively. She will be given an epidural anesthesia, and outlet forceps may be indicated to shorten the second stage of labor. Answer 2 is not correct. Breathing shallowly and rapidly will cause respiratory alkalosis. Answer 3 is not correct. Sitting on the side of the bed is not an appropriate action during second stage labor. Second stage labor is the expulsion stage. Answer 4 is not correct. Sometimes mothers do dose between contractions in second stage. However, answer 1 is the priority instruction that the nurse should give this mother.

28. (4) Always make sure the airway is clear first. Apgar scoring is not the LPN's responsibility, and it is not the highest priority. Checking heart rate and applying identification bracelets are secondary to clearing the airway.

29. (3) He receives two points for respiratory effort because he is crying. He receives two points for his heartbeat because it is over 100. He receives one point for acrocyanosis (blue extremities). He receives two points for reflexes because he resists the suction catheters. He receives one point instead of two because his arms are extended instead of flexed. He receives 8 points out of the maximum score of 10 points.

30. (2) The Apgar score assesses the infant on respiratory effort, heart rate, color, reflexes, and muscle tone. These indicate his adaptation to extrauterine life. The purpose of the Apgar score is not to evaluate the effectiveness of labor and delivery, assess respiratory distress syndrome, or give an estimate of gestational age of the infant.

31. (3) Chills occur frequently after the administration of a regional anesthetic such as Carbocaine. A spinal anesthesia does not usually cause the client to be dizzy and light-headed. Fever and rash are not likely to occur after spinal anesthesia.

32. (3) Lochia can accumulate under the buttocks. It cannot be accurately observed in a supine position. The nurse assesses the fundus every 15 minutes and massages it only when it is soft. Vital signs will be q 15 minutes, not every hour. The client will not get up to void this soon after delivery.

33. (2) A distended bladder may interfere with involution of the uterus and cause excessive bleeding. The nurse will observe for appropriate bonding behaviors and maternal relaxation and maternal knowledge of newborn behavior but the most important is assessment for bladder distention (because that could cause uterine relaxation and hemorrhage).

34. (1) This woman is in premature labor. Ritodrine is used to suppress uterine activity. Note that answers 1 and 3 are opposites. Usually when there are opposites, one of the opposites is the correct answer. It would not be logical to enhance contractions in a woman who is not at term. Ritodrine is not an analgesic and does not increase fetal oxygenation.

35. (2) Abruptio placenta causes hemorrhage, either apparent or concealed. The nurse must observe for hypovolemic shock. Jaundice is not seen with placenta abruptio. Convulsions occur with eclampsia or pregnancy-induced hypertension. The client who is hemorrhaging will develop shock, not hypertension. Note the opposites; shock is low blood pressure and hypertension is high blood pressure. The answer is likely to be one of the opposites.

The Postpartal Client

PHYSIOLOGICAL CHANGES IN THE POSTPARTAL PERIOD

Vascular System

A. Increase in blood fibrinogen may be contributing factor in increased incidence of thrombophlebitis
B. Increase in leukocytes
C. Hct and Hgb should not vary significantly from labor.
D. During pregnancy, body carries approximately two additional liters of blood that are eliminated by renal system and diaphoresis within first two weeks postpartum; heavy sweating, particularly night sweats, are common

Reproductive System

A. Uterus evaluated for firmness and position:
   1. Should be halfway between umbilicus and symphysis pubis immediately after delivery
   2. Within next 12 hours, rises to umbilicus or one finger breadth above
   3. Rapidly begins to decrease in size and descends one a day

4. By fifth postpartum day, fundus is approximately 4–5 finger breadths below umbilicus and weighs about 1 lb. compared to 2 lb. immediately after delivery
5. By tenth postpartum day, uterus descended into true pelvis
6. By six weeks, uterus should be completely involuted
7. The inside endometrium is healing from a "wide gaping wound" to normal without even a scar.

B. Cervix begins to regenerate and heal immediately; by end of first week, one finger can barely be admitted; cervix never regains nulliparous appearance, but internal os closes completely
C. Vagina is relaxed and edematous following delivery.
D. Episiotomy must be inspected closely; should appear intact, stitches barely visible with no redness or swelling; sutures usually absorbable; condition of episiotomy must be charted

Abdominal Wall

A. Muscles soft and flabby, but return to normal by about six weeks if mother has maintained good tone during pregnancy and works to regain muscle tone afterward
B. Stretch marks or striae gradivarum caused by the rupture of elastic fibers in skin may appear brownish or red.
C. Rectus muscle may show marked separation; exercise and diet thought to help prevent this

Lochia

A. Lochia rubra occurs during first two to four days and consists of blood from placental site, shreds of membranes and decidua, vernix, lanugo, and meconium.
B. Lochia serosa: by fourth day, lochia turns brownish or dark red color, has fleshy odor; is composed of blood, wound exudate, leukocytes and erythrocytes, shreds of decidua, cervical mucous, and microorganisms; lasts 4–10 days
C. Lochia alba appears after 10th day; whitish-yellow, may last 3–6 weeks; small clots normal, large clots or unusual tissue may be reported
D. When client is lying and then stands, she often has a "gush" of blood that has pooled in the vagina.
E. Prolonged lochia rubra indicates slowed involution, perhaps a retained placenta.
F. Foul odor usually indicates infection.

Breasts

A. Pregnancy hormones (estrogen, progesterone, and chorionic somatomammotropin) prepare breasts for lactation.

B. Immediately after placental separation, prolactin levels increase to begin milk production.

Perineum

Examine episiotomy for REEDA: redness, edema, ecchymosis, discharge, and approximation.

Urinary System

A. Rids body of excess fluid; major diuresis occurs during first few days after delivery
B. Full bladder main cause of uterine atony
C. Encourage client to void; catheterize if unable to void

Vital Signs

A. Bradycardia often present
B. Temperature:
   1. Slight elevation normal on day of delivery
   2. Elevation of 100.4°F or greater after 48 hours usually indicative of infection

Gastrointestinal System

A. Constipation
B. May be nausea and vomiting after delivery or hunger
C. Common nursing diagnoses (see Table 15.30)
D. Nursing management:
   1. Teaching in relation to Rubin's phases
      a. "Taking In" phase:
         (1) Woman is dependent
         (2) Lasts for 1–2 days after delivery
         (3) Needs physical support
         (4) Need to talk about labor and delivery to integrate experience
      b. "Taking Hold" phase:
         (1) Mother very receptive to teaching about self and baby
         (2) Starts by third day
         (3) Identifies need for knowledge
         (4) "Baby Blues" common; mother may cry for no reason; hormonal shifts thought to play a role
      c. "Letting Go":
         (1) Resumes normal life with infant and other activities
         (2) Occurs two or more weeks after delivery
         (3) Mother fatigued and often feels overwhelmed
B. Comfort measures
   1. Cramping; Anaprox, ibuprofen, narcotics, heat
   2. Perineum:
      a. Ice for the first 24 hours
      b. Sitz bath after 24 hours

    c. Teach mother to cleanse after voiding or bowel movement.

C. Keep bladder empty either by voiding or by catheterization if woman is unable to void.

E. Encourage parent-infant attachment
  1. Bonding:
    a. Claiming: identifying ways in which baby looks or acts like family members
    b. Identification: establishing baby's unique nature (naming)
    c. Attachment facilitated by positive feedback between baby and caregivers
  2. Sensual responses enhance adaptation to parenthood:
    a. Touch; from fingertip to open palm to enfolding
    b. Eye to eye contact
    c. Voice: parents await baby's first cry; babies respond to higher-pitched voice
    d. Odor: babies quickly identify their own mother's breast milk by odor
    e. Entrainment: babies move in rhythm to patterns of adult speech
    f. Biorhythm: babies respond to maternal heartbeats

F. Rest and exercise:
  1. Try to organize care to give rest time.
  2. Begin exercise slowly.

G. Teach infant care:
  1. Clothing
  2. Feeding
  3. Characteristics of normal newborn
  4. Bathing and care of cord and circumcision if present
  5. Signs of illness

H. Breast care:
  1. If not breastfeeding, supportive bra for 1–2 weeks; apply ice if engorged
  2. If breastfeeding:
    a. Supply and demand; increased nursing causes increased milk production
    b. Positioning: tummy to tummy, use pillows, football hold to help keep pressure off sore abdomen; baby's mouth on areola, not nipple
    c. Timing: minimum 5–7 min. on a side, every 1–3 hours; baby should nurse 10–12 times in 24 hours
    d. Prevent/treat sore nipples by air drying, use of colostrum, or Vitamin E oil to keep nipples soft
    e. Prevent mastitis: cleanse with water, empty breasts, avoid plastic liners, nurse frequently

I. Discharge planning:
  1. Return check-up four to six weeks postpartum
  2. Contraception: sexual relations resume 4–6 weeks after delivery
  3. Menstruation: returns in 6–8 weeks if not breastfeeding; breastfeeding mother may or may not menstruate

COMPLICATIONS

Hemorrhage

A. Major cause of maternal death
B. Causes:
  1. Uterine atony
    a. Most common cause of early hemorrhage
    b. Women most at risk are those who had an over-distended uterus such as with twins or a complicated or precipitous delivery
  2. Lacerations
  3. Retained placenta often causes late hemorrhage
C. Interventions:
  1. Check the fundus frequently for firmness and massage if not firm.
  2. Check the perineum frequently for bleeding; apply ice to perineum first 24 hours after delivery.
  3. Oxytocin I.V., Methergine I.M. or P.O. after delivery to keep uterus firm

Infection

A. Major risk factors:
  1. Premature rupture of membranes (PROM)
  2. Cesarean delivery
  3. Birth trauma
  4. Maternal anemia
  5. Retained placenta
B. Signs and symptoms:
  1. Temperature of 100.4°F or greater for two consecutive days after first 24 hours
  2. Pelvic pain
  3. Foul-smelling lochia
  4. Burning upon urination
  5. Chills, malaise, increased pulse, increased white count
  6. Cultures positive for organisms
C. Interventions:
  1. Encourage fluids to 3,000 ml/day.
  2. Administer antibiotics.
  3. Semi-Fowler's to high-Fowler's position to promote drainage

Thrombophlebitis

A. Increased risk postpartum due to increased amount of fibrinogen after delivery
B. Assessment findings:
  1. Positive Homan's sign
  2. Redness, pain, and edema in leg
C. Interventions:
  1. Bed rest with leg elevated
  2. Moist heat
  3. Do not massage, because this may make the thrombus into an embolus and cause a pulmonary embolus.
  4. Analgesics if needed

5. Heparin to prevent formation of new clots
6. Antibiotics may be indicated if pelvic thrombus with temperature elevation

Mastitis

A. Bacteria enters through cracks in nipples
B. Assessment findings include redness and tenderness of breasts and flu-like symptoms
C. Interventions:
   1. Antibiotics
   2. Analgesics
   3. Frequent nursing or pumping

Postpartum depression

A. Goes beyond "Baby Blues;" lasts for several weeks or longer
B. Mother is unable to assume normal activities.
C. May need psychiatric care, especially if psychosis is evident
D. Make appropriate referral.

Sample Questions

1. A woman who had a normal vaginal delivery two hours ago has just arrived on the postpartum floor. Vital signs are normal. When assessing her uterus, the nurse notes that it is boggy. What should be the nurse's initial intervention?
   1. Massage the uterus.
   2. Report to the charge nurse.
   3. Contact the doctor stat.
   4. Continue to assess it frequently.
2. The nurse is caring for a woman who had a normal vaginal delivery two hours ago and has just arrived on the postpartum floor. Two hours later her uterus is displaced to the right. What is the most likely explanation for this?
   1. A fibroid tumor
   2. A full bladder
   3. An increase in interstitial fluid
   4. Retained placental fragments
3. The day after delivery, a new mother asks why her milk is so creamy and yellow. What is the best response for the nurse to make?
   1. "I wouldn't worry about it."
   2. "This is normal. It will soon turn to real milk."
   3. "You're coming along fine."
   4. "You haven't gotten your milk in yet."
4. A new mother is in the first period of adjustment following birth called the taking-in phase. What type of maternal behavior would the nurse expect her to exhibit?
   1. Passivity and dependence
   2. Preoccupation with baby's needs
   3. Independence
   4. Resuming control of life

5. A new mother has decided not to breastfeed her baby. Which statement indicates the best understanding of the management of engorgement?
   1. "I will stand with my back to the shower."
   2. "I will take a sitz bath every day."
   3. "I will apply a warm compress to my breasts three times a day."
   4. "I will drink a lot of liquids for the next few days."
6. A new mother is about to be discharged from the hospital. Which statement made by a new mother indicates a need for more instruction?
   1. "I will use my old diaphragm for contraception."
   2. "I have an appointment for my six-week check up."
   3. "My mother will be helping me with the children for the next two weeks."
   4. "I plan to go back to my job as a secretary in six weeks."
7. A woman who delivered today by cesarean delivery asks the nurse, "How come my baby has such a round head? My other baby's head was not so round, and she was more red." What is the best response for the nurse to make?
   1. "Each baby is different. It is not a good idea to compare your children."
   2. "Were forceps used when your older child was delivered?"
   3. "Babies born by cesarean have rounder heads because they do not go through the birth canal."
   4. "A round head is a sign the baby is very intelligent. Your child should do very well in school."
8. A new mother is checking the list of supplies she will need at home for care of the newborn. She asks the nurse why she needs rubbing alcohol. What is the best response for the nurse to make?
   1. "Rubbing alcohol is good for the baby's skin. You should apply it to his body three times a day."
   2. "Apply the rubbing alcohol to the baby's circumcision to speed healing."
   3. "Wipe his bottom off with alcohol after each bowel movement."
   4. "Clean his cord stump with alcohol each time you change his diaper."
9. A woman is admitted to the postpartum unit two hours after delivery of a baby. What action is especially important because the membranes were ruptured for 28 hours before delivery?
   1. Monitor her temperature every two hours.
   2. Provide perineal care with zephiran every four hours.
   3. Maintain a strict perineal pad count.
   4. Have the mother take a sitz bath four times a day.

10. The nurse is caring for a woman who delivered a baby three hours ago. The woman pulls the emergency call light and says she is bleeding all over the bed. The nurse enters the room and sees the blood-soaked bed. What is the best initial action for the nurse to take?
    1. Assess and massage the fundus if soft.
    2. Take vital signs.
    3. Place the client in sharp Trendelenburg position.
    4. Notify the physician immediately.

11. Methergine 5 mg qid is ordered for a postpartum client. An hour after taking the drug, the woman complains of uterine cramping. What is the best explanation for the nurse to give her?
    1. "This is an unfortunate side effect, but you need the medicine."
    2. "The cramping is uncomfortable, but it is a sign that the drug is keeping your uterus contracted so you won't bleed too much."
    3. "Since you are experiencing cramps, I'll ask the doctor to discontinue the drug."
    4. "The cramping should decrease soon. If it does not, let me know. I'll see if the doctor will decrease the dosage."

12. The nurse is caring for a woman who had a post partum hemorrhage. Which of the following facts about her delivery most likely contributed to her hemorrhage?
    1. The baby weighed 10 lb 6 oz.
    2. She received pitocin after delivery of the placenta.
    3. She delivered 10 days after her due date.
    4. Her second stage of labor lasted an hour.

13. A woman who has just delivered has chosen to bottle feed. What should the nurse teach her about breast care?
    1. "Take long warm showers, allowing the shower to hit your breasts."
    2. "Massage your breasts every three hours to increase circulation."
    3. "Wear a supportive bra, and do not handle your breasts."
    4. "Hold the baby away from your chest so he will not smell the breast milk."

14. The nurse is observing a new mother for good maternal infant attachment. Which observation would be a sign of inappropriate attachment?
    1. Calling the baby "little bit."
    2. Holding the baby in "en face" position.
    3. Telling the baby "You look just like your Daddy."
    4. Continually saying, "I'm too tired to hold the baby."

15. A woman who had a cesarean section tells the nurse, "I guess I flunked natural childbirth because I had to have a cesarean." This statement is most indicative of which phase of postpartum adjustment?
    1. Taking in
    2. Working through
    3. Taking hold
    4. Letting go

16. Six hours after delivery, the nurse notes that a woman's fundus is two finger breadths above the umbilicus and deviated to the right of the midline. What is the most likely cause of this finding?
    1. Retained placental fragments
    2. Bladder distention
    3. Normal involution
    4. Second degree uterine atony

17. Which area of health teaching will a new mother be most responsive to during the taking-in phase of the postpartum period?
    1. Family planning
    2. Newborn care
    3. Community support groups
    4. Perineal care

18. On the first day after a cesarean section, the client is ambulating. She is uncomfortable and asks the nurse, "Why am I being made to walk so soon after surgery?" What is the nurse's best response?
    1. "You can get to hold your baby more quickly if you walk around."
    2. "Early walking keeps the blood from pooling in your legs and prevents blood clots."
    3. "Walking early will prevent your wound from opening."
    4. "Early walking helps lower the incidence of wound infection."

19. A pregnant woman tells the nurse that she is planning to breastfeed because "You don't have to take contraceptives until you wean the baby." What is the best response for the nurse?
    1. "Lactation does suppress ovulation, so you are not likely to get pregnant."
    2. "You will not get pregnant until you start to menstruate again."
    3. "When a woman is breastfeeding, she may not menstruate although she may ovulate. It is best to use some type of birth control."
    4. "You will find that you won't be interested in resuming sexual activity until after you wean the baby."

20. A new mother who has been breastfeeding her infant for six weeks calls the nurse at the doctor's office and says her right nipple is cracked and sore, she has a temperature, and feels as though she had the flu. How should the nurse respond to the woman?
    1. "Try putting warm compresses over your right breast."
    2. "Immediately stop nursing and apply cold compresses to your breasts."
    3. "Come to see the physician. You may need medication to help."
    4. "Reduce the time the baby nurses on your right breast, and call again if the breast is not better in two days."

Answers and Rationales

1. (1) The initial response is to massage the uterus. Most of the time, massaging the uterus will cause it to firm up immediately. If it does not respond to massage by becoming firm, then the practical nurse should report it to the charge nurse or contact the physician. The nurse will continue to assess frequently after massaging the fundus. Note that the question asked for the initial intervention.

2. (2) A full bladder causes the uterus to be elevated above the umbilicus and displaced to the right. A fibroid tumor, if present, would not cause a change in position of the uterus in a two-hour time period. Interstitial fluid does not accumulate in the uterus and could not cause the uterine position change. Retained placental fragments would cause an increase in vaginal bleeding or a boggy fundus, but not displacement of the fundus.

3. (2) The client is describing colostrum. Milk comes in about 72 hours after delivery. Answers 1 and 3 do not address the question asked by the mother. Answer 4 is technically accurate but does not give as much information and reassurance as Answer 2.

4. (1) The taking-in period is characterized by passivity and dependence. The mother relives her labor and integrates it into her being. Preoccupation with the baby's needs and reasserting independence are characteristic of the taking-hold phase, which follows the taking-in phase. Resuming control of life is characteristic of the letting-go phase.

5. (1) Standing with her back to the shower will keep the warm water from stimulating milk production. Cool compresses will help with engorgement; warm compresses stimulate milk flow. A sitz bath is indicated for an episiotomy. It is not related to the care of the breasts. Pushing fluids will encourage milk production.

6. (1) A woman should be resized for a diaphragm after the birth of a baby. The old one may no longer be the correct size. The resizing will occur after involution is completed, usually at her six-week checkup. If sexual activity is resumed before that time, another means of contraception (such as the condom) should be used if she does not wish to get pregnant. All of the other responses are good responses.

7. (3) Babies born by cesarean delivery do not have molded heads because they have not passed through the pelvis and the birth canal. The other responses are not helpful. Answer 1 does not address the questions. Forceps can cause distinctive marks on the head. A round head is not a sign of intelligence.

8. (4) Alcohol is used to dry the cord. The other answers are not correct and are contraindicated. Alcohol is too drying to apply to the skin. Alcohol is not applied to the circumcision; it would cause great pain. Petrolatum (Vaseline) gauze is applied to the circumcision. The baby's bottom should not be wiped with alcohol because it will cause drying of the skin.

9. (1) Temperature over 100.4°F after the second day usually indicates infection. Infection is the most frequent maternal complication after prolonged rupture of the membranes. Zephiran perineal care is not a current practice and is not related to prolonged rupture of the membranes. A strict perineal pad count is not necessary. Sitz baths are a comfort measure for a sore perineum and are not related to prolonged rupture of the membranes.

10. (1) The biggest cause of postpartum hemorrhage is uterine atony. Always assess and massage the fundus first. Taking vital signs and notifying the physician will be done after the nurse massages the fundus. The client will not be placed in the Trendelenburg position.

11. (2) This response explains the drug's action to the client. Methergine is an oxytocic drug that helps the uterus to contract and prevents postpartum bleeding. Answer 1 is not correct because it does not give the mother the information she needs to understand why she is cramping. Answers 3 and 4 are not accurate.

12. (1) An over-stretched uterus is subject to hemorrhage. A large baby causes additional stretching of the uterus. Answer 2 is not correct. Pitocin contracts the uterus and decreases hemorrhage. It is also standard procedure following delivery. Answer 3 is not correct. Delivering after the due date itself does not increase postpartum hemorrhage. However, the large baby does. Answer 4 is not correct. An hour second stage is normal.

13. (3) Decreasing stimulation will decrease milk production. Hot showers and massaging breasts stimulates milk production. The baby should be held close to the chest regardless of the feeding method.

14. (4) This may mean she is rejecting the baby. Nicknames, holding the baby in "en face" position (so the mother can look at the baby's face) and seeing family resemblance are positive signs of attachment.

15. (1) By discussing her experience, she is bringing it into reality. This is characteristic of the taking-in phase. The taking-hold phase is when the mother tries to reassert her control of the family, and letting-go is when the baby is integrated into the family. Working through is not one of the phases of postpartum adjustment.

16. (2) Bladder distention causes uterine displacement, which interferes with involution and may lead to postpartum hemorrhage. With normal involution, the fundus would be at or slightly above the umbilicus and in the midline. Retained placental fragments and uterine atony would cause excessive bleeding.

17 (4) During the taking-in phase, the mother is more self-centered. She will be most responsive to perineal care. She will be most responsive to family planning and newborn care during the taking-hold phase. Awareness of community support groups would be in the taking-hold or letting-go phase.

18 (2) Early walking helps to prevent thrombophlebitis. She does not have to walk in order to hold her baby. Walking does not prevent dehiscence or wound infection.

19. (3) The bottle-feeding mother's ovulation and menstrual cycle has been noted to occur as early as 36 days; the breastfeeding mother's, as early as 39 days. Lactation sometimes, but not always, suppresses ovulation. A nursing mother may ovulate and not menstruate, so another method of contraception is recommended. Lactation does not have an effect on sexual desire. Breastfeeding is not a reliable method of contraception.

20. (3) The data suggest that the mother has mastitis. Antibiotics may be a part of the treatment. She should be seen by the physician. Warm compresses might be helpful, but the woman needs to be seen by the physician. Cold compresses are not indicated for infection. She will probably not need to stop nursing or reduce feeding on that breast.

Normal Newborn

TRANSITION TO EXTRAUTERINE LIFE

Respiratory

A. First breath:
   1. Pulmonary resistance drops rapidly.
   2. Mucous and meconium, if present, can be inhaled.
B. Respirations irregular in depth, rate, rhythm; 30–60 breaths/min.
C. Newborns are obligate nose breathers; they breathe through their noses.
D. Blocked nares is called choanal atresia and is an emergency.
E. Adequate levels of surfactants (lecithin and sphingomyelin) provide mature lung function and prevent alveolar collapse and respiratory distress syndrome.

Cardiovascular

A. Pulse normally irregular at 120–150 and increases in rate and irregularity with physical stimulation
B. Peripheral extremities bluish color first 24 hrs (acrocyanosis)
C. Foramen ovale (opening between atria) and ductus arteriosus (opening between pulmonary artery and aorta) are functionally closed; permanent closure by three to four months
D. Ductus venous (opening between the umbilical vein and the inferior vena cava) closes when the cord is clamped
E. Cord should contain two umbilical arteries and one umbilical vein
F. Absence of normal flora in intestine results in lower levels of vitamin K (necessary for blood clotting); vitamin K injection is given on the first day to prevent bleeding

Temperature

A. Newborn has unstable heat-regulating system
B. Body temperature influenced by environmental temperature
C. Dry infant immediately after birth, wrap warmly, cover head (head is major source of heat loss), and place in a warm area.
D. Newborn is unable to shiver.
E. Infection may be manifested by hypo- or hyperthermia.
F. Cold stress increases oxygen consumption and may lead to metabolic acidosis and respiratory distress.

Genitourinary

A. Newborn must begin to eliminate own waste; first voiding within 24 hours
B. Voidings frequent and urine dilute; infant unable to concentrate urine until three months old
C. Pinkish-red stain may be seen on diaper due to deposits of uric acid crystals.

Gastrointestinal

A. Newborn can't move food from lips to pharynx; must have suck-swallow reflex to ingest milk by mouth
B. Immature cardiac sphincter may allow reflux of food when burped; place infant on right side after eating to prevent regurgitation.
C. Stools:
   1. First stool is meconium: sticky, greenish-black; 8–24 hours after birth

2. First week transitional stools: loose, greenish-yellow
3. After first week, depends on feeding:
   a. Breastfed are loose and golden yellow
   b. Formula-fed are formed and pale yellow

Immunologic

A. Newborn has passive acquired immunity from IgG from the mother and receives additional antibodies in colostrum and breast milk.
B. Infant develops its own antibodies during the first three months but is at risk for infection during the first six weeks.

Neurologic

A. Myelin sheath only beginning to form; body functions and responses to stimuli are carried out chiefly by the midbrain and reflexes of the spinal cord
B. Reflexes: grasp, Moro, (startle) tonic neck, Babinski, rooting, blinking
C. Periods of Reactivity:
   1. First (birth through first half hour): newborn is alert with good sucking reflex; respirations and heart beat irregular
   2. Second (4–8 hours after birth): may regurgitate mucus, pass meconium, and suck well
   3. Equilibrium usually achieved by eight hours of age
D. Sleep and hunger cycles:
   1. Newborn sleeps about 17 hours a day
   2. Breastfed infants may nurse every two to three hours.
   3. Bottle-fed infants may be fed every three to four hours.
E. Special senses:
   1. Touch: most highly developed; infant responds to touch from moment of birth
   2. Sight:
      a. Gazes at objects
      b. Uncoordinated eye movements
      c. Preference for black and white and geometric shapes
   3. Hearing:
      a. Hears at 24 weeks gestation
      b. Prefers sound of human voices
   4. Taste:
      a. Sense of taste established at birth
      b. Prefers sweet-tasting liquids
   5. Smell: newborn can identify own mother's milk by the odor

Integumentary

A. Large surface area for heat and water loss
B. Skin breaks down easily; entrance for microorganisms

Hepatic System

A. Liver is immature and unable to break down bilirubin
B. Infant has increased bilirubin at birth; during first week there is a further breakdown of hemoglobin, thereby increasing bilirubin; immature liver can't handle this, so jaundice appears on skin and sclera and urine becomes dark and infant becomes sluggish and anorexic
C. Bilirubin increases about the second day for a few days; normal by seventh day; called physiologic jaundice
D. Medications given less frequently because liver is immature
E. Management of physiologic jaundice:
   1. Increase water intake.
   2. Place under a bili light.
   3. Shield eyes while under the light.
   4. If jaundice occurs before two days or if bilirubin level is above 18–20 mg/100 ml, there is another cause such as ABO or Rh incompatibility.

ASSESSMENT OF NEWBORN

Physical Assessment

A. Length and weight:
   1. Average length 18–22 in (45.7–55.9 cm)
   2. Average weight 6–8 1/2 lbs. (2,700–3,850 Gms)
B. Head
   1. Fontanels
      a. Anterior:
         (1) Diamond-shaped
         (2) Junction of two parietal and two frontal bones
         (3) .8–1.2 in (2–3 cm) wide and 1.2–1.6 in (3–4 cm) long
         (4) Closes at 12–18 months
      b. Posterior:
         (1) Triangular shape
         (2) Located between occipital and parietal bones
         (3) Closes by end of second month
      c. Both should be flat and open
   2. Head should turn freely from side to side; if rigid sternocleidomastoid muscle, may have been injured during delivery
   3. Head circumference proportionately large (1/4 total length):
      a. Average 13–14 in (33–35.5 cm)
      b. May need to remeasure in a few days if baby has significant molding or caput succadaneum
   4. Caput succadaneum:
      a. Swelling or edema of the presenting portion of the scalp
      b. Swelling crosses suture lines
      c. Usually disappears by day three

5. Cephalohematoma:
   a. Accumulation of blood between the periosteum and the flat skull bone
   b. Mass is soft, irreducible, and fluctuating
   c. Does not cross suture lines
   d. Does not increase with crying
   e. Aspiration NOT done because of danger of infection; will resolve in time

C. Ears:
   1. Should be even with canthi of eyes; low-set ears suggest abnormalities such as Down's syndrome
   2. Cartilage should be present and firm.

D. Eyes:
   1. May be irritated by medications used to prevent ophthalmia; some edema and discharge is normal
   2. Color is slate blue

E. Chest circumference: average 3/4 in. (1.9 cm) less than head

F. Skin:
   1. Skin thickens with gestational age; post-mature infants may have dry and peeling skin
   2. Lanugo:
      a. Slight downy distribution of fine hair over body; most evident on shoulders, back, extremities
      b. Begins to appear at 16 weeks gestation
      c. Begins to disappear after 32nd week
      d. Premature infants have more lanugo than full-term infants.
   3. Vernix caseosa:
      a. Cheese-like, greasy yellow-white substance covering skin consisting of secretions of sebaceous glands and epithelial cells
      b. Heaviest in folds of the skin and between labia
   4. Milia:
      a. Tiny white papillae on nose and chin related to obstruction of sebaceous glands
      b. Disappears in 1–2 weeks
   5. Hemangiomas
      a. Pink spots on upper eyelids, between eyebrows, and on nose, upper lip, and back of neck
      b. Related to birth trauma and disappear spontaneously
   6. Mongolian spots:
      a. Slate-colored spots on buttocks or lower back in blacks, Asians, and darker-skinned infants
      b. No treatment; disappear by school age

G. Umbilical stump:
   1. Begins to shrink and disappear soon after birth
   2. Sloughs off between six and 10 days; may take up to three weeks
   3. Examine closely for first 24 hours for signs of bleeding

4. Clean with alcohol at each diaper change
5. Slight bleeding when cord detaches is normal

H. Genitalia:
   1. Male
      a. Testes descended or in inguinal canal; usually descend at eight months gestation; undescended testicles (cryptorchidism) surgical correction done by six years of age; cryptorchidism more common in premature babies
      b. Rugae over scrotum
      c. Meatus at tip of penis
   2. Female:
      a. Genitalia slightly swollen; related to mother's hormone level
      b. Blood-tinged mucous (pseudomenstruation) from vagina for first week due to maternal hormones
      c. Vernix between labia

I. Legs:
   1. Bowed
   2. No click or displacement of head of femur observed when hips flexed and abducted

J. Feet:
   1. Flat
   2. Soles covered with creases in fully mature infant

K. Muscle tone:
   1. Infant stays flexed most of the time; premature infant usually in extension
   2. Occasional transient tremors of mouth and chin normal
   3. Newborn can turn head from side to side in prone position
   4. Needs head supported when held erect or lifted

L. Nervous system:
   1. Very immature at birth
   2. Reflexes present at birth:
      a. Blinking: stimulated when infant is subjected to a bright light
      b. Coughing and sneezing: protective mechanism which clears the respiratory tract
      c. Yawn: allows infant to get more O_2
      d. Rooting: infant turns head to the side when his cheek is touched; allows baby to find nipple
      e. Grasp: infant will grasp any object put in hand; hold it briefly and then drop it; disappears by third month
      f. Startle (Moro): aroused by sudden loud noise or loss of support; infant draws legs up with soles of feet turned toward each other, arms extended into embrace position, and body in fixed and rigid position; demonstrates awareness of equilibrium; disappears at eight weeks

M. Motor activity:
   1. Movements are rapid, varied, are diffuse.

2. Whole body is involved in an activity.
3. Responses aroused by a generalized state, such as hunger, pain, or discomfort
4. Despite the infant's lack of strength and inability to control them, the infant's muscles should be firm and slightly resistant to pressure.

N. Nursing diagnoses (see Table 15.31)

Table 15.31 Nursing Diagnoses Related to the Normal Newborn

- Ineffective breathing pattern
- Imbalanced fluid volume
- Imbalanced nutrition
- Ineffective breastfeeding
- Urinary retention
- Impaired parenting
- Risk for aspiration
- Constipation
- Diarrhea
- Ineffective thermoregulation
- Impaired gas exchange

O. Management of Newborn infant
1. Care in Nursery
   a. Keep the infant warm.
   b. Administer medications as ordered:
      (1) 0.5% erythromycin or 1% tetracycline into conjunctival sac to prevent ophthalmia neonatorum
      (2) Vitamin K to prevent bleeding; infant does not manufacture vitamin K in intestinal tract until bacteria are present; infant is born with a sterile gut
      (3) Hepatitis B vaccine in first 12 hours
   c. Measure height and weight.
   d. After temperature stabilized, bathe and dress newborn
   e. Daily care routine:
      (1) Weight
      (2) Vital signs (temperature, apical pulse, respirations) at least every shift
      (3) Suction if needed; mucus may be present
      (4) Daily bath if ordered
      (5) Skin care of diaper area with each diaper change; teach parents
      (6) Start feedings; may start with sterile water or glucose water before formula offered; record daily intake
      (7) Record stools and voidings
      (8) Wipe umbilical cord with alcohol with each diaper change to help dry cord; teach parents
   f. Care of circumcision:
      (1) Discuss option with parents
      (2) Signed permit if circumcision to be performed

      (3) Assess for hemorrhage, infection after procedure
      (4) Apply petroleum gauze to penis if ordered; teach parents how to care for circumcision
   g. Tests:
      (1) Phenylketonuria (PKU) Guthrie test and thyroid; done 24 hours after first milk feeding and again in 4–6 weeks
      (2) Dextrostix/Accucheck in all babies at risk for hypoglycemia
   h. Teach parents general care of newborn; feeding, burping, bathing, dressing, and cord and circumcision care
   i. Promote attachment by involving parents in care of newborn

HIGH RISK NEWBORN

Prematurity

A. Gestational age of less than 37 weeks, regardless of weight; weight usually less than 2,500 g (5 1/2 lb)
B. Causes include maternal age (young or old), smoking, poor nutrition, placental problems, pregnancy-induced hypertension, and fetal factors such as multiple pregnancy or infection
C. Physical assessment:
   1. Thin, translucent skin; visible red vessels give red appearance
   2. Neurologic immaturity:
      a. Scarf sign: draw one arm across chest until resistance is felt; note relation of elbow to midline of chest; resistance increases with advancing gestational age. In premature infant, elbow will be well past midline
      b. Lack of reflexes and poor muscle tone
   3. Respiratory system:
      a. Infant has insufficient surfactant
      b. Periods of apnea
      c. Retractions, nasal flaring, grunting, seesaw pattern of breathing
      d. Cyanosis
      e. Increased respiratory rate: above 60/min.
      f. Week, feeble cry
   4. May have petechiae or bleeding at injection sites caused by fragile capillaries and prolonged prothrombin time
   5. Genitals:
      a. Lack pigment
      b. Males: testes may not have descended, no rugae or pigment
      c. Females: labia do not cover enlarged clitoris
   6. No baby fat
   7. Ear lobes: soft, less cartilage

8. Cardiovascular: patent ductus arteriosus and persistent fetal circulation may be present
C. Nursing diagnoses (see Table 15.32)

Table 15.32 Nursing Diagnoses Related to the Premature Infant

- Risk for aspiration related to immobility and increased secretions
- Risk for infection related to vulnerability of infant, lack of normal flora, environmental hazards, open wounds (umbilical cord, circumcision), and invasive lines
- Risk for impaired skin integrity related to susceptibility to nosocomial infections secondary to lack of normal skin flora
- Ineffective thermoregulation related to newborn transition to extrauterine environment
- Ineffective infant feeding pattern related to lethargy secondary to prematurity
- Risk for colonic constipation related to decreased intestinal motility and immobility
- Risk for impaired respiratory function related to increased oropharyngeal secretions

D. Management:
1. Monitor respirations every 1–2 hours; goal is less than 60/min.
2. Administer oxygen as ordered:
   a. Check levels frequently.
   b. High levels of oxygen cause retrolental fibroplasia (blindness) in the infant.
3. Assess breath sounds to assess lung expansion.
4. Gently rub back and feet to promote breathing.
5. Suction as needed.
6. Reposition every 1–2 hours to promote lung expansion and prevent exhaustion of the infant.
7. Maintain body temperature and prevent cold stress.
8. Observe for signs of infection; premature infants have fewer antibodies than term babies and are more susceptible to infection.
9. Feed infant as ordered:
   a. If sucking reflex absent or poor feeding may be by gavage
   b. Use "preemie" nipple (a soft nipple that decreases the work of feeding) if bottle feeding.
10. Record intake and output.
11. Measure and record daily weights; premature infants at high risk for dehydration and electrolyte imbalance
12. Monitor blood gases, electrolytes; glucose and bilirubin levels
13. Organize care to minimize the infant's energy expenditures.
14. Observe potential bleeding sites (umbilicus, injection sites) because these babies have lower levels of clotting factors.
15. Involve parents in care of infant whenever possible; explain care to parents.
16. Observe for complications frequently seen:
    a. Hypothermia
    b. Hypoglycemia
    c. Hypocalcemia
    d. Hyperbilirubinemia
    e. Birth trauma
    f. Sepsis
    g. Intracranial hemorrhage
    h. Necrotizing enterocolitis
    i. Apnea

Small for Gestational Age (SGA/Dysmature)

A. Birth weight in the lowest 10th percentile at birth
B. Caused by placental insufficiency; often related to:
1. Pregnancy-induced hypertension
2. Multiple gestation
3. Poor nutrition
4. Smoking, drugs, alcohol
5. Adolescent pregnancy
C. Assessment findings:
1. Skin: loose and dry, little fat, little muscle mass
2. Small body makes skull look larger than normal
3. Sunken abdomen
4. Thin, dry umbilical cord
5. Wide skull sutures
6. Respiratory distress
7. Hypoglycemia
8. Weak cry, lethargic
D. Nursing diagnoses (see Table 15.32)
E. Interventions: similar to those for premature infant

Large for Gestational Age (LGA)

A. Caused by maternal diabetes, postdates infant
B. Complications:
1. Birth trauma: fractured clavicle
2. Hypoglycemia
3. Polycythemia
4. If mother is diabetic, infant is at same risk as premature infant and receives premature infant care; even though large in size, lungs are usually immature
C. Nursing diagnoses (see Table 15.31)
D. Nursing care similar to newborn care; premature infant care if related to maternal diabetes

Postmature Infant

A. Born after the completion of 42 weeks of pregnancy
B. Primary problem is placenta becomes less efficient

C. Assessment findings:
1. Vernix and lanugo completely disappeared
2. If placenta functions well, infant will be large.
3. If poor placental perfusion, skin is dry, cracked, and looks like parchment; hard nails, and skin color is yellow to green from meconium staining
4. Infant looks old; very little subcutaneous fat
D. Nursing diagnoses (see Tables 15.31 and 15.32)
E. Nursing care similar to care of premature infant

Neonatal Respiratory Distress Syndrome

A. Respiratory distress syndrome (RDS) occurs in infants with immature lungs and is thought to be caused by insufficient surfactant.
B. Assessment findings:
1. Tachypnea (over 60/min.)
2. Nasal flaring, expiratory grunt, retractions, cyanosis, chin lag
3. Tachycardia
4. Hypothermia
5. Decreased activity level
6. Elevated carbon dioxide levels
7. Metabolic acidosis
C. Nursing diagnoses (see Table 15.33)
D. Interventions:
1. Maintain infant's body temperature at 97.6°F (36.2°C); body temperatures too high or too low require increased oxygen.
2. Provide adequate caloric intake to prevent the breakdown of tissues; usually IV glucose in addition to gradual increase in feedings, may be administered by gavage; sucking requires hard work
3. Plan care to reduce amount of handling and energy expenditure.
4. Administer oxygen therapy as ordered:
   a. Monitor oxygen concentration every 2–4 hours; maintain oxygen concentration at less than 40% if possible to prevent retrolental fibroplasia (blindness).

Table 15.33 Nursing Diagnoses Related to Respiratory Distress Syndrome

- Activity intolerance related to insufficient oxygenation of tissues secondary to impaired respirations
- Risk for infection related to vulnerability of infant, lack of normal flora, environmental hazards (parents, personnel), and open wounds (umbilical cord, circumcision)
- Risk for impaired skin integrity related to susceptibility to nosocomial infections secondary to lack of normal skin flora
In addition, nursing diagnoses related to the premature infant are appropriate.

---

b. Oxygen can be given by hood, nasal prongs, intubation, mask, ventilator.
c. Oxygen should be warmed and humidified.
d. Monitor blood gases.
5. Suctioning: PRN for not more than five seconds, being careful not to damage nasal mucosa

Rh and ABO Incompatibility (Erythroblastosis Fetalis)

A. Incompatibility occurs when mother is Rh negative and baby is Rh positive or when the mother is type O and the baby is type A, B, or AB.
B. Red blood cell destruction causes anemia and hyperbilirubinemia, which can lead to brain damage.
C. Physiology:
1. When mother is Rh negative and father is Rh positive, 65% of infants will be Rh positive.
2. Mother is sensitized by passage of fetal Rh positive RBCs through placenta either at time of placental separation at delivery or during pregnancy if there is a leak or break in the membrane.
3. Stimulates mother's immune system to produce anti-Rh antibodies that attack fetal RBCs and cause hemolysis (breakdown of RBCs)
4. Next pregnancy, maternal anti-Rh antibodies cross placenta and attack fetal RBCs, causing hemolytic disease of the newborn.
5. ABO incompatibility has same underlying mechanism; mother is type O and infant is A, B, or AB; reaction is less severe than Rh incompatibility.
D. Diagnostic tests:
1. Indirect Coombs' test (tests for anti-Rh antibodies in mother's circulation) performed at first prenatal visit and at 28 weeks. If indirect Coombs is negative at 28 weeks, a small dose of RhoGam is given to prevent sensitization in the third trimester.
2. Direct Coombs' test done on cord blood at delivery to determine presence of anti-Rh antibodies on fetal RBCs. If both indirect and direct Coombs' tests are negative, mother is given Rhogam to prevent antibody development and to assure that the next pregnancy will not be affected.
E. Assessment findings:
1. Jaundice and pallor within 24–36 hours
2. Anemia
3. Enlarged placenta
4. Edema and ascites
5. Kernicterus (brain damage from high levels of unconjugated bilirubin) can occur
F. Nursing diagnoses (see Table 15.34)

Table 15.34 Nursing Diagnoses Related to Rh and ABO Incompatibility

- Diagnoses in Table 15.31
- Risk for impaired corneal tissue integrity related to phototherapy light and continuous wearing of eyepads
- Risk for impaired skin integrity related to diarrhea, urinary excretions of bilirubin, and exposure to phototherapy light

G. Interventions:
  1. Administer RhoGam within 72 hours of delivery for Rh-negative mothers who have negative Coombs tests; nothing comparable for ABO incompatibility.
  2. Monitor infants carefully for jaundice.
  3. Implement phototherapy as ordered to increase the conjugation of bilirubin and prevent levels of bilirubin from becoming dangerously high.
     a. Remove clothes from infant; diaper minimally to allow maximum exposure to light.
     b. Cover eyes to prevent damage to retinas.
     c. Change infant's position every two hours to maximize exposure.
     d. Monitor temperature carefully.
     e. Remove from phototherapy for feeding; hold to provide human contact.
     f. Provide extra fluids to help excrete bilirubin.
     g. Observe skin for signs of irritation.
  4. Assist with exchange transfusion if ordered:
     a. Keep infant warm and restrained.
     b. Check blood for correct identification.
     c. Have oxygen and suction equipment available.
     d. Aspirate infant's stomach to prevent vomiting and aspiration.
     e. Obtain baseline vital signs and monitor every 15 minutes during the procedure.
     f. Assess infant after transfusion for cold stress and bleeding and check vital signs.
     g. Keep umbilical cord moist in case further transfusions are needed.

Hypoglycemia of the Newborn

A. Leading cause of preventable brain damage
B. Occurs frequently in infants born to diabetic mothers; may occur in other infants as well
C. Assessment findings:
  1. Lethargy
  2. Irritability; "jittery," tremors
  3. Pallor
  4. Irregular respirations; respiratory distress
  5. Poor feeding

  6. Blood glucose levels below 45 mg/dl (20 mg/dl in premature infants) using Dextristix
D. Nursing diagnoses:
  1. Nursing diagnoses (see Table 15.31)
  2. Risk for deficient fluid volume related to increased urinary excretion and osmotic diuresis
E. Interventions:
  1. Monitor blood glucose on any baby at risk: S.G.A., L.G.A., I.D.D.M. in mother, prematures.
  2. Feed: breast, 5 or 10% glucose water or formula
  3. If no improvement or if infant unable to suck, IV glucose is administered.
  4. Care as for a premature infant.

Sepsis

A. Sepsis is very serious; infant cannot localize infection.
B. Risk increased with prolonged rupture of membranes, maternal fever, or infection at delivery.
C. Assessment findings:
  1. Symptoms are often subtle.
  2. Temperature changes
  3. Behavioral changes: lethargy, irritability
  4. Poor feeding
  5. Vomiting
  6. Diarrhea
  7. Increased white blood cell (newborn has WBC up to 30,000 at birth, then drops)
  8. Sepsis workup: culture of spinal fluid, blood, any lesions, crevices, orifices, urine (suprapubic tap)
D. Nursing diagnoses (see Tables 15.31 and 15.32)
E. Interventions:
  1. Perform cultures as ordered.
  2. IV antibiotics
  3. Prevent heat loss.
  4. Maintain hydration.
  5. Administer oxygen if ordered.
  6. Weigh daily.
  7. Monitor closely.

Infant Born to Addicted Mother

A. Substance may be any addicting substance such as alcohol, heroin, or morphine.
B. Mother may have taken dose of addictive substance at beginning of labor, delaying withdrawal symptoms for 12–24 hours.
C. Assessment findings:
  1. Infants born to alcohol-abusing mothers exhibit fetal alcohol syndrome.
     a. Facial anomalies
     b. Fine motor dysfunction
     c. Genital anomalies (especially girls)
     d. Cardiac defects
     e. May be SGA

2. Irritability an early symptom
3. Sneezing and nasal stuffiness
4. High-pitched cry
5. Tremors
6. Respiratory distress, tachypnea, excessive secretions
7. Feeding problems
8. Other signs of withdrawal: sneezing, sweating, yawning, short sleep, frantic sucking
D. Nursing diagnoses (see Table 15.35)

Table 15.35 Nursing Diagnoses for Infant Born to Addicted Mother

- Risk for impaired skin integrity related to generalized diaphoresis and marked rigidity
- Diarrhea related to increased peristalsis secondary to hyperirritability
- Disturbed sleep pattern related to hyperirritability
- Risk for injury related to frantic sucking of fists
- Risk for injury related to uncontrolled tremors or tonic-clonic movements
- Disturbed sensory perception related to hypersensitivity to environmental stimuli
- Ineffective infant feeding pattern related to lethargy

E. Interventions:
1. Prevent over-stimulation to reduce seizures.
2. Swaddle, hold firmly.
3. Monitor vital signs, intake, and output.
4. Suction as needed.
5. Feed frequently in small amounts.
6. Provide careful skin care.
7. Administer anticonvulsants if ordered.

Necrotizing Enterocolitis

A. An ischemic attack to the intestine resulting in thrombosis and infarction of the affected bowel; may be caused by anything that causes blood to be shunted away from the intestine to the heart and brain (for example, fetal distress, low Apgar scores, RDS, prematurity, neonatal shock)
B. Usually occurs about four days of age
C. May result in bowel perforation and death
D. Assessment findings:
1. Infant in a high risk group
2. Findings relating to sepsis:
   a. Elevated temperature
   b. Apnea, labored breathing
   c. Cardiovascular collapse
   d. Lethargy or irritability
3. Gastrointestinal symptoms:
   a. Abdominal distention and tenderness
   b. Vomiting or increased gastric residual
   c. Poor feeding
   d. Stools test positive for blood.

e. X-rays show air in bowel, adynamic ileus, and thickening of the bowel wall.
E. Nursing diagnoses (see Tables 15.32 and 15.36)

Table 15.36 Nursing Diagnoses Related to Necrotizing Enterocolitis

- Risk for impaired skin integrity related to edema and immobility
- Diarrhea related to intestinal irritation secondary to infecting organism
- Risk for injury related to tonic-clonic movements and hematopoietic insufficiency
- Ineffective thermoregulation related to newborn transition to extrauterine environment
- Constipation related to decreased intestinal motility and immobility

---

F. Interventions:
1. Oral feedings discontinued; insert nasogastric tube
2. Do not use diapers to prevent possible trauma to abdomen.
3. Fluids and electrolytes as ordered to maintain acid-base balance
4. Antibiotics as ordered

Phenylketonuria

A. Autosomal recessive disorder in which there is an error of metabolism in which infant does not have ability to metabolize phenylalanine to tyrosine
B. Phenylalanine is in almost all proteins.
C. High levels of phenylalanine affect brain cells, causing mental retardation; danger to the infant is immediate.
D. Diagnostic tests:
1. Guthrie test (blood test) done after infant has ingested protein (breast milk or formula) for at least 24 hours.
2. Secondary screening:
   a. Done about six weeks
   b. Test fresh urine with Phenistix, which changes color.
3. Tests mandatory in most states to facilitate early detection and treatment
E. Assessment findings:
1. Phenylalanine levels above 8 mg/dl
2. Newborn appears normal; often fair with decreased pigmentation
3. Untreated PKU can cause failure to thrive, vomiting, eczema; brain involvement obvious by about six months
F. Interventions:
1. Restrict protein intake; substitute low phenylalanine formula (Lofenalac)
2. Teach parents about special diet which will be maintained throughout childhood

Sample Questions

1. At three hours of age, a term newborn seems jittery and has a weak and high-pitched cry and irregular respirations. The nurse suspects that the infant may have which of the following?
   1. Hypoglycemia
   2. Hypercalcemia
   3. Hypervolemia
   4. Hypothyroidism
2. The mother of a newborn is breastfeeding her infant on the delivery table. How can the nurse best assist her?
   1. Touch the infant's cheek adjacent to the nipple to elicit the rooting reflex.
   2. Leave the mother and baby alone and allow the infant to nurse as long as desired.
   3. Position the infant to grasp the nipple so as to express milk.
   4. Give the infant a bottle first to evaluate the baby's ability to suck.
3. Parents of a newborn note petechiae on the newborn's face and neck. The nurse should tell them that this is a result of which of the following?
   1. Increased intravascular pressure during delivery
   2. Decreased vitamin K level in the newborn infant
   3. A rash called erythema toxicum
   4. Excessive superficial capillaries
4. A newborn has a total body response to noise or movement that is distressing to her parents. What should the nurse tell the parents about this response?
   1. It is a reflexive response that indicates normal development.
   2. It is a voluntary response that indicates insecurity in a new environment.
   3. It is an automatic response that may indicate that the baby is hungry.
   4. It is an involuntary response that will remain for the first year of life.
5. When changing her newborn infant, a mother notices a reddened area on the infant's buttocks. How should the nurse respond?
   1. Have staff nurses instead of the mother change the infant.
   2. Use both lotion and powder to protect the area.
   3. Encourage the mother to cleanse and change the infant more frequently.
   4. Notify the physician and request an order for a topical ointment.
6. A woman, 32 weeks gestation, delivers a 3-pound, 8-ounce baby boy two hours after arriving at the hospital. What is the baby at risk for because of his gestational age?
   1. Mental retardation and seizures
   2. Hypothermia and respiratory distress
   3. Acrocyanosis and decreased lanugo
   4. Patent ductus arteriosus and pneumonia
7. Orders for a premature infant are for nipple feedings or gavage. What assessment findings are necessary before nipple feedings are given?
   1. The baby must have a respiratory rate of 20–30 and heart rate of 110–130.
   2. The baby must be alert and rooting.
   3. Sucking and gag reflexes must be present.
   4. Weight and temperature must be stable.
8. The mother of a 3-pound preterm infant has expressed a desire to breastfeed her baby. Because of his prematurity, she expresses fear that she can't. What is the best response for the nurse to make?
   1. "The baby won't be able to nurse for several weeks, but you can try at that time."
   2. "Breast milk does not have enough calories for premature babies."
   3. "You must be very disappointed that he is so small. Special formula is necessary. Perhaps you can nurse your next baby."
   4. "Breast milk is very good for premature babies. Even if he is not strong enough to nurse now, we will help you pump your breasts and give him the milk."
9. The mother of a term newborn born two hours ago asks the nurse why the baby's hands and feet are blue. What information should the nurse include when responding?
   1. Blue hands and feet can indicate possible heart defects.
   2. This is normal in newborns for the first 24 hours.
   3. This pattern of coloration is more common in infants who will eventually have darker skin color.
   4. Once the baby's temperature is stabilized, the hands and feet will warm up and be less blue.
10. A newborn is thought to have toxoplasmosis. The nurse explains to the family that toxoplasmosis is most likely to have been transmitted to the infant in which manner?
    1. Through a blood transfusion given to the mother
    2. Through breast milk during breastfeeding
    3. By contact with the maternal genitals during birth
    4. It crosses the placenta during pregnancy.
11. A newborn infant is with his mother, who is a diabetic. He appeared pink and alert and his temperature was stable when he left the nursery 15 minutes ago. His mother calls the nurse and says, "Look at his legs." The nurse observes spontaneous jerky movements. What is the best INITIAL action for the nurse to take?
    1. Tell his mother that this is normal behavior for a newborn.
    2. Tell the mother to feed him his glucose water now.
    3. Do a Dextrostix test on the infant.
    4. Take the baby back to the nursery and observe him for other behaviors and neurologic symptoms.

12. The nurse is caring for a premature infant. Immediately after arrival in the nursery, which nursing action is essential?
    1. Take the rectal temperature.
    2. Examine for anomalies.
    3. Check the airway for patency.
    4. Cleanse the skin of vernix.

13. A baby boy was born at 2:45 a.m. after a 35-week gestation. He weighed 1,170 grams. Upon admission to the premature nursery, he had slight respiratory distress, nasal flaring, grunting, intercostal retractions, and slight cyanosis. Apgar score at 1 minute was 4 and at 5 minutes was 6. Apical pulse 164, respirations 44, axillary temperature 96°F. What was the most likely cause of the baby's cyanosis?
    1. Increased serum concentration of bilirubin
    2. Inadequate oxygenation of arterial blood
    3. Excessive number of red blood cells
    4. Lack of subcutaneous fatty tissue

14. When assessing a newborn's need for oxygen, which should the nurse assess because it is the best indicator?
    1. Respiratory rate
    2. Skin color
    3. Pulse rate
    4. Arterial pO$_2$

15. On the evening of the second day after birth, the nurse notes that an infant appears icteric. What is the most likely cause?
    1. Rupture of a great number of fragile red cells in a short period of time
    2. Inflammatory obstruction of hepatic bile ducts and resorption of pigments
    3. Extravasation of blood from ruptured capillaries into subcutaneous tissue
    4. Faulty melanin metabolism due to absence of enzymes for normal protein synthesis

16. On the evening of the second day after birth, an infant was observed to be icteric, so he was exposed to blue light. What is the purpose of the blue light?
    1. To stimulate increased formation of vitamin K in the skin
    2. To enhance pigment breakdown by increasing body temperature
    3. To convert indirect bilirubin to a less toxic compound
    4. To increase brain electrical activity by stimulating the optic nerve

17. A young woman delivered her first baby this morning. She asks the nurse why the top of the baby's head is so soft and doesn't seem to have any bone. What should the nurse include when responding to the mother?
    1. This soft spot is called a fontanel and is normal; it makes delivery easier.
    2. It is a condition that occurs in some babies and will disappear within a few days.
    3. The physician is monitoring the infant for any problems which might occur with this common defect.
    4. It is called caput succadaneum and is caused by bleeding under the scalp during birth.

18. Which finding, if present, would suggest to the nurse that the infant was not at term when born?
    1. The scrotum has rugae.
    2. Testicles are not descended.
    3. Scanty vernix
    4. Sparse lanugo

19. The nurse is preparing a three-day-old infant for discharge from the hospital. When checking the record for completeness, the nurse checks to see that the infant has had which of the following?
    1. DTP and polio immunizations
    2. MMR immunization and tuberculin test
    3. Pneumococcal vaccine and HIV test
    4. Hepatitis B vaccine and PKU test

20. The physician has told the parents that their child probably has phenylketonuria. The parents ask the nurse what special needs the child will have. What should the nurse include in the response?
    1. The baby will most likely not develop normally for longer than six months and will die in a few years.
    2. The baby will have a special formula and cannot eat protein foods during childhood.
    3. Special feeding techniques are necessary until the child has surgery.
    4. The baby will not be able to void normally and will need to be catheterized frequently.

Answers and Rationales

1. (1) Being jittery and having a weak and high-pitched cry and irregular respirations are classic symptoms of hypoglycemia.

2. (1) The rooting reflex is stimulated when the cheek next to the breast is gently stroked. Answer 2 is not correct. The nurse should not leave the mother and baby alone until the nurse is confident that mother and baby are doing well. The infant should not nurse long enough to cause sore nipples. Answer 3 is not correct. The infant should grasp the areola, not the nipple. Answer 4 is not correct. Giving a bottle first would serve no purpose and might interfere with nursing.

3. (1) Increased intravascular pressure during delivery can cause petechiae. These will quickly disappear. Decreased vitamin K level in the infant might predispose the infant to bleeding from the umbilical cord but does not cause petechiae on the face and neck. Erythema toxicum is a generalized rash sometimes seen in newborns. It is not limited to the face and neck. Petechiae are not a result of excessive superficial capillaries.

4. (1) The response described is the startle reflex and is normal in newborns. It lasts only a few months.

5. (3) More frequent changing and cleaning of the area should help to prevent diaper rash. The mother should learn how to care for her baby and should be encouraged to change the infant. Using both lotion and powder would create a caked mess. The description in the question suggests a diaper rash. There is no need to contact the physician. The nurse will, of course, record the observation on the client's record.

6. (2) A premature infant lacks fat cells and is not able to alter body temperature. He has decreased surfactant and is apt to develop respiratory distress. Mental retardation and seizures are possible later complications of prematurity. Acrocyanosis is normal. Decreased lanugo is seen at term; a premature infant has more lanugo. Patent ductus arteriosus is not specifically related to prematurity. Pneumonia is not specifically related to prematurity.

7. (3) Before an infant can be given nipple feedings, he/she must have sucking and gag reflexes to prevent aspiration. The respiratory rate and heart rate given in answer 1 are below those of term infants and are totally unrealistic. A baby who is alert and rooting but does not have sucking and gag reflexes should not be given nipple feedings. Stable weight and temperature are not requirements for nipple feeding.

8. (4) This response helps to reinforce the mother's positive feelings as well as giving correct information. Answer 1 denies the mother's feelings and does not give correct information. Answers 2 and 3 are not correct. Breast milk is the best food for premature babies.

9. (2) Acrocyanosis or blue hands and feet is normal for the first 24 hours of life and is thought to be related to the establishment of circulation after delivery. Acrocyanosis in the first 24 hours does not suggest heart defects. Continuing acrocyanosis might. Bluish discoloration over the lower back and buttocks are called Mongolian spots and are typical in infants with more pigment in their skin. Acrocyanosis is not related to the regulation of temperature as much as it is related to the establishment of nonfetal circulatory patterns.

10. (4) Toxoplasmosis is transmitted from the mother to the baby through the placenta. The mother most likely acquired it from cat feces or eating raw meat. The mother could contract HIV or hepatitis from a blood transfusion. HIV could then affect the fetus. HIV can probably be transmitted through breast milk. Gonorrhea, chlamydia, and herpes can all be picked up by the infant during the birth process.

11. (3) The nurse needs more data on which to make an assessment. Dextrostix will test for blood sugar. The baby of a diabetic mother is apt to develop hypoglycemia. If the blood sugar is 35 mg/dl or less, he will be given glucose water and the physician will be notified. Jerky movements of the extremities are not normal and suggest hypoglycemia.

12. (3) The airway should be checked for patency immediately. Removing vernix is not a high priority. The temperature will be monitored, but this is not the highest priority. The nurse will check for anomalies, but this is not the highest priority. When the infant is stable, it will be bathed, and bloody material will be removed. Vernix is good for the skin.

13. (2) Cyanosis is indicative of inadequate oxygenation. Increased bilirubin would be evidenced by jaundice. It is normal for newborns to have excessive red blood cells. This does not cause cyanosis. Lack of subcutaneous fatty tissue is common in premature infants and causes poor temperature regulation.

14. 4) Arterial pO_2 is the best indicator of oxygen levels. Respiratory rate, skin color, and pulse rate can be affected by factors other than oxygenation. They are indicators but are not the most reliable.

15. (1) Red blood cells of premature infants are fragile and break down rapidly, causing an increase in bilirubin, which causes icterus or jaundice. The timing is key. Jaundice occurring after 49 hours is usually physiologic jaundice. Jaundice presenting at birth or within the first 24 hours is usually pathologic in nature. Obstruction of hepatic bile ducts would be a pathologic cause of jaundice and would occur earlier. Answer 3 is not realistic. This might cause a bruising appearance but not jaundice. Answer 4 makes no sense.

16. (3) The bili light or blue light enhances the breakdown of indirect bilirubin to a less-toxic compound. Vitamin K is not made in the skin, it is made in the intestines. Vitamin D is absorbed by the skin. Increasing temperature does not enhance pigment breakdown. The eyes are covered when the blue light is used to protect the eyes against damage.

17. (1) The mother appears to be describing the anterior fontanel, or soft spot, which occurs in all babies. The skull bones are not completely fused, allowing molding of the head during the birth process. This should close between 12 and 18 months. It is a normal condition occurring in all babies and is not a defect. Caput succadaneum is a swelling that may occur on the head following delivery. It crosses suture lines and is due to bleeding under the scalp during birth. It is normal and disappears in a few days. This is not what is described in the question.

18. (2) Testicles normally descend into the scrotum at eight months gestation. An infant born prior to that time will have undescended testicles. A term infant will have rugae on the scrotum. Vernix and lanugo are less with a term infant than with a premature infant.

19. (4) Hepatitis B vaccine is given within the first 12 hours after birth. A PKU test is done when the infant has had milk feedings for 24 hours. DTP and polio immunizations are usually started at two months of age. MMR is given at 15 months. A tuberculin test is usually done at one year. Pneumococcal vaccine is not routinely given to infants. Newborns are not routinely tested for HIV.

20. (2) Phenylketonuria is a disorder of purine metabolism in which phenylalanine is not metabolized properly and builds up in the blood and brain and causes severe mental retardation if not treated promptly. The treatment is to avoid foods containing phenylalanine. The child will have a special formula (Lofenalac) and cannot eat protein-containing foods. If diagnosed early and if the proper diet is followed, the child should do well.

Chapter 16

Pediatrics

GROWTH AND DEVELOPMENT

Terms

A. Growth: increase in body size
B. Development: increase in functional capacity
C. Maturation: the inborn, genetic transmitted capacity for development in all areas
D. Learning: the process by which one gains specific knowledge or skill and acquires a habit or attitude

Developmental Principles

A. General to specific: gross motor to fine motor progression of growth and development
B. Cephalocaudal: head to toe progression of growth and development
C. Proximodistal: center, outward progression of growth and development
D. Simple to complex

FIRST YEAR OF LIFE

A. Developmental periods:
   1. Freud:
      a. 0–6 months: oral passive; development of id; biologic pleasure principle
      b. 7–18 months: oral aggressive; teething; oral satisfaction of needs by mother decreases tension
   2. Erickson: birth to 1 year; trust versus mistrust; infant learns to trust when needs for food, comfort, and so on are met
   3. Piaget: 0–2 years; sensorimotor (reflexes, repetition of acts)
B. Growth:
   1. Doubles birth weight by 5–6 months
   2. Triples birth weight by one year
   3. Height is one and one-half times birth length by one year
   4. Rapid myelinization
C. Play: solitary

Infant: One to Four Months

A. Growth and development:
   1. Gains about 5–7 oz. weekly; weighs 8–13 lbs.
   2. Grows about 1 inch/month; head circumference increases by 1/2 inch for first six months; posterior fontanel closes about two months
   3. Pulse 100–150; respiration 30–40; B.P. 80s/40s
   4. Most neonatal reflexes disappear by four months; Babinski continues up to one year.
   5. Salivation and tears develop.
   6. Uses limbs simultaneously but not separately
   7. Starts to roll over (3 months)
   8. Turns head to side when prone
   9. Holds head erect in prone position (3 months)
   10. Sits if supported (3 months)
   11. Pushes feet against hard surface to move (3–4 months)
   12. Hitches: scoots backwards when sitting (3–4 months)
   13. Strong grasp (diminishes after 3 months when grasp reflex disappears)
B. Language:
   1. Communicates through crying, gurgling
   2. Quiet vowel sounds
C. Play: solitary
   1. Smiles at comforting person
   2. Plays with hands and fingers
   3. Reaches for objects; uses crib mobile
   4. Attends to voices
   5. Follows moving person when supine/enjoys supine position
   6. Brings feet to mouth
   7. Responds to more than one person at a time
   8. Rakes with whole hand to try to pick up small objects
   9. Reaches for and pats mirror
   10. Shakes rattle vigorously back and forth
   11. Needs to be held for warmth and security
D. Eating patterns/nutrition:
   1. Breast milk or iron-fortified commercial formula
   2. Two to 4 oz. every 2–4 hours—gradually increase to 6 oz. every 4–5 hours
   3. Hold and cuddle during feeding.
   4. Do not prop bottles and discourage infant cereals too early.
   5. Strong extrusion reflex (tongue) makes nipple feeding primary nutritive technique; pushes out with tongue when spoon put in mouth

Infant: Five to Six Months

A. Growth and development:
   1. Gains 3–5 oz./week
   2. Grows 1/2 inch/month
   3. Pulse 100–150; respiration 30; B.P. 91/50–30
   4. Eruption of one or two lower incisors
   5. Rolls over completely
   6. Improves binocular vision and hand-eye coordination
   7. Pulls self to sitting position
   8. Holds head steady when sitting
   9. Sits alone for short periods; leans forward (6 months)
B. Language: "ah-goo" sound occurs; babbling begins
C. Play: solitary
   1. Reaches for objects with flexed fingers
   2. Looks for objects when they are dropped
   3. Transfers objects from hand-to-hand at six months
   4. Bangs with objects held in hands
   5. Enjoys making lip noises
   6. Concentrates on inspection and exploration of toys
   7. Enjoys gross motor activity: being sat up, rolling over
   8. Cradle gym
   9. Teething beads
D. Eating patterns/nutrition:
   1. Continue breast milk or formula
   2. Six to 8 oz., 4–5 times daily
   3. May begin dry, iron-fortified infant cereal, approx. 2 Tbs. daily
      a. Mix cereal with milk to form a paste consistency and warm it slightly.
      b. Start with rice cereal, adding single grain types gradually and mixed grain last.
      c. Expect much cereal to be pushed out by tongue; scoop up and refeed.

Infant: Seven to Nine Months

A. Growth and development:
   1. Gains 3–5 oz./week and grows 1/2 inch/month
   2. Pulse 100–150; respiration 30; B.P. 90/40+ age in months
   3. Palmar grasp developed
   4. Teething: eruption of upper central incisors
   5. Hand-mouth coordination
   6. Probes with index finger
   7. Sits erect without support
   8. Pulls self to standing by holding onto crib side
   9. Crawls or creeps by 9 months
B. Language:
   1. Social babbling in interaction with others
   2. "Da-da" occurs before "ma-ma"
C. Play: solitary
   1. Picks up objects with both hands; holds bottle
   2. Preference for use of one hand
   3. Feeds self a cracker

4. Spoon and cup, nesting measuring cups, cereal bowl encourage learning to feed self
5. Peek-a-boo
6. Bouncing seats
7. Rubber blocks, plastic bells, balls
8. Small ball encourages locomotion
9. Stranger anxiety
10. Begins to test limits

D. Eating patterns/nutrition:
1. Breast milk or commercial formula
2. 24–32 oz. daily
3. Should still be held for feeding
4. Chewing replaces sucking.
5. Begins weaning process; addition of supplemental foods fed via spoon or cup
6. Discourage bottle in bed; give fluids in non-spill infant cup.
7. Two servings of iron-fortified cereal daily
8. Start apple or non-citrus fruit juice; 1–2 oz. and increase to 4 oz. daily
9. Offer juice in cup and large finger foods.
10. Begin strained fruits, vegetables, meats, whole cow's milk after 7 months of age.
11. Introduce one new food per week.
12. Avoid egg white, citrus, tomatoes, strawberries, corn syrup, seafood, spices, and chocolate.
13. Avoid honey as a sweetener.

Infant: Ten to Twelve Months

A. Growth and development:
1. Gains 3–5 oz./week; triples birth weight at 12 months
2. Grows 1/2 inch/month; height 29–30 inches—up 50% since birth
3. Head and chest circumference equal (18 1/2 inches); anterior fontanel almost closed
4. Pulse 80–150; respiration 30; B.P. 90/47+ age in months
5. Six teeth (central upper and lower lateral incisors)
6. Sits alone steadily

7. Hitches backward when sitting
8. Stands alone momentarily
9. Cruises (walks sideways while holding on to things)
10. Turning of feet and bowing of legs normal
11. Bowel and bladder patterns more regular (1–2 stools/day; dry diaper longer than 1–2 hours)
12. Uses jargon; uses da-da, ma-ma, and may use one other word
13. Imitates animal sounds; recognizes some objects by name (12 months)

B. Play: solitary:
1. Releases objects at will; on request (11 months)
2. Explores, feels, and pulls
3. Makes marks on paper
4. Repeats action that attracts attention
5. Waves bye-bye (10 months)
6. Clings to caregiver in strange situations but explores familiar surroundings in sight of caregiver
7. Exhibits frustration when restricted
8. Plays pat-a-cake and interactive games
9. Looks at pictures in book; learns what objects do
10. Toys of choice: blocks, balls, bright-colored rings, boxes and baskets, plastic bottles and containers, kiddie car propelled by feet

C. Eating patterns/nutrition:
1. Continue breast milk or commercial formula.
2. Gradually decrease the amount to 18–24 oz. daily.
3. Continue iron-fortified infant cereals.
4. Begin providing more textured food—finely chopped table or junior foods.
5. Start three meals per day; pattern of eating
6. Introduce small finger foods (for example, cheese cubes, and peeled/diced peaches).
7. Avoid high-fat foods (for example, fried foods, gravy, and bacon).

D. See Table 16.1.

Table 16.1 Summary of Growth and Development Milestones in First Year of Life

Age by the end of	Gross Motor	Fine Motor	Language	Personal-Social
First Quarter (3 months)	Rolls over	Grasps/shakes rattle	Squeals	Smiles spontaneously
Second Quarter (6 months)	Sits alone	Passes cube hand-to-hand	Polysyllabic vowel sounds	Shows interest in strange stimuli
Third Quarter (9 months)	Crawls/creeps	Picks up objects with both hands	Imitative/repetitive speech; "da-da" and "ma-ma"	Begins stranger anxiety/ definite social attachment
Fourth Quarter (12 months)	Stands alone	Neat pincer grasp	Recognizes some objects by name	Explores away from caregiver in familiar surroundings

TODDLER: ONE TO THREE YEARS

Overview

A. Developmental periods:
   1. Freud:
      a. Eighteen months—three years: anal (toilet training)
      b. Projection of feelings onto others
      c. Elimination and retention as ways to control and inhibit
   2. Erikson: autonomy versus shame and doubt
   3. Piaget:
      a. Two to four years: pre-operational
      b. No cause and effect reasoning
      c. Magical thinking
B. Growth and development:
   1. Growth begins to slow; average weight gain 4–6 pounds
   2. Legs elongate rather than trunk; height slows; grows three inches

Fifteen Months

A. Growth and development:
   1. Pulse 80–150; respiration 26–30; B.P. 91/56
   2. Walks alone at 12–15 months
   3. Creeps upstairs
B. Language:
   1. Vocalizes wants; responds to simple commands
   2. Uses 4–6 words, responds with no even if agreeing
C. Play: parallel:
   1. Builds a tower of two blocks
   2. Throws objects and picks them up again
   3. Pokes fingers in holes
   4. Opens boxes
   5. Points to desired objects
   6. Pats pictures in book; turns pages
   7. Indicates when diaper is wet
   8. Likes seeing people
   9. Simple fit together toys
   10. Toys of choice: balls, clothes pins, boxes, blocks, water toys, soft toys, stack toys
D. Eating patterns/nutrition
   1. Holds a cup; becoming more steady but spills
   2. Grasps a spoon and puts it in the dish; spills frequently
   3. Nutritional needs (see Table 16.2)

Eighteen Months

A. Growth and development:
   1. Pulse 80–150; respiration 26–30; B.P. 91/56
   2. Anterior fontanel closed
   3. Abdomen protrudes
   4. Walks and runs with a wide stance; seldom falls
   5. Walks sideways and backwards

Table 16.2 Toddler Nutritional Needs (12–30 Month Summary)

- Caloric need: 1300 Kcal/day
- Begin whole milk and completely wean from bottle.
- Limit milk intake to 16 to 24 oz. daily; low-fat or skim milk only after age 2 years (child needs fatty acids for growth; skim milk increases renal solute load)
- Two servings per day of iron-fortified infant cereals with other breads/cereals
- Gradually change to table foods such as canned fruits, well-cooked ground meats, drained tuna, custard, puddings.
- Avoid spicy food and mixed foods (stews or casseroles); toddlers are picky eaters and tolerate spicy foods poorly.
- Expect "food jags".
- Avoid small round or hard foods; choking is still a high risk.
- Expect a decreased appetite; diffuse power struggles; don't force child to eat.
- Offer nutritious between-meal snacks like cheeses, crackers, fruit; small nutritious snacks ensure nutritional balance in spite of their decreased intake.
- Avoid new food introduction when a toddler is hospitalized for short term.

   6. Climbs stairs and on furniture
   7. Seats himself on a small chair/pushes light furniture around room
   8. Short attention span/gets into everything
   9. Peak of thumb sucking
B. Language:
   1. Knows 10 words/adjective and noun phrases
   2. Calls for mother
C. Play: parallel:
   1. Pulls a toy behind him
   2. Throws ball into box; puts blocks into hole
   3. Scribbles; differentiates between straight and circular strokes
   4. Builds tower of three blocks
   5. Temper tantrums start
   6. Smears stool
   7. Has favorite toy or blanket
   8. Hugs doll or teddy bear
   9. Needs variety of activities
   10. Toys of choice: pull toys, stuffed toys, sturdy books with large pictures, pots and pans, drum, sand toys
D. Eating patterns/nutrition:
   1. Drinks from cup with little spilling
   2. Nutritional needs (see Table 16.2)

Twenty-Four Months

A. Growth and development:
   1. Weighs 26–28 pounds
   2. 32–33 inches tall (gain 3–4 inches in second year)
   3. Pulse 80–120; respiration 20–35; B.P. 92/56
   4. 16 temporary teeth; will get two-year molars soon
   5. Abdomen protrudes less than at 18 months

6. More grown up, gait steady
7. Jumps crudely
8. Walks up and down stairs with both feet on one step at a time, holding onto railing or wall
9. Obeys simple commands; does not ask for help, "Me do it"
10. Helps undress self
11. Temper tantrums continue
12. Does not know right from wrong
13. Fears parents leaving
B. Language:
   1. 300-word vocabulary
   2. Uses pronouns, no jargon
   3. 3–4 word sentences
C. Play: parallel:
   1. Builds tower of five or more blocks
   2. Turns doorknob
   3. Scribbles in a more controlled way
   4. Treats other children as physical objects
   5. Possessive; enjoys manipulating play materials
   6. Mimics parents in play
   7. Can put toys away
   8. Many bedtime demands, rituals; favorite toy to bed
   9. Toys of choice: pounding sets, slate, clay, paints, pulls blocks in wagon, doll carriage, doll furniture
D. Eating patterns/nutrition:
   1. Drinks well from small glass
   2. Uses spoon without spilling
   3. Nutritional needs (see Table 16.2)

Thirty Months

A. Growth and development:
   1. Pulse 70–110; respiration 20–35; B.P. 92/56
   2. Full set of 20 deciduous teeth
   3. Knows self as separate person
   4. Walks on tiptoe
   5. Copies horizontal or vertical lines—O or X
   6. Temper tantrums (continue)
   7. Toilet training if not before
B. Language
C. Play
   1. Parallel play; does not share, dawdles
   2. Stacks seven or eight blocks
   3. Play accompanied by constant talking; spontaneous, often rhythmical and repetitive
   4. Toys of choice: same as 24 months; likes household equipment, simple puzzles, sand and water play, tea parties with mud pies, painting, large beads to string
D. Eating patterns/nutrition:
   1. Fine motor skills improving so can feed self better
   2. Encourage independence in eating.

PRESCHOOLER: (THREE TO FIVE YEARS)

Overview

A. Developmental period:
   1. Freud
      a. 3–6 years
      b. Phallic: love of opposite sex parent
      c. Ego development
   2. Erickson:
      a. 3-6 years
      b. Initiative versus guilt
   3. Piaget:
      a. 2–4 years: pre-operational (preconceptual); no cause and effect reasoning; egocentrism
      b. 4–7 years: intuitive/pre-operational (beginning of causation)
B. Growth:
   1. Slow growth: 4–6 lbs/year; 3–5 inches/year
   2. 4 years: 40 inches, 40 lbs; double birth length
C. Vital signs: pulse 70–110; respiration 24–28; B.P. 90–100/56–60
D. Play: associative

Three Years Old

A. Growth and development:
   1. Weight—33 pounds; height—37 inches
   2. Tells when going to bathroom; occasional accident when playing
   3. Nighttime bowel and bladder control
   4. Walks backwards
   5. Climbs stairs with alternate feet
   6. Jumps from low step
   7. Pedals tricycle
   8. Swings
   9. Undresses; helps with dressing
   10. Washes hands; feeds self
   11. Brushes own teeth
B. Language:
   1. 900-word vocabulary
   2. Uses understandable language; some sounds experimental
   3. Some adjectives and adverbs; uses plurals
   4. Simple sentences
   5. Repeats sentence of six syllables
   6. Monologue; doesn't care if anyone listens
   7. Talks to self and imaginary playmate
   8. Knows first and last names
   9. Names figures in pictures
   10. Repeats three numbers
   11. Sings simple songs
C. Play:
   1. Solitary and parallel play with increasing social play in shifting groups of two or three
   2. Can wait turn and share

3. Can catch ball with arms extended
4. Pours liquid from pitcher
5. Hits large peg on board with hammer
6. Can build a tower of 9–10 blocks
7. Imitates a bridge
8. Copies circle or cross
9. Begins to use scissors (blunt)
10. Strings large beads
11. Simple puzzles (trial and error approach)
12. Tries to draw picture and name it
13. Dress-up play
14. Swings with trapeze
15. Likes fairy tales
16. Plays house
17. Frequently changes activity
18. Acts out nursery rhymes and stories
19. Acts out dumping and hauling
20. Toys of choice: crayons and paper, tricycle, spool toys

D. Eating patterns/nutrition (see Table 16.3)

Table 16.3 Preschooler Nutritional Needs (3–5 Year Summary)

- Caloric need: 1800 Kcal/day
- Diet from food pyramid; rule of thumb for serving size: 1 tablespoon for each food served for each year of age
- Quality over quantity; adjust to child's appetite
- Age 3–4 developmentally not ready to sit through long meal quietly
- Age 5–6 able to dine socially with decent table manners
- Limit fat to three daily servings to meet calorie needs
- Limit sweets and high fat/high salt foods to 1–2 daily servings to prevent excess weight gain
- Use substitute nutritious foods (yogurt, raisins, ice cream) in place of sweet desserts
- Fluoride supplements to prevent tooth decay

E. Mental and emotional characteristics:
1. Knows he is a separate person
2. Knows own sex and sex differences
3. Resists commands but can be distracted and will respond to suggestions
4. Can ask for help
5. Desire to please; friendly
6. Sense of humor
7. Uses language, rather than physical activity, to communicate
8. Imaginative
9. Can sacrifice immediate pleasure for promise of future gain
10. Can follow simple directions; does minor errands
11. Knows today; little comprehension of past and future
12. Attention span of 10–20 minutes

Four Years Old

A. Growth and development:
1. Weight 30–40 pounds; height 40 inches (double birth length)

2. Independent toilet habits (wants door shut for self but wants to be in bathroom with others); asks many questions about defecation
3. Runs easily
4. Skips clumsily
5. Hops on one leg
6. Aggressive physical activity
7. Heel-toe walk
8. Walks a plank
9. Climbs stairs without holding on to rail
10. Climbs and jumps without difficulty
11. Enjoys motor stunts and gross gesturing
12. Likes new activities
13. Can touch end of nose with forefinger
14. Dresses and undresses self except ties and zippers; can button
15. Catches ball thrown at five feet
16. Has concept of birthdays—knows his and his age
17. Loves parties and holidays
18. Concept of time; knows day of week
19. Attention span of 20 minutes

B. Language:
1. 1,500-word vocabulary
2. Concrete speech
3. Uses
4. Imitates and plays with words
5. Talks in sentences
6. Uses plurals and understands prepositions
7. Talks incessantly; asks many questions
8. Exaggerates, boasts, tattles
9. Uses profanity for attention
10. Combines reality and fantasy in stories
11. Likes to sing
12. Calls people names

C. Play:
1. Associative play; plays in groups of two or three
2. Puts toys away when reminded
3. Imaginative and dramatic play; plays house
4. Imaginary playmate; projects feelings and deeds onto others or imaginary playmate
5. May run away from home
6. Suggests and accepts turns; apt to be bossy
7. Dress up
8. Helps with household tasks
9. Silly; may be bossy
10. May be so busy playing he forgets to go to the bathroom
11. Poor space perception
12. Sand and water play
13. Draws, paints, colors
14. Combines blocks with furniture
15. Toys of choice: kite, paper weaving, sewing cards, paper airplanes

D. Eating patterns/nutrition (see Table 16.3)
E. Mental/emotional characteristics:
1. Counts to five; repeats four numbers
2. Knows which line is longer
3. Names one or more colors

4. Imaginary playmate of same sex and age
5. Seeks reassurance
6. Interested in things being funny; likes puns

Five Years Old

A. Growth and development:
   1. Weight—40–45 pounds; height—46–52 inches
   2. Vision—20/50 or 20/40
   3. Begins to lose baby teeth
   4. No longer tells when going to the bathroom
   5. Self-conscious about exposing self
   6. Separate bathrooms for boys and girls
   7. Voids four to six times during waking hours; occasional nighttime accident
   8. Runs with skill, speed, agility, and plays games simultaneously
   9. Jumps from 3–4 steps
   10. Balances self on toes; dances with rhythm
   11. Jumps rope
   12. Roller skates
   13. Hops and skips on alternate feet
   14. Getting adult curve to spine
   15. May tie shoelaces
   16. Uses hands to catch ball (not arms)
   17. Copies triangle or diamond from model
   18. Puzzles done quickly and smoothly
   19. Prints first name and some other letters
   20. Draws person
B. Language:
   1. 2,100-word vocabulary
   2. Meaningful sentences
   3. Talks constantly
   4. Repeats sentences of 12 or more syllables
   5. Asks searching questions
   6. Can tell a long story dramatically; adds to reality
   7. Sings relatively well
   8. Counts to 10
   9. Knows four colors; red, green, blue, yellow
C. Play:
   1. More graceful in play
   2. Puts toys away by self
   3. More realistic in play; less interested in fairy tales
   4. Restrained but creative
   5. Associative play; groups of 5–6
   6. Generous with toys
   7. Dramatic play about every event
   8. Play continues from day to day
   9. Rhythmic motion to music
   10. Tools and equipment of adults; sewing, carpentry
   11. Cuts out pictures
   12. Likes to run and jump, play with bicycle, wagon, sled, and skates
   13. Toys of choice: jump rope, cars, trucks, fad figures; beanie babies, and so on and mechanical toys
D. Eating patterns/nutrition (see Table 16.3)
E. Mental/emotional characteristics:
   1. Tells name and address
   2. Increasing independence
   3. Admits when needs help
   4. Improves uses of symbol system; concept formation
   5. Repeats long sentences accurately
   6. Can carry plot in story
   7. Defines objects in terms of use
   8. Less imaginative; seeks reality
   9. Asks details
   10. Can be reasoned with logically
   11. Begins to understand money
   12. Does more chores with confidence
   13. Interested in relatives
   14. Understands week as unit of time
   15. Knows day of week, month, and date
   16. Adults seen as changeless

SCHOOL-AGED CHILD

Overview

A. Developmental periods:
   1. Freud:
      a. 6–12 years; latent
      b. Sexual drive repressed; socialization occurs
      c. Superego and morality development
   2. Erikson:
      a. 6–12 years
      b. Industry versus inferiority
   3. Piaget:
      a. 4–7 years: intuitive/pre-operational (beginning of causation)
      b. 7–11 years; concrete operations
B. Growth:
   1. Slow growth
   2. No longer thin and wary in appearance
   3. Doubles weight during this period
   4. Permanent teeth
   5. Refinement of fine motor skills; basic neuromuscular mechanisms developed by age six
   6. Vision 20/20 by age 6–7
   7. Second teeth appear; year molars by 6–7 years; then 4 teeth/year for seven years; most permanent teeth by age 12
   8. Secondary sex characteristics appear: girls 10–12 years; boys 12–14 years
C. Vital signs: pulse 70–100; respiration 18–30; BP 95–108/ 56–68
D. Play:
   1. Cooperative
   2. Likes rules
   3. Team play

Six Years Old

A. Behavioral characteristics:
   1. Self-centered
   2. Temper outbursts release tension

3. Behavioral extremes: impulsive or dawdles; loving or antagonistic
4. Difficulty making decisions; needs reminders
5. Verbally aggressive but easily insulted
6. Intense concentration for a short time, then abruptly stops activity
7. Security of routines and rituals essential
8. Series of three commands followed
9. Praise and recognition needed

B. Body image development:
1. Self centered
2. Likes to be in control of self, situations, and possessions
3. Knows right from left hand
4. Regresses occasionally with baby talk or earlier behavior
5. Plays at being someone else to clarify sense of self and others
6. Interested in marriage and reproduction
7. May indulge in sex play
8. Draws man with hands, neck, clothing, and six identifiable parts

C. Eating patterns/nutrition (see Table 16.4):
1. Large appetite; likes snacks
2. Awkward at table; likes to eat with fingers
3. Dawdles
4. Better manners away from home

Table 16.4 School Age Nutritional Needs (6–12 Years Summary)

- Calorie needs: 2,100 Kcal/day (7–10 years) 2,400 Kcal/day (11–12 years)
- Diet from pyramid food groups with gradual portion increase
- Avoid excess fat, desserts, and "junk" foods
- Protein and calorie needs increase as the child grows.
- Teaching about foods is well received in this age group.

Eight Years Old

A. Behavioral characteristics:
1. Expansive personality but fluctuating behavior
2. Robust, energetic
3. Impatient
4. Affectionate to parents
5. Hero worship
6. Responds better to suggestions than commands
7. Feelings easily hurt
8. Gradually accepts inhibitions and limits

B. Body image development:
1. Ready for physical contact in play; teach self-defense mechanisms
2. Aware of sex differences; curious about another's body
3. Asks questions about marriage and reproduction
4. Same-sex playmates preferred; will play with opposite sex if no one else around

5. More independent and self-controlled; dependable, responsible
6. Loyal to home and parents
7. More involved with peers
8. Own interests subordinated to group demands and adult authority
9. Critical of own and other's behavior
10. Concerned about fairness; willing to take own share of blame
11. More aware of society

C. Eating patterns/nutrition:
1. Large appetite
2. Enjoys trying new foods
3. Handles utensils skillfully
4. Better table manners away from home

Ten Years Old

A. Behavioral characteristics:
1. More adult-like and posed, especially girls
2. More self-directive, independent
3. Organized and rapid in work; budgets time and energy
4. Suggestions followed better than requests, but obedient
5. Family activities and care of younger siblings, especially below school age, enjoyed
6. Aware of individual differences among people but does not like to be singled out in a group
7. Hero worship of adult
8. Loyal to group; has a best friend
9. Preoccupied with right and wrong
10. Better able to play by the rules
11. Critical sense of justice; accepts immediate punishment for wrongdoing
12. Liberal ideas of social justice and welfare
13. Strong desire to help animals and people
14. Identifies with parents
15. Sense of leadership

B. Body image development:
1. Relatively content and confident of self
2. Perfected most small motor movements
3. Wants privacy for self but peeks at the other sex
4. Asks some questions about sexual matters again; investigates own sexual organs
5. Girls show beginning prepubertal changes

C. Eating patterns/nutrition (see Table 16.4):
1. Goes on eating sprees; likes sweet foods
2. Criticizes parent's table manners at times
3. Has lapses in control of table manners at times
4. Enjoys cooking

Twelve Years Old

A. Behavioral characteristics:
1. Self-contained, self-competent, tactful, kind, reasonable, less self-centered
2. Outgoing, eager to please, enthusiastic

3. Sense of humor
4. Sensitive to feelings of others
5. Wants to be treated like an adult; sometimes behaves childlike
6. Tolerant of self and others
7. Peer groups and best friends important
8. Ethical sense more realistic than idealistic
9. Decisions about ethical questions based on consequences
10. Less tempted to do wrong; basically truthful
11. Self-disciplined, accepts just discipline
12. Enthusiastic about community projects
B. Body image development:
  1. Growth spurt, changes in appearance
  2. Muscular control almost equal to adult
  3. Group important
  4. Begins to accept and find self as unique person
  5. Feels joy of life with mature understanding
C. Eating patterns/nutrition:
  1. Large appetite
  2. Adult table manners
  3. Participates in table discussion in adult-like manner

ADOLESCENCE

Developmental Period

A. Freud: genital:
  1. 12–20 years
  2. Sexual pleasure through genitals
  3. Becomes independent of parents, responsible for self
  4. Develops sexual identity, ability to love and work
B. Erickson:
  1. 12–20 years
  2. Identity versus role confusion
  3. Develops sense of self; preparation for adult roles versus doubts relating to sexual identity
C. Piaget:
  1. 11–15 years
  2. Formal operations
  3. Reality; abstract thought

Physiologic Aspects: Growth and Development

A. Males grow 4–12 inches and gain 15–65 pounds in a period of a couple of years.
B. Females grow 2–8 inches and gain 15–35 pounds in a period of a couple of years.
C. Skeletal system grows faster than supporting muscle; clumsy and awkward

D. Heart and lungs grow more slowly; fatigue and increased needs for rest and sleep
E. Girls stop growing sooner; rapid epiphyseal closure because of increasing estrogen levels
F. Ovulation and onset of regular menses in girls
G. Spermatogenesis and nocturnal emissions occur in boys
H. Vital signs reach adult level
I. Sebaceous glands become very active, causing acne
J. Sweat glands over entire body, which were nonfunctional in childhood, now become more active

Cognitive and Language Aspects

A. Time when the mind has the greatest ability to acquire and utilize knowledge
B. Imaginative thinking
C. Setting up structure for adult thinking

Psychosocial Aspects

A. Peer group has five stages:
  1. Unisexual; preadolescent group
  2. Unisexual but mixing with groups of opposite sex
  3. Heterosexual
  4. Heterosexual with paired couples
  5. Paired couples; going steady or engaged; several couples sharing activities but disintegration of total group
B. Mood swings and extremes of behavior
C. Swings from independent behaviors to dependent behaviors
D. Parent-child relationship changes from one of protection and dependency to mutual affectionate equality
E. Relationship problems occur, including rejection of the parents as the adolescent tries to achieve independence and the parents continue to place some checks on the process.
F. Nutritional needs (see Table 16.5)

Table 16.5 Adolescent Nutritional Needs (Adolescence)

- Calorie needs: males need 3,000 Kcal/day; females need 2,200–2,400 Kcal/day
- Always hungry
- Sharply increased needs for protein and calcium; quart of milk/day
- Males need more B vitamins.
- Females need more iron.
- Choice of foods influenced by peers
- Provide written materials/visual aids when teaching about diet.

REACTION TO HOSPITALIZATION/SEPARATION

Infant

A. Little awareness in early infancy
B. Stranger anxiety starts at 6–8 months; wants parent

Toddler

A. Protest:
   1. Cries loudly when parents leave
   2. Normal response; comfort child
B. Despair:
   1. Sits in a corner and sucks thumb or blanket; does not cry
   2. Child needs comforting; more serious than protest
C. Denial:
   1. Ignores parents when they visit and goes to the nurse
   2. Comfort child and reassure parents that child is just trying to avoid being hurt again when they leave.

Preschooler

A. Separation anxiety; fears separation from parents
B. Fear of loss of body control and bodily injury; has just gained control of bowel and bladder; fears losing it

School Age

A. Separation anxiety; fears separation from parents
B. Fear of mutilation

Adolescents

A. Fear of separation from peers
B. Fear of loss of body control
C. Fear of pain
D. Loss of identity

GROWTH AND DEVELOPMENT ISSUES

Communicable Diseases

A. Prevention of disease:
   1. Immunization schedule (see Table 16.6)
   2. If immunization schedule is interrupted, child does not need to start over; give next immunization due.
   3. For children not immunized by age 7, recommended immunizations are given in the same sequencing.
   4. If immunization status of child is unknown, the child should be considered at risk for disease and immunized appropriately.
   5. Contraindications for immunization:
     a. Anaphylactic reaction to a vaccine; give no more doses of that vaccine
     b. Anaphylactic reaction to a vaccine constituent such as eggs; give no vaccines containing that substance
     c. Moderate or severe illness even if the child does not have a fever
     d. Immunocompromised persons should not receive live vaccines.

B. Management of children with communicable diseases:
   1. If the child has symptoms of a communicable disease, keep the child out of school and away from other children.
   2. Institute appropriate precautions to prevent the spread of the disease; most childhood diseases are spread by respiratory secretions.
   3. Chicken pox: keep child home from school until lesions are all crusted over; child is communicable just before rash starts and as long as there are any fluid-filled vesicles.
   4. Diseases caused by a virus are treated symptomatically; bacteria-caused diseases are treated with the appropriate antibiotic.

C. Tuberculin testing:
   1. Tuberculin skin test is the most practical method for screening for tuberculosis.
   2. Tuberculin skin test can be done at the same time as immunizations.
   3. Testing is recommended at 12–15 months of age, before starting school at 4–6 years, in adolescence (14–16 years), and whenever a person has contact with a person who has tuberculosis; testing may be done yearly in areas with a high incidence of tuberculosis.
   4. Procedure:
     a. 0.1 ml PPD tuberculin injected intradermally into forearm
     b. Read 48–72 hours after injection.
     c. 10 mm or more induration indicates a positive reaction; redness does not indicate a positive reaction.
   5. Positive reaction indicates client has antibodies to tuberculosis:
     a. The most likely reason for antibody production is exposure to the tuberculosis organism.
     b. Persons who have had the BCG vaccine may have a positive skin test.
     c. Positive skin test does not prove individual has tuberculosis.
     d. Positive skin test will be followed by X-ray and sputum test.

Table 16.6 Recommended Childhood Immunization Schedule (From Centers of Disease Control and Prevention, United States, January to December 2001)

Vaccine	Birth	1 mo	2 mo	4 mo	6 mo	12 mo	15 mo	18 mo	24 mo	4–6 mo	11–12 mo	14–18 mo
									Age			
Hepatitis B	Hep B #1											
		Hep B #2			Hep B #3						Hep B	
Diphtheria tetanus toxids, and pertussis		DTaP	DTaP	DTaP		DTaP				DTaP	Td	
H. influenzea type b		Hib	Hib	Hib	Hib							
Inactivated polio--		IPV	IPV	IPV						IPV		
Pneumococcal conjugate		PCV	PCV	PCV	PCV							
Measles-Mumps-Rubella					MMR					MMR	MMR	
Varicella					Var						Var	
Hepatitis A									Hep A in selected area			

 Range of recommended ages for vaccination.

 Vaccines to be given if previously recommended doses were missed or were given earlier than the recommended minimum age.

Recommended in selected states and/or regions.

Failure to Thrive

A. Physical and developmental retardation in infants and small children; usually related to disruptive maternal-child relationship
B. Must rule out physical diseases such as cystic fibrosis and malabsorption syndromes
C. Assessment findings:
  1. Child fails to gain weight and is persistently below fifth percentile on growth charts
  2. Below-normal achievement in fine and gross motor, social-adaptive, and language skills
  3. Sleep disturbances
  4. Feeding problems; rumination (voluntary regurgitation and reswallowing)
  5. Disturbed maternal-infant interaction patterns: mother may not hold and cuddle infant frequently; may not respond to infant's signals for hunger and need for contact
D. Nursing diagnoses (see Table 16.7)

E. Interventions:
  1. Provide consistent care: same caregiver should care for child whenever possible.
  2. Teach parents how to feed child correctly.
  3. Involve parents in care of child.
  4. Nurse should model loving, caring behaviors toward child.
  5. Make sure that referrals to appropriate community agencies have been made.

Child Abuse (See Psychiatric Nursing)

Sudden Infant Death Syndrome (SIDS)

A. Sudden and unexpected death of an apparently healthy infant, not explained by careful postmortem studies; usually occurs between birth and 9 months with peak incidence at 3 to 5 months
B. Cause is unknown at the present time.
C. Assessment findings:

Table 16.7 Nursing Diagnoses Related to Failure to Thrive

- Imbalanced nutrition: less than body requirements related to inadequate intake secondary to lack of emotional and sensory stimulation or lack of knowledge of caregiver
- Delayed growth and development related to inadequate caretaking, indifference, multiple caretakers, or environmental and stimulation deficiencies
- Disturbed sleep pattern related to anxiety and apprehension secondary to parental deprivation
- Disturbed sensory perception related to history of insufficient sensory input from primary caregiver
- Impaired parenting related to insufficient knowledge of parenting skills, impaired caregiver, impaired child, lack of support system, lack of role model, relationship problems, unrealistic expectations for child, or unmet psychological needs
- Impaired home maintenance management related to difficulty of caregiver with maintaining a safe home environment
- Deficient knowledge regarding pathophysiology of condition, nutritional needs, growth/development expectations, and parenting skills related to lack of information or misinformation or misinterpretation of information
- Risk for ineffective management of therapeutic regiment related to insufficient knowledge of growth and development requirements, feeding guidelines, risk for child abuse, parenting skills, and community agencies

1. Usually occurs during sleep with no evidence of struggle; death is silent.
2. Incidence is higher in preterm infants, twins, triplets, and low-birth-weight infants.
3. Infant with abnormalities in respiration, feeding, and those with neurological symptoms have higher incidence.
4. Some studies show a higher incidence in infants who are positioned on their abdomen.
5. Some studies show a higher incidence in infants in homes where cigarette smoking occurs.

D. Interventions:
   1. Resuscitation is usually unsuccessful because death is silent and child has usually been dead for some time when discovered.
   2. Support of family is essential:
      a. Provide private area for family.
      b. Prepare family for appearance of infant (cold, may be discolored due to settling of blood after death).
      c. Allow family to hold and rock infant if desired; facilitates reality of death, allows time to say good-bye, and helps grieving process.
   3. Emphasize that baby's death was not their fault.
   4. Be sure that appropriate support referrals are made (clergy, SIDS support groups, and so on).

Death and Dying

A. Parental response:
   1. Parents initially express grief in response to the anticipated loss of a child.
   2. Parents will be at different stages of grief response at different times during child's illness.
   3. Death or anticipated death of child a very stressful event; often places severe strain on marriage and family relationships.
   4. Parents who have lost a child experience intense grief for a long period of time.
B. Child's response to death depends on age of child:
   1. Infants and toddlers:
      a. Live only in the present
      b. Do not understand concept of death as end of life as we know it
      c. May sense sadness in others
      d. Toddlers may feel guilty for making others sad (due to magical thinking).
   2. Preschoolers:
      a. Think of death as temporary; like sleep or separation
      b. Very concrete thinkers; use the word "dead" but do not understand the finality of death
      c. May make statements such as, "Who will take care of me when I die?" or "Will you come and visit me after I am dead?"
      d. May regress in behavior
   3. School-age:
      a. Have concept of time, cause and effect, and irreversibility of death but may still question it
      b. Fear pain, mutilation, and abandonment
      c. Interested in death ceremony
      d. Often feel death is punishment
      e. Sometimes personify death as the "boogey man"
      f. May know they are going to die; are comforted by having parents and loved ones with them
   4. Adolescents:
      a. Think about the future they will not be able to participate in
      b. Often express anger at impending death; sometimes find it difficult to talk about death
      c. May want to leave a legacy; want the world to know they were here
      d. May want to plan their own funeral

Poisonings

A. Poisonings occur most frequently in toddlers and suicidal adolescents; most ingestions are acute; most poisonings are preventable.

B. General interventions:
  1. Emergency care: Airway, Breathing, Circulation
  2. Identify what substance ingested and how much ingested
  3. Remove the poison from the body:
     a. Induce emesis:
        (1) Do not induce vomiting if child is unconscious or a caustic substance was ingested (toilet bowl cleaner, dishwasher detergent) or petroleum distillate (kerosene, roach spray, furniture polish)
        (2) Syrup of ipecac:
           (a) 30 cc for teens; 15 cc for child; 10 cc for infant
           (b) Follow with 100–200 cc of water.
           (c) Repeat in 20–30 min. if there is no response.
     b. Gastric lavage:
        (1) Largest tube that will pass through esophagus is used.
        (2) Aspirate gastric contents.
        (3) Use water or half normal saline.
        (4) Aspirate until returns clear.
  4. Reduce the effect of the poison:
     a. Activated charcoal:
        (1) Minimizes absorption by binding toxins
        (2) Give after vomiting with ipecac.
        (3) 5–10 gm for each gram of drug ingested
        (4) Mix charcoal with water to make a syrup that can be given by mouth or NG tube.
     b. Specific antidote if there is one
  5. Eliminate the absorbed poison:
     a. Force diuresis.
     b. Dialysis
     c. Exchange transfusion
  6. Teach parents to childproof environment.
  7. Follow-up psychiatric care for suicide attempt
C. Nursing diagnoses (see Table 16.8)
D. Aspirin ingestion:
  1. Information:
     a. Toxicity begins at doses of 50–100 mg/kg

     b. Additional substances may be in aspirin products and create additional problems.
     c. Peak effect of aspirin is 2–4 hours; lasts eight hours
     d. Aspirin causes CNS stimulation, fluid and electrolyte loss, respiratory alkalosis, metabolic acidosis, and impaired glucose metabolism.
  2. Assessment findings:
     a. Hyperventilation, hyperpyrexia, hyperglycemia, tinnitus, headache, bleeding
     b. Vomiting, sweating, dehydration
     c. Decreased LOC, confusion, seizures, coma
  3. Interventions:
     a. As above
     b. Monitor for latent effects if time-release capsules
     c. Hemodialysis may be indicated.
     d. IV therapy may be indicated.
E. Acetaminophen ingestion:
  1. Assessment findings:
     a. Vague and nonspecific initially; nausea and vomiting, anorexia, sweating
     b. Jaundice, liver tenderness, increase in liver enzymes, abdominal pain
     c. Progresses to hepatic failure
  2. Intervention
     a. Emesis or lavage
     b. Do NOT use activated charcoal because it will bind the antidote.
     c. Antidote: acetylcysteine (mucomyst) lessens liver damage if given within 16 hours of ingestion
F. Lead Poisoning:
  1. Causes:
     a. Most common source is lead-based paint used in homes prior to 1950.
     b. Lead is also in dust on the streets from leaded gas.
     c. Pica (strange appetite, eating paint chips) in toddlers and preschoolers leads to lead poisoning.
  2. Lead is absorbed through the GI tract and pulmonary system and deposited in bone, soft tissue, and blood; excretion is via urine, feces, and sweat.
  3. Assessment findings:
     a. Abdominal complaints including colicky pain, constipation, anorexia, vomiting, and/or weight loss
     b. Pallor, listlessness, fatigue
     c. Clumsiness, irritability, loss of coordination, ataxia, seizures
     d. Encephalopathy
     e. Lead in blood: lead levels of 5–30 mg/dL not dangerous; symptoms appear above 70 mg/d
  4. Nursing diagnoses (see Table 16.9)

Table 16.8 Nursing Diagnoses Related to Accidental Poisonings

- Risk for poisoning related to presence of toxic substance, immature judgment of child
- Risk for injury related to presence of toxic substance
- Fear/anxiety related to sudden hospitalization and treatment
- Interrupted family processes related to sudden hospitalization and emergency aspects of illness

Table 16.9 Nursing Diagnoses Related to Lead Poisoning

Acute:
- Risk for trauma related to loss of coordination, altered level of consciousness, clonic or tonic muscle activity, and neurological damage
- Risk for fluid volume deficit related to excessive vomiting, diarrhea, or decreased intake
- Deficient knowledge regarding sources of lead and prevention of poisoning related to lack of information or misinterpretation of information

Chronic:
- Imbalanced nutrition, less than body requirements related to decreased intake due to chemically induced changes in the gastrointestinal tract
- Disturbed thought processes related to deposition of lead in central nervous system and brain tissue
- Chronic pain related to deposition of lead in soft tissues and bone

5. Interventions:
   a. Chelating agents (dimercaprol [BAL in oil] edate calcium disodium [Calcium EDTA]) to bind the lead and remove it
   b. Eliminate sources of lead in the environment.

Sample Questions

1. A three-month-old infant is admitted. Upon admission, the nurse assesses her developmental status as appropriate for age. Which of the following would the client be least likely able to do?
   1. Smile in response to mother's face
   2. Reach for shiny objects but miss them
   3. Hold head erect and steady
   4. Sit with slight support

2. A three-month-old infant is doing well after the repair of a cleft lip. The nurse wants to provide the client with appropriate stimulation. What is the best toy for the nurse to provide?
   1. Colorful rattle
   2. String of large beads
   3. Mobile with a music box
   4. Teddy bear with button eyes

3. Which toys would be best for a five-month-old infant who has infantile eczema?
   1. Soft, washable toys
   2. Stuffed toys
   3. Puzzles and games
   4. Toy cars

4. Which diversion would be appropriate for the nurse to plan to use with an eight-month-old infant?
   1. A colorful mobile
   2. Large blocks to stack
   3. A colorful rattle
   4. A game of peek-a-boo

5. Which activity would best occupy a 12-month-old child while the nurse is interviewing the parents?
   1. String of large snap beads and a large plastic bowl
   2. Riding toy
   3. Several small puzzles
   4. Paste, paper, and scissors

6. An 18-month-old is admitted for a repeat cardiac catheterization. The parents are continuously present and do everything for the child: dress him, feed him, even play for him. The nurse wants to prepare the child and the parents for the procedure. Which should be included in the care plan?
   1. Give the child simple explanations.
   2. Talk with the parents to assess their knowledge and how they can help with the child's care.
   3. No specific action will be necessary because the child and family have been through a cardiac catheterization previously.
   4. Ask the parents to stay away as much as possible because they upset the child.

7. In planning care for an 18-month-old, the nurse would expect him to be able to do which of the following?
   1. Button his shirt and tie his shoes
   2. Feed himself and drink from a cup
   3. Cut with scissors
   4. Walk up and down stairs

8. The mother of a two-year-old child asks the nurse how to cope with the child's frequent temper tantrums when he does not get what he wants immediately. What information should the nurse include when responding?
   1. As long as the child is safe, ignore him during the tantrum.
   2. If the child's demands are reasonable, give him part of what he wants.
   3. Spank the child if the tantrum continues for more than five minutes.
   4. Explain to the child why he cannot have what he wants and promise him a reward when he stops crying.

9. A three-year-old is admitted to the pediatric unit for diagnostic tests. His mother is discussing the child's hospitalization with the nurse. She is concerned about staying with this child and caring for her other two children at home. Which suggestion to the mother will most help the child adjust to being in the hospital?
   1. Do not visit the child until discharge so that your child won't cry when you leave.
   2. Spend the night in the hospital with your child.
   3. Bring your child's favorite teddy bear and security blanket to the hospital.

4. Buy your child a gift to let the child know you care deeply.
10. The parents of a three-year-old are leaving for the evening. Which behavior would the nurse expect the child to exhibit?
    1. Wave good-bye to the parents
    2. Cry when the parents leave
    3. Hide his/her head under the covers
    4. Ask to go to the playroom
11. When planning outdoor play activities for a normal four-year-old child, which activity is most appropriate?
    1. Two-wheeled bike
    2. Sandbox
    3. Climbing trees
    4. Push toy lawn mower
12. A five-year-old had major surgery several days ago and is allowed to be up. When planning diversion activity, which action by the nurse is most appropriate?
    1. Give the child a book to read.
    2. Play a board game with the child.
    3. Encourage the child to play house with other children.
    4. Turn on the television so the child can watch cartoons.
13. A six-year-old is admitted for a tonsillectomy. Considering the child's age, which of the following would be the most important to include in a pre-operative physical assessment?
    1. Characteristics of tongue, gum, or lip sores
    2. Any sign of tonsilar inflammation
    3. The number and location of any loose teeth
    4. The location and presence of tenderness in any swollen lymph nodes
14. A six-year-old child is in the terminal stage of leukemia. The child appears helpless and afraid. How can the nurse best help the child?
    1. Allow the child to make the major decisions for her care.
    2. Make all decisions for the child.
    3. Discuss with the child the fears that dying children usually have.
    4. Discuss with the child the reasons for her fears.
15. The nurse is preparing a six-year-old for cardiac surgery. Which pre-operative teaching technique is most appropriate?
    1. Have the child practice procedures that will be performed post-operatively, such as coughing and deep breathing.
    2. Arrange for the child to tour the operating room and surgical ICU.
    3. Encourage the child to draw pictures illustrating the operation.
    4. Arrange for the child to discuss heart surgery and post-operative events with a group of children who have undergone heart surgery.
16. A 10-year-old girl is being treated for rheumatic fever. Which would be an appropriate activity while she is on bed rest?
    1. Stringing large wooden beads
    2. Engaging in a pillow fight
    3. Making craft items from felt
    4. Watching television
17. A 10-year-old who is immobilized in a cast following an accident has been squirting other children and the staff with a syringe filled with water. The nurse wants to provide other activities to help him express his aggression. Which activity would be most appropriate?
    1. Cranking a wind-up toy
    2. Pounding clay
    3. Putting charts together
    4. Writing a story
18. An 11-year-old boy is admitted to the pediatric unit in traction with a fractured femur sustained in a motorcycle accident. His uncle, who was driving the cycle when the accident occurred, received only minor injuries. The child tells the nurse that his uncle was not to blame for the accident. He is "the best motorcycle rider in the world." The nurse interprets this to mean that the child is exhibiting which defense mechanism?
    1. Denial
    2. Repression
    3. Hero worship
    4. Fantasy
19. The nurse is planning care for an 11-year-old who has a fractured femur and is in traction. Which activity would be most appropriate?
    1. Dramatizing with puppets
    2. Building with popsicle sticks
    3. Watching television
    4. Coloring with crayons or colored pencils
20. A two-year-old is hospitalized for a fractured femur. During his first two days in the hospital, he lies quietly, sucks his thumb, and does not cry. Which is the best interpretation of his behavior?
    1. He has made a good adjustment to being in the hospital.
    2. He is comfortable with the nurses caring for him.
    3. He is experiencing anxiety.
    4. He does not have a good relationship with his parents.
21. A hospitalized two-and-a-half-year-old has a temper tantrum while her mother is bathing her. Her mother asks the nurse how she should handle this behavior. Which information should be included in the nurse's reply?
    1. Temper tantrums in a hospitalized child indicate regression.
    2. Tantrums suggest a poorly developed sense of trust.
    3. Discipline is necessary when a child has a temper tantrum.
    4. This behavior is a normal response to limit setting in a child of this age.
22. A three-year-old resists going to bed at night. Her mother asks the nurse what she should say

to her. Which response should the nurse suggest to the mother as most appropriate?
1. "I don't love you anymore because you don't know how to listen."
2. "All good children go to bed on time."
3. "If you go to sleep now, I'll take you to the zoo tomorrow."
4. "Here is your blanket. It's time to go to sleep."

23. An eight-year-old is terminally ill. Considering the child's age, which statement would you most expect the child to make?
1. "After I'm dead, will you come visit me?"
2. "Who will take care of me when I am dead?"
3. "Will it hurt me when I die?"
4. "Can you help me do a videotape about dying from leukemia?"

24. A father has brought his four-month-old daughter to the well-baby clinic. Which statement he makes is greatest cause for concern to the nurse?
1. "She cannot sit up by herself."
2. "She does not hold the rattle as well as she did at first."
3. "She does not follow objects with her eyes."
4. "She spits up after a feeding."

25. A three-year-old has all of the following abilities. Which did he acquire most recently?
1. Walking
2. Throwing a large ball
3. Riding a tricycle
4. Stating his name

26. The mother of a two-year-old calls the doctor's office because her child swallowed "the rest of the bottle of adult aspirin" about a half hour ago. The nurse determines that there were about 15 tablets left in the bottle. What initial assessment findings are consistent with aspirin ingestion?
1. Bradypnea and pallor
2. Hyperventilation and hyperpyrexia
3. Subnormal temperature and bleeding
4. Melena and bradycardia

27. A toddler who has swallowed several adult aspirin is admitted to the emergency room. When admitted, the child is breathing but is difficult to arouse. What is the immediate priority of care?
1. Administration of syrup of ipecac
2. Cardiopulmonary resuscitation
3. Ventilatory support
4. Gastric lavage

28. A six-month-old is being seen for a well-baby visit. The child has received all immunizations as recommended so far. What immunizations does the nurse expect to give at this visit?
1. DTP, MMR, IPV
2. DTP, hepatitis B, HIB
3. HIB, IPV, varicella
4. MMR, hepatitis B, HIB

29. The mother of a six-year-old who has chicken pox asks the nurse when the child can go back to school. What information should be included in the nurse's response? The child is contagious
1. Until all signs of the disease are gone.
2. As long as the child has scabs.
3. As long as there are fluid-filled vesicles.
4. Until the rash and fever are gone.

30. A two-year-old child is in for an annual examination. Which comment by the mother alerts the nurse to a risk for lead poisoning?
1. "Why does he eat paint off the window sills?"
2. "Will his temper tantrums ever stop?"
3. "I haven't been able to toilet train him yet."
4. "He is such a messy eater."

Answers and Rationales

1. (4) Sitting with slight support would be expected in a child of 5 months. All of the other tasks are appropriate for this age.

2. (3) Anything that can be put in the mouth is inappropriate for a child with cleft lip repair. A rattle and beads can go in the mouth. Button eyes are a hazard for any infant because they may swallow them. A mobile with a music box is appropriate for a three-month-old who lays in a crib, and this item cannot be put in the mouth. Note that a colorful rattle is also age-appropriate but not condition-appropriate.

3. (1) Soft, washable toys of smooth, nonallergenic material should be used. Stuffed toys are contraindicated. Puzzles and games are not age-appropriate. Toy cars could be used for scratching and should be avoided. Toy cars are also not age-appropriate.

4. (4) Peek-a-boo is appropriate for an eight-month-old. Peek-a-boo helps the infant with the concept of object permanence; things that are out of sight do exist. An eight-month-old can sit up; once an infant can sit up, the mobiles should be removed as they can strangle an infant who might try to stand up. An eight-month-old infant cannot stack large blocks yet. A colorful rattle is more appropriate for a younger infant.

5. (1) Stringing large beads is appropriate for 12 months. Note that the beads are large and therefore not subject to being swallowed. A riding toy and small puzzles would be more appropriate for a toddler. Paste, paper, and scissors are appropriate for a preschooler when used with supervision.

6. (2) An 18-month-old child cannot understand explanations. The nurse needs to assess the patient's knowledge and base teaching on that assessment. The nurse should not assume that no teaching is needed just because the child

has had the procedure before. There is no data to indicate that the parents upset the child. They do appear to be smothering the child, but at this time the child would probably be more miserable without the parents. The nurse may want to teach parents about growth and development needs of the toddler.

7. (2) An 18-month-old should be able to feed himself and drink from a cup. He may be messy. A five- or six-year-old can usually button a shirt and tie shoes. Cutting with scissors is appropriate for a preschool child. A two-year-old can go up and down stairs with both feet on the same step, and a three-year-old child can go up and down stairs by alternating feet.

8. (1) Temper tantrums are common and normal in a two-year-old because he is developing autonomy. As long as the child is safe, he should be ignored. Giving in to the child's demands is likely to reinforce the negative behavior and create a long-term pattern of behavior. The nurse should not recommend to the parents that they spank a child. Promising a reward to stop crying is bribing the child and should not be recommended. A two-year-old who is having a temper tantrum is not likely to listen to explanations.

9. (3) The child's teddy bear and security blanket will help to give the child a sense of security. Spending the night would be ideal, but it may not be possible for this mother with two children at home. It is part of the normal separation reaction for a three-year-old to be upset when the mother leaves. The parents should visit even if the child cries when they leave. Buying a gift will provide less security than bringing the child's favorite comfort items to the hospital.

10. (2) It is normal for a three-year-old to cry when the parents leave. The child will probably not wave good-bye even though he/she is able to. The child is not likely to hide under the covers. The child will likely be too upset to ask to go to the playroom.

11. (2) A sandbox is appropriate for outdoor play. A four-year-old is too young for a two-wheeled bike or for climbing a tree without strict supervision. He is probably past the age of pushing a toy lawn mower, which is more appropriate for a toddler.

12. (3) Five-year-old children like cooperative play, such as playing house. The other activities are solitary activities. Note that the child is several days post surgery. Most five-year-olds are not able to read a book by themselves. Playing a board game with a child is not wrong, but it is a solitary activity. Most five-year-olds would prefer to play with other children. There is almost always a better alternative than turning on the television. This child is several days post

surgery and is able to be up and play with others.

13. (3) A six-year-old is apt to be loosing baby teeth. This is an important consideration when anesthesia is to be administered and the child will be intubated. The nurse should assess for loose teeth in any school-age child who is admitted for surgery or other procedures requiring intubation of any kind.

14. (4) By discussing with the child the reasons for the child's fears, the child will feel less afraid and less abnormal. Discussion of fears should be individualized. The child is not old enough to make care decisions. The child should, however, be given some input into the care plan. The child might decide which site the nurse will use for an injection but not whether or not the medication will be given. The parents will make those decisions.

15. (1) A six-year-old learns best by doing. A six-year-old can not conceptualize what he/she cannot see. Touring the operating room and surgical ICU can be very frightening for a six-year-old. Drawing pictures of the procedure would be more appropriate post-operatively, when the nurse may want to help him in understanding what happened to him. Drawing pictures is a good way to express feelings that a six-year-old cannot put into words. It is more appropriate post-operatively. Group discussion is more appropriate for an adolescent. A six-year-old does not have the verbal skills to participate in and learn from a discussion group.

16. (3) Craft work allows her to accomplish something while meeting her needs for rest. Industry is the developmental task for school-age children. The joint pains with rheumatic fever tend to be in the large joints, not the small ones, so craft work utilizing finger activity would probably not be painful. Stringing large wooden beads is appropriate for younger children. Pillow fighting requires too much energy for a child on bed rest and is not appropriate for a hospital environment. Watching television is a solitary activity with no sense of accomplishment.

17. (2) Pounding movements allow for the expression of aggression. The other activities would not allow for an expression of aggression. The scenario describes a child who is expressing aggression in a very physical manner. This child is not likely to respond well to writing a story. Writing a story could be used to help a child express aggression, but pounding clay is more appropriate given the child's aggressive behavior.

18. (3) Hero worship is very common among school-age children. Denial would be manifested by saying that his leg really is not broken. Repression is putting an upsetting or

guilt-laden experience deep in the unconscious mind. This behavior does not suggest repression. Fantasy is living in a make-believe world. This boy shows no evidence of living in a make-believe world.

19. (2) Building with popsicle sticks will foster his sense of industry and can be done while he is in bed in traction. Puppets and coloring would be more appropriate for younger children. Watching television will not promote his development, although it can be used as diversion occasionally.

20. (3) The child's behavior is typical of the despair phase of toddler responses to anxiety. The child should cry. Lying quietly, sucking his thumb, and saying nothing are suggestive of severe anxiety, a bad adjustment to the hospital, and no comfort with the nurses. This anxiety response does not suggest a poor relationship with his parents. In fact, his severe separation anxiety may be because he is so close to his parents.

21. (4) Temper tantrums are a normal response to limit setting in a two-year-old child. Answer 1 might be correct if the child were older. However, temper tantrums in a two-year-old child do not indicate regression; rather, they are normal for this age. Tantrums are not suggestive of a poorly developed sense of trust; they are normal. Ignoring the tantrum is preferable to discipline when a two-year-old has a tantrum.

22. (4) The best response is to simply state that it is time for sleep and to give the child their security blanket or toy. Answer 1, telling the child that she isn't loved because she won't listen, is not therapeutic. Answer 2 implies that if you don't go to bed on time, you are not a good child. This is not a good suggestion to implant in a child. Answer 3 is bribery and is not appropriate.

23. (3) An eight-year-old is concerned about pain and mutilation. An eight-year-old has an understanding that death is the end of life as we know it and would be unlikely to respond with Answers 1 or 2. Answers 1 and 2 are typical of a preschooler. Answer 4 is typical of an adolescent who wants to leave a legacy.

24. (3) A four-month-old should follow objects with her eyes. A four-month-old is not likely to be able to sit up by herself. This behavior is seen at six months of age. Not being able to hold the rattle as well as she did at first is typical of the time after the loss of the grasp reflex and before pincer movement is established. Most

newborn reflexes are gone by about four months of age. Spitting up after a feeding is normal four-month-old behavior.

25. (3) Riding a tricycle is three-year-old behavior. Remember "three years, three wheels." Children start to walk at about one year of age. Throwing a large ball and stating his name are two-year-old behaviors. Remember to use developmental trends when determining the most recently acquired behavior: head to tail and simple to complex. Look for a complex lower-body behavior.

26. (2) The child will have an elevated body temperature. Contrary to what you might expect, metabolism is increased following aspirin overdose. The child will be hot and flushed. Hyperpyrexia means high temperature. The child will be in metabolic acidosis from the acid load of the aspirin. Compensation for metabolic acidosis is rapid, deep breathing. The first choice is incorrect; the child will be hyperventilating and will be flushed, not pale. The third choice is not correct, the temperature will be high, not low. Bleeding may occur following aspirin ingestion, but not initially. The fourth choice is not correct. Melena is hidden blood in the stool. It will take some time for a GI bleed to develop and pass through the stool. Bradycardia will not be present. The child will have tachycardia.

27. (4) Since the child is breathing, there is no need for CPR or ventilatory support. Because the child is difficult to arouse, gastric lavage rather than syrup of ipecac will be given.

28. (2) At six months of age, the nurse would expect to administer the third DTP, the third hepatitis B, and the third Hemophilus influenza B (HIB) immunizations. MMR (measles, mumps, and rubella) is not given until 15 months of age. IPV is given at two months and four months and then again at 18 months and preschool. Varicella vaccine is given between the ages of one year and 12 years.

29. (3) Chicken pox is contagious as long as there are fluid-filled vesicles. Scabs are not contagious. The child will have scabs for a while. The fever may be down, but if there are fluid-filled vesicles, the child is contagious.

30. (1) Eating paint is one of the major risk factors for lead poisoning. Temper tantrums are normal in a two-year-old. Most two-year-olds are not toilet trained. Most two-year-olds are messy eaters.

Conditions Related to the Cardiovascular System

CONGENITAL HEART DEFECTS

Hemodynamics

A. Fetal circulation (see Figure 16.1):
  1. Ductus venosus carries oxygenated blood from placenta to inferior vena cava; partially bypasses liver; obliterated when umbilical cord is ligated
  2. Ductus arteriosus bypasses lungs by shunting blood from pulmonary artery to aorta
  3. Foramen ovale connects right and left atria to bypass lungs
B. Newborn circulation:
  1. At first breath, lungs expand—increasing blood flow to the pulmonary system.
  2. Pulmonary vascular resistance decreases, and systemic vascular resistance increases.
  3. Result of above two events is closure of the ductus arteriosus and closure of the foramen ovale
C. Defect develops between second and 10th weeks of gestation; possible etiologic factors

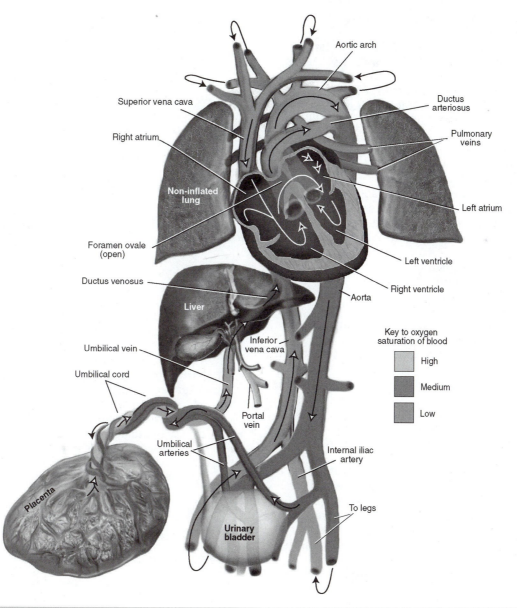

Figure 16.1 Fetal Circulation

include intrauterine infections, radiation, drugs (unknown in 90% or more of cases).

D. Occurs four to 10 times in every 1,000 live births and is the major cause of deaths other than prematurity in the first year

Defects Causing Increase in Pulmonary Blood Flow

Patent Ductus Arteriosus (See Figure 16.2)

A. Failure of the open channel between the pulmonary artery and aorta (normal prenatally) to close after birth
B. Assessment findings:
   1. May be asymptomatic
   2. Growth impairment
   3. Left ventricular hypertrophy
   4. "Machinery murmur"
   5. Wide pulse pressure
C. Nursing diagnoses (see Table 16.10)
D. Interventions:
   1. Treated by surgical ligation of patent ductus, usually before child is two years old
   2. Premature infant may respond to indomethacin (prostaglandin inhibitor) to medically close ductus; may still require surgery
E. Nursing care:
   1. Pre-operative:
      a. Obtain baseline data.
      b. Locate peripheral pulses; note rates, quality, and presence or absence.
      c. Reduce the separation from parents.
      d. Allow the child and parents to express fears.
      e. Prepare for the surgery in age-appropriate ways.
   2. Post-operative:
      a. Maintain a patent airway.
      b. Monitor vital signs, including peripheral pulses.
      c. Monitor intake and output with specific gravity.
      d. Check BUN, creatinine to assess kidney function
      e. Daily weights
      f. Fluid requirements; maintain balance between overload and hypovolemia
      g. Respiratory care:
         (1) Turn, cough and deep breathe
         (2) Chest tubes for clients who have had cardiac surgery
      h. Monitor neurologic status by assessing the LOC and doing neuro checks: pupils, motor response, and response to stimuli.
      i. Provide for adequate nutrition as ordered.
      j. Provide for rest as ordered.
      k. Reduce stress of intensive care environment.
      l. Give parents/siblings and significant others support: follow-up and home care assistance.
      m. Teach parents and family members about medications, physical care, and other therapies that may be ordered.

Atrial Septal Defect (See Figure 16.2)

A. Hole in atria, allowing left to right shunting of oxygenated blood
B. Assessment findings:
   1. Soft, blowing systolic murmur
   2. Thin child
   3. Frequent episodes of pulmonary inflammatory disease
   4. Poor exercise tolerance
   5. Ventricular hypertrophy
   6. Cardiac cath shows increased oxygen content of R atrium
C. Nursing diagnoses (see Table 16.10)
D. Interventions:
   1. Treated by open heart surgery with direct closure of defect or suturing of plastic prosthesis usually before school age to lower risk of CHF/pulmonary vascular obstruction
   2. Nursing care same as patent ductus arteriorsus

Ventricular Septal Defect (See Figure 16.2)

A. Hole between the right and left ventricles, allowing left to right shunting of blood
B. Assessment findings:
   1. Small, low defects may be asymptomatic
   2. Systolic murmur
   3. Tachypnea
   4. Growth failure
   5. Feeding problems
   6. Left ventricular hypertrophy
   7. Cardiac cath shows higher oxygen content in R ventricle than R atrium
C. Nursing diagnoses (see Table 16.10)
D. Interventions:
   1. Treated with open heart surgery; direct closure or suturing a plastic prosthesis in place usually within the first year of life to prevent progressive respiratory disease
   2. Nursing interventions same as patent ductus arteriorsus

Defect Causing Obstruction to Pulmonary Blood Flow

Coarctation of the Aorta (See Figure 16.2)

A. Obstruction to the flow of blood through the constricted segments causes increased left ventricular pressure and workload; extensive

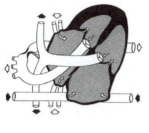

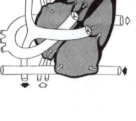

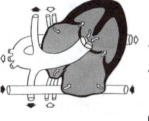

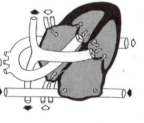

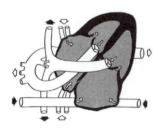

Patent Ductus Arteriosus

The patent ductus arteriosus is a vascular connection that, during fetal life, short-circuits the pulmonary vascular bed and directs blood from the pulmonary artery to the aorta. Functional closure of the ductus normally occurs soon after birth. If the ductus remains patent after birth, the direction of blood flow in the ductus is reversed by the higher pressure in the aorta.

Tetralogy of Fallot

Tetralogy of Fallot is characterized by the combination of four defects: 1) pulmonary stenosis, 2) ventricular septal defect, 3) overriding aorta, and 4) hypertrophy of right ventricle. It is the most common defect causing cyanosis in patients surviving beyond two years of age. The severity of symptoms depends on the degree of pulmonary stenosis, the size of the ventricular septal defect, and the degree to which the aorta overrides the septal defect.

Ventricular Septal Defects

A ventricular septal defect is an abnormal opening between the right and left ventricle. Ventricular septal defects vary in size and may occur in either the membranous or muscular portion of the ventricular septum. Due to higher pressure in the left ventricle, a shunting of blood from the left to right ventricle occurs during systole. If pulmonary vascular resistance produces pulmonary hypertension, the shunt of blood is then reversed from the right to the left ventricle, with cyanosis resulting.

Complete Transposition of Great Vessels

This anomaly is an embryologic defect caused by a straight division of the bulbar trunk without normal spiraling. As a result, the aorta originates from the right ventricle and the pulmonary artery from the left ventricle. An abnormal communication between the two circulations must be present to sustain life.

Truncus Arteriosus

Truncus arteriosus is a retention of the embryologic bulbar trunk. It results from the failure of normal septation and division of this trunk into an aorta and pulmonary artery. This single arterial trunk overrides the ventricles and receives blood from them through a ventricular septal defect. The entire pulmonary and systemic circulation is supplied from this common arterial trunk.

Subaortic Stenosis

In many instances, the stenosis is valvular with thickening and fusion of the cusps. Subaortic stenosis is caused by a fibrous ring below the aortic valve in the outflow tract of the left ventricle. At times, both valvular and subaortic stenosis exist in combination. The obstruction presents an increased work load for the normal output of the left ventricular blood and results in left ventricular enlargement.

Coarctation of the Aorta

Coarctation of the aorta is characterized by a narrowed aortic lumen. It exists as a preductal or postductal obstruction, depending on the position of the obstruction in relation to the ductus arteriosus. Coarctations exist with great variation in anatomical features. The lesion produces an obstruction to the flow of blood through the aorta, causing an increased left ventricular pressure and work load.

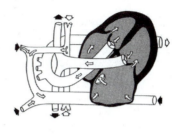

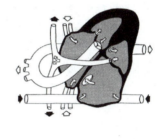

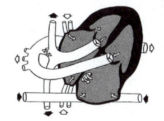

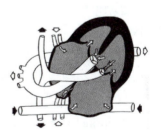

Atrial Septal Defects

An atrial septal defect is an abnormal opening between the right and left atria. Basically, three types of abnormalities result from incorrect development of the atrial septum. An incompetent foramen ovale is the most common defect. The high ostium secundum defect results from abnormal blood returning from the lungs, flows into the left ventricle, and is propelled into the systemic circulation. Improper development of the septum primum produces a basal opening known as an ostium primum defect, frequently involving the atrioventricular valves. In general, left to right shunting of blood occurs in all atrial septal defects.

Tricuspid Atresia

Tricuspid valvular atresia is characterized by a small right ventricle, large left ventricle, and usually a diminished pulmonary circulation. Blood from the right atrium passes through an atrial septal defect into the left atrium, mixes with oxygenated blood returning from the lungs, flows into the left ventricle, and is propelled into the systemic circulation. The lungs may receive blood through one of three routes: 1) a small ventricular septal defect, 2) patent ductus arteriosus, and 3) bronchial vessels.

Anomalous Venous Return

Oxygenated blood returning from the lungs is carried abnormally to the right side of the heart by one or more pulmonary veins emptying directly, or indirectly through venous channels, into the right atrium. Partial anomalous return of the pulmonary veins to the right atrium functions the same as an atrial septal defect. In complete anomalous return of the pulmonary veins, an interatrial communication is necessary for survival.

Figure 16.2 Congenital heart abnormalities

Table 16.10 Nursing Diagnoses Related to Heart Defects

- Activity intolerance related to insufficient oxygenation secondary to heart defects
- Risk for imbalanced nutrition: less than body requirements related to inadequate sucking, fatigue, and dyspnea
- Risk for infection related to debilitated physical status
- Risk for delayed growth and development related to impaired ability to achieve developmental tasks due to inadequate oxygen and nutrients, social isolation
- Risk for ineffective management of therapeutic regimen related to insufficient knowledge of condition, prevention of infection, signs and symptoms of complications, digoxin therapy, nutrition requirements, and community services
- Self-care deficit related to limitations imposed by illness
- Caregiver role strain related to multiple, ongoing care needs secondary to restrictions imposed by disease and treatments
- Disturbed body image related to activity intolerance; feeling different
- Deficient knowledge related to unfamiliarity with diagnosis/treatment
- Interrupted family process related to situational crisis

collateral circulation bypasses coarcted area to supply lower extremities with blood

B. Assessment findings:
   1. Hypertension in upper extremities with decreased blood pressure in lower extremities (before age 2, BP in arms is equal to BP in legs; after 2 years, BP in arms > BP in legs)
   2. Weak or absent pulses in lower extremities
   3. Systolic murmur
   4. Congestive heart failure
   5. Fatigue, headaches, leg cramps
   6. Left ventricular hypertrophy
   7. May be asymptomatic
C. Nursing diagnoses (see Table 16.10)
D. Interventions:
   1. Treatment is surgical resection of the coarcted area with direct anastamosis when possible or a vessel graft within first two years of life (lowers risk of hypertension at rest and exercise and induced systematic hypertension)
   2. Nursing care (same as patent ductus arteriosus)

Defect Causing Decrease in Pulmonary Blood Flow

Tetralogy of Fallot

A. Four defects:
   1. Pulmonary stenosis causes obstruction to R ventricular outflow.
   2. R ventricular hypertrophy is caused by pulmonary stenosis.
   3. Ventricular septal defect; allows for outflow of blood and causes right to left shunt

   4. Overriding aorta; aorta overrides the ventricular septal opening, allowing blood from both left and right ventricles to enter aorta and causing unoxygenated blood to enter systemic circulation
B. Assessment findings:
   1. Cyanosis that increases with physical exertion; "blue spells," "tet spells"
   2. Clubbing of fingers and toes: an increase in capillary supply and soft tissue fibrosis due to peripheral hypoxemia
   3. Systolic murmur
   4. Paroxysmal attacks of dyspnea with loss of consciousness (syncope)
   5. Squatting increases intraabdominal pressure, promoting venous return.
   6. Growth retardation
   7. Protrusion of chest due to R ventricular hypertrophy
   8. Ductus arteriosus patent or surgically opened
   9. Cardiac cath shows elevated R ventricular pressure; as catheter passes pulmonary stenosis, there is a sudden fall in pressure
   10. X-ray studies show "boot-shaped" heart
C. Nursing diagnoses (see Table 16.10)
D. Interventions:
   1. Surgery to allow oxygenated blood into systemic circulation
   2. Surgery may be done in stages or a total repair completed
   3. Nursing care (same as patent ductus arteriosus)

Defect Causing Mixed Blood Flow

Transposition of the Great Vessels (See Figure 16.2)

A. The aorta originates from the R ventricle, and the pulmonary artery originates from the L ventricle.
B. Incompatible with life unless other defects such as atrial septal defect and patent ductus are present to connect arterial and venous circulations
C. Assessment findings:
   1. Deep cyanosis at birth
   2. Early clubbing of fingers and toes
   3. Poor growth and development
   4. Tachypnea
   5. Fatigue
   6. Anoxic, paroxysmal, dyspneic attacks
   7. Right ventricular hypertrophy
   8. Congestive heart failure
   9. No murmurs
D. Nursing diagnoses (see Table 16.10)
E. Interventions:
   1. Immediate surgery
   2. Nursing care: see above

Complications

A. Congestive heart failure:
   1. Failure of the heart to meet the demands of the body
   2. Both right-sided and left-sided failure are simultaneously manifested.
   3. Assessment findings:
      a. Tachycardia even during rest; slight exertion dramatically increases rate; sleep heart rate > 160 bpm in infants
      b. Tachypnea; respiratory rate > 60 bpm in infants
      c. Dyspnea; caused by decrease in lung distensibility
      d. Diaphoresis; may or may not be present; seen on the head
      e. Hepatomegaly; late sign
      f. Edema; late sign: pulmonary occurs first, peripheral occurs later
   4. Nursing diagnoses (see Table 16.11)

Table 16.11 Nursing Diagnoses Related to Congestive Heart Failure

- Decreased cardiac output related to structure defect/myocardial dysfunction
- Ineffective breathing patterns related to pulmonary congestion
- Risk for infection related to pulmonary congestion/reduced defenses
- Imbalanced nutrition: less than body requirements related to circulatory impairment/fatigue
- Delayed growth and development related to cardiac inefficiency
- Activity intolerance related to imbalance between oxygen demand and supply
- Ineffective health maintenance related to disease process; medical therapy
- Deficient knowledge regarding disease, medications, dietary needs, and activity restrictions
- Risk for interrupted family process

   5. Interventions:
      a. Administer digitalis preparations as ordered:
         (1) Digitalis slows conduction in the heart and decreases the heart rate, increases contractility, and enhances renal perfusion (increases diuresis).
         (2) Side effects include nausea and vomiting, diarrhea, anorexia, visual disturbances, bradycardia, and/or dysrhythmias.
         (3) Monitor serum digoxin levels (range from 0.8 to 2.0 mcg/L); hold digoxin if levels are elevated.
         (4) Monitor serum potassium (digoxin toxicity occurs more quickly when serum potassium is low).
         (5) Monitor pulse rate; do not give if pulse is below written heart rate order.
         (6) Hold digoxin if apical pulse < 90–110 bpm (young child/infant); < 70 bpm (older child).
         (7) Optimally, calculate dose in mg, mcg, and ml with another RN.
         (8) No infant should ever receive more than 1 ml (50 mcg or 0.05 mg) per dose.
      b. Administer diuretics as ordered:
         (1) Given to reduce venous and systemic congestion
         (2) Used to treat acute episodes and for long term therapy
         (3) Weigh daily.
         (4) Keep an intake and output record.
         (5) Monitor electrolytes; side effects of diuretics are hypokalemia and hypovolemia.
         (6) Provide high-potassium foods.
      c. Administer morphine for sedation as ordered.
      d. Reduce energy expenditure:
         (1) Prevent crying.
         (2) Position in upright/semi-Fowler's position.
         (3) Use a large-holed, soft nipple for feeding.
      e. Allow child to squat/side lie with knees flexed to chest to increase blood flow to lungs.
      f. Administer oxygen as ordered prn.

B. Subacute endocarditis:
   1. Inflammation of endocardium; may be caused by staphylococcus aureus, streptococcus viridous; candida albicans
   2. Assessment findings:
      a. History of dental work or invasive procedure; portals of entry may be oral (dental work), urinary tract, heart (cardiac cath), bloodstream (central lines)
      b. Fever
      c. Malaise
      d. Night sweats
      e. Weight loss
      f. Elevated sedimentation rate, anemia, positive blood cultures
   3. Nursing diagnoses (see Table 16.11)
   4. Intervention:
      a. Administer antibiotics as ordered.
      b. Antibiotics may be ordered to prevent disease prior to and after dental work or other invasive procedures in persons at risk.

C. Cerebral thrombosis:
   1. Occurs frequently in children with cardiac defects due to increased blood viscosity
   2. Assessment findings:
      a. Irritability and restlessness
      b. Paralysis
   3. Nursing diagnoses (see cerebral vascular accident in Neurology section, Table 9.7)

4. Interventions:
   a. Fluids; adequate but not overload
   b. Oxygen as ordered
   c. Anticoagulants as ordered
D. Cerebral damage due to inadequate blood flow to brain
   1. Assessment findings:
      a. Irritability
      b. Generalized weakness
      c. Slurred speech
      d. Unequal pupils
   2. Interventions:
      a. Try to prevent by keeping child controlled and oxygenated
      b. Supportive care once it occurs

RHEUMATIC FEVER

A. An autoimmune inflammatory disorder that involves the heart, joints, connective tissue, and the central nervous system; seems to run in families; peaks in school-age children; prognosis depends on degree of heart damage
B. Assessment findings:
   1. History of beta hemolytic streptococcus infection within 1–4 weeks; antigenic markers for strep toxin closely resemble markers for heart valves; this resemblance causes antibodies made against the strep to also attack heart valves
   2. Jones criteria (major symptoms):
      a. Carditis: seen in 50% of all patients
         (1) Aschoff bodies (areas of inflammation and degeneration around heart valves, pericardium, and myocardium)
         (2) Valvular insufficiency of mitral and aortic valves
         (3) Cardiomegaly
         (4) Shortness of breath
         (5) Hepatomegaly
         (6) Edema
      b. Migratory polyarthritis:
         (1) Large joints become red, swollen, and painful
         (2) Synovial fluid is sterile
      c. Chorea (Sydenham's chorea, St. Vitus' dance): central nervous system disorder characterized by abrupt, purposeless, involuntary muscular movements
         (1) Gradual, insidious onset; starts with personality change or clumsiness
         (2) Occurs most often in girls, age 6–11
         (3) May occur months after infection
         (4) Movements increase with excitement
         (5) Lasts 1–3 months
      d. Subcutaneous nodules:
         (1) Usually a sign of severe disease
         (2) Occur with active carditis
         (3) Firm, nontender nodes on bony prominences of joint
         (4) Lasts for weeks
      e. Erythema marginatum:
         (1) Transient, nonpruritic rash starting with central red patches that expand
         (2) Results in series of irregular patches with red, raised margins and pale centers
   3. Minor symptoms:
      a. Reliable history of fever
      b. Recent history of strep infection
      c. Diagnostic tests:
         (1) Elevated sedimentation rate (ESR), anti-streptolysin O (ASO) titre and C-reactive protein (positive)
         (2) ECG changes
C. Nursing diagnosis (see Table 16.11)
D. Interventions:
   1. Penicillin administered:
      a. Given during acute phase to control strep infection
      b. Given prophylactically for several years (until age 20 or for five years, whichever is longer) after recovery from rheumatic fever to prevent future damage to heart
      c. Additional penicillin given before surgery or tooth extractions
   2. Salicylates for analgesic, anti-inflammatory, antipyretic effects
   3. Steroids for anti-inflammatory action
   4. Decrease cardiac workload; bed rest until lab studies return to normal:
      a. Provide age-appropriate diversionary activities
      b. Arrange for homebound education

KAWASAKI DISEASE (MUCOCUTANEOUS LYMPH NODE SYNDROME)

A. Identified in Japan in 1961; etiology unknown; non-communicable; cause may be environmental toxins, infections origin, or immunologic process
B. Assessment findings: five or six diagnostic criteria constitute the disease:
   1. Fever for five or more days
   2. Bilateral ocular conjunctivitis
   3. Oropharyngeal changes ("strawberry tongue"; fissured/crusted lips; erythema in throat/mouth)
   4. Peripheral extremity changes (skin on fingers and toes peels two weeks after illness; transverse grooves on fingernails 2–3 months after illness)
   5. Trunk rash
   6. Cervical lymph node swelling

7. Other symptoms include photophobia, arthritis; diarrhea, pneumonia, and malaise.
8. Most severe consequence is cardiac damage.
9. Diagnostic tests:
   a. Elevated ESR and C-reactive protein
   b. Two weeks into the illness, CBC, platelet, ESR, and cardiac studies show thrombocytosis.
C. Nursing diagnoses (see Table 16.12)

Table 16.12 Nursing Diagnoses Related to Kawasaki's Disease

- Ineffective tissue profusion: cardiac and peripheral related to disease process
- Hyperthermia related to disease process
- Impaired skin integrity related to erythema/skin sloughing (palms, soles)
- Impaired comfort (pain/pruritis) related to edema/skin irritation
- Risk for imbalanced nutrition: less than body requirements related to anorexia due to sore mouth/malaise
- Fear/anxiety related to prognosis/tests

D. Interventions:
1. Aspirin therapy for antipyretic, anti-inflammatory effect (especially on cardiac vessels)
2. Alleviate symptoms.
3. Prevent/lessen cardiac complications.
4. Provide symptom relief.
5. Adequately hydrate; monitor intake and output.
6. Maintain intact skin.
7. Range of motion exercises
8. Monitor the cardiac status.
9. Support the child and family.

Sample Questions

1. A six-year-old has Tetralogy of Fallot. He is being admitted for surgery. The nurse knows that which problem is not associated with Tetralogy of Fallot?
   1. Severe atrial septal defect
   2. Pulmonary stenosis
   3. Right ventricular hypertrophy
   4. Overriding aorta

2. A six-year-old with Tetralogy of Fallot is being admitted for surgery. While the nurse is orienting the child to the unit, the child suddenly squats with the arms thrown over the knees and knees drawn up to the chest. What is the best immediate nursing action?
   1. Observe and assist if needed.
   2. Place the child in a lying position.
   3. Call for help and return the child to the room.
   4. Assist the child to a standing position.

3. A six-year-old with Tetralogy of Fallot is being admitted for surgery. What is most important to teach the child during the pre-operative period?
   1. Strict hand washing technique
   2. How to cough and deep-breathe
   3. The importance of drinking plenty of fluids
   4. Positions of comfort

4. A six-year-old with Tetralogy of Fallot has open heart surgery. The septal defect was closed, and the pulmonic valve was replaced. When the child returns to the unit, he has oxygen, IVs, and closed chest drainage. How should the nurse position the chest bottles?
   1. Above the level of the bed
   2. At the level of the heart
   3. Below the level of the bed
   4. With the first two bottles above the third

5. A parent brings a three-week-old infant to the clinic. The parent states that the baby does not eat very well. She takes 45 cc of formula in 45 minutes and gets "tired and sweaty" when eating. The nurse observes the baby sleeping in the parent's arms. Her color is pink, and the child is breathing without difficulty. What is the best response for the nurse to make?
   1. "It's normal for an infant to get tired while feeding. That will go away as the child gets older."
   2. "It's normal for an infant to get tired while feeding. You could try feeding the baby smaller amounts of formula more frequently."
   3. "This could be a sign of a health problem. Does your baby's skin color change while eating?"
   4. "This could be a sign of a health problem. How does your baby's behavior compare with your other children when they were that age?"

6. The nurse is explaining cardiac catheterization to the parents of a child. The nurse explains to the parents that information about which of the following can be obtained during cardiac catheterization?
   1. Oxygen levels in the chambers of the heart
   2. Pulmonary vascularization
   3. Presence of abdominal aortic aneurysm
   4. Activity tolerance

7. The nurse is caring for a toddler who is six hours post cardiac catheterization. The nurse is administering antibiotics. The child's mother asks why the child needs to have antibiotics. The nurse's response should indicate that antibiotics are given to the client to prevent which type of infection?
   1. Urinary tract infection
   2. Pneumonia
   3. Otitis media
   4. Endocarditis

8. The nurse is caring for a toddler with a cardiac defect who has had several episodes of congestive heart failure in the past few months. Which data would be the most useful to the nurse in assessing the child's current congestive heart failure?
   1. The degree of clubbing of the child's fingers and toes
   2. Amount of fluid and food intake
   3. Recent fluctuations in weight
   4. The degree of sacral edema

9. A child with a cyanotic heart defect has an elevated hematocrit. What is the most likely cause of the elevated hematocrit?
   1. Chronic infection
   2. Recent dehydration
   3. Increased cardiac output
   4. Chronic oxygen deficiency

10. The nurse is administering the daily digoxin dose of .035 mg to a 10-month-old child. Before administering the dose, the nurse takes the child's apical pulse and it is 85. Which of the following interpretations of these data is most accurate?
    1. The child has just awakened, and the heart action is slowest in the morning.
    2. This is a normal rate for a 10-month-old child.
    3. The child may be going into heart block due to digoxin toxicity.
    4. The child's potassium level needs to be evaluated.

11. The nurse is discussing dietary needs of a child with a serious heart defect. The child is being treated with digoxin and hydrochlorothiazide (Hydrodiuril). The nurse should stress the importance of giving the child which of these foods?
    1. Cheese and ice cream
    2. Finger foods such as hot dogs
    3. Apricots and bananas
    4. Four glasses of whole milk per day

12. A child with a cyanotic heart defect has a hypoxic episode. What should the nurse do for the child at this time?
    1. Administer prn oxygen and position the child in the squat position.
    2. Position the child side-lying and give the ordered morphine.
    3. Ask the parents to leave and start oxygen.
    4. Give oxygen and notify the physician.

13. The nurse notes that a child who has had a serious heart condition since birth does not do the expected activities for that age. The child's mother says, "I worry constantly about my child. I don't let the older children or the neighbor kids play with my child very much. I try to make things as easy for my child as I can." What is the best interpretation of this data?
    1. The child is physically incapable due to his cardiac defect.
    2. The child's mother is overprotective and allows the child few challenges to develop skills.
    3. The child is probably mentally retarded from the effects of continual hypoxia.
    4. The child has regressed due to the effects of hospitalization.

14. Ten days after cardiac surgery an 18-month-old is recovering well. The child is alert and fairly active and is playing well with the parents. Discharge is planned soon. The nurse notes that the parents are still very reluctant to allow the child to do anything without help. What is the best initial action for the nurse to take?
    1. Reemphasize the need for autonomy in toddlers.
    2. Provide opportunities for autonomy when the parents are not present.
    3. Reassess the parent's needs and concerns.
    4. Discuss the success of the surgery and how well the child is doing.

15. Sodium salicylate is prescribed for a child with rheumatic fever. What should the nurse assess the child for because the child is on this medication?
    1. Tinnitus and nausea
    2. Dermatitis and blurred vision
    3. Unconsciousness and acetone odor of breath
    4. Chills and elevation of temperature

Answers and Rationales

1. (1) Atrial septal defect is not associated with Tetralogy of Fallot. The four defects are pulmonary stenosis, which causes right ventricular hypertrophy, ventricular septal defect, and overriding aorta.

2. (1) The squatting position will help the child with tetralogy to have better hemodynamics. It increases intraabdominal pressure and increases pulmonary blood flow. Placing the child in a lying or standing position will increase his symptoms and be counterproductive. It is not necessary to call for help because this is not an emergency situation.

3. (2) The child will have to learn to cough and deep-breathe post-operatively. Studies demonstrate that pre-operative teaching makes it easier for the client to perform coughing and deep-breathing exercises in the post-operative period. The nurses will do strict hand washing, not the client. Fluids will likely be restricted post-operatively. It is important to teach the client about positions of comfort, but it is more important to teach the child how to deep-breathe and cough.

4. (3) Chest bottles are always positioned below bed level to prevent the reflux of material into the chest cavity.

5. (3) Activity intolerance related to feeding is often a key sign of a serious cardiac problem in an infant. Taking only 45 cc of formula in 45 minutes at three weeks of age probably indicates difficulty sucking. This is definitely not normal. The fact that the infant's color is pink at rest does not tell you what happens during exertion, such as with eating. Asking about skin color during feeding is a good first question to ask. Answers 1 and 2 are incorrect because they interpret the infant's behavior as normal, which it is not. Answer 4 is not correct. It does identify the behavior as abnormal but suggests comparing it to the child's siblings. This is not the appropriate question to ask to get the most information.

6. (1) The catheter is passed into the chambers of the heart, and oxygen levels can be measured. The cardiac catheter does not assess pulmonary vascularization. Coronary arteries can be visualized, however. An abdominal aortic aneurysm is diagnosed with an arteriogram, not a cardiac catheterization. A cardiac catheterization gives information about the heart structures but does not give information about activity tolerance.

7. (4) During a cardiac catheterization, a catheter is inserted into the heart; the infection that the client is most at risk for is, therefore, endocarditis. Urinary tract infection, pneumonia, and otitis media are not related to a client undergoing a cardiac catheterization.

8. (3) Weight is the best indicator of fluid balance. Congestive heart failure causes fluid retention. Sacral edema is positionally dependent. Weight will give a better indication of the child's status. Clubbing of the fingers and toes is an indication of chronic hypoxemia, not the status of his current congestive heart failure. Fluid and food intake is a general indicator of his status and is not particularly related to his current congestive heart failure.

9. (4) The body tries to compensate for chronic oxygen deficiency by making additional red cells to transport oxygen. The additional red cells increase the hematocrit, which is the percent of blood that is RBCs. Chronic infection is more likely to cause anemia. Recent dehydration will cause an elevated hematocrit because there is less fluid in the blood. However, there is no indication that the child is dehydrated, and we are told that he has a cyanotic heart defect, which makes him chronically hypoxic. Therefore, answer 4 is better than answer 2. Answer 3, increased cardiac output, is also incorrect. Increased cardiac output does not cause an elevated hematocrit.

10. (3) A pulse below 100 in a 10-month-old child who is taking digoxin most likely indicates digoxin toxicity. The nurse should withhold the medication and notify the physician. The normal pulse for this age is about 120 or a little more at rest. The pulse rate does not tell us that the child needs to have his/her potassium level checked. If the child is also taking Lasix or another potassium-depleting diuretic, then the potassium should be checked.

11. (3) The child should be on a sodium-restricted diet with high-potassium foods because he is taking Hydrodiuril, a potassium-depleting diuretic. Apricots and bananas are low in sodium and high in potassium. Cheese and ice cream are high in sodium. Hot dogs are high in sodium. Whole milk is high in sodium. Not only is potassium needed, but excessive sodium should be avoided because those with severe heart defects are prone to fluid retention.

12. (1) The knee-chest or squat position increases intraabdominal pressure and increases blood flow to the lungs. Oxygen is also indicated because the child is hypoxic. Positioning on the side is not appropriate because it will not improve the blood flow to the lungs. There is no need to ask the parents to leave. In fact, they need to know how to handle these episodes if they are not yet comfortable doing so. Children with cyanotic heart defects have hypoxic episodes fairly regularly. Positioning in the squat position is more important at this time than notifying the physician.

13 (2) The child's mother does not let the child play with others and appears to do everything for the child. She seems to be overprotective. Most children with heart defects are capable of doing most age-appropriate activities. There is no evidence to support that the child is mentally retarded. There is no data to support that the child has regressed.

14. (3) Before the nurse can teach the parents, it will be necessary to reassess their needs and concerns. The question asks for the best *initial* action. Initially, the nurse should assess. Later, the nurse may emphasize the toddler's need for autonomy. The nurse may provide the child with opportunities to develop autonomy, although it would be better to teach the parents. The nurse may also discuss the success of the surgery and how well the child is doing, but this is not the initial action.

15. (1) Tinnitus and nausea are signs of toxicity to salicylate drugs.

Respiratory and Eyes, Ears, Nose, and Throat (EENT) Conditions

TONSILLITIS (NOT USUALLY HOSPITALIZED)

A. Inflammation of tonsils often as a result of a viral or bacterial pharyngitis:
   1. Ten to 15% of cases are caused by group A beta-hemolytic streptococci.
   2. Tonsils aid in protecting the body from infection.
B. Assessment findings:
   1. Enlarged, red tonsils; fevers
   2. Sore throat, difficulty swallowing, mouth breathing, snoring
   3. White patches of exudate on tonsilar pillars; enlarged cervical lymph nodes
C. Nursing diagnoses (see Table 16.13)
D. Interventions:
   1. Comfort measures and symptomatic relief:
      a. Cool mist vaporizer
      b. Salt water gargles, throat lozenges
      c. Acetaminophen
   2. Antibiotics for bacterial infection, usually penicillin or erythromycin
   3. Surgery: removal of tonsils alone/or with adenoids

TONSILLECTOMY/ ADENOIDECTOMY

A. Indications for surgery:
   1. Recurrent tonsillitis, peritonsillar abscess
   2. Airway or esophageal obstruction
B. Nursing diagnoses (see Table 16.14)
C. Pre-operative interventions:
   1. Bleeding and clotting times to assure safety because hemorrhage is a common complication
   2. Assess the child for infection; surgery is not done during an acute episode.
   3. Prepare child for surgery in ways appropriate to age.
D. Post-operative interventions:
   1. Position child prone or side-lying to facilitate drainage of secretions.
   2. Do not suction unless absolutely necessary; suctioning removes clots forming at the surgical site.
   3. Provide ice collar for pain; medicate as ordered.
   4. Observe for signs of hemorrhage: biggest risk is first 48 hours and 5–7 days post surgery.
      a. Frequent swallowing; child complains of "trickle in throat"
      b. Persistent, bright-red emesis
      c. Oozing from suture line
      d. Tachycardia and signs of shock
   5. Acetaminophen for pain (no aspirin); involve child/parent in pain assessment
   6. Diet:
      a. Cool, clear, non-citrus, non-red fluids when awake and alert
      b. No milk products at first because milk increases mucous in throat
      c. Fluids essential
      d. Advance diet as tolerated: no roughage, acidic foods, milk products; progress from soft to bland to regular.
   7. Activity:
      a. Keep child quiet for several days
      b. Child may return to school 1–2 weeks after surgery.
      c. Scab falls off in 7–10 days; instruct parents to watch for bleeding and call physician if any questions.

Table 16.13 Nursing Diagnoses Related to Tonsillitis

- Acute pain related to inflammation of tonsils
- Hyperthermia related to inflammation
- Deficient knowledge regarding cause, transmission, treatment, and potential complications
- Risk for deficient fluid volume related to inadequate fluid intake secondary to pain

Table 16.14 Nursing Diagnoses Related to Tonsillectomy/Adenoidectomy

- Risk for injury (hemorrhage/increased body temperature) related to surgical trauma
- Deficient fluid volume related to pre-op NPO/fluid loss through post-op emesis
- Acute pain related to surgical trauma
- Deficient knowledge (parent) related to home care/medical follow-up
- Risk for ineffective airway clearance related to sedation, secretions/blood in oropharynx, vomiting
- Anxiety related to separation from parents, unfamiliar surroundings, and perceived threat of pain or abandonment

UPPER RESPIRATORY INFECTIONS (URI)

A. Common cold; usually viral; incubation period is only two days
B. Assessment findings:
   1. Nasal congestion (mild) to dyspnea (severe sign); the younger the child, the more potential for airway difficulty; infants are nose breathers
   2. Rhinorrhea (runny nose)
   3. Low-grade fever
C. Nursing diagnoses (see Table 16.15)
D. Interventions:
   1. Antipyretic such as acetaminophen
   2. Decongestants
   3. Humidity; may be croup tent or cool mist vaporizer
   4. Suction infant with bulb syringe to keep airway patent (infants are nose breathers).
   5. Increase fluids to loosen secretions and restore fluid lost due to fever and rapid breathing.
   6. Frequently assess the airway.

EPIGLOTITTIS

A. Potentially life-threatening infection of epiglottis and surrounding structures caused by H. Influenzae, type B; affecting children from 1–8 years of age; it onsets rapidly and quickly progresses to respiratory arrest
B. Assessment findings:
   1. Severe sore throat
   2. Drooling
   3. Dysphagia
   4. Muffled voice
   5. Child sits upright with mouth open and tongue protruding ("sniffing position").
   6. Fever
   7. Tachycardia
   8. Labored respirations
   9. Elevated WBC
   10. Lateral neck X-ray shows "knife" sign, indicating a swollen epiglottis.
C. Nursing diagnoses (see Table 16.16)
D. Interventions:
   1. Airway; mist tent with oxygen
   2. Tracheostomy or endotracheal tube if needed; anticipate need for artificial airway

Table 16.15 Nursing Diagnoses Related to Upper Respiratory Infection

- Risk for ineffective airway clearance related to secretions
- Risk for ineffective breathing patterns related to secretions, fever
- Hyperthermia related to infectious process
- Risk for deficient fluid volume related to fluid losses from rapid breathing and decreased intake of fluids

   3. IV antibiotics
   4. Sedation if child too anxious
   5. Avoid direct examination of epiglottis because it may precipitate spasm and obstruction.
   6. Assess airway frequently.
   7. Keep child calm.

LARYNGOTRACHEOBRONCHITIS (CROUP)

A. Viral infection that usually starts as URI and proceeds to lower respiratory tract; primarily affects children from 1–3 years of age
B. Assessment findings:
   1. URI
   2. Hoarseness
   3. Brassy cough
   4. Inspiratory stridor
   5. Low grade fever
   6. Increasing distress
   7. WBC normal
C. Nursing diagnoses (see Table 16.16)

Table 16.16 Nursing Diagnoses Related to Epiglottis/Croup

- Ineffective airway clearance related to laryngeal obstruction
- Risk for transmission of infection related to bacterial/viral organisms
- Risk for deficient fluid volume related to excess loss/swallowing difficulty/increased metabolic demands
- Anxiety related to health status change/environmental threats (therapy; hospitalization)
- Deficient knowledge related to home care/recurrence (croup)

D. Interventions:
   1. Keep airway clear
      a. Oral or nasotracheal intubation for moderate hypoxia
      b. Oxygen at low concentration to relieve mild hypoxia
   2. NPO
   3. IV fluids
   4. Mist tent with oxygen
   5. Care of child in a croup tent:
      a. Croup tent contains humidity and oxygen.
      b. Toys should be objects that will not create static electricity or sparks.
         (1) Avoid wool, synthetics, and things with metal and moving parts.
         (2) Toys made of cotton are appropriate.
      c. Change the child's clothing when it becomes wet.
      d. If child is removed from croup tent for feeding, flood the tent with oxygen before returning the child to the tent.

6. Antibiotics only if secondary bacterial infection present
7. Child may vomit large amounts of mucous; reassure parents that this is normal.
8. Keep child calm.
9. Teach family how to care for child if croup recurs; close bathroom door and run shower to create high humidity environment.

OTITIS MEDIA

A. Bacterial or viral infection of the middle ear commonly occurring in young children
B. Risk factors:
   1. Occurs more frequently in young children because the eustachian tube is shorter, wider, and straighter
   2. Infants who are positioned primarily in the supine position
   3. Infants who go to sleep with milk or juice in their mouths
   4. Infants and children who are immunocompromised
C. Assessment findings:
   1. Fever often, but not always present
   2. Increased irritability
   3. Pulling, tugging, or rubbing the ear
   4. URI
   5. Vomiting and diarrhea often, but not always present
   6. Bulging of tympanic membrane
D. Nursing diagnoses (see Table 16.17)
E. Interventions:
   1. Antibiotics; instruct parents to give all of antibiotic
   2. Decongestants to relieve eustachian tube obstruction
   3. Analgesics (acetaminophen)
   4. Myringotomy with insertion of pereustachian (PE) tubes:
      a. Nursing diagnoses (see Table 16.17)
      b. Interventions:
         (1) Use ear plugs if showering or washing child's hair; no diving
         (2) Tubes fall out for no reason.

Table 16.17 Nursing Diagnoses Related to Otitis Media

- Acute pain related to inflammation in ear
- Risk for deficient fluid volume related to decreased intake and fluid losses due to vomiting and fever

Nursing Diagnoses Related to Myringotomy with PE Tube Insertion:

- Risk for injury (hemorrhage) related to surgical trauma
- Risk for deficient fluid volume related to pre-op NPO/loss via emesis (post-op)
- Acute pain related to surgical trauma
- Deficient knowledge related to home care/medication follow-up

c. Complications:
   (1) Mastoiditis
   (2) Meningitis
   (3) Hearing loss
5. When administering ear drops, pull ear lobe up and back for older children and down and back for infants

ASTHMA (REACTIVE AIRWAY DISEASE)

A. Obstructive disease of the lower respiratory tract; often caused by an allergic reaction to an environmental allergen, foods, inhalants, infection, vigorous activity, or emotions
B. Pathophysiology:
   1. Immunologic/allergic reaction results in histamine release, which produces three main airway responses:
      a. Edema of mucous membranes
      b. Spasm of the smooth muscle of bronchi and bronchioles
      c. Accumulation of tenacious secretions
   2. Status asthmaticus occurs when there is little response to treatment and when symptoms persist.
C. Assessment findings:
   1. Family history of allergies
   2. Patient history of eczema
   3. Respiratory distress; shortness of breath
   4. Expiratory wheeze, prolonged expiratory phase, air trapping (barrel chest if chronic)
   5. Use of accessory muscles
   6. Irritability (from hypoxia)
   7. Diaphoresis
   8. Change in sensorium if severe attack
   9. Thick, tenacious mucous
D. Nursing diagnoses (see Table 16.18)
E. Interventions:
   1. Bronchodilators to relieve bronchospasm:
      a. IV Theophylline: check pulse and blood pressure
      b. Epinephrine in emergency room
      c. Metaproterenol (Alupent), isoetharine (Bronkosol)
   2. IV corticosteroids to relieve inflammation and edema

Table 16.18 Nursing Diagnoses Related to Asthma

- Ineffective airway clearance related to bronchospasm
- Impaired gas exchange related to air trapping
- Activity intolerance related to dyspnea
- Deficient fluid volume related to tachypnea/dyspnea/increased metabolic demand
- Anxiety related to change in health status/environment change
- Ineffective airway clearance related to status asthmaticus
- Deficient knowledge regarding diagnosis, treatment, and home care
- Fear related to breathlessness and recurrence

3. Expectorants (acetylcysteine [Mucomyst] to decrease congestion)
4. Antibiotics if infection is present
5. Sedatives if anxiety is severe
6. Cromolyn sodium: not used during acute attack; inhaled; inhibits histamine release in lungs and prevents further attacks
7. Physical therapy
8. Allergy testing/sensitization
9. High Fowler's position
10. Oxygen
11. Humidification/hydration to loosen secretions
12. Chest percussion and postural drainage when bronchodilation improves
13. Modify environment:
    a. Good ventilation
    b. Stay indoors when grass is being cut or pollen count is high.
    c. Use damp dusting to reduce allergens.
    d. Avoid rugs, draperies, or curtains, and stuffed animals.
    e. Avoid natural fibers: wool and feathers.
14. Swimming is a good form of moderate exercise.
15. Breathing exercises

CYSTIC FIBROSIS (MUCOVISCIDOSIS)

A. Dysfunction of the exocrine glands: mucous-producing glands of the respiratory tract, GI tract, pancreas, sweat glands, salivary glands; transmitted as an autosomal recessive trait; most common lethal genetic disease among caucasians in the United States and Europe; no test to detect carriers
B. Pathophysiology:
   1. Secretions from mucous glands are thick, causing obstruction and fibrosis of tissue.
   2. Sweat and saliva are high in sodium chloride.
   3. Pancreas:
      a. Obstruction of the pancreatic ducts and eventual fibrosis and atrophy of the pancreas leads to little or no release of enzymes: lipase, amylase, and trypsin.
      b. Malabsorption of fats and proteins due to no enzymes
      c. Unabsorbed food residues excreted in the stool produce steatorrhea.
      d. Failure to thrive due to loss of nutrients and inability to absorb fat-soluble vitamins
   4. Respiratory tract:
      a. Increased production of secretions cause obstruction of airway, air trapping, and atelectasis
      b. Cor pulmonale

5. Reproductive system:
   a. Males are sterile.
   b. Females: conception difficult but possible
   c. Pregnancy causes increased stress on respiratory system of mother.
6. Liver: some patients have cirrhosis/ portal hypertension
7. Ultimately fatal: average age of death is 20 years; 95% die from lung problem
C. Assessment findings:
   1. Failure to thrive
   2. Bulky, pale, frothy, foul-smelling stools
   3. Meconium ileus in newborns
   4. Rectal prolapse due to greasy stools
   5. Protruding abdomen with atrophy or extremities and buttocks
   6. Voracious appetite
   7. Anemia
   8. Respiratory distress
   9. Clubbing of digits
   10. Decreased exercise tolerance
   11. Frequent productive cough and infections
   12. Chest X-ray reveals atelectasis, infiltrations, and emphysemic changes.
   13. Abnormal pulmonary function studies
   14. ABGs show respiratory acidosis.
   15. Hyponatremia/heat exhaustion in hot weather
   16. Salty taste to sweat
   17. Sweat test shows increased NaCl in sweat
D. Nursing diagnoses (see Table 16.19)

Table 16.19 Nursing Diagnoses Related to Cystic Fibrosis

- Ineffective airway clearance related to thick mucous
- Ineffective breathing patterns related to thick mucous and concurrent infection
- Imbalanced nutrition: less than body requirements related to poor intestinal absorption of nutrients
- Decreased cardiac output related to lung congestion
- Activity intolerance related to respiratory compromise
- Disturbed sleep pattern related to excessive secretions and difficulty breathing
- Anxiety related to chronic disease
- Compromised family coping related to chronic nature of disease and intense home therapy
- Deficient knowledge regarding nature of treatments and medications to be administered at home

E. Interventions:
   1. Pancreatic enzymes with meals
   2. High calorie, high carbohydrate, high protein, normal fat diet
   3. Multivitamins; administer fat-soluble vitamins (A, D, E, and K) in water-soluble form
   4. Antibiotics: ongoing, low-dose prophylaxis
   5. Expectorants, mucolytics
   6. Percussion and postural drainage qid

7. Breathing exercises
8. Aerosol treatments
9. Avoid cough suppressants and antihistamines.
10. Genetic counseling

Sample Questions

1. The nurse makes an initial assessment of a four-year-old admitted with possible epiglottitis. Which observation is most suggestive of epiglottitis?
   1. Low-grade fever
   2. Retching
   3. Excessive drooling
   4. Substernal retractions
2. Which nursing action could be life-threatening for a child with epiglottitis?
   1. Examining the child's throat with a tongue blade
   2. Placing the child in a semi-Fowler's position
   3. Maintaining high humidity
   4. Obtaining a nasopharyngeal culture
3. Which factor would most likely be a cause of epiglottitis?
   1. Acquiring the child's first puppy, the day before the onset of symptoms
   2. Exposure to the parainfluenza virus
   3. Exposure to Hemophilus influenza, type B
   4. Frequent upper respiratory infections as an infant
4. The nurse is caring for a child who has epiglottitis. What position would the child be most likely to assume?
   1. Squatting
   2. Sitting upright and leaning forward, supporting self with hands
   3. Crouching on hands and knees and rocking back and forth
   4. Knee-chest position
5. The nurse is assessing a child who has epiglottitis and is having respiratory difficulty. Which is the nurse most likely to assess in the child?
   1. Flaring of the nares; cyanosis; lethargy
   2. Diminished breath sounds bilaterally; easily agitated
   3. Scattered rales throughout lung fields; anxious and frightened
   4. Mouth open with a protruding tongue; inspiratory stridor
6. Which is the most important goal of nursing care in the management of a child with epiglottitis?
   1. Preventing the spread of infection from the epiglottis throughout the respiratory tract
   2. Reduction of high fever and prevention of hyperthermia
   3. Maintaining a patent airway
   4. Maintaining him in an atmosphere of high humidity with oxygen

7. Which is the most important nursing action when caring for a child with epiglottitis?
   1. Cardiac monitoring
   2. Blood pressure monitoring
   3. Temperature monitoring
   4. Monitoring intravenous infusion
8. A five-year-old is admitted with his first asthma attack. Which would have been least likely to have precipitated his asthma attack?
   1. A new puppy in the house
   2. A visit from his uncle who smokes cigars
   3. An unusually early snowstorm
   4. Eating fresh fruit salad
9. During aminophylline infusion, a child becomes restless, nauseated, and his blood pressure drops. What is the appropriate nursing response to these findings?
   1. Because these are common side effects of the drug, which will pass when the infusion is completed, simply chart the response.
   2. Stop the infusion immediately and notify the physician or charge nurse, because the symptoms are suggestive of an adverse response to aminophylline.
   3. Continue to monitor the child, because the symptoms are probably related to the child's illness because they are not commonly associated with aminophylline.
   4. Continue to monitor the child, because these are expected responses to aminophylline.
10. It is important to teach the parents of a child with asthma about the disease and its long-term management. Teaching play techniques such as blowing cotton balls or ping pong balls across a table are good for him. Which is the best explanation for this play technique?
    1. It decreases expiratory pressure.
    2. It provides for an extended expiratory phase of respiration.
    3. It promotes a fuller expansion of the thoracic cavity during inspiration.
    4. It develops the accessory muscles of respiration.
11. After having chronic sore throats and repeated absences from school over the past year, a six-year-old has been admitted to the pediatric unit for a tonsillectomy. Which would be the most important information to obtain in a pre-operative health history?
    1. Evidence of bleeding tendencies
    2. Parent's responses to anesthesia, especially adverse reactions
    3. Child's perception of the surgical procedure
    4. Frequency and type of bacterial tonsilar infections
12. A six-year-old has just returned from having a tonsillectomy. The child's condition is stable but the child remains quite drowsy. How should the nurse position this child?
    1. On her back with head elevated 30 degrees
    2. High-Fowler's

3. Semi-prone
4. Trendelenburg
13. The nurse is caring for a child who had a tonsillectomy this morning. The child is observed to be swallowing continuously. What is the most appropriate initial nursing action?
    1. Administer acetaminophen for pain.
    2. Place an ice collar around her throat.
    3. Call the surgeon immediately.
    4. Encourage the child to suck on ice chips.
14. The nurse is caring for a six-year-old who had a tonsillectomy this morning. Once the child is fully awake and alert, which liquid is the best to offer her?
    1. A cherry popsicle
    2. Apple juice
    3. Orange juice
    4. Cranberry juice
15. A 10-year-old has had diagnosed bronchial asthma for three years. The child has been admitted to the pediatric unit in acute respiratory distress. Which would be most characteristic of the child's asthmatic attack upon admission?
    1. Expiratory wheezing
    2. Inspiratory stridor
    3. Cyanotic nail beds
    4. Prolonged inspiratory phase
16. A child is admitted with asthma. Which aspects of the health history would be most closely associated with asthma?
    1. The child's grandfather died of emphysema at age 76.
    2. The child's grandmother died of lung cancer.
    3. The child had respiratory distress syndrome following premature birth.
    4. The child had eczema as an infant and toddler.
17. A stat dose of epinephrine is ordered for a child with asthma. How should the nurse administer the epinephrine?
    1. Intramuscular
    2. Sublingual
    3. Subcutaneous
    4. Nebulization
18. A child with an asthma attack has received epinephrine. The child is also to receive isoproteronol (Isuprel) via intermittent positive pressure breathing. When should the isoproteronol be given in relation to the epinephrine?
    1. Isoproteronol should be given 30 minutes prior to the administration of epinephrine.
    2. Isoproteronol should never be given in conjunction with epinephrine. Check with the physician.
    3. Isoproteronol should not be given within one hour after the administration of epinephrine.
    4. Isoproteronol should be given at the same time as epinephrine for maximum benefit.
19. A child is having an asthma attack. The nurse places the child in high-Fowler's position for which of the following reasons?
    1. To prevent the aspiration of mucous
    2. To visualize abnormal inspiratory excursion
    3. To prevent atelectasis
    4. To relieve dyspnea
20. A thirteen-month-old is diagnosed with croup and placed in a croup tent. Which toy is most appropriate for the nurse to give the child?
    1. A doll made of cotton
    2. A music box
    3. A soft fuzzy toy made of synthetic materials
    4. A wind-up bunny
21. The nurse is caring for a five-year-old who has cystic fibrosis. What should the nurse do to help the child manage secretions and avoid respiratory distress?
    1. Administer continuous oxygen therapy.
    2. Perform chest physiotherapy every four hours.
    3. Administer pancreatic enzymes as ordered.
    4. Encourage a diet high in calories.
22. The nurse is to administer pancreatic enzymes to an eight-month-old who has cystic fibrosis. When should this medication be administered?
    1. A half hour before meals
    2. With meals
    3. An hour after meals
    4. Between meals
23. A ten-month-old is being treated for otitis media. What is the most important nursing action to prevent recurrence of the infection?
    1. Administer acetaminophen as ordered.
    2. Encourage the parents to maintain a smoke-free home environment.
    3. Explain to the parents that they must give the child all of the prescribed antibiotic therapy.
    4. Encourage the parents to bottle-feed the child in an upright position.
24. The nurse is caring for a six-month-old infant who is in a croup tent. The child's mother calls and tells the nurse that the child's clothes are all wet. What is the best action for the nurse to take?
    1. Explain to the mother that this is normal because the croup tent has high humidity.
    2. Change the child's clothing.
    3. Cover the child with a dry blanket.
    4. Remove the child from the croup tent until his clothes are dry.
25. A five-year-old has cystic fibrosis. What is best to offer the child on a hot summer day?
    1. Kool-aid
    2. Ice cream
    3. Lemonade
    4. Broth

Answers and Rationales

1. (3) Excessive drooling is a sign of epiglottitis. A child with epiglottitis is apt to have a high fever. Retching is not typical. Retractions could occur if respiratory distress were great enough, but drooling is the hallmark of epiglottitis.

2. (1) Examining the child's throat with a tongue blade may cause the epiglottis to become so irritated that it will close off completely and obstruct the airway. The child should be placed in a semi- to high-Fowler's position. Humidity is not a problem. A nasopharyngeal culture would not cause problems. The nurse should get a throat culture, however.

3. (3) H. Influenza is the usual causative agent of epiglottitis. A puppy would be more apt to cause asthma than epiglottitis.

4. (2) Sitting upright and leaning forward, supporting self with hands, is the position typically assumed by children with epiglottitis. It helps to promote the airway and drainage of secretions. Squatting is more typically seen in children who have cyanotic heart defects.

5. (4) The child with an edematous glottis will keep his mouth open with his tongue protruding to increase free movement in the pharynx. In the presence of potential laryngeal obstruction, laryngeal stridor can be heard especially during inspiration. Rales and diminished breath sounds are more typical of croup. Cyanosis is typical of late-stage, extremely critical respiratory distress.

6. (3) In a child with epiglottitis the first signs of difficulty in breathing can progress to severe inspiratory distress or complete airway obstruction in a matter of minutes or hours. The child usually has a high fever, but airway takes precedence. High humidity may also be appropriate, but the highest priority is maintaining an airway.

7. (1) Regular monitoring of cardiac rate is essential, because a rapidly rising heart rate is an initial indication of hypoxia and impending obstruction of the airway. The blood pressure and temperature may well be monitored, but they are not the most important. An IV will be monitored, if present, but is not the highest priority.

8. (4) Pets, smoke, and changes in temperature can all precipitate asthma. A fruit salad is least likely to precipitate an asthma attack. It is possible that someone could be allergic to something in a fruit salad, but these are not common asthma triggers.

9. (2) These are symptoms of an adverse response to aminophylline. The IV should be stopped and the physician notified immediately. The child may be going into shock.

10. (2) Blowing will extend the expiratory phase of respiration and help the child with asthma exhale more completely. Blowing ping pong balls is exhalation, not inhalation. It does not develop accessory muscles of respiration.

11. (1) The most common and serious complication following tonsillectomy is hemorrhage. The nurse should ask about bleeding tendencies. Information about any familial adverse responses may be nice to know but is not as important as information about the child's tendency to bleed. The child's perception of the surgery is also nice to know but is not the most important information. The frequency and type of tonsil infections is nice to know but not essential.

12. (3) Because the child is sleepy, the child should be semi-prone to prevent aspiration in case the child vomits. When the child is alert, he/she can be in semi-Fowler's. Trendelenburg position is contraindicated because it would cause more swelling in the operative area.

13. (3) Continual swallowing indicates bleeding. The surgeon should be notified at once. None of the other responses is appropriate. The child may be hemorrhaging.

14. (2) The child needs clear, cold liquids that are not red and are not citrus. Red would make it difficult to determine if vomitus was blood or juice.

15. (1) Bronchial constriction occurs in asthma. This increases the airway resistance to airflow. The respiratory difficulty is accentuated during expiration, when the bronchi are supposed to contract and shorten, as opposed to inspiration, when the bronchi are dilating and elongating. Inspiratory stridor is characteristic of croup. Note that answers 2 and 4 both deal with the inspiratory phase. Asthma affects the expiratory phase.

16. (4) Asthma is an allergic condition and frequently follows eczema, also an allergic condition. Relatives having emphysema or lung cancer is not usually related to childhood asthma. Respiratory distress syndrome as an infant does not predispose the child to asthma.

17. (3) Epinephrine is a rapid-acting drug of short duration. The subcutaneous route is the most effective for rapid relief of respiratory distress. The stat dose is not given intramuscular, sublingual, or by nebulizer.

18. (3) The side effects of epinephrine (tachycardia, rise in blood pressure, tremors, weakness, and nausea) are potentiated by isoproteronol. Therefore, when given concurrently, isoproteronol should not be given within one hour after administration of epinephrine.

19. (4) By providing for maximum ventilatory efficiency, the high-Fowler's position increases the oxygen supply to the lungs and helps to relieve dyspnea. This is most important for the

asthmatic child who is experiencing a diminished ventilatory capacity.

20. (1) The major concern regarding toys for a child in a croup tent is that there not be any chance of static electricity or a spark, because the croup tent contains oxygen. Cotton does not create static electricity. Wool and synthetic materials create static electricity. A wind-up toy could create a spark.

21. (2) Chest physiotherapy aids in loosening secretions throughout the respiratory tract. Oxygen therapy does not loosen secretions and may be contraindicated, because many children with cystic fibrosis experience carbon dioxide retention and respiratory depression with too high levels of oxygen. Pancreatic enzymes will be given to this child, but to improve the absorption of nutrients, not to facilitate respiratory effort. A diet high in calories is appropriate for a child with cystic fibrosis. However, it does not facilitate respiratory effort.

22. (2) Pancreatic enzymes should be given with meals. They can be mixed with applesauce. The purpose of the enzymes is to help with the digestion and absorption of nutrients. Therefore, they must be given when the child is having food.

23. (3) The child should receive all of the antibiotic medication. Parents are apt to stop giving it to the child when he/she begins to feel better. This encourages recurrence of the infection that may be resistant to antibiotic therapy. Acetaminophen may be given to the infant, but it is for pain and does not prevent recurrence of the infection. There is some evidence that children who live around smokers have a higher incidence of otitis media. This teaching is relevant but not the most important. Children who go to sleep with milk or juice in their mouths after feeding have a higher incidence of otitis media, but this is not the most important nursing action to prevent recurrence of infection.

24. (2) A croup tent is high humidity, and the child's clothes will get wet. When they do, they should be changed so that the child will not get chilled. It is appropriate to explain this to the mother, but the best response is to change the child. Covering the child will not prevent chilling. The nurse should not remove the child from the croup tent just because his clothing is wet.

25. (4) The child with cystic fibrosis has a problem with chloride metabolism and loses excessive amounts of salt in sweat. The child should be given something with high amounts of sodium, such as broth. Ice cream contains some sodium, but not as much as broth. Kool-Aid and lemonade contain no sodium.

Pediatric Conditions Related to the Neurosensory System

SPINA BIFIDA (MYELODYSPLASIA)

A. Pathophysiology:
  1. Failure of posterior vertebral arches to fuse during embryonic development
  2. Neural tube defects associated with folic acid deficiency; many cases of unknown cause
  3. Defects may be in the lower thoracic, lumbar, or sacral area (85%) or in the upper thoracic and cervical areas (15%).
  4. Usually associated with other neurological defects such as hydrocephalus
B. Types (see Figure 16.3):
  1. Spina bifida occulta:
    a. Spinal cord and meninges remain in the normal anatomical position; they do not protrude
    b. Defect may not be visible, or there may be a dimple or a small tuft of hair on the spine
    c. Child is often asymptomatic; may have slight neuromuscular deficit
  2. Spina bifida cystica:
    a. Meningocele:
      (1) Sac formed by meninges filled with spinal fluid protrudes through the opening in the spinal canal; sac is covered with thin skin
      (2) No nerves in sac
      (3) No motor or sensory loss
      (4) Good prognosis after surgery
    b. Meningomyelocele/myelomeningocele:
      (1) Same as meningocele except there are nerves in the sac
      (2) Sensory and motor deficit below the level of the lesion

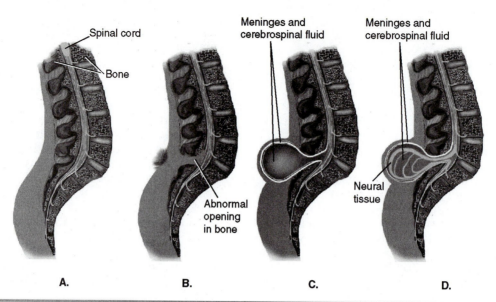

Figure 16.3 Spinal Column Defects: A. Normal Spine, B. Spina Bifida Occulata, C. Spina Bifida with meningocele, D Spina Bifida with myelomeningocele

(3) Most children (80%) have multiple handicaps such as lower body paralysis and bowel and bladder dysfunction

B. Assessment findings:
  1. Can be detected with amniocentesis with a 98% accuracy; increased alphafetoprotein (AFP) level prior to 18th week of gestation
  2. Ultrasound during pregnancy shows fetal spinal defect and sac
  3. Sac on spine as described above
  4. Loss of bowel and bladder functions; check for urinary and fecal dribbling
  5. Flaccid paralysis of lower extremities; may have club foot or congenital hip

C. Nursing diagnosis: myelomeningocele (see Table 16.20)

D. Interventions:
  1. Surgical closure of defect, usually within 48 hours of birth
  2. Shunt if hydrocephalus present
  3. Antibiotics to prevent infection
  4. Pre-operative nursing care:
     a. Keep baby in prone position to prevent pressure on sac.
     b. Prevent sac infection; cover sac with sterile, moist saline 4×4's.
     c. Place small pad under lower portion of legs to prevent deformities.
     d. Give perineal care to prevent contamination of sac.
  5. Post-operative nursing care:
     a. Check for signs of shock or hemorrhage.
     b. Keep dressings free of urine and feces.
     c. Keep infant in prone position.
     d. Measure head circumference for evidence of hydrocephalus.

Table 16.20 Nursing Diagnoses Related to Myelomeningocele

- Risk for infection related to presence of meningeal sac and infective organisms
- Risk for trauma related to delicate spinal sac
- Risk for impaired skin integrity related to meningeal sac, motor sensory impairment, and orthopedic appliances
- Interrupted family process related to situational crisis
- Chronic constipation related to effects of spinal cord disorder on anal sphincter
- Urinary retention related to effects of spinal cord injury on bladder function
- Self-care deficit related to sensory-motor impairments
- Impaired physical mobility related to lower limb impairments
- Parental grieving related to birth of infant with defects
- Risk for ineffective therapeutic regimen management related to lack of knowledge of condition, home care, orthopedic appliances, self-catheterization, activity program, and community services

     e. Monitor musculoskeletal movement.
     f. Use intermittent urinary catheterization to manage neurogenic bladder.
  6. Anticholinergic drugs to increase bladder capacity and lower intravesicular pressure
  7. Immobilization (casts, braces, traction) for defects of hips, knees, or feet

HYDROCEPHALUS

A. Increased amount of cerebrospinal fluid within the ventricles of the brain may be caused by obstruction of CSF flow, overproduction or inadequate reabsorption of CSF, congenital malformations, or may be secondary to injury, infection, or tumor

B. Types:
1. Noncommunicating: flow of CSF from ventricles to subarachnoid space is obstructed
2. Communicating: flow is not obstructed, but CSF is inadequately reabsorbed in subarachnoid space

C. Assessment findings:
1. Infant:
   a. Increased head circumference
   b. Tense bulging anterior fontanel
   c. Separation of cranial sutures
   d. Distended scalp veins
   e. High pitched cry
   f. Feeding problems
   g. Vomiting
   h. Irritability
   i. Discomfort when held
   j. Downward rotation of eyes ("setting sun" sign—sclera visible above iris)
   k. Opisthotonos (spine hyperflexed with posterior of head near or actually touching heels)
2. Older child:
   a. Signs of increased intracranial pressure: headache, nausea, and vomiting
   b. Diplopia, blurred vision
   c. Behavioral changes
   d. Decreased motor function
   e. Decreased LOC
   f. Seizures
3. Diagnostic tests: CAT scan

D. Nursing diagnoses (see Table 16.21)

Table 16.21 Nursing Diagnoses Related to Hydrocephalus

- Risk for infection related to surgically-implanted drainage system (shunt)
- Risk for impaired skin integrity related to paralysis; pressure areas; anal sphincter relaxation
- Ineffective cerebral tissue perfusion related to decreased arterial/venous blood flow caused by compression of brain tissue.
- Disturbed sensory perceptions: visual related to pressure on sensory/motor nerves
- Impaired physical mobility related neuromuscular impairment, decreased muscle strength, and impaired coordination
- Risk for injury related to inability to support large head and strain on neck
- Risk for impaired nutrition: less than body requirements related to vomiting secondary to cerebral compression and irritability
- Risk for ineffective therapeutic regiment management related to insufficient knowledge of condition, home care, signs and symptoms of infection, increased intracranial pressure, and emergency treatment of shunt
- Interrupted family process related to situational crisis.

E. Interventions:
1. Shunt: insertion of a flexible tube into the lateral ventricle of the brain; catheter is then threaded under the skin and the distal end positioned in the peritoneum (most common) or the right atrium; a subcutaneous pump may be attached to keep it patent
2. Pre-operative nursing care:
   a. Measure head circumference
   b. Monitor for ICP
3. Post-operative nursing care:
   a. Vital signs
   b. Check for hemorrhage
   c. Neuro assessment
   d. Keep shunt patent:
      (1) Position child on non-operative side
      (2) Pump shunt
      (3) Monitor for ICP
      (4) Monitor for infection
      (5) Position flat or with head only slightly elevated
   e. Assess for return of bowel sounds
   f. Teach parent care of shunt, follow-up care, community resources

BRAIN TUMORS

A. Pathophysiology:
1. Space occupying mass in the brain tissue, either benign or malignant, with peak incidence in 3–7-year-old boys
2. Second most common type of cancer in children
3. Two-thirds of brain tumors in children are beneath the tentorium.

B. Assessment findings:
1. Signs of ICP:
   a. Morning headache
   b. Projectile vomiting
   c. Personality changes
   d. Diplopia
   e. Papilledema; late sign
   f. Elevated BP with decreased pulse
   g. Cranial enlargement
2. Focal signs and symptoms:
   a. Ataxia in cerebellar tumors
   b. Decrease in muscle strength
   c. Head tilt in posterior fossa tumors
   d. Ocular signs:
      (1) Nystagmus on the same side as the infratentorial lesion
      (2) Diplopia/strabismus
      (3) Visual field deficit
3. Focal disturbances, papilledema, optic nerve atrophy, blindness
4. Symptoms depend on the location and type of tumor.
5. Decrease in school performance
6. Skull X-ray shows tumor

7. CT scan, MRI show location of tumor
8. EEG shows seizure activity
C. Nursing diagnoses (see Table 16.22)

Table 16.22 Nursing Diagnoses Related to Brain Tumors

- Risk for injury related to growing tumor
- Risk for injury, infection, related to surgery
- Acute pain related to surgical procedure/tumor pressure
- Risk for deficient fluid volume related to medications/hypermetabolic state, vomiting
- Anxiety related to situational crisis
- Disturbed self-concept related to medical-surgical therapies; inability to perform activities of daily living
- Self-care deficit related to sensory/neuromuscular impairment interfering with ability to perform tasks
- Impaired physical mobility related to sensory-motor impairment
- Disturbed thought processes related to altered circulation to brain tissue or destruction of brain tissue
- Interrupted family processes related to a child with critical surgery for a life-threatening disease

D. Interventions:
1. Radiation
2. Chemotherapy
3. Surgery:
   a. Remove a tumor
   b. After trauma
   c. Aspiration of an abscess
   d. Insertion of a shunt
4. Pre-operative nursing care:
   a. Prepare child in age-appropriate way
   b. Prepare child and parents for complications from surgery
   c. Monitor for changes in vital signs and neurologic status.
   d. Safety: side rails, ambulation, and so on
   e. Comfort measures; analgesics
5. Post-operative nursing care:
   a. Monitor vital signs and neurologic status.
   b. Use hypothermia blanket if markedly elevated temperature.
   c. Observe dressing for discharge: CSF is colorless and positive for glucose.
   d. Close or cover eyes, apply ice, instill saline drops or artificial tears.
   e. Take seizure precautions.
   f. Position carefully: varies with procedure; infratentorial lesions usually flat position.
   g. Maintain fluid and electrolyte balance; intake and output.
   h. Provide emotional support for child and family.

REYE'S SYNDROME

A. Acute, potentially fatal disease of childhood characterized by severe edema of the brain and increased intracranial pressure, hypoglycemia,
and fatty infiltration and dysfunction of the liver; etiology unknown but almost always associated with a viral infection; may be associated with aspirin administration in a viral infection

B. Assessment findings:
1. Child is recovering from a viral infection during which he was given aspirin.
2. Stage I: sudden onset of persistent vomiting, fatigue, and listlessness
3. Stage II: personality and behavior changes; disorientation; confusion; hyperreflexia
4. Stage III: coma, decorticate posturing
5. Stage IV: deeper coma, decerebrate rigidity
6. Stage V: seizures, absent DTRs (deep tendon reflexes), respiratory reflexes; flaccid paralysis
7. Increased free fatty acids
8. Elevated ammonia levels
9. Impaired liver function
10. Brain swelling

C. Nursing diagnoses (see Table 16.23)

Table 16.23 Nursing Diagnoses Related to Reye's Syndrome

- Disturbed thought process related to progressive encephalopathy
- Risk for injury related to disease process, cerebral edema
- Decreased cardiac output related to myocardial effect, side effects of medication
- Risk for deficient fluid volume related to NPO, diuretic use, glucose requirements
- Risk for impaired gas exchange related to complications from prolonged ventilatory support
- Anxiety related to course of disease, uncertain prognosis
- Interrupted family processes related to a child with a life threatening illness
- Risk for trauma related to generalized weakness, reduced coordination, and cognitive deficits
- Ineffective breathing pattern related to decreased energy and fatigue, cognitive impairment, tracheobronchial obstruction, inflammatory process, and aspiration pneumonia
- Risk for infection related to invasive monitoring devices

D. Interventions:
1. Stage I: Assess Hydration Status: monitor skin turgor, mucous membranes, intake and output, urine specific gravity, monitor IV therapy
2. Stage I–V: Assess Neurologic Status: monitor LOC, pupils, extremity movement, motor coordination; seizures
3. Stage II–V:
   a. Assess respiratory status.
   b. Assess circulatory status.
   c. Support the child and family.

BACTERIAL MENINGITIS

A. Infection of the meninges caused by organisms such as Haemophilus influenzae type B,

Streptococcus pneumoniae, Escerichia coli, and Neisseria meningitidis
B. Assessment findings:
1. Neonates:
   a. Poor sucking
   b. Weak cry
   c. Lethargy
2. Infants and young children:
   a. Fever
   b. Poor feeding
   c. Irritability
3. Children and adolescents:
   a. Rapid onset with fever, chills, headache, and vomiting
   b. Alterations in sensorium or seizure
   c. Signs of meningeal irritation:
      (1) Nuchal rigidity followed by severe hyperextension
      (2) Opisthotonos: head and heels bent backward and body arched forward
      (3) Brudzinski's sign: flexion at the hip and knee in response to forward flexion of the neck
      (4) Kernig's sign: contraction or pain in the hamstring muscle when attempting to extend the leg when the hip is flexed
   d. Petechial rash or joint involvement
4. Lumbar puncture shows increased pressure of CSF and elevated WBC and protein, decreased glucose, and culture positive for specific organism
C. Nursing diagnoses (see Table 16.24)
D. Interventions:
1. Administer antibiotics as ordered.
2. Maintain the child in respiratory isolation.
3. Monitor vital signs and LOC for signs of increased intracranial pressure.
4. Assess for signs of meningeal irritation, such as a stiff neck and change in LOC.
5. Keep child in darkened room with minimal stimuli to help prevent seizures
6. Prevent complications of immobility; do ROM, skin care, and so on.
7. Identify contacts who may need prophylactic antibiotic therapy.

CEREBRAL PALSY

A. Neuromuscular disorder resulting from anoxia to the brain before, during, or after birth
B. Assessment findings:
1. Spasticity: exaggerated hyperactive reflexes; poorly coordinated movements
2. Poor speech
3. Athetosis: constant involuntary, purposeless, slow, writhing movements except when asleep
4. Ataxia: disturbance in equilibrium
5. Tremor
6. Rigidity
7. Associated problems:
   a. Mental retardation in 18–50% of cases
   b. Hearing loss (13% of cases)
   c. Defective speech (75% of cases)
   d. Dental anomalies from muscle contractures
   e. Visual disabilities (28% of cases)
   f. Disturbance of body image, touch, perception
C. Nursing diagnoses (see Table 16.25)
D. Interventions:
1. Antianxiety drugs
2. Skeletal muscle relaxants
3. Local nerve blocks
4. Physical, occupational, speech, and hearing therapy
5. Surgery: muscle and tendon releasing

Table 16.24 Nursing Diagnoses Related to Meningitis

- Risk for injury related to seizures
- Impaired comfort related to headache, nuchal rigidity, and muscle aches
- Impaired physical mobility related to intravenous infusions, nuchal rigidity, and restraints
- Risk for impaired skin integrity related to immobility
- Risk for infection transmission related to contagious nature of organism
- Risk for impaired oral mucous membrane related to dehydration and impaired ability to perform mouth care
- Risk for imbalanced nutrition: less than body requirements related to anorexia, nausea, and vomiting
- Risk for impaired respiratory function related to immobility
- Hyperthermia related to infectious process
- Risk for disturbed cerebral tissue perfusion related to cerebral edema
- Interrupted family processes related to critical nature of disease and uncertain prognosis
- Anxiety related to treatments, environment, and risk of death.
- Risk for ineffective therapeutic regimen management related to insufficient knowledge of condition, treatments, and possible complications

Table 16.25 Nursing Diagnoses Related to Cerebral Palsy

- Impaired physical mobility related to neuromuscular impairment
- Risk for injury related to physical disability, neuromuscular impairment, and perceptual and cognitive impairment
- Fatigue related to increased energy expenditure
- Impaired verbal communication related to facial muscle involvement
- Bathing/hygiene, dressing/grooming, feeding, toileting self-care deficits related to physical disability
- Disturbed body image related to perception of disability
- Interrupted family processes related to a child with a lifelong disability
- Risk for deficient fluid volume related to difficulty obtaining or swallowing fluids
- Ineffective family coping related to permanent and severe nature of condition

6. Assistance with activities of daily living (ADL); nutrition, elimination, sleep-rest, activity
7. Safety
8. Teaching and support for child and parents

TAY-SACHS DISEASE

A. Degenerative brain disease caused by absence of hexosaminidase A from all body tissues; transmitted through an autosomal recessive gene occurring in persons of Eastern European Jewish ancestry
B. Fatal with death by four years of age
C. Assessment findings:
   1. Normal growth and development for two to six months
   2. Progressive lethargy after two to six months
   3. Baby stops skill development and loses skills.
   4. Loss of vision
   5. Hyperreflexia, decerebrate posturing, dysphagia, seizures
   6. Eating difficulties
   7. Classic cherry-red spot on the macula
   8. Enzyme tests in blood, amniotic fluid, or WBC
D. Nursing diagnoses (see Table 16.26)
E. Interventions:
   1. Receive no treatment; supportive care only.
   2. Help the parents cope with long-term care and grief.
   3. Receive genetic counseling and psychologic follow-up.

CONJUNCTIVITIS (PINK EYE)

A. Infection of the membrane covering the anterior surface of the eye globe and inner surface of the eyelid; may be bacterial, viral, or allergic
B. Assessment findings:
   1. Tearing eye
   2. Reddened conjunctiva

Table 16.26 Nursing Diagnoses Related to Tay Sachs Disease

- Delayed growth and development related to effects of physical condition
- Disturbed sensory perceptions: visual related to neurological deterioration of the optic nerve
- Anticipatory grieving (family) related to expected death of infant
- Powerlessness (family) related to absence of therapeutic interventions for this fatal disease
- Risk for spiritual distress related to expected death of infant
- Ineffective family coping related to situational crisis

3. Sensitivity to light
4. Eyelids stick shut with crusty exudate
C. Nursing diagnoses (see Table 16.27)

Table 16.27 Nursing Diagnoses Related to Conjunctivitis

- Risk for infection transmission related to lack of knowledge regarding handwashing technique and age of child
- Impaired comfort related to inflammation in eye, sensitivity to light

D. Interventions:
   1. Administer ophthalmic antibiotic, steroid, and anesthetic ointments as ordered.
      a. Apply from inner to outer canthus of eye.
      b. Do not let container touch eye.
   2. Teach client and family how to prevent spread of infection:
      a. Bacterial and viral forms very contagious: must be out of school until antibiotics have been taken for 24–48 hours.
      b. Teach child not to share pillows, tissues, or toys.
      c. Teach child and family good hand-washing techniques.
      d. Teach the family when and how to administer medications.

Sample Questions

1. Which assessment finding in a 10-month-old indicates a need for further neurologic evaluation?
   1. Inability to crawl
   2. Speaking only 2–4 words
   3. Inability to sit up without support
   4. Presence of crude pincer grasp
2. What should the nurse do to protect a child from injury during a seizure?
   1. Restrain the child's arms and legs.
   2. Place a tongue blade in the child's mouth.
   3. Place a pillow under the child's head.
   4. Provide a waterproof pad for the bed.
3. The nurse is teaching the parents of a child who has cerebral palsy to feed a child. What position is best to recommend?
   1. A normal eating position and provide stabilization of the jaw
   2. A semi-reclining position
   3. Upright while using a nasogastric or gastrostomy tube
   4. Hyperextension of the neck
4. A one-year-old child is admitted to the pediatric unit with the diagnosis of bacterial meningitis. Which room should the nurse assign to this child?

1. A room with a two-year-old who had surgery for a hernia repair
2. A room with a one-year-old child who has pneumonia
3. A room with a two-year-old who has cerebral palsy
4. A private room with no roommates

5. The nurse is caring for an infant who is admitted with bacterial meningitis. What is the first priority when providing nursing care for this child?
   1. Administer ordered antibiotics as soon as possible.
   2. Keep the room quiet and dim.
   3. Explain all procedures to the parents.
   4. Begin low-flow oxygen via mask.

6. A newborn has a myelomeningocele. What is the most important nursing action prior to surgery?
   1. Turn the infant every two hours.
   2. Encourage holding and cuddling by the parents.
   3. Apply sterile, moist, nonadherent dressings over the lesion.
   4. Administer pain medication every 3–4 hours.

7. A three-year-old is being seen in the neurology clinic for a routine visit. The child had a repair of a myelomeningocele shortly after birth. The child's mother asks the nurse when she can accomplish bladder training. What is the best reply?
   1. "You need to take your child to the bathroom every two hours."
   2. "We will teach you how to do intermittent, clean catheterization."
   3. "Continue to diaper the child until school age."
   4. "Your child needs to learn how to do self-catheterization."

8. Which assessment regularly performed on newborns and infants will do most to help with early identification of infants who might have hydrocephalus?
   1. Head circumference
   2. Weight measurement
   3. Length measurement
   4. Presence of reflexes

9. How should the nurse position a four-month-old infant who has hydrocephalus?
   1. Side lying
   2. Sitting up in an infant seat
   3. Alternating prone and supine
   4. Left Sims

10. The parents of a child who has otitis media ask the nurse why the doctor told them to give the child acetaminophen instead of aspirin. What should the nurse include when answering?
    1. Acetaminophen is more effective against ear pain than aspirin.
    2. Acetaminophen is better at reducing temperature than aspirin.
    3. Aspirin may cause gastritis in children.
    4. Aspirin is thought to cause Reye's syndrome, a very serious disease.

11. The parents of a child who is newly diagnosed with Tay-Sachs disease ask the nurse if they have more children could they be affected. Which information should be included when responding to the parents?
    1. Boys are more likely to inherit the disease than girls.
    2. Tay-Sachs is not inherited, so there is little chance other children will have it.
    3. There is a one-in-four chance that each pregnancy will result in a child who has the disease.
    4. Fifty percent of the girls will have the disease.

12. When planning care for an infant who has Tay-Sachs, the nurse knows that the care is aimed at which of the following?
    1. Providing supportive care until the child dies
    2. Preventing spread of the disease to others
    3. Curing the underlying problem so the child will grow normally
    4. Providing for maximum development of the child

13. An infant is born with a meningomyelocele. How should the nurse position the infant before surgery?
    1. Prone with a pillow under the legs
    2. Supine with head elevated
    3. Sidelying with a pillow at the back
    4. Semi-Fowler's with a small pillow

14. The parents of a two-year-old who has meningitis ask the nurse why the lights are dim in the child's room even in the day time. What information should the nurse include in the answer?
    1. Rest is essential, and a dimly lit room promotes rest.
    2. The child is sensitive to light and may develop seizures.
    3. The IV medications are very sensitive to light.
    4. Light could cause severe damage to the eyes and possible blindness.

15. A six-year-old child is brought to the doctor's office with crusts on the eyelid and a very red conjunctiva. The doctor prescribes antibiotic eye drops. The child's mother asks the nurse if the child can go back to school this afternoon. How should the nurse respond?
    1. Teach the child not to touch his eyes, and take him back to school.
    2. He should stay out of school today but can go back tomorrow.
    3. He should stay out of school for a week because it usually takes a week for the condition to clear.
    4. This condition is very contagious. The child should stay out of school for the next two days.

16. The nurse is administering eye drops to a child who has conjunctivitis. Where should the eye drops be placed?
    1. On the pupil
    2. In the conjunctival sac
    3. By the inner canthus
    4. On the sclera
17. The nurse is caring for a five-month-old infant who had a craniotomy following a head injury. Which observation the LPN/LVN makes should be reported to the charge nurse?
    1. Respirations of 38
    2. Difficulty arousing the baby from a nap
    3. Pulse rate of 120
    4. The baby cannot sit up by herself.
18. The nurse is caring for a child who has cerebral palsy. The nurse notes that the child does not writhe when sleeping but is in constant motion when awake. How should the nurse interpret this observation?
    1. The child should be encouraged to do something productive so she will not think about writhing.
    2. This indicates that the child could control the movements if she wanted to. A behavior modification program may be effective.
    3. This is typical of cerebral palsy. The nurse should assist the child with ADL as needed.
    4. The child should be sedated much of the time to prevent the dangerous writhing that occurs during waking.
19. A ten-year-old tells his neighbor, a nurse, that his eyes were "stuck together" this morning when he woke up. The nurse notes that his eyes are red and the conjunctiva is inflamed. What should the nurse neighbor recommend to the boy's mother?
    1. Tell his mother that he may have a contagious disease and should be seen by his doctor today.
    2. Encourage the mother to make an appointment to see the eye doctor.
    3. Suggest to the mother that the boy go to school today but make an appointment with the doctor if the condition does not clear up soon.
    4. Explain to the boy that he should wash his face and eyes with a wash cloth as soon as he wakes up.
20. The nurse is caring for an infant who has had surgery for a meningomyelocele. When thinking of long-term care needs, which understanding is most accurate?
    1. The surgery corrects the defect, and the infant should develop normally.
    2. The infant will probably have lower body paralysis and bowel and bladder dysfunction.

3. The infant should develop normally physically but is likely to have some degree of mental retardation.
4. The surgery may need to be repeated if the condition recurs.

Answers and Rationales

1. (3) A child who is 10 months of age should have been sitting without support for several months. This sign indicates a developmental lag and the need for further assessment. The ability to crawl is usually acquired between 9 and 12 months. Saying 2–4 words is normal for a child of 10 months. The development of the pincer grasp is refined by 11 months of age. It is normal for a 10-month-old child to use a crude pincer grasp.

2. (3) Placing a pillow under the head, using padded side rails, and removing sharp or hard objects from the immediate area all provide for the safety of a child who is having a seizure. No restraints or force should be used during a seizure. Nothing should be put in the mouth of a person who is having a seizure. Although having a waterproof mattress or pad would prevent the bed from being soiled, it has nothing to do with the child's safety.

3. (1) Upright with stabilization of the jaw is important, because jaw control is often lacking in a child with cerebral palsy. Feeding in a semireclining position does not promote swallowing. A child with cerebral palsy does not usually need tube feeding or a gastrostomy. Hyperextending the neck may interfere with swallowing.

4. (4) Bacterial meningitis is infectious. The child should be placed in a private room with respiratory precautions.

5. (1) The first priority is to begin antibiotics as soon as possible. The more quickly antibiotics are started, the better the child's prognosis. The nurse will keep the room quiet and dim and will explain actions to the parents. However, these actions are not as high of a priority as administering the antibiotics. Oxygen is administered only if the child's respiratory status is impaired.

6. (3) It is important to prevent the defect from becoming dry and cracked and allowing microorganisms to enter. Infants with myelomeningocele remain in a prone position to prevent excessive pressure or tension on the defect. In most cases, infants with myelomeningocele cannot be held and cuddled as other babies are. The parents should stroke

and touch the infant even if they cannot hold him or her. The infant is not usually in pain.

7. (2) Parents should be taught intermittent, clean catheterization. Parents can begin using this procedure at the age when unaffected children are toilet trained (about 3 years). Children who have myelomeningocele do not usually have bowel and bladder control, so taking him to the bathroom would serve no purpose. The child does not need to wear diapers until he goes to school. He should be as normal as possible. A three-year-old child is not old enough to learn self-catheterization techniques. He will learn when he is older and has better motor coordination and understanding of the procedure.

8. (1) Head circumference is the most important tool in early identification of hydrocephalus. Head circumference is measured at birth and at all well-baby visits. Measurements above the norm will be seen in infants with hydrocephalus. Weight and length do not have any connection with hydrocephalus. An infant with severe hydrocephalus may have abnormal reflexes, but head circumference will do the most to help with the early identification of infants who might have hydrocephalus.

9. (2) The infant with hydrocephalus should be positioned sitting up in an infant seat to promote drainage as much as possible and reduce intracranial pressure. Side lying, Sims, prone, and supine are not indicated. These positions would increase intracranial pressure.

10. (4) Aspirin given to children, especially those who may have a viral infection, is associated with the development of Reye's syndrome, a very serious problem affecting the brain and the liver that is often fatal. Therefore, we do not give aspirin to children. Acetaminophen is nearly as effective as aspirin in relieving pain and fever; it is not more effective. Aspirin can cause gastritis in anyone, but that is not the reason why we do not give it to children.

11. (3) Tay-Sachs is an autosomal, recessive condition. That means that both parents must have the gene and that there is a one-in-four chance with every pregnancy that the child will have the condition. The disease is not X-linked, so it is not seen more frequently in boys. Hemophilia is X-linked.

12. (1) There is no cure for Tay-Sachs. The child is missing the enzyme hexosaminidase A, which is necessary for all tissues. The child will become blind and lose any skills that he may have developed and will eventually die. There is no cure and no way to stop the progress of the disease. The disease is not communicable; it is genetic. The parents will need genetic counseling, but that is not the goal of care for the child.

13. (1) Infants with meningomyelocele should be positioned prone with a pillow under the lower legs. Every effort is made to avoid putting pressure on the sac. Breaking the sac would likely cause the infant to develop meningitis. All of the other position choices would put pressure on the sac.

14. (2) The child is sensitive to light and may develop seizures. A dimly lit room reduces the chance that seizures will occur. The child does need rest, but that is not the reason for a dimly lit room. The other answer choices are not correct.

15. (4) The condition described is probably pink eye, and it is very contagious. Once antibiotic treatment is started, the child should stay out of school for 24–48 hours.

16. (2) Eye drops should be placed in the conjunctival sac. Gentle pressure should be applied to the inner canthus to prevent the eye drops from entering the tear ducts and causing a runny nose.

17. (2) Difficulty arousing the child from a nap suggests a change in level of consciousness, a cardinal sign of increased intracranial pressure, and should be reported immediately to the charge nurse. The other findings are all normal for a five-month-old infant.

18. (3) Children with cerebral palsy who have athetoid movements are in constant motion during waking hours but move much less during sleep. The nurse should assist the child with ADLs as needed. The child cannot control these movements. The child should not be sedated constantly.

19. (1) The symptoms suggest conjunctivitis or "pink eye," which is very contagious. The child should not go to school and should be seen by his physician today. Conjunctivitis is treated by the pediatrician or primary care physician and does not require an eye doctor.

20. (2) Infants who have meningomyelocele usually have lower body paralysis and bowel and bladder dysfunction. The surgery closes the defect, but when the spinal nerves are in the sac, there is usually permanent damage. Unless there is associated hydrocephalus, the infant may well have normal mental development.

Pediatric Conditions Related to the Gastrointestinal System

CLEFT LIP

A. Failure of maxillary processes to fuse with nasal processes; familial disorder with a higher incidence among Caucasians
B. Assessment findings:
  1. Facial abnormality visible at birth
  2. Difficulty sucking; unable to form airtight seal around nipple
C. Nursing diagnoses (see Table 16.28)
D. Interventions:
  1. Surgical correction:
    a. Usually done at age 6–12 weeks (to prepare gums for eruption of teeth; promote parent-child bonding)
    b. Steri-strips or Logan bar to take tension off suture line
    c. Elbow restraints to keep child from touching suture line
  2. Speech therapy, dental care, audiologist care (prone to otitis media)
  3. Pre-operative nursing care:
    a. Establish and maintain airway.
    b. Problems with sucking, speech; incorporate parents in care
    c. Feeding problems: use Breck feeder, large-holed nipple, or rubber-tipped syringe
    d. Feed in upright position.
    e. Burp frequently because these babies swallow air when sucking.
    f. Observe for ear infections; watch for ear pulling, fever.
    g. Provide emotional support of infant and family.
    h. Role model touching and cuddling infant.
    i. Elbow restraints: allows infant to become accustomed to arm restraint prior to surgery
  4. Post-operative nursing care:
    a. Maintain airway.
    b. Monitor vital signs.
    c. Sedate if necessary to prevent crying and damage to suture line.
    d. Provide emotional support for infant/parents.
    e. Prevent infection: clean suture line after feeding with saline, peroxide, or water to remove crusts and prevent scarring.
    f. Infant should not suck; use Breck feeder or asepto syringe.
    g. Use elbow restraints: Remove one at a time for passive ROM and infant stimulation
    h. Assess pain; medicate prn.
    i. Change position; do not allow child to lie prone.
    j. Be alert to developmental needs.

Table 16.28 Nursing Diagnoses Related to Cleft Lip and Palate

- Risk for aspiration related to impaired sucking
- Impaired physical mobility related to restricted activity secondary to use of restraints
- Risk for impaired verbal communication related to impaired muscle development, insufficient palate function, faulty dentition, or hearing loss
- Risk for ineffective therapeutic regimen management related to insufficient knowledge of condition, feeding and suctioning techniques, surgical site care, risks for otitis media, and referral to speech therapist

Post-operative:
- Risk for trauma related to surgical site
- Risk for aspiration related to surgical site
- Imbalanced nutrition: less than body requirements related to difficult ingestion
- Risk for impaired skin integrity related to mouth secretions and/or restraining devices
- Interrupted family process related to situational crisis

CLEFT PALATE

A. Failure of palatine processes to fuse; roof of mouth communicates with nasopharynx
B. Assessment findings:
  1. Facial abnormality may accompany this defect
  2. Difficulty sucking; cannot form airtight seal around nipple—if accompanied by cleft lip
  3. Milk escapes through nose
  4. Difficulty swallowing
  5. Frequent infections; otitis media, URI
  6. Abdominal distention due to swallowed air
C. Nursing diagnoses (see Table 16.28)
D. Interventions:
  1. Surgical correction at age 1–2 years; prior to speech development
  2. Pre-operative nursing care:
    a. Maintain airway.
    b. Feed using Breck feeder, large-holed nipple, or rubber-tipped syringe.

c. Feed in upright position.
d. Prevent infection.
e. Support infant and parents.
f. Use elbow restraints pre-operative.
3. Post-operative nursing care:
a. Airway; position on side for drainage
b. Have suction available but use only in emergency.
c. Prevent injury or trauma to suture line:
   (1) Use cups only; no bottles.
   (2) No straws, popsicle sticks, or anything that goes into the mouth
   (3) Soft toys
   (4) Elbow restraints
d. Provide liquid diet progressing to soft and then regular.
e. Cleanse suture line with water after each feeding.
f. Hold and cuddle baby.
g. Provide for developmental needs.

ESOPHAGEAL DEFECTS

A. Pathophysiology (see Figure 16.4):
1. Esophageal atresia: Esophagus ends in a blind pouch with no connection to the stomach
2. Tracheoesophageal fistula (TEF): open connection between trachea and esophagus
3. Esophageal atresia with TEF: esophagus ends in a blind pouch; stomach, end of esophagus connects with trachea
4. These deformities found more often in low birth weight infants and are often associated with polyhydramnios

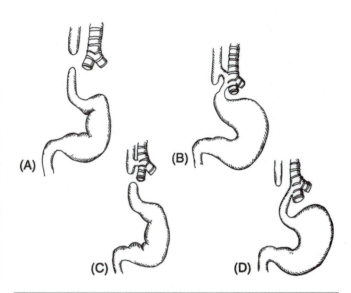

Figure 16.4 Esophageal Defects: (A) Esophageal Atresia, (B) (C) (D) Esophageal Atresia with tracheoesophageal Fistual.

Table 16.29 Nursing Diagnoses Related to Esophageal Disorders

- Ineffective airway clearance related to abnormal structure
- Impaired swallowing related to abnormal structure
- Risk for injury related to surgical procedure
- Interrupted family process related to situational crisis
- Risk for imbalanced nutrition: less than body requirements related to inability to swallow
- Risk for ineffective therapeutic regimen management related to insufficient knowledge of condition and management of gastrostomy tube.

B. Assessment findings:
1. Esophageal atresia:
   a. Polyhydramnios in mother because baby cannot swallow amniotic fluid
   b. Nasogastric tube cannot be passed
   c. Drooling and salivation
   d. Immediate regurgitation of undigested formula or milk when fed
   e. Choking and intermittent cyanosis
2. TEF:
   a. Normal swallowing but some food/mucous crosses fistula, causing choking and intermittent cyanosis
   b. Distended abdomen from inhaled air crossing fistula into stomach
   c. Aspiration pneumonia from reflux of gastric secretions into trachea
3. Esophageal atresia with TEF:
   a. All findings seen with esophageal atresia
   b. Distended abdomen from inhaled air crossing fistula into stomach
   c. Aspiration pneumonia from reflux of gastric secretions into trachea
4. Fluoroscopy with contrast dye shows type of defect
C. Nursing diagnoses (see Table 16.29)
D. Interventions:
1. Surgery to tie off fistula
2. Gastrostomy for feeding
3. Corrective surgery when child is older if possible
4. Antibiotics to prevent infections
5. Keep airway open
6. Position with head elevated 30°
7. Chest tube care after surgery
8. Provide pacifier to meet sucking needs
9. Teach family care of child with gastrostomy tube
10. Teach family signs of respiratory distress and how to suction infant

PYLORIC STENOSIS

A. Hypertrophy of pyloric sphincter causing stenosis and obstruction; occurs five in 1000 live births; more common in Caucasian, first born, full-term boys; may be familial

B. Assessment findings:
   1. Olive-sized bulge under right rib cage
   2. Insidious vomiting that occurs 2–3 weeks after birth and increases in intensity until it is forceful and projectile (no bile); no nausea, wants to eat again
   3. Peristaltic waves from L to R during and after feeding
   4. Failure to thrive
   5. Dehydration: sunken fontanels, poor skin turgor, decreased urine output, lack of tears
   6. Metabolic alkalosis
   7. Decreased sodium and potassium, elevated hematocrit
   8. Barium swallow shows narrowing of pylorus
C. Nursing diagnoses (see Table 16.30)

Table 16.30 Nursing Diagnoses Related to Pyloric Stenosis

- Risk for deficient fluid volume related to persistent/recurrent emesis
- Imbalanced nutrition: less than body requirements related to emesis
- Interrupted family process related to situational crisis: anxiety about feeding; home care/medical therapies (ongoing)

D. Interventions:
   1. Nonsurgical: thickened feedings
   2. Surgery: pyloromyotomy (Fredet-Ramstedt procedure)
   3. Pre-operative care:
      a. Fluids and electrolytes to correct dehydration and metabolic alkalosis
      b. NPO with NG tube in place to decompress intestine
      c. Fowler's position
      d. IV therapy to rehydrate
      e. Minimize handling.
      f. Intake and output, daily weights, urine specific gravity
   4. Post-operative care:
      a. NPO with parenteral fluids; oral fluids begun 4–6 hours after surgery
      b. Upright position after feeding
      c. Vital signs
      d. Position on right side to prevent aspiration
      e. NG tube until bowel sounds return
      f. Monitor incision for hemorrhage, infection; keep diaper below incision
      g. Intake and output; daily weights
      h. Parental support, teaching

GASTROESOPHAGEAL REFLUX (GER)

A. Return of stomach contents into esophagus above relaxed esophageal sphincter; no known cause

B. Assessment findings:
   1. Vomiting
   2. Weight loss
   3. Irritability
   4. Complications:
      a. Respiratory: apnea, aspiration
      b. Gastrointestinal: esophagitis, bleeding
   5. Barium esophageal/acid reflux test (pH probe over 24 hours)
C. Nursing diagnoses (see Table 16.29)
D. Interventions:
   1. Maintain adequate nutrition.
   2. Monitor for complications.
   3. Position upright during feeding.
   4. Elevate head of bed 30–60 degrees for 30 minutes after feeding.
   5. Maintain minimal stimulation after feeding.
   6. Thicken feeding with rice cereal/small frequent feedings.
   7. Instruct parents about feeding techniques and to monitor for complications (respiratory signs; home apnea monitoring).

HIRSCHSPRUNG'S DISEASE (CONGENITAL AGANGLIONIC MEGACOLON)

A. Absence of autonomic parasympathetic ganglion cells in a portion of the large colon (usually occurs 4–25 cm proximal to anus) resulting in decreased motility in that portion of the colon and signs of functional obstruction; when stool enters the affected part of the colon, lack of peristalsis causes it to remain there until additional stool pushes it through; colon dilates as stool is impacted; familial disease, more common in boys; associated with Down's syndrome
B. Assessment findings:
   1. Newborn: failure to pass meconium stool within 24 hours of birth
   2. Older child: recurrent abdominal distention, chronic constipation with ribbon-like stools, diarrhea, bile-stained emesis
   3. Weight loss; failure to grow
   4. Volvulus (twisting of bowel) due to fecal stagnation
C. Nursing diagnoses (see Table 16.31)

Table 16.31 Nursing Diagnoses Related to Hirschsprung's Disease

- Imbalanced nutrition: less than body requirements related to decreased appetite/poor absorption in bowel
- Chronic constipation related to disease process
- Risk for ineffective therapeutic regimen management related to insufficient knowledge in managing pre- and post-op bowel regimens

D. Interventions:
   1. Stool softeners
   2. Isotonic enemas
   3. Low-residue diet; TPN if needed
   4. Surgery:
      a. Palliative: loop or double-barrel colostomy
      b. Corrective: abdominal-perineal pull through, bowel containing ganglia is pulled down and anastamosed to rectum
   5. Colostomy care
   6. Teach parents colostomy care/follow-up needs

INTUSSUSCEPTION

A. Telescoping of bowel into itself, usually at the ileocecal valve, causing edema, obstruction, and possible necrosis of the bowel; occurs at 3–12 months; is three times more common in males and is often associated with cystic fibrosis or celiac disease
B. Assessment findings:
   1. Sharp, shrill cry
   2. Severe abdominal pain; pulls legs up
   3. Vomiting bile-stained fluid
   4. Currant jelly stool (contains bloody mucous)
C. Nursing diagnosis (see Table 16.32)
D. Interventions:
   1. Barium enema to reduce telescoping
   2. Surgery if barium unsuccessful or if peritonitis
   3. Fluid and electrolyte balance
   4. Observe for peritonitis.
   5. Routine post-op nursing care

IMPERFORATE ANUS

A. Incomplete anal development resulting in blind pouch; associated with difficulty swallowing and tolerating feedings; color changes during feeding; recurrent urinary tract infections
B. Assessment findings:
   1. Failure to pass meconium
   2. Difficulty inserting rectal thermometer
C. Nursing diagnoses (see Table 16.33)
D. Interventions:
   1. Sigmoidostomy
   2. Manual dilation

Table 16.32 Nursing Diagnoses Related to Intussusception

- Deficient fluid volume related to excessive loss of fluid (emesis)
- Risk for injury related to hemorrhage/infection
- Acute pain related to decreased circulation to bowel

Table 16.33 Nursing Diagnoses Related to Imperforate Anus

- Impaired skin integrity related to surgical repair
- Bowel incontinence related to colostomy

   3. Anastamosis later
   4. Administer prophylactic antibiotics as ordered.
   5. Keep suture lines clean.
   6. Post-op position side lying to decrease tension
   7. Teach patients home care related to ostomy care.

CELIAC DISEASE

A. Malabsorption syndrome characterized by intolerance of gluten (found in rye, oats, wheat, barley); familial disease, found more often in Caucasians
B. Assessment findings:
   1. Steatorrhea: frothy, pale, bulky, foul-smelling, greasy stools
   2. Chronic diarrhea in infancy and toddlerhood
   3. Failure to thrive
   4. Distended abdomen, muscle wasting
   5. Abdominal pain, irritability, listlessness
   6. Vomiting
   7. Vitamin A, D, E, and K deficiency
   8. Normal pancreatic enzymes and sweat test (rule out Cystic Fibrosis)
   9. Jejunal and duodenal biopsies show characteristic atrophy of mucosa
C. Nursing diagnoses (see Table 16.34)

Table 16.34 Nursing Diagnoses Related to Celiac Disease

- Imbalanced nutrition: less than body requirements related to malabsorption
- Risk for injury related to celiac crisis
- Interrupted family processes related to a child with a chronic illness
- Anxiety related to chronic disease
- Ineffective family coping related to chronic nature of disease and intense home therapy
- Deficient knowledge regarding nature of treatments and medications to be administered at home

D. Interventions:
   1. Gluten-free diet: avoid barley, rye, oats, and wheat (called a BROW diet)
   2. TPN if severely malnourished
   3. Fat-soluble vitamins must be given in water-soluble form.

HERNIAS

A. Protrusion of an organ through the structures that normally contain it; most common hernias in children are inguinal and umbilical
B. Assessment findings:
  1. Umbilical hernia: protrusion of part of the intestine at the umbilicus; seen as a bulge at the umbilicus, particularly when the child cries or strains
  2. Inguinal hernia: protrusion at the inguinal ring; may be seen in male infants who have undescended testicle
C. Nursing diagnoses: same as routine pre- and post-operative diagnoses
D. Interventions:
  1. Surgery
  2. Post-operative nursing care:
    a. Consider child's developmental level; fear of mutilation common in school-age children
    b. Care of surgical site
    c. Vital signs
    d. Parental support
    e. Observe for bladder retention following inguinal hernia repair.
    f. Observe for paralytic ileus.
    g. Observe for infections (3–5 days).
    h. Observe for shock and hemorrhage.

GASTROENTERITIS

A. Results from increased rate of peristalsis causing watery, acidic stools to be forcefully expelled; can be serious in young children; causes include bacteria (salmonella, shigella, staph); virus; allergy; dietary
B. Assessment findings:
  1. Dehydration:
    a. Sunken eyes
    b. Depressed anterior fontanel
    c. Oliguria
    d. Weight loss
    e. Poor tissue turgor
    f. Dry mucous membranes
    g. Thirst
    h. Temperature
  2. Listlessness
  3. Unstable fluid and electrolyte balance
  4. Susceptibility to infection
C. Nursing diagnoses (see Table 16.35)
D. Interventions:
  1. Get careful history, including possible sources of food poisoning and other sources of infection—skin or lungs.
  2. NPO with parenteral fluids
  3. Antibiotics
  4. Vitamins
  5. Diet:
    a. Oral electrolytes such as Pedialyte
    b. Glucose water

Table 16.35 Nursing Diagnoses Related to Gastroenteritis

- Deficient fluid volume related to active losses in stools
- Risk for impaired skin integrity related to frequent, loose stools
- Risk for infection related to presence of infectious organisms
- Interrupted family processes related to a child with a serious illness
- Impaired comfort related to abdominal cramping, diarrhea, and vomiting
- Imbalanced nutrition: less than body requirements related to diarrhea

    c. 1/4–1/2 strength formula
    d. Gradual introduction of fluids and solids
  6. Isolate child until cause is known; may be very contagious.
  7. Monitor stools.
  8. Maintain intake and output.
  9. Daily weight, specific gravity of urine
  10. Check sensorium.
  11. Monitor for secondary infection.

PARASITIC WORMS

A. Parasites live in, on, or at the expense of the host; pinworms and roundworms are most common in this country.
B. Assessment findings:
  1. Pinworms:
    a. Anal itching, irritation
    b. Disturbed sleep
    c. Eggs enter mouth from dirty fingers of child; adult worm leaves intestine and lays eggs in anus; child scratches, gets eggs on fingers and into mouth
    d. Scotch tape test for diagnosis
  2. Roundworms:
    a. Colic, abdominal pain, lack of appetite, weight loss
    b. Eggs laid in host and passed out in feces; after worms have been ingested, egg batches are laid; larvae in host invade lymphatics and venules of mesentery and migrate to liver, lungs, and heart; larvae from lungs reach the host's epiglottis and are swallowed; cycle repeats
C. Nursing diagnoses (see Table 16.36)
D. Interventions:
  1. Drug treatment depends on type of worm:
    a. Mebendazole (Vermox) and pyrantel pamoate (Antiminth, Pin-Rid) used to treat pinworms and roundworms
    b. Thiabendazole (Mintezol) used to treat roundworms and other worms
  2. Teach parents to launder clothing, bed linens, and towels in hot water.

Table 16.36 Nursing Diagnoses Related to Parasites

- Risk for imbalanced nutrition: less than body requirements related to anorexia, nausea, vomiting, and deprivation of host nutrients by parasites
- Impaired skin integrity related to pruritus secondary to emergence of parasites (pinworms) onto perianal skin, lytic necrosis, and tissue digestion
- Diarrhea related to parasitic irritation to intestinal mucosa
- Acute pain related to parasitic invasion of small intestines
- Risk for infection transmission related to contagious nature of parasites
- Risk for ineffective therapeutic regimen management related to insufficient knowledge of condition, mode of transmission, and prevention of infection
- Interrupted family processes related to a child with an infestation

3. Clean toilets with disinfectant.
4. Whole family is usually treated because parasites are very communicable

Sample Questions

1. The nurse is teaching the mother of a newborn who has a cleft lip and palate to feed the infant. Which would be least appropriate to include?
   1. Place the tip of the asepto at the front of the baby's mouth so that the baby can suck.
   2. Rinse the mouth with sterile water after each feeding to minimize infections.
   3. Feed the baby in an upright position and bubble frequently to reduce air in the stomach.
   4. Apply lanolin to lips to reduce dryness associated with mouth breathing.

2. The mother of a two-month-old infant with a cleft lip and palate calls the clinic. She tells the nurse that the baby has a temperature of 102°, has been turning her head from side to side, and has been eating poorly. What should the nurse advise?
   1. Clean the baby's ears with warm water.
   2. Give the baby infant Tylenol 0.3 cc and call back in four hours after taking her temperature.
   3. Bring the baby into the clinic for evaluation.
   4. Give the baby 4 ounces of water and retake her temperature in one hour.

3. A three-month-old infant is hospitalized for repair of a cleft lip. Following surgery, the baby returns to the unit with a Logan bow in place. The baby is awake and beginning to whimper. The baby's color is pink and pulse is 120 with respirations of 38. An IV is ordered in the baby's right hand at 15 cc per hour. The fluid is not infusing well. Her right hand is edematous. The jacket restraint has loosened, and one arm has partially come out. What is the priority nursing action?

1. Recheck the baby's vital signs.
2. Check the baby's IV site for infiltration.
3. Check to see if the baby has voided.
4. Replace the restraints securely.

4. Following surgery for repair of a cleft lip, it is important to prevent excessive crying by the infant. What should the nurse do to accomplish this?
   1. Give the baby a pacifier to meet his/her sucking needs.
   2. Place the baby in the usual sleeping position, which is on the abdomen.
   3. Ask the baby's mother to stay and hold the child.
   4. Request a special nurse to hold the infant.

5. The nurse is doing discharge planning and establishing long-term goals for an infant who had a cleft lip repair. The baby also has a cleft palate. Which long-term goal is most appropriate and necessary for this child?
   1. Prevent joint contractures.
   2. Promote adequate speech.
   3. Promote bowel regularity.
   4. Prevent infection of surgical incision.

6. The nurse is caring for an eight-month-old infant who has had diarrhea for two days. Which is the most useful in assessing the degree of dehydration?
   1. Number of stools
   2. Skin turgor
   3. Mucous membranes
   4. Daily weight

7. An infant who has severe diarrhea and dehydration is hospitalized and is NPO. Intravenous fluids are ordered. What is the immediate goal of care?
   1. Restoration of intravascular volume
   2. Prevention of further diarrhea
   3. Promotion of skin integrity
   4. Maintenance of normal growth and development

8. The nurse is caring for a nine-month-old infant who is allowed only clear fluids. What are the most appropriate liquids for the nurse to offer?
   1. 7-Up and ginger ale
   2. Pedialyte and glucose water
   3. Half-strength formula
   4. Tea and clear broth

9. The nurse is caring for an infant who is being treated for severe diarrhea. 24 hours after admission, the diet is advanced from NPO to clear liquids. After clear liquids are started, the baby has four stools in two hours. What should the nurse do?
   1. Continue oral feedings.
   2. Take the pulse, temperature, and respirations.
   3. Stop feeding the child orally.
   4. Weigh the child.

10. A 12-month-old who was diagnosed at birth as having Hirschsprung's disease has been maintained at home under conservative

treatment. The parents have brought the child to the clinic for a well-baby examination. After interviewing the child's parents, the nurse concludes that an appropriate treatment regime is being followed. Which of the following would indicate this?
1. Use of tap water enemas and a low-residue diet
2. Use of soap suds enema and a high-fiber diet
3. Use of isotonic saline enemas and a high-fiber diet
4. Use of isotonic saline enemas and a low-residue diet

11. A three-month-old is admitted to the pediatric unit with a diagnosis of Hirschsprung's disease. What is most important when monitoring the infant's status?
1. Weigh the infant every morning.
2. Maintain intake and output records.
3. Measure abdominal girth every four hours.
4. Check serum electrolyte levels.

12. An infant who has Hirschsprung's disease is scheduled for surgery. Which explanation should the nurse include when discussing the upcoming surgery with the parents?
1. They will need to learn colostomy care because the child will have a permanent colostomy.
2. The baby will have tap water enemas until clear before the surgery.
3. The baby will have a temporary colostomy to allow the bowel time to heal.
4. They will need to learn how to administer gastrostomy feedings while the colostomy is present.

13. A five-week-old infant is seen in the physician's office for gastroesophageal reflux. What should the nurse suggest to the parents regarding feeding practices?
1. Dilute the formula to facilitate better absorption.
2. Position the child at a 30°-45° angle after feedings.
3. Change from milk-based formula to soy-based formula.
4. Delay burping to prevent vomiting.

14. Which assessment finding would the nurse expect in an infant diagnosed with pyloric stenosis?
1. Abdominal rigidity
2. Ribbon-like stools
3. Visible waves of peristalsis
4. Rectal prolapse

15. An infant has had frequent episodes of green, mucous-containing stools. The nursing assessment reveals that the infant has dry mucous membranes, poor skin turgor, and an absence of tearing. Based on these data, what is the most appropriate nursing diagnosis?
1. Impaired skin integrity related to irritation caused by frequent, loose stools

2. Deficient fluid volume related to frequent, loose stools
3. Impaired comfort related to abdominal cramping and diarrhea
4. Imbalanced nutrition: less than body requirements related to diarrhea

16. The nurse is caring for an infant admitted with diarrhea, poor skin turgor, and dry mucous membranes. Which laboratory data would cause the nurse the most concern?
1. Sodium 140 mmol/l
2. Urine specific gravity 1.035
3. Hematocrit 38%
4. Potassium 4 mmol/l

17. Following surgery for pyloric stenosis, a five-week-old infant is started on glucose water. When will infant formula be started?
1. Following the return of bowel sounds
2. After vital signs are stable
3. When the infant is able to retain clear liquids
4. When there is no evidence of diarrhea

18. The nurse is feeding a newborn infant glucose water. Which finding would make the nurse suspect the infant has esophageal atresia?
1. The infant has projectile vomiting.
2. The infant sucks very slowly.
3. The infant seems fatigued after only a few sucks.
4. The infant chokes after taking a few sucks of water.

19. The parents of an infant who has esophageal atresia ask the nurse how the baby will eat. Which response by the nurse is most accurate?
1. "A tube will be passed from the nose to the stomach."
2. "The doctor will place a tube through the abdomen into the baby's stomach."
3. "Your baby will be given nutrients through a vein."
4. "Your baby can tolerate small feedings given frequently."

20. The nurse is teaching the parents of a child who has celiac disease about the dietary modifications that need to be made. Which foods, if selected by the parents, indicate an understanding of the child's dietary needs?
1. Toast, orange juice, and an egg
2. Rice cake, milk, and a banana
3. Crackers, apple juice, and a hot dog
4. Hamburger, grape juice, and fries

Answers and Rationales

1. (1) The asepto should be placed in the unaffected side of the baby's mouth and back far enough to encourage swallowing. All of the other answers are correct. The baby's mouth should be rinsed with saline after each feeding to minimize the chance of infection. The baby

should be held in an upright position and bubbled or burped frequently because the baby tends to swallow air. The baby with a cleft palate is a mouth breather and will have dry lips. Applying lanolin is appropriate.

2. (3) The symptoms suggest ear infection. A child with an ear infection needs to be seen by a physician and probably treated with an antibiotics. Children with cleft palate are very susceptible to infections and need to be treated promptly to reduce the chance of hearing loss from recurrent ear infections.

3. (4) Priority care following cleft lip repair is to keep the child from pulling at the lip repair site. The IV is probably infiltrated. Further assessment of the IV should be done after the restraint has been replaced. The vital signs are normal. Checking to see if the baby has voided is not a priority measure.

4. (3) Having the mother hold the infant would be most comforting to the infant. A child with cleft lip repair cannot have a pacifier and cannot be on the abdomen. A special nurse is not necessary; the mother will do very well.

5. (2) Promoting speech is a very important long-term goal for a child who has a cleft palate, because speech problems are common. Immobilization following a cleft lip repair is brief. Preventing joint contractures is not a long-term goal. Preventing infection at the surgical site is also a short-term goal.

6. (4) Daily weights are the best indicator of fluid balance. The number of stools gives an indication of fluid loss but is not the best indicator of fluid balance. Skin turgor and assessing mucous membranes are helpful, but daily weights are the best indicator of fluid balance.

7. (1) Restoration of intravascular volume is the immediate goal. This will prevent life-threatening fluid and electrolyte imbalances. The others are goals but are not immediate.

8. (2) Pedialyte and glucose water are appropriate. The infant needs clear liquids, and these are age appropriate. Pedialyte gives electrolytes, and glucose water gives sugar. A nine-month-old infant does not drink carbonated beverages such as 7-Up and ginger ale. Half-strength formula is not a clear liquid. Tea is not appropriate for an infant and broth is too salty for an infant.

9 (3) The bowel still needs rest. Stop the feedings, and notify the charge nurse or the physician. Taking vital signs and weighing the child do not address the issue, which is that oral feedings stimulate diarrhea—indicating the bowel is still irritable and needs further rest.

10 (4) The child should be receiving isotonic saline enemas. Repeated tap water or a soap suds enemas would cause fluid and electrolyte imbalances. A low-residue diet is indicated because the child has no peristalsis. High-fiber diets are contraindicated.

11. (3) In Hirschsprung's disease, a lack of peristalsis in the lower colon causes accumulation of intestinal contents, distention of the bowel, and possible obstruction. Measuring abdominal girth is most important. The other actions are not wrong, but they are not the most important.

12. (3) The baby will have a temporary colostomy to allow the bowel time to heal and return to normal functioning. The usual surgery for Hirschsprung's disease involves a temporary colostomy, not a permanent colostomy. The child will receive enemas prior to surgery, but they will be saline enemas, not tap water enemas. Tap water enemas cause fluid shifts. A gastrostomy tube is unlikely after surgery. Following recovery from anesthesia, the child should return to oral intake and normal feedings.

13. (2) Small, frequent feedings followed by positioning at a 30°–45° angle have been found to prevent gastric distention and vomiting in the infant with gastroesophageal reflux. Diluting the formula is not appropriate. Infants with gastroesophageal reflux do not have a problem with the absorption of nutrients. Gastroesophageal reflux is not related to milk intolerance, so a change in formula is not indicated. Delaying burping can aggravate gastroesophageal reflux. An infant with gastroesophageal reflux needs frequent burping to prevent reflux.

14. (3) Visible waves of peristalsis moving from left to right across the epigastrum are usually seen in infants with pyloric stenosis. Abdominal rigidity is not typical of pyloric stenosis. Ribbon-like stools might be seen in the child with Hirschsprung's disease. The child with pyloric stenosis will have small, rabbit pellet stools. Rectal prolapse is seen in children with cystic fibrosis.

15. (2) The data presented (dry mucous membranes, poor skin turgor, no tearing) suggest a deficient fluid volume related to frequent stools. Impaired skin integrity is a possibility with frequent stooling, but there are no data to confirm this. Pain related to cramping is a possibility, but there are no data to confirm this. Imbalanced nutrition: less than body requirements is also a possibility, but there are no data to confirm this.

16. (2) A urine-specific gravity of 1.035 indicates dehydration. Normal range for an infant is 1.002–1.030. The normal sodium level is 135–146 mmol/l. The normal hematocrit for an infant is 28%–42%. The normal potassium for an infant is 3.5–6 mmol/l.

17. (3) Once the infant retains small, frequent feedings of glucose for 24 hours, the nurse may begin small, frequent feedings of formula until

the infant returns to a normal feeding schedule. Answer 1 is not correct, because bowel sounds need to be present before starting clear liquids. A decrease in bowel sounds is not normally a problem in the child who has undergone surgical correction for pyloric stenosis, because the surgery does not enter the stomach itself but rather the pyloric muscle. Answer 2 is not correct, because vital signs do not directly affect the initiation of infant formula. Answer 4 is not correct. The absence of diarrhea is not the criterion for beginning formula.

18. (4) With esophageal atresia, the esophagus ends in a blind pouch. The infant will choke after a few sucks of water because it has no place to go. Projectile vomiting, especially at the age of 2 or 3 weeks, is suggestive of pyloric stenosis. Slow sucking and fatigue with sucking would be more suggestive of cardiac problems.

19. (2) Infants with esophageal atresia will need a gastrostomy tube because the esophagus ends in a blind pouch. There is no connection between the esophagus and the stomach, so a nasogastric tube cannot be passed. Intravenous or TPN feedings are not indicated. Gastrostomy tube feedings are much safer. Because there is no connection between the esophagus and the stomach, the infant cannot have anything by mouth.

20. (2) There is nothing in this choice that contains barley, rye, oats, or wheat, which all contain gluten. Toast, crackers, and hamburger rolls all contain wheat, which has gluten, and is not allowed in a child who has celiac disease and cannot tolerate gluten.

Pediatric Conditions Related to the Genitourinary System

URINARY TRACT INFECTION (SEE CHAPTER 11)

Exstrophy of the Bladder

A. Congenital condition in which the abdominal and anterior walls of the bladder did not fuse during embryological development. The anterior surface of the bladder lies open on the abdominal wall.
B. Assessment findings:
   1. Associated structural changes often seen:
      a. Prolapsed rectum
      b. Inguinal hernia
      c. Split symphisus
      d. Rotated hips
   2. Associated anomalies:
      a. Epispadias
      b. Cleft scrotum or clitoris
      c. Undescended testicles
      d. Downward deflection of penis
C. Nursing diagnoses (see Table 16.37)
D. Interventions:
   1. Two-stage reconstruction surgery; possible urinary diversion; done at 3–6 months
   2. Provide bladder care; prevent infections:
      a. Keep area as clean as possible to prevent skin breakdown and infection.
      b. Cover exposed bladder with petrolatum gauze; wash with mild soap and water.
      c. Keep diaper loose fitting.
   3. Teach parent appropriate home care:
      a. Provide activities to foster development of child.
      b. Avoid activities that might cause trauma and infection, such as sandboxes.

Table 16.37 Nursing Diagnoses Related to Exstrophy of the Bladder
- Risk for infection related to exposed bladder
- Impaired skin integrity related to exposed bladder/urinary incontinence
- Disturbed body image related to perception of being "different"/surgical repair delayed due to staging
- Interrupted family process related to situational crisis

CRYPTORCHIDISM

A. Unilateral or bilateral undescended testicle; testicles descend at eight months' gestation; premature male infants have undescended testicles; most descend spontaneously before puberty

Table 16.38 Nursing Diagnoses Related to Cryptorchidism

- Risk for sexual dysfunction related to undescended testicles
- Fear related to concerns about body mutilation
- Risk for impaired skin integrity related to sutures post-operatively

Table 16.39 Nursing Diagnoses for Hypospadias (Post-operative)

- Risk for deficient fluid volume related to NPO status/nausea and vomiting
- Impaired urinary elimination patterns related to surgical trauma/catheter clamping and removal
- Impaired comfort (pain) related to surgical procedure
- Risk for injury and infection/catheter dislocation related to surgical trauma/improper taping/placement of catheter

B. Assessment findings:
  1. Scrotal sack empty when palpated
  2. Usually one-sided; painless
C. Nursing diagnosis (see Table 16.38)
D. Interventions:
  1. Treatment remains controversial; testes in abdomen past five years of age may cause sterility due to increased body temperature
  2. Chorionic gonadotropin can be given for a 6–8 week trial if not descended by age 8 or 9
  3. Orchiopexy: surgical pulling down of testes done by age 6
  4. Nursing care after orchiopexy:
    a. Do not disturb tension mechanism; in place for one week.
    b. Avoid contamination of incision.
    c. Support child/family; psychosocial implications.

HYPOSPADIAS

A. Urethral opening located along ventral surface of penis; epispadias: urethral opening is along the dorsal surface of the penis; chordee (ventral curvature of penis) often associated with it, causing constriction
B. Assessment findings:
  1. Urinary meatus misplaced
  2. Foreskin on dorsum gives penile tip a hooded appearance
  3. Inability to make straight stream of urine (psychosocial implications)
  4. Some infants have increased urinary tract infections due to urinary retention.
  5. Some concern about later fertility due to location of urethral opening
C. Nursing diagnosis (see Table 16.39)
D. Interventions:
  1. No treatment for mild defects

Table 16.40 Nursing Diagnoses Related to Enuresis

- Maturational enuresis related to stressors, inattention to bladder cues, lack of motivation, small bladder capacity, attention-seeking behavior
- Disturbed self-esteem related to embarrassment and/or ridicule by others

  2. Do not circumcise, because tissue may be needed for later repair.
  3. Surgical repair at three years
  4. Prevent infection in the post-operative period.
  5. Assess adequacy of voiding in the post-operative period.
  6. Assess pain control and administer analgesics as ordered post-operative.

NEPHROTIC SYNDROME (SEE CHAPTER 11)

ACUTE GLOMERULONEPHRITIS (SEE CHAPTER 11)

ENURESIS

A. Involuntary discharge of urine, especially during the night, beyond the age when bladder control should have been achieved (four years); may be primary (children who have never achieved control) or secondary (children who have developed control and lose it)
B. Assessment findings:
  1. History of repeated episodes of bedwetting
  2. Normal physical examination
C. Nursing diagnoses (see Table 16.40)
D. Interventions:
  1. Bladder retention exercises
  2. Avoid fluids after the evening meal.
  3. Bed alarm devices
  4. Drug therapy:
    a. Vasopressin (antidiuretic hormone) nasal spray at bedtime
    b. Tricyclic antidepressants: imipramine HCl (Tofranil)
    c. Anticholinergics

WILM'S TUMOR (NEPHROBLASTOMA)

A. Large, encapsulated tumor that develops in renal parenchyma; originates during fetal life from undifferentiated tissues and becomes manifest at 1–3 years of age; prognosis good if no metastases

Table 16.41 Nursing Diagnoses Related to Wilm's Tumor

- Risk for injury: rupture of tumor/hemorrhage/hypertension related to growing tumor/renal involvement
- Constipation related to medications/nutrition
- Anxiety related to threat to or change in environment/health status
- Interrupted family process related to situational crisis

B. Assessment findings:
  1. Stage I: limited to kidney
  2. Stage II: tumor extends beyond kidney but is completely encapsulated
  3. Stage III: tumor confined to abdomen
  4. Stage IV: tumor has metastasized to lung, liver, bone, or brain
  5. Stage V: bilateral renal involvement at diagnosis
  6. Mother notices mass while bathing child
  7. Hypertension, hematuria, anemia
  8. IVP reveals mass
C. Nursing diagnoses (see Table 16.41)
D. Interventions:
  1. Nephrectomy with removal of tumor performed within 24–48 hours of diagnosis
  2. Post-surgical radiation in stages II, II, IV
  3. Post-surgical chemotherapy—vincristine and Daunorubicin, Doxorubicin
  4. DO NOT PALPATE ABDOMEN before surgery to avoid dissemination of cancer cells.
  5. Handle child carefully.

Sample Questions

1. A three-year-old child is admitted with a diagnosis of nephrotic syndrome. Which signs and symptoms would the nurse expect the parents to report when the child is admitted?
   1. Jaundiced skin and pale stools
   2. Blood in the urine and high fever
   3. Chest pain and shortness of breath
   4. Puffy eyes and weight gain
2. Which assessment by the nurse would best indicate that a child with nephrotic syndrome is responding appropriately to treatment?
   1. The child has more energy.
   2. The child's pulse rate increases.
   3. The child's appetite improves.
   4. The child weighs less.
3. A three-year-old is admitted with a tentative diagnosis of Wilm's tumor. What nursing action is essential because of the diagnosis?
   1. Avoid palpating the abdomen.
   2. Encourage the child to eat adequately.
   3. Give emotional support to the parents.
   4. Keep the child on strict bed rest.

4. A three-year-old is brought to the physician's office by the parent. The parent states that the child was completely toilet trained but has been "having accidents" recently. The parent also tells the nurse that the child is voiding more often than usual and that the urine has a strong odor. What is the best response by the nurse?
   1. "These could be symptoms of a urinary tract infection. We should obtain a urine specimen for analysis."
   2. "Many preschool children regress when something stressful happens. Has your child been under any stress lately?"
   3. "Accidents like these are not unusual. You have nothing to worry about as long as your child does not have a fever."
   4. "This is very unusual. Your child will probably need to be hospitalized to receive intravenous antibiotics."
5. A four-year-old has been admitted to the nursing unit with a diagnosis of nephrotic syndrome. The symptoms include generalized edema with weight gain, hypoproteinemia, hyperlipidemia, hypotension, and decreased urine output. In developing a nursing care plan for this child, which nursing diagnosis would be highest priority?
   1. Risk for imbalanced nutrition: less than body requirements related to protein loss and poor appetite
   2. Infection related to edema secondary to nephrotic syndrome
   3. Fluid volume excess related to nephrotic syndrome
   4. Disturbed body image related to edema
6. The nurse is caring for an infant born with exstrophy of the bladder. What will be included in the care of this infant?
   1. Give continuous saline irrigations of the exposed bladder.
   2. Cover the exposed bladder with petrolatum gauze.
   3. Insert an indwelling catheter.
   4. Apply a tight-fitting, super-absorbent diaper.
7. A five-year-old had an orchiopexy this morning. Which nursing action is essential?
   1. Tell the parents not to disturb the tension mechanism until the physician removes it in a week or 10 days.
   2. Explain to the parents that the child has a good chance of being sterile.
   3. Teach the parents how to help the child with leg exercises.
   4. Encourage the parents to join a support group related to the child's condition.
8. The parents of a newborn with hypospadias ask the nurse why the doctor told them the baby could not be circumcised. What is the best response?
   1. The infant is not stable enough for the procedure.

2. The deformity makes circumcision impossible.
3. The foreskin will need to be used later to repair the defect.
4. Circumcision is not currently recommended for most infants.

9. A two-year-old has just been diagnosed with a Wilm's tumor. Surgery is recommended. The parents tell the nurse that they feel they are being pushed into surgery and wonder if they should wait and get more opinions. What information is essential for the nurse to include when responding to the parents?
   1. Surgery is one of several options for treating a Wilm's tumor.
   2. Surgery is an essential part of the treatment for Wilm's tumor and must be done immediately.
   3. Surgery can be safely delayed for up to a year after diagnosis.
   4. Wilm's tumor has been successfully treated by chemotherapy and radiation therapy.

10. The parents of a five-year-old ask the nurse in the doctor's office what they should do about their child who is still wetting the bed several nights a week. In addition to reporting this to the physician, what suggestion should be included in the nurse's discussion with the parents?
   1. Do not give the child anything to drink after the evening meal.
   2. Have the child wear diapers to bed.
   3. Suggest that they promise the child a sleepover party if the child stays dry for two weeks.
   4. Punish the child each time he wets the bed.

Answers and Rationales

1. (4) Nephrotic syndrome is characterized by proteinuria, hypoalbuminemia, and fluid retention with significant edema. Answer 1 suggests liver or gall bladder disease. Answer 2 is more suggestive of acute glomerulonephritis than nephrotic syndrome. Answer 3 is not likely. A child with renal failure and resulting pulmonary edema could experience these symptoms, but that is not likely at this point in the disease process.

2. (4) Diuretics and steroids will have been prescribed. The goal is to decrease edema. This will be demonstrated by a weight loss. He may feel better and have an improved appetite, but weight loss is a better indicator of the specific goal of therapy for a child with nephrotic syndrome.

3. (1) It is essential not to palpate the abdomen because this may cause the encapsulated tumor to spread. Emotional support to the parents and encouraging the child to eat well are nice but not of the highest priority. Strict bed rest is probably not indicated, although the child will not be allowed to run around.

4. (1) The symptoms described (frequency, urgency, and a strong odor to urine) are those of a urinary tract infection. A urinalysis is indicated. It is true that preschool children may regress when they are under stress. However, that does not explain the frequency and the strong odor of the urine. While a recently toilet-trained child may have an occasional "accident," recurring episodes should be further investigated. Not all persons with a UTI have a fever. If the child does have a UTI as suspected, the treatment is usually oral antimicrobial agents. There is no data to suggest that this child needs to be hospitalized.

5. (3) The symptoms described all suggest fluid overload, which is characteristic of nephrotic syndrome. This must be corrected as quickly as possible to prevent further problems. The child probably already has altered nutrition rather than simply being at risk for it. However, fluid overload is a higher priority. The child is at risk for infection because of the hypoalbuminemia, but there is no evidence to support that the child already has an infection. The child may develop a disturbed body image related to edema. Again, there is no evidence to suggest that the child has a disturbed body image. Even if the child did, fluid volume excess would take priority.

6. (2) Exstrophy of the bladder is when the bladder lies open on the abdominal wall. The exposed bladder should be covered with petrolatum gauze to help prevent skin damage from constant exposure to urine. Continuous saline irrigations are not appropriate. An indwelling catheter would serve no purpose, because the bladder is on the abdominal wall. Diapers should be applied loosely to prevent irritation of the site.

7. (1) An orchiopexy is the surgical procedure done to bring an undescended testicle into the scrotal sac. The key care following this procedure, which may be done on an outpatient basis, is not to disturb the tension mechanism (a "button" in the scrotum that keeps the testicle from going back up into the abdomen) until the physician removes it in 7–10 days. Children who have the surgery by five years of age are not usually sterile. Waiting longer increases the risk of sterility. The child will not probably need leg exercises following this outpatient surgery. This is not a condition that has or needs a support group. Cryptorchidism (undescended testicle) is quite common and sometimes corrects itself. If it

doesn't, the surgery (orchiopexy) is safe and simple.

8. (3) Hypospadias is when the urethral opening is on the ventral side of the penis. Surgical repair is likely at about three years of age. The foreskin is the perfect repair tissue. Hypospadias does not cause the infant to be unstable. Circumcision will be done when the surgery is done at age three. Male circumcision is a choice that the parents make. The American Academy of Pediatrics states that it is not necessary but is optional and may slightly reduce the risk of urinary tract infections in infant boys.

9. (2) A Wilm's tumor is an encapsulated tumor on the kidney. Surgery is an essential part of the treatment. There is no option. In addition, the child may receive radiation and or chemotherapy. Surgery must be done immediately before the tumor spreads or the capsule breaks.

10. (1) Not giving the child anything to drink after the evening meal helps, particularly if the child is a sound sleeper. Cola-type beverages have a diuretic effect. Wearing diapers is not appropriate for a five-year-old. That would be devastating to the child's self esteem. Bribing the child by promising a sleepover party is not appropriate. The child should not be punished for wetting the bed. This usually makes the situation worse. Of course, the nurse will report the mother's concerns to the physician and encourage the mother to discuss it with the physician.

Pediatric Conditions Related to the Musculoskeletal System

CONGENITAL HIP DYSPLASIA

A. Displacement of the head of the femur from the acetabulum; present at birth but may not be diagnosed immediately; occurs more commonly in girls and may be associated with spina bifida; The cause is unknown.
B. Assessment findings:
   1. Classic diagnostic signs:
      a. Shortening of affected limb
      b. Asymmetry of gluteal folds
      c. Limited abduction
   2. Ortolani's maneuver (with infant in supine position, bend knees and place thumbs on bent knees, fingers at hip joint; bring femurs 90° to hip, then abduct); with dislocation, there is a palpable click where the head of the femur snaps over edge of acetabulum (see Figure 16.5)
C. Nursing diagnoses (see Table 16.42)
D. Interventions:
   1. Goal is to enlarge and deepen the socket by pressure; the earlier treatment that is initiated, the shorter and less traumatic it will be.
   2. Position hip in abduction with the head of the femur in the acetabulum; methods include Pavlik harness or Frejka pillow splint and triple diapering (see Figure 16.6)
   3. If conservative measures unsuccessful, traction and hip spica cast or surgery may be done

4. Care for child who is immobilized:
   a. Provide stimulation.
   b. Give traction care.
   c. Give cast care.
   d. Teach for home care/follow-up.

CONGENITAL CLUBFOOT: TALIPES

A. A deformity in which the infant is born with the foot twisted out of normal position
B. Types:
   1. Varus (inward rotation): bottoms of feet face each other; would walk on ankles if not corrected
   2. Valgus (outward rotation): would walk on inner ankles if not corrected
   3. Calcaneous (upward rotation): would walk on heels if not corrected
   4. Equinas (downward rotation): would walk on toes if not corrected
   5. Most common type is talipes equinovarus (see Figure 16.7)
C. Assessment findings: foot cannot be manipulated with passive exercise into normal position.
D. Nursing diagnoses (see Table 16.43)
E. Interventions:
   1. Casting in infancy (before child starts to walk); cast changed periodically to change angle of foot

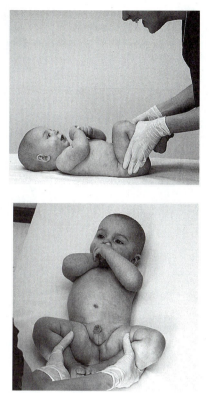

Figure 16.5 Ortolani's Maneuver.

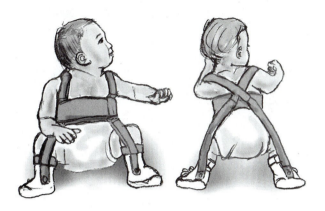

Figure 16.6 Treatment for congenital hip dysplasia

Table 16.42 Nursing Diagnoses Related to Congenital Hip Dysplasia

- Impaired physical mobility related to correction device
- Risk for impairment of skin integrity related to correction device
- Interrupted family process related to situational crisis

Table 16.43 Nursing Diagnoses Related to Club Foot

- Risk for trauma
- Risk for impaired skin integrity related to pressure of casts
- Impaired physical mobility
- Disturbed body image
- Deficient diversional activity
- Interrupted family process related to care of child with congenital defect
- Risk for ineffective therapeutic regimen management related to insufficient knowledge of cast care and signs and symptoms of complications

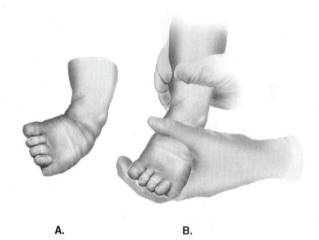

A.   **B.**

Figure 16.7 A. Talipes Equinovarus (Clubfoot). B. If the foot can be moved toward midline, the twisting is positional rather than congenital.

LEGG-CALVE PERTHES DISEASE

A. Aseptic necrosis of femoral head due to disturbance of circulation to the area; affects boys 4–10 years
B. Pathophysiology:
   1. Initial stage: similar to transient synovitis
   2. Avascular stage: diagnosis often made at this stage
   3. Revascularization stage: regeneration of vascular and connective tissue
   4. Regeneration stage: formation of new bone
C. Assessment findings:
   1. Limp, limitation of movement
   2. Pain in groin, hip, and referred to knee; often difficult for child to localize pain
   3. X-ray shows opaque ossification center of head of femur (softened in avascular stage).
D. Nursing diagnoses (see Table 16.44)

2. Denis-Brown splint (metal bar with shoes attached to the bar at a specific angle) worn when sleeping
3. Surgery followed by casting indicated in some cases
4. Cast care (See Chapter 12)
5. Assess the toes for adequate circulation.
6. Provide skin care.
7. Teach family care of child in a cast.

Table 16.44 Nursing Diagnoses Related to Legg-Calve Perthes Disease

- Pain related to joint dysfunction
- Risk for impaired skin integrity related to immobilization devices
- Self-care deficits related to pain and immobilization devices
- Risk for injury related to musculoskeletal impairment, unaccustomed use of appliance
- Risk for disuse syndrome related to immobilization
- Interrupted family processes related to child with temporary but extended disability
- Risk for ineffective therapeutic regimen management related to insufficient knowledge of disease and treatments

E. Interventions:
1. Bed rest with traction followed by an abduction brace to minimize deformity while the healing process takes place
2. Possible surgery
3. Diversionary activities

SCOLIOSIS

A. Lateral curvature of the spine seen most often in adolescent girls
B. Types:
1. Functional/nonstructural; C curve:
   a. Due to posture
   b. Can be corrected voluntarily; disappears when the child lies down
   c. Treated with posture exercises
2. Structural/progressive; S curve of spine:
   a. Idiopathic; tends to run in families
   b. Structural change in spine; does not disappear with position changes
C. Assessment findings (structural):
1. Curve does not straighten when child bends forward with knees straight and arms hanging down to feet (see Figure 16.8)
2. Uneven bra strap marks
3. Uneven hips
4. Uneven shoulders
5. Asymmetry of rib cage
6. X-ray shows curvature
D. Nursing diagnoses (see Table 16.45)
E. Interventions:
1. Stretching exercises of the spine for mild curvatures
2. Milwaukee brace worn 23 hours/day for three years
3. Plaster jacket cast
4. Halo-pelvic or halo-femoral traction
5. Check pressure points when brace is worn
6. Adjust diet for decreased activity
7. Spinal fusion with insertion of Harrington rod:
   a. Spinal fusion and installation of a permanent steel rod along spine used for moderate to severe curvatures

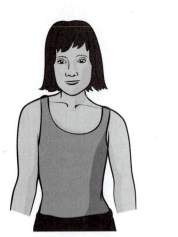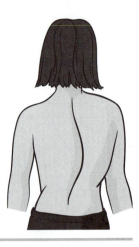

Figure 16.8 Structural Scoliosis

Table 16.45 Nursing Diagnoses Related to Structural Scoliosis

- Risk for injury related to unaccustomed brace
- Risk for impaired skin integrity related to corrective device
- Disturbed body image related to perception of defect in body structure
- Impaired physical mobility related to restricted movement secondary to brace
- Risk for noncompliance related to chronicity and complexity of treatment regimen
- Risk for ineffective therapeutic regimen management related to insufficient knowledge of condition, treatment, exercises, follow-up care, and community services

   b. Usually results in increase in height—positive body image change
   c. General pre- and post-op care for laminectomy
   d. Log roll
   e. Do not raise head of bed
   f. Help with adapting home environment to allow for privacy yet interaction with family
   g. Discuss alternate education methods.

MUSCULAR DYSTROPHY

A. A group of genetically determined, painless, degenerative muscle diseases in children that cause progressive muscle weakness and atrophy
B. Most common type is Duchenne (pseudohypertrophic):
1. Transmitted as X-linked recessive (mothers pass it to sons)
2. Usually manifests in first four years of life
C. Assessment findings:
1. Pelvic girdle weakness; child waddles and falls

2. Grower's sign; child uses hands to push up from the floor
3. Scoliosis from weakness of shoulder girdle
4. Contractures and hypertrophy of muscles
5. Muscle biopsy shows changes
6. EMG shows decreased function
7. Elevated muscle enzymes, especially CPK
D. Nursing diagnoses (see Table 16.46)

Table 16.46 Nursing Diagnoses Related to Muscular Dystrophy

- Impaired physical mobility related to musculoskeletal weakness
- Delayed growth and development related to effects of physical disability
- Risk for imbalanced nutrition: less than body requirements related to impaired sucking ability in the infant
- Risk for imbalanced nutrition: more than body requirements related to sedentary lifestyle
- Risk for injury related to inability to control movements
- Self-care deficits related to sensory-motor impairments
- Impaired verbal communication related to impaired ability to speak words secondary to facial muscle involvement
- Ineffective family coping related to situational crisis/emotional conflicts about hereditary nature of condition and prolonged disability that exhausts family's resources
- Grieving (parental) related to progressive, terminal nature of disease

E. Interventions:
1. Keep child as active as possible within the limits of his disease.
2. Plan diet to prevent obesity.
3. Support child and parents.
4. Reevaluate child's capacities continually; will need increasing assistance with mobility and ADL.
5. Provide diversionary activities; child's mind is not affected; fingers are the last muscles to be affected.
6. Provide information about community services and support groups.

JUVENILE RHEUMATOID ARTHRITIS

A. Several types of rheumatoid arthritis affect children. See Chapter 12 for more information.

Lyme Disease

A. A disease affecting the skin, nervous system, and joints caused by the spirochete Borrelia burgdorferi and transmitted by a deer tick
B. Assessment findings:
1. History of deer tick bite
2. Tick bite surrounded by circular rash: "bull's eye rash"
3. Blood tests available, but client often treated on basis of history and findings

4. Stage I:
   a. Skin rash starting 3–32 days past tick bite and lasting three weeks; rash usually on thighs, buttock, axilla
   b. Systemic symptoms include malaise, fatigue, headache, stiff neck, fever, and joint pains
5. Stage II:
   a. Late disease symptoms may occur months to years after the initial disease.
   b. Neurologic symptoms such as facial palsies, sensory losses, focal weaknesses, and cardiac dysrhythmias
   c. Arthritis involving multiple joints
C. Nursing diagnoses (see Table 16.47)

Table 16.47 Nursing Diagnoses Related to Lyme Disease

1. Impaired comfort related to systemic effects of toxins, presence of rash, urticaria, and joint swelling
2. Fatigue related to increased energy requirements, altered body chemistry, and discomfort
3. Risk for decreased cardiac output related to alterations in cardiac rate/rhythm; conduction

D. Interventions:
1. Antibiotics given for 10–21 days if detected early; longer course necessary if treatment started late in disease
2. Teach how to prevent disease:
   a. Wear long pants, long sleeves, and high socks when walking in grassy or wooded areas.
   b. Use insect repellents for skin and clothing.
   c. Check carefully for ticks after possible exposure.
   d. Remove tick by pulling straight out with tweezers.
   e. Do not crush ticks with your fingers.

BONE TUMORS

Osteogenic Sarcoma

A. Primary bone tumor arising from the mesenchymal cells and characterized by formation of osteoid (immature bones); invades ends of long bones, most frequently distal end of femur or proximal end of tibia and can metastasize to the lungs; occurs more often in boys between ages of 10 and 20
B. Assessment findings:
1. Insidious pain increasing with activity, gradually becoming more severe
2. Tender mass, warm to touch, limitation of movement
3. Pathologic fractures
C. Nursing diagnoses (see Table 16.48)

Table 16.48 Nursing Diagnoses Related to Bone Cancer

- Grieving related to loss of limb
- Impaired physical mobility related to amputation of lower extremity
- Acute pain related to surgical procedure and disease process
- Disturbed body image related to loss of limb
- Interrupted family processes related to having a child with a lifelong disability, traumatic therapy, and possible death

D. Interventions
   1. Surgery:
      a. Amputation
      b. Temporary prosthesis used immediately after surgery
      c. Permanent one usually fitted a few weeks later
   2. Administer radiation only in areas where tumor is not accessible to surgery.
   3. Prepare child for surgery in age-appropriate ways.
   4. Reassure child and family that phantom pain will subside.

Ewing's Sarcoma

A. Primary tumor arising from cells in bone marrow; invades bone longitudinally, destroying bone tissue; no new bone formation; affects femur; may metastasize to lungs
B. Assessment findings:
   1. Pain and swelling
   2. Palpable mass, tender and warm to touch
   3. 15–35% have metastasis at diagnosis
C. Nursing diagnoses (see Table 16.48)
D. Interventions:
   1. High dose radiation
   2. Chemotherapy
   3. Exercise of limb to maintain function
   4. Avoid activities causing added stress to the affected limb.
   5. Administer analgesics as needed.

Sample Questions

1. A 13-month-old has just been placed in a hip spica cast to correct a congenital anomaly. Which nursing actions should be included in the plan of care?
   1. Turn the child no more than every four hours to minimize manipulation of the wet cast.
   2. Use only fingertips when moving the child to prevent indentations in the cast.
   3. Assess and document neurovascular function at least every two hours.
   4. Use a hair dryer to speed the cast drying process.

2. A 13-year-old has just arrived on the nursing care unit from the Post Anesthesia Care Unit. This morning, the child underwent a surgical spinal fusion procedure that included the placement of Harrington rods for the treatment of scoliosis. After receiving a report from the PACU nurse, which action should the nurse perform first?
   1. Assess the pain level and administer analgesics as needed.
   2. Offer clear liquids to ensure adequate hydration.
   3. Drain the Hemovac and record the output on the intake and output record.
   4. Notify the child's parents of his/her arrival on the unit.

3. A newborn has been diagnosed as having mild hip dysplasia. The mother asks the nurse why the physician told her to "triple diaper" the baby. What should the nurse include when responding?
   1. It is important that there be no contamination of the area.
   2. Extra diapers will abduct the hips and help to put the hip in the socket correctly.
   3. Triple diapers cause the baby's legs to be sharply flexed and realign the hip.
   4. Hip dysplasia can cause abnormal stooling.

4. A six-month-old is placed in bilateral leg casts because she has talipes equinovarus. The mother asks how to bathe the baby. What should the nurse tell the mother?
   1. "Bathe the baby as you usually do."
   2. "Put the baby's buttocks in the bath water, but try to keep the feet out of the water."
   3. "Sponge bathe your baby until the casts are removed."
   4. "Give the baby a bath in the baby bath tub, but limit the time in the water."

5. The nurse is providing home care for an eight-year-old boy who has Legg-Calve Perthes Disease. The boy asks the nurse to let him get out of bed to go to walk to the bathroom. What should the nurse do?
   1. Allow the child to get up and walk to the bathroom.
   2. Explain to him that he must stay in bed so that his hip can heal.
   3. Allow him up to the bathroom if he has no pain.
   4. Encourage his mother to talk with the physician about his desire to be out of bed.

6. The nurse has been asked to set up a program to screen children for scoliosis. What age group should the nurse screen?

1. Preschoolers
2. Six-to-eight year olds
3. Junior high students
4. College-age students

7. A 12-year-old girl has been diagnosed with scoliosis and is placed in a Milwaukee brace. What instruction should the nurse give about the brace?
   1. "Put the brace on underneath all of your clothes."
   2. "Wear the brace only when you are exercising."
   3. "Wear the brace only when you are in bed or resting."
   4. "Put an undershirt on before putting the brace on."

8. The nurse is caring for a child who has Duchenne's muscular dystrophy. What understanding is correct about the progress of the disease?
   1. The disease is controllable with aggressive treatment.
   2. Most children will die of something else before they die of muscular dystrophy.
   3. Brothers of children with muscular dystrophy should be evaluated for the disease.
   4. Muscular dystrophy causes its victims to become incoherent and often violent.

9. The nurse is caring for a child who is diagnosed as having Lyme disease. The mother asks how the child got this disease. Which explanation about Lyme disease is correct?
   1. It is transmitted by a mosquito.
   2. It is inherited through a recessive gene.
   3. It is caused by a deer tick bite.
   4. It is caused by contact with the oil from plant leaves.

10. The nurse is caring for a child who has Lyme disease and one who has rheumatoid arthritis. What problem are they most likely to have in common?
    1. Joint pain
    2. High fever
    3. Risk for urinary tract infection
    4. Risk for cardiac dysrhythmias

Answers and Rationales

1. (3) Neurovascular function must be assessed every two hours. The child should be turned at least every two hours to prevent skin damage and to facilitate cast drying. Fingertips should be avoided when handling a wet cast because they can leave indentations on a wet cast. The nurse should palm the cast. A hair dryer should not be used to dry the cast. This causes the cast to dry from the outside in and may leave the inside wet and soft.

2. (1) Pain management is a high priority. The child probably is not taking liquids at this time. Even if she is taking clear liquids, pain management is a higher priority. The nurse may drain the Hemovac, but that is not the highest priority. The nurse will notify the child's parents, but pain management is of a higher priority.

3. (2) The treatment for hip dysplasia is abduction. Triple diapers are the easiest way to abduct the hips in mild cases. If that is not successful, then a pillow splint or harness can be used. There is no open wound with hip dysplasia and no worry about contamination of the area. Hip dysplasia does not cause abnormal stooling. Triple diapers do not cause increased flexion; they actually cause less flexion. Less flexion is recommended for children with hip dysplasia.

4. (3) The baby who has bilateral casts should not be placed in water but should receive a sponge bath. Answers 2 and 3 put the baby in water and are not correct. The nurse should not tell the mother to bathe the baby as usual without knowing what the usual is. By six months of age, most babies are being bathed in a baby bath tub. This is not appropriate when there are casts.

5. (2) Legg-Calve Perthes Disease is avascular necrosis of the hip. The primary goal is to keep the child on bed rest to allow the hip to heal. New bone will regenerate. There is great risk of permanent damage if the child bears weight on the damaged hip. The child will be on bed rest and will probably be in traction to keep the bed properly aligned. The child often has pain, which needs to be controlled, but the absence of pain does not mean that he can get out of bed. The mother can talk with the physician, but the nurse should understand that the usual treatment involves keeping the child off the affected hip.

6. (3) Junior high girls are the target group for screening for scoliosis.

7. (4) An undershirt should be worn under the brace to prevent skin injury from the brace. The brace is worn 23 hours a day for three years.

8. (3) Duchenne's muscular dystrophy is an X-linked disease. Therefore, it appears in boys. It would be appropriate to assess brothers of children with muscular dystrophy for the condition. The disease is not controllable and will eventually kill its victims. Muscular dystrophy does not affect the mental status of those who have it; it is a muscular problem.

9. (3) Lyme disease is transmitted by the bite of the deer tick. Malaria is transmitted by a mosquito. The mosquito that carries malaria does not live in the United States. Lyme disease is not inherited. Poison ivy is caused by contact with the oil in plant leaves.

10. (1) Both Lyme disease and rheumatoid arthritis case joint pain, which can be severe. High fever is not characteristic of either condition. A urinary tract infection is not characteristic of either condition. The child with stage II Lyme disease is at risk for cardiac dysrhythmias due to the nerve involvement that may occur. The child with rheumatoid arthritis is not at risk for cardiac dysrhythmias.

Pediatric Conditions Related to the Endocrine System

DIABETES MELLITUS

A. Hyperglycemia resulting from a lack of insulin; chronic, systemic disease characterized by disorders in the metabolism of carbohydrates, fat, and protein that eventually produces structural abnormalities in various tissues and organs
B. Onset of Type I, insulin-dependent diabetes is often in childhood
C. Assessment findings same as adult (see Chapter 13):
   1. Rapid onset
   2. Polyuria, polydipsia, polyphagia
   3. Fatigue, weight loss
   4. Ketoacidosis
D. Nursing diagnoses same as adults (see Chapter 13)
E. Interventions: same as adult (see Chapter 13):
   1. Insulin
   2. Dietary management
   3. Exercise
   4. Teach child and family about management of disease; make child as independent as possible for child's age.
   5. Children may have difficulty adjusting their diet, insulin, and exercise with sports and episodic activities.
   6. Periods of rapid growth may make insulin adjustment more difficult.

CONGENITAL HYPOTHYROIDISM (CRETINISM)

A. Arrested physical and mental development with dystrophy of the bones and soft tissues due to a congenital lack of thyroid hormone due to absence or hypofunction of thyroid gland

B. Assessment findings:
   1. Neonatal screening blood test (mandatory in some states)
   2. Newborn has maternal thyroid hormones that last up to three months; if infant is not treated, symptoms occur after this age
   3. Large head, puffy eyes
   4. Short limbs, short neck
   5. Thick and protruding tongue that may interfere with breathing and feeding
   6. Delayed dentition
   7. Hypotonia, lack of coordination
   8. Low levels of T_3 and T_4
   9. Low body temperature, cool extremities
   10. Dry skin
   11. Developmental delays
   12. Mental retardation
C. Nursing diagnoses (see Table 16.49)
D. Interventions:
   1. Thyroid hormone replacement for life can result in normal growth and mental development; without treatment, delayed growth and development will occur after three months.
   2. Teach family importance of daily doses of thyroid hormone and vitamin D.

Table 16.49 Nursing Diagnoses Related to Congenital Hypothyroidism (Cretinism)

- Imbalanced nutrition: more than body requirements related to slowed metabolic rate
- Activity intolerance related to insufficient oxygen secondary to slowed metabolic rate
- Chronic constipation related to decreased peristalsis secondary to slowed metabolic rate and decreased activity
- Impaired skin integrity related to edema and dryness of skin secondary to decreased metabolic rate
- Disturbed body image related to short stature and protruding tongue
- Risk for ineffective therapeutic regiment management related to insufficient knowledge of condition, treatment regiment, dietary management, and pharmacologic therapy

HYPOPITUITARISM (PITUITARY DWARFISM)

A. Hyposecretion of growth hormone by the anterior pituitary; may be of unknown cause or there may be a craniopharyngioma
B. Assessment findings:
1. Child normal size at birth but falls below third percentile by the end of the first year
2. Child well proportioned but may be underweight for height
3. Underdeveloped jaw, teeth positioned abnormally
4. High voice
5. Delayed puberty
6. X-rays show delayed closing of bones
7. Normal intelligence
C. Interventions:
1. Administration of growth hormone; availability is limited and cost is high
2. Interact with the child according to chronological age, not appearance.
3. Support child and parents.

HYPERPITUITARISM (GIGANTISM)

A. Hypersecretion of growth hormone by the anterior pituitary, usually caused by a tumor in the anterior pituitary
B. Assessment findings:
1. Height above maximum percentiles
2. Hands and feet especially large; coarse facial features
3. Particularly noticeable at puberty
4. Signs of increased intracranial pressure may be present if caused by a tumor.
C. Management:
1. Surgery to remove tumor
2. Radiation therapy if there is no tumor
3. Record height and head circumference.
4. Care for child who has surgery or radiation.
5. Assist the child in interacting with peers in a normal manner.

Sample Questions

1. Which of the following children would most likely be diagnosed with pituitary dwarfism?
   1. A 13-month-old who weighs 21 pounds
   2. A 4-year-old who is 41 inches tall
   3. A 9-year-old who has no permanent teeth
   4. A 15-year-old girl who has not begun to menstruate
2. A five-year-old has been diagnosed with congenital hypopituitarism. Which should be included when teaching the parents about this child's condition?

1. You will probably need to give him subcutaneous injections of human growth hormone three to seven times a week at bedtime.
2. Your child is unlikely to achieve normal intelligence and will probably need special schooling.
3. All the other children in the family should be evaluated to see if they have any of the same signs of the condition.
4. Your child is likely to have emotional problems related to growth retardation and should be referred to a psychiatrist soon.

3. The nurse at a summer camp for diabetics is assisting a 15-year-old with adjusting her daily insulin dosage. Which factor will have the greatest impact on insulin needs?
   1. The weather forecast calls for high temperature and high humidity.
   2. Activities scheduled for the day include a hike in the woods, swim time, and tennis.
   3. The girl started her period the previous evening.
   4. Daily insulin dose should never be changed, because consistency is important.

4. The nurse is working at a summer camp for diabetic children. A seven-year-old comes to the nurse complaining of dizziness and nausea. It is a warm day and the child has just returned from horseback riding, followed by a walk back from the stables. The nurse notes that the child is sweaty. Which action should the nurse take first?
   1. Give the child a cool drink of water.
   2. Give the child three units of regular insulin and observe for a response.
   3. Give the child three crackers to eat and observe for a response.
   4. Have the child rest in the infirmary and reevaluate in 20 minutes.

5. A four-year-old has recently been diagnosed with Insulin Dependent Diabetes Mellitus (IDDM). The parents tell the nurse that they do not understand much about diabetes. Which is the best way to explain IDDM to them?
   1. IDDM is an inborn error of metabolism that makes the child unable to burn fatty acids without insulin requirements.
   2. IDDM is a genetic disorder that makes the child unable to metabolize protein without insulin supplements.
   3. IDDM is a deficiency in the secretion of insulin by the pancreas, which makes the child unable to metabolize carbohydrates without insulin supplements.
   4. IDDM is a problem that occurs when children eat too many sweets early in life and then are unable to metabolize sugar without insulin supplements.

6. A one-month-old is seen in the clinic and is diagnosed as having congenital

hypothyroidism (cretinism). Her parents ask the nurse if their child will be normal. What is the best response for the nurse?
1. Your child will need to take medication for life but has a good chance of normal development because of the early detection.
2. Cretinism causes both physical delay and mental retardation in the vast majority of children with the condition.
3. There is no way to tell at this point if there is permanent damage; your child will need continual evaluation.
4. Your child will need to take medication until puberty is completed; if there are no serious problems by then, your child should be perfectly normal.

Answers and Rationales

1. (3) Delayed dentition is a sign of hypopituitarism or pituitary dwarfism due to a lack of growth hormone. Permanent teeth should begin to erupt around age 5. A 13-month-old that weighs 21 pounds is within the normal range. A 4-year-old who is 41 inches tall is within the normal range. Menarche normally occurs between 10 1/2 and 15 1/2 years of age. This child is within normal limits.

2. (1) Human growth hormone is the treatment for primary hypopituitarism. Three to seven times a week is usual. Bedtime is the best time to give it, because that closely simulates the body's normal production. A child with hypopituitarism should achieve normal intelligence. Endocrine workups of children who have no signs of disease are not necessary. While emotional difficulties relating to this condition are possible and the family should be alerted to that possibility, referral to a psychiatrist at this time seems premature.

3. (2) Increase in exercise will affect the insulin dose the most. Heat and humidity might have some effect. Diabetics are taught to adjust their insulin dose within ranges. An adolescent needs to learn how to do this.

4. (3) The symptoms suggest hypoglycemia, which should be treated with food. Fluids such as juice or milk that contain carbohydrates should be given to treat hypoglycemia, not plain water. Insulin should not be given because the symptoms suggest hypoglycemia, not hyperglycemia. Having him rest for 20 minutes without treating hypoglycemia will make it worse. Rest following the treatment of hypoglycemia is appropriate.

5. (3) IDDM is a lack of insulin secretion by the pancreas which makes the child unable to metabolize carbohydrates without additional insulin. IDDM is not a metabolic error and fatty acids are not primarily affected. IDDM is not a genetic disorder, although there may be a hereditary predisposition to the condition, and proteins are not primarily affected. IDDM is not caused by eating too many sweets early in life.

6. (1) Because the child is one month old, there is a good chance that she will develop normally. Maternal thyroid circulates for the first three months. If the child is started on treatment within the first three months of life, there is a good chance for normal development. Untreated cretinism will cause delays in physical and mental development. This child is being treated early, so answer 2 is not correct. Answer 3 is not correct. She will be continually evaluated but should be normal because of treatment is being started early. Answer 4 is not correct. She will need to take medication for the rest of her life.

Pediatric Conditions Related to the Integumentary System

BURNS (SEE CHAPTER 14)

A. Children are proportioned differently, so the Rule of Nines is not accurate and needs to be modified; the head of a small child is 18–19%, the trunk is 32%, each leg is 15%, and each arm is 9 1/2%.

B. Burns in infants and toddlers are often due to spills, such as pulling a dish of boiling hot water off the stove. Burns in older children are more apt to be flame burns.

C. A greater proportion of an infant's body weight is water than an adult's; therefore, fluid losses such as those occurring in burns are a serious problem for infants and small children.

IMPETIGO

A. An infection of the outer layers of the skin usually caused by Group A Beta streptococcus or Staphylococcus Aureus that is common in toddlers and preschoolers and is very contagious
B. Assessment findings:
1. Macules, papules, and vesicles that rupture, causing a superficial, moist erosion
2. Moist area dries and a yellow crust forms
3. Found most commonly on face, axillae, and extremities
4. Spreads from one part of the body to another
5. Pruritus
C. Nursing diagnoses (see Table 16.50)

Table 16.50 Nursing Diagnoses Related to Impetigo

- Impaired skin integrity related to lesions and pruritus
- Acute pain related to inflammation and pruritus
- Risk for secondary infection related to broken skin
- Risk for infection transmission related to contagious nature of the organism
- Risk for ineffective therapeutic regimen management related to insufficient knowledge of condition, prevention, treatment, and skin care

D. Interventions:
1. Topical and systemic antibiotics
2. Antibiotic ointment may also be applied under fingernails to help prevent spread of disease
3. Soften skin and crusts with Burrow's solution compresses
4. Remove crusts gently.
5. Cover draining lesions to prevent the spread of infection.
6. Teach client and family regarding medication and hygiene

RINGWORM (TINEA)

A. Fungal infection of the skin; may be in head, axilla, groin, arms, legs, feet (athlete's foot)
B. Assessment findings:
1. Reddish patches that may be scaly or blistered
2. May damage hair shafts
3. Itching and soreness
4. Detected by Wood's lamp, which fluoresces green at the base of the affected hair shaft)
C. Nursing diagnoses (see Table 16.51)
D. Interventions:
1. Antifungal drugs such as Griseofulvin by mouth or topical antifungals

Table 16.51 Nursing Diagnoses Related to Ringworm (Tinea)

- Impaired skin integrity related to fungal infection of the dermis
- Deficient knowledge regarding infectious nature, therapy, and self-care needs related to lack of information
- Risk for infection transmission related to contagious nature of fungus

2. Teach prevention by good hygiene; thorough drying after washing (fungi like moist places, such as between the toes)
3. If recurring infections, check pets for infection; can be transmitted from cats and dogs to humans

PEDICULOSIS (LICE)

A. A common parasitic infection of the hair usually spread by close contact or by objects such as combs, hats, scarves, and so on
B. Assessment findings:
1. White eggs (nits) firmly attached to base of hair shafts; nits do not disappear when hair is combed; they stick to the hair shaft.
2. Itching
3. Excoriation due to scratching
C. Nursing diagnoses (see Table 16.52)

Table 16.52 Nursing Diagnoses Related to Pediculosis (Lice)

- Risk for infection related to lesions
- Impaired comfort related to pruritus
- Risk for infection transmission related to insufficient knowledge of modes of transmission
- Risk for ineffective therapeutic regimen management related to insufficient resources, repeated infections

D. Interventions:
1. Shampoo such as Kwell; must be repeated in a week to kill the lice
2. Comb the hair with a fine-tooth comb to remove the nits.
3. Wash clothes, bed linens, hats; disinfect or discard combs, hair brushes that client has used.
4. Teach client and family not to share combs, hair brushes, hats, scarves, head phones, and so on.
5. Teach family how to check for pediculosis.

POISON IVY

A. Contact dermatitis caused by exposure to the oils in the poison ivy plant, a trailing three leafed plant

B. Assessment findings:
1. Rash usually develops 24–48 hours after exposure to oils on leaves or stems of poison ivy plant.
2. Rash is followed by fluid-filled blisters which break, ooze, and then become crusty.
3. Severe itching occurs.

C. Nursing diagnoses (see Table 16.53)

Table 16.53 Nursing Diagnoses Related to Poison Ivy

- Impaired comfort related to pruritus
- Risk for infection related to lesions
- Risk for secondary infection related to broken skin
- Risk for ineffective therapeutic regimen management related to insufficient knowledge of condition, prevention, treatment, and skin care

D. Interventions:
1. Antihistamines and corticosteroids
2. Topical agents to help with itching
3. Teach client how to identify plants (three leaves).
4. Teach client to wash with soap and water after any possible contact with plant.
5. Teach client to wash clothing after possible exposure.
6. Dogs and cats can carry oil from the plant on their fur and cause a reaction in persons who are sensitive to the oils.

CHILDHOOD ECZEMA

A. Allergic skin reaction occurring in infants; is often the first sign of allergic predisposition in children; respiratory allergies often develop later

B. Assessment findings:
1. Redness and itching
2. Papules and vesicles followed by oozing and weeping and crusts
3. Most common sites are face, neck, and insides of elbows and knees; can cover the entire body
4. Dry skin
5. Rash often associated with certain foods

C. Nursing diagnoses (see Table 16.54)

Table 16.54 Nursing Diagnoses Related to Eczema

- Impaired skin integrity related to lesions and itching
- Impaired comfort related to itching
- Risk for infection related to broken skin and tissue trauma
- Risk for social isolation related to appearance and fear of negative reactions from others
- Risk for ineffective therapeutic regimen management related to insufficient knowledge of condition and treatment

D. Interventions:
1. Topical steroids
2. Antihistamines
3. Coal tar preparations
4. Medicated or colloid baths
5. Avoid heat and sweating; keep skin dry because moisture aggravates the condition.
6. Elimination diet:
   a. Remove all solid foods from diet, giving formula only
   b. If symptoms disappear after three days, add one food group every three days to see if symptoms reappear
   c. Withdraw suspected food to see if symptoms disappear; reintroduce food to see if symptoms appear (challenge test).
7. Assess items in contact with child's skin; avoid wool, perfumed soaps, lotions
8. Avoid frequent baths:
   a. Add Alpha Keri to bath to lubricate skin
   b. Provide lubricant immediately after bath
   c. Pat dry; do not rub
   d. Avoid soap in bath because it dries the skin
9. Use cotton clothing; no wool
10. Keep child's nails short to reduce scratching and secondary infection
11. Use gloves, mitts, or elbow restraints if needed to prevent scratching
12. Apply wet saline or Burrow's solution compresses

Sample Questions

1. A child is seen in the physician's office for a crusty lesion at the corners of his mouth. The lesion has a yellow crust. The arms and legs also have similar lesions. The physician diagnoses impetigo and prescribes an antibiotic. What teaching is appropriate for the nurse who is working with the child and parents?
   1. Help the parents understand the need for an elimination diet.
   2. Instruct the parents to put antibiotic ointment under the fingernails as well as on the lesions.
   3. Describe what the poison ivy plant looks like.
   4. Inform the parents not to let the child share a comb or a hat with anyone.

2. The mother of a child who has ringworm asks what kind of worm the child has. How should the nurse respond?
   1. Ringworm is caused by a fungus, not a worm. The lesion often takes the form a circle or ring.

2. The same worm that causes pinworms can cause ringworm. Good handwashing is essential to prevent spreading.
3. The worm is often on plants and leaves, such as those that cause poison ivy.
4. Worms that are on house plants and common garden plants can cause ringworm.

3. The mother of a child who has pediculosis says that she plans to use kerosene to wash the child's hair just like her grandmother did for her. What is the best response for the nurse?
   1. "Your grandmother was a wise woman. Kerosene is the major ingredient in the special shampoo we recommend."
   2. "Kerosene will work, but the shampoo we recommend is less irritating."
   3. "Kerosene can cause serious injury to your child. Try using the shampoos which are not dangerous."
   4. "Your grandmother was not a physician. Please do what the doctor recommends."

4. A five-year-old child keeps developing poison ivy. The child's mother insists that the child has not been near any poison ivy plants since the first outbreak several weeks ago. What question should the nurse ask the mother?
   1. "Has your child been eating any particular food that might be associated with outbreaks?"
   2. "Does your child scratch the blisters and touch the liquid that comes out?"
   3. "Does your child ever share combs or hats with other children?"
   4. "Do you have a cat or a dog that goes outdoors?"

5. A 10-month-old infant is hospitalized with severe eczema. The child has elbow restraints applied. When should the elbow restraints be removed?
   1. They should not be removed until the lesions have healed.

2. When someone is holding the baby
3. Once a shift to check for circulation
4. When the baby is asleep

Answers and Rationales

1. (2) Impetigo is usually caused by staph or strep, causes severe itching, and is often spread from one site to the other by scratching. Putting antibiotic ointment underneath the fingernails helps to prevent the child from spreading from one part of his body to another. An elimination diet is appropriate for a child who has eczema. Impetigo is not caused by poison ivy. Pediculosis (head lice) is spread by sharing combs and hats.
2. (1) Ringworm is caused by a fungus, not a worm. It is often called ringworm because the lesion is often in the shape of circle or ring and looks as if a worm was burrowing under the surface.
3. (3) Kerosene is an old folk remedy for pediculosis. It is very irritating to the scalp and the fumes are very dangerous for the child, to say nothing of the risk of fire. Kerosene should not be used.
4. (4) Cats and dogs may run through poison ivy and get the oil on their fur. A susceptible child who pats or hugs the animal may develop the allergic response. Allergic response to foods is associated with eczema, not poison ivy. Pediculosis or head lice is spread by sharing combs or hats. Poison ivy is not spread by the liquid that oozes out of the blisters.
5. (2) The restraints can be removed when someone is holding the baby. They do need to be removed to check for circulation at least every two hours. The baby could scratch when asleep, so the restraints need to be on during sleep.

Chapter 17

The Mental Health Client

BASIC CONCEPTS

THERAPEUTIC COMMUNICATION

A. Therapeutic communication utilizes the principles of communication in a goal-directed, professional framework.
B. Therapeutic communication techniques (see Table 17.1)
C. Initial communication:
    1. Goal is to open communication.
    2. Empathy and restatement/reflection
D. Barriers to communication (Table 17.2)

PHASES IN NURSE–PATIENT (CLIENT) RELATIONSHIP

A. Initiation or orientation phase:
    1. Establish boundaries of relationship:
        a. Purpose
        b. Place, length, and time of meetings
    2. Identify problems.
    3. Assess anxiety levels of self and the client.
    4. Identify expectations.
B. Continuation or active working phase:
    1. Acceptance of each other
    2. Use therapeutic and problem-solving techniques.
    3. Assess and evaluate problems continuously.
    4. Focus on increasing the client's independence and decreasing reliance on the nurse.
    5. Goal is for client to confront and work through his problems
C. Termination phase:
    1. Plan for end of therapy early in the relationship.

Table 17.1 Therapeutic Communication Techniques

Technique	Example
1. Silence	Sitting quietly with a client
2. Offering self	"I will stay with you."
3. Clarifying	Client: "Nobody here likes me." Nurse: "Who is it that you think doesn't like you?"
4. Restatement/Reflection	Client: "I didn't sleep well last night." Nurse: "You didn't sleep well last night." Client: "Nurse, do you think I am going to die? Nurse: "Do you think you are going to die?"
5. Giving information	Client: "Where is the bathroom?" Nurse: "Second door on the left."
6. Focusing and exploring	"You said you were upset about your mother's visit. What is it that upset you?"
7. Empathy	"It must be difficult to be away from your family."

Table 17.2 Barriers to Communication

Block	Example	Rationale
1. Advising	"If I were you, I would . . ." "I think you should join AA."	Goal is for client to make his own decisions.
2. Approval/disapproval	"You did the right thing when you put your mother in the nursing home." "I would not do it like that."	Goal is for client to make his own decisions; nurse should not be the authority figure.
3. Devaluing client's feelings	"Don't be concerned. It is only a small scar." "Don't be so sad. Every one gets depressed."	Opinion is conveyed that client's feelings are not important.
4. Focus on nurse	"I know what you mean. I had a baby last year. When I was in labor . . ."	Therapeutic communication focuses on the client.
5. Requesting an explanation	"Why are you upset?"	Puts client on the defensive; better to ask who, what, when, and where questions.
6. Clichés and false reassurance	"Everything will be all right." "Every cloud has a silver lining."	Nurse does not know if things will be all right; implies nurse does not understand; does not think client's feelings are important.
7. Defending	Client: "What kind of nurses are working here? You're all stupid!" Nurse: "All of our nurses are highly qualified."	Nurse acts defensively; implies client's feelings are unjustified; reinforces client's unhappy feelings; better to be empathetic.
8. Changing the subject	Client: "I'm scared I'm going to die during my operation." Nurse: "Look at the pretty flowers that came."	Tells client it is not safe to discuss feelings with the nurse.

Table 17.3 Erikson's Developmental Stages

Stage	Task	Example
Infancy (0–2 years)	Trust versus Mistrust	Feeding, diapering
Early childhood (2–3 years)	Autonomy versus shame and doubt	Toileting, eating, dressing, walking
Late childhood (3–5 years)	Initiative versus Guilt	Help make cookies
School age (6–12 years)	Industry versus Inferiority	Joins same-sex clubs, collects things
Adolescence (12–20 years)	Identity versus Role Diffusion	"Who am I?"
Young adulthood (18–25 years)	Intimacy versus Isolation	Careers, marriage
Adulthood (25–65 years)	Generativity versus Stagnation	Family, community, church leadership roles
Later adulthood (retirement)	Integrity versus Despair	Accomplishment versus hopelessness, depression

2. Maintain initially defined boundaries.
3. Anticipate problems of termination:
   a. Client dependence on nurse
   b. Previous traumatic separations
4. Discuss client's feelings about separation.

THEORETICAL MODELS

Psychoanalytical Model (Freud)

A. Believes repressed childhood trauma is the cause of conflicts in later life
B. Structures of the mind:
   1. Id: contains the instinctual, primitive drives
   2. Ego: mediates demands of primitive id, and self-critical superego.
   3. Superego: conscience, perfection, morality
   4. Conscious: awareness of self when awake
   5. Unconscious: memories and thoughts which do not enter the conscious
C. Stages of psychosexual development:
   1. Oral   0–1 yrs Infancy
   2. Anal   1–3 yrs Toddler
   3. Phallic (Oedipal) 3–6 yrs Preschool
   4. Latency   6–12 yrs School
   5. Genital   12–18 yrs Adolescent

D. Interventions:
   1. Treatment goal is to bring into the conscious mind conflicts which are unconscious.
   2. Techniques used by psychiatrist include free association and dream analysis.

Psychosocial Developmental Model: Erikson

A. Each life stage has psychosocial tasks that need to be accomplished.
B. Stages and tasks (see Table 17.3)
C. Interventions: goal of treatment is to bring the individual through the stages to the appropriate level.

Basic Human Needs (Maslow)

A. There is a hierarchy of needs, and needs are fulfilled in a progressive order from physiologic and safety through self actualization.
B. Hierarchy of needs (see Figure 17.1):
   1. Physiologic: air, food, water, sleep
   2. Safety: avoiding harm, feeling secure, preventing injury

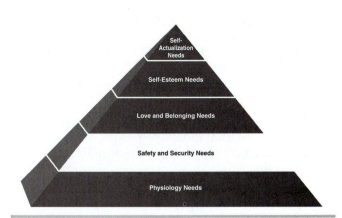

Figure 17.1 Maslow's Hierarchy of Needs

    3. Love and belonging: group identity, being cared about, caring for
    4. Self esteem: self confidence, self acceptance
    5. Self actualization: self knowledge, satisfying interpersonal relationships, stress management
C. Treatment:
    1. Goal is to fulfill needs in a progressive manner
    2. Nursing considerations
      a. Hierarchy of needs used as a basis for assessment
      b. Help client fulfill needs to relieve stress
      c. Help client advance through stages
      d. Help client develop new behaviors to reduce stress and prevent recurrence of dysfunction

Behavior Modification

A. Behavior can be changed by applying the stimulus response learning theory: The behavior that is rewarded is most apt to be repeated.
B. Interventions:
    1. Reinforcement of a behavior increases the probability of a behavior recurring:
      a. Positive reinforcement: using food, privileges, praise as rewards for desired behavior
      b. Negative reinforcement: ignoring, leaving, or removing privilege when undesired behavior occurs
    2. Punishment decreases the probability of a behavior recurring.
    3. Desensitization: Frequent exposure to increasing doses decreases anxiety and increases coping mechanisms
C. Behavior modification used for a variety of conditions, including:
    1. Children, adolescents
    2. Anxiety disorders
    3. Eating disorders
    4. Personality disorders
    5. Schizophrenia

D. Nursing interventions:
    1. Assess behavior.
    2. Provide reinforcers consistently (key to effectiveness of the program).
    3. Evaluate the effectiveness of the program.

Community Mental Health Model

A. Mental illness is seen as a reaction to stress; the goal is to keep the client in the community.
B. Interventions:
    1. Primary prevention: maintenance and promotion of health; teaching client how to prevent illness
    2. Secondary prevention: early diagnosis and treatment; dealing with the here and now crisis; partial hospitalization
    3. Tertiary prevention: follow up to avoid permanent disability following a crisis

TYPES OF INTERVENTIONS

Crisis Intervention

A. A type of therapy aimed at immediate intervention in an acute episode or crisis in which the individual is unable to cope alone
B. A crisis exists when a threat to the individual is so great that usual coping mechanisms are ineffective.
C. Principles of intervention:
    1. Determine level of functioning.
    2. Determine event causing crisis.
    3. Assess past coping mechanisms.
    4. Focus on the problem, not the causes.
    5. Give support and empathy.
    6. Help the client use strengths and positive coping skills.
    7. Evaluate and encourage use of situational supports
    8. Intervention is short term: 6–8 weeks.

Group Therapy

A. A process in which group interactions are designed to cause improvement in symptoms or behavior
B. Types of groups:
    1. Structured group:
      a. Group has predetermined goals.
      b. Leader retains control.
      c. Factual material is presented in a clear and specific format.
    2. Unstructured group:
      a. Responsibility for goals is shared by group and leader.
      b. Leader is nondirective.
      c. Discussion topic reflects concerns of group members.
      d. The emphasis is on feelings, not facts.
      e. The group makes decisions.

C. Principles related to group therapy:
1. Support: Members gain support from others by sharing.
2. Verbalization: Members express feelings; group reinforces appropriate communication.
3. Change: Members have opportunity to try out new, more adaptive behaviors in group setting.
4. Focus is on the here and now.

Self-Help Groups

A. Groups of lay persons who have a common problem and give each other support as they deal with the problem
B. Examples:
1. Alcoholics Anonymous (AA): all members are alcoholics; very successful in helping alcoholics stay sober using 12-step recovery program
2. Narcotics Anonymous (NA): all members are addicted to drugs; uses same 12-step program as AA
3. Alanon: 12-step program for families of alcoholics
4. Alateen: 12-step program for children of alcoholics
5. Overeaters Anonymous: 12-step program for persons who overeat

6. Reach for Recovery: persons who have had mastectomies
7. Mended Hearts: persons who have had heart surgery

Family Therapy

A. A form of group therapy based on the premise that it is the total family rather than the identified client that is dysfunctional
B. Concepts:
1. Identified patient is the member with obvious symptoms
2. Changes in one member cause changes in how the family functions.
3. Family involvement is necessary in all treatment.
C. Used often when children are in therapy

Milieu Therapy

A. Management of the client's environment to promote a positive living experience
B. Concepts:
1. Patients take as much responsibility as possible.
2. Client government: meetings with clients and staff to promote therapeutic environment
3. The environment in the facility is as close as possible to the "real world" and has the potential for therapeutic value.

Psychiatric Mental Health Problems

ANXIETY

General Concepts

A. Tension in response to a perceived physical or psychological threat
B. Assessment findings:
1. Physical: sympathetic nervous system, "fight or flight" response
   a. Dry mouth
   b. Elevated pulse, BP, respirations
   c. Hyperventilation
   d. Diarrhea
   e. Nausea
   f. Increased urination
   g. Diaphoresis
   h. Insomnia
   i. Fatigue
   j. Irritability and tenseness
   k. Sexual dysfunction

2. Psychological:
   a. Fear
   b. Sense of impending doom
   c. Feeling of helplessness
   d. Insecurity
   e. Low self confidence
   f. Anger
   g. Guilt
C. Levels of anxiety (see Table 17.4)
D. Coping mechanisms (defense mechanisms):
1. An unconscious mental process or coping pattern that lessens the anxiety associated with a situation or an internal conflict and protects the person from mental discomfort; all people use defense mechanisms to decrease anxiety; excessive use may result in maladaptive responses
2. Types of mechanisms (see Table 17.5)

Table 17.4 Levels of Anxiety

Level	Physiologic Response	Cognitive Function	Behavioral Response	Nursing Care
Mild	Minimum muscle tension	Broad perceptual field	Can deal with change, restless, irritable, can learn	Listen; nurse calm
Moderate	Increased tension, headache, fatigue, butterflies	Narrowed perceptual field	Focus on immediate events	Nurse discusses in a calm, rational manner
Severe	Increased BP, TPR, dry mouth, diaphoresis, conversions, somatic symptoms	Greatly narrowed perceptual field, connections between details not perceived	Feels threatened; increased physical activity	Very calm; brief information; reassurance
Panic	Sometimes hypotensive, poor motor coordination, pale, cool, clammy, hyperventilation	Perceptual field closed, details out of proportion; logical thinking impaired, feeling of dread	Helpless; may strike physically or withdraw; voice high	Isolate from stimuli; stay with client

Table 17.5 Defense Mechanisms

Mechanism	Description
Repression	Unconscious forgetting: the exclusion of unacceptable ideas, fantasies, or feelings from the consciousness; the repressed material cannot be recalled but may show up in disguised form in dreams or other associations; mechanism involved in anxiety disorders
Suppression	Conscious, deliberate forgetting of unacceptable impulses or thoughts
Compensation	Covering up for a weakness by emphasizing a desirable trait; a poor athlete becomes an outstanding scholar
Denial	Refusal to face reality; protects ego; denial of an illness
Displacement	Discharging pent-up feelings from one object to a less dangerous object; a person may be angry at her boss and kick the dog or slam the door rather than yell at the boss
Fantasy	Gratification by imaginary achievements and wishful thinking; children's play
Fixation	The persistence into later life of interests and behavior patterns appropriate to an earlier age
Identification	The process of taking on the desirable attributes in personalities of other people one admires; the child mimics mother or father; important for superego development
Introjection	A type of identification in which there is symbolic incorporation of a loved or hated object, belief system, or value into the individual's own ego structure; there is no assimilation as in identification; being around depressed people makes the person depressed
Insulation	Withdrawal into passivity; becoming inaccessible in order to avoid further threatening circumstances; the individual may appear cold and indifferent to his surroundings; a rape victim who refuses to talk about what happened
Isolation	Excluding certain ideas, attitudes, or feelings from awareness; separating feelings from intellect; emotions are put in a locked-tight compartment; a person talks about his wife's serious illness with no display of emotion
Projection	Attributing one's own undesirable traits to someone else. After being punished, the child says to the parent: "You hate me."; seen in paranoia.
Rationalization	Person offers a good excuse for his behavior instead of giving the true reason; "I failed the test because it was a bad test."; used very frequently
Reaction formation	Prevention of dangerous feelings and desires from being expressed by exaggerating the opposite attitude; the legislator who promotes anti-homosexual laws and is later found to be homosexual
Regression	Resorting to an earlier developmental level in order to deal with reality; frequently seen during a physical illness; a child who is toilet trained will have "accidents" while hospitalized
Sublimation	A primitive or unacceptable tendency is redirected into socially acceptable channels; a person is very aggressive and becomes a boxer and earns millions; a person loves to view the human body naked and paints it
Substitution	The replacement of a highly valued, unacceptable object with an object that is more acceptable to the ego
Symbolization	Use of an idea or object by the conscious mind to represent another actual event or object; obsessive thoughts and behavior such as hand washing means cleaning or purification
Undoing	Performance of a specific action that is considered to be the opposite of a previous unacceptable action; this action is felt to neutralize or "undo" the original action; frequent hand washing will undo obsessive thoughts; one of the mechanisms in obsessive-compulsive behavior

E. Nursing diagnoses related to anxiety disorders (see Table 17.6)

F. Antianxiety medications:
1. Agents and dosage (see Table 17.7)
2. Side effects and nursing interventions (see Table 17.8)

a. Most side effects relate to central nervous system depression and anticholinergic effects

b. Antianxiety agents also have the potential for tolerance, dependence, and abuse and therefore should be given on a short-term basis

3. Teaching for clients taking antianxiety agents:
   a. Do not abruptly stop medication.
   b. Do not take with other CNS depressants, such as alcohol.
   c. Be aware of the risk when taking it during pregnancy.
   d. Drug effects last for several days after the last dose.
   e. Withdrawal symptoms: insomnia, headaches, anorexia, blurred vision, anxiety

Table 17.6 Nursing Diagnoses Related to Anxiety Disorders

- Anxiety related to irrational thoughts or guilt
- Disturbed sleep pattern related to psychological stress and irrational thoughts
- Ineffective individual coping related to ineffective coping mechanisms
- Impaired social interactions related to effects of behavior and low self concept
- Risk for ineffective family coping related to temporary family disorganization and role changes
- Risk for ineffective management of therapeutic regimen related to insufficient knowledge of condition and pharmacological therapy

ANXIETY DISORDERS

Disorders characterized by fear that is out of proportion to external events

Panic Attacks

A. Sudden onset of intense apprehension
B. Assessment findings:
   1. Dyspnea
   2. Palpitations
   3. Chest pain
   4. Dizziness and faintness
   5. Fear of dying or going crazy; feels out of control
   6. Choking sensation
   7. Depersonalization

Table 17.7 Antianxiety Medications

Class	Generic Name	Trade Name	Daily Dose
Benzodiazepine	alprazolam	Xanax	0.5–4 mg
	chlordiazepoxide	Librium	15–100 mg
	clonazepam	Klonopin	0.5–10 mg
	diazepam	Valium	2–40 mg
	lorazepam	Ativan	2–4 mg
	oxazepam	Serax	15–90 mg
	prazepam	Centrax	20–60 mg
Sedative/hypnotic	flurazepam	Dalmane	15–60 mg
	triazolam	Halcion	0.25–0.5 mg
Antihistamine	diphenhydramine	Benadryl	50–100 mg
	hydroxyzine	Vistaril	75–200 mg
Anxiolytic	buspirone	Buspar	10–40 mg
Barbiturates	secobarbital	Seconal	100–200 mg
	phenobarbital	Luminal	100–200 mg

Table 17.8 Antianxiety Medications: Side Effects and Nursing Care

Side Effects	Nursing Interventions
CNS depression Dizziness	Safety; don't drive until adjusted to medications
	Don't give other CNS depressants, such as alcohol.
Paradoxical excitement	Discontinue.
Dependence	Withdraw slowly.
Tolerance	Observe for proper use; withdraw slowly.
Depression	Decrease the dose.
Hypotension	
	Monitor BP; teach safety when changing positions.
Decreased Pulse and respirations	Monitor pulse and respirations.
Dry mouth	Fluids, hard candy
Nausea	Give with meals.
Constipation	High-fiber diet.
Urinary retention	Monitor intake and output.
Irregular menses	Reassure that irregularity is related to medication

C. Nursing diagnoses (see Table 17.6)
D. Interventions:
1. Give antianxiety medications.
2. Have the client take deep breaths.
3. Do not focus on the attack.
4. Distract the client.
5. Have client use paper bag if hyperventilating to correct respiratory alkalosis.
6. Remove stimuli.
7. Stay with the client.

Phobias

A. Intense, irrational fear reactions to objects or situations
B. Common types:
1. Acrophobia: fear of heights
2. Agoraphobia: fear of open or public spaces—fear of marketplace
3. Claustrophobia: fear of closed places
C. Nursing diagnoses (see Table 17.6)
D. Defense mechanisms frequently utilized:
1. Repression
2. Displacement
E. Interventions:
1. Antianxiety medications
2. Discuss fears.
3. Allow client to make decisions about activities of daily living (ADL) such as eating, sleeping, working
4. Gradual desensitization
5. Behavior modification
6. Relaxation
7. Individual and group psychotherapy
8. Milieu therapy

Obsessive Compulsive Disorder (OCD)

A. Presence of obsession (uncontrollable, recurring thoughts) or compulsion (a ritualistic act done in an attempt to relieve the anxiety related to the thoughts or to make the thoughts go away)
B. Assessment findings:
1. Performing a repetitive action, often hand washing, to relieve guilt
2. Feelings of inferiority
3. Self-hatred
4. Rigidity
5. Difficulty with decision making
C. Defense mechanisms frequently utilized:
1. Repression
2. Displacement
3. Undoing
D. Nursing diagnoses (see Table 17.6)
E. Interventions:
1. Medications:
   a. Antianxiety
   b. Clomipramine (Anafranil): a tricyclic antidepressant that is effective in OCD
2. Distract client; engage in alternate activities with client

3. Do not interrupt rituals.
4. Allow time to complete rituals; gradually decrease time and frequency.
5. Desensitization
6. Behavior modification
7. Provide physical protection from repetitive acts; skin care for compulsive washers.
8. Help client express feelings and concerns in socially acceptable ways
9. Individual and group psychotherapy

Post Traumatic Stress Disorder (PTSD)

A. Anxiety neurosis resulting from severe external stress that is beyond what is usual or tolerable for most people, such as war, natural disaster, or fire
B. Assessment findings:
1. Severe anxiety
2. Inability to function or concentrate
3. Sleep disturbance, nightmares
4. Anger
5. Hypervigilance
6. Exaggerated startle response
7. Flashbacks
8. Poor interpersonal relationships
C. Nursing diagnoses (see Table 17.6)
D. Interventions:
1. Prevention by encouraging discussion of feelings when major stress exists
2. Crisis intervention during acute stage
3. Antianxiety medications for short-term use
4. Encourage client to express feelings
5. Be nonjudgmental when client does express feelings or describes the horrors of the trauma
6. Help client feel safe and worthwhile
7. Family therapy
8. Psychotherapy
9. Relaxation therapy
10. Desensitization

Somatoform Disorders

A. Somatic behaviors that may involve any organ system whose etiologies are in part related to emotional factors
B. Somatization disorder:
1. Client presents with multiple, recurrent physical complaints for which medical attention has been sought but for which there is no organic reason.
2. Symptoms onset before age 30.
3. Symptoms last for several years.
C. Conversion disorder:
1. Dysfunction of an organ of special meaning to the person; however, there is no organic damage
2. Assessment findings:
   a. Voluntary nervous system involved
   b. Little concern about symptoms: "la belle indifference"

   c. Usually one major symptom; arm or leg paralysis, loss of sight, speech, hearing
   d. Organ involved is related to the underlying stress
   e. Primary gain is suppressing conflict
   f. Secondary gain is sympathy or getting out of unpleasant activities

D. Hypochondriasis:
  1. An exaggerated concern with one's physical health while having no organic pathological condition or loss of function; concern persists in spite of medical assurance that there is no health problem
  2. Assessment findings:
    a. Multiple symptoms
    b. Seeks medical care; sees many doctors

E. Nursing diagnoses for somatoform disorders (see Table 17.6)

F. Interventions for somatoform disorders:
  1. Do not focus on physical symptoms.
  2. Encourage the expression of feelings.
  3. Discourage secondary gains.
  4. Help client learn alternatives for dealing with stress.

EATING DISORDERS

Anorexia Nervosa

A. Compulsive resistance to eating, intense fear of being obese:
  1. Loss of weight in excess of 25%
  2. Five to 20% of those with anorexia nervosa die from it.
  3. Affects primarily females from 13 to 35 years; can occur in men

B. Causes:
  1. Controlling family
  2. Low self-esteem
  3. Societal emphasis on thinness

C. Assessment findings (see Table 17.9):
  1. Skeletal muscle atrophy, emaciated
  2. Loss of fatty tissue
  3. Hypotension
  4. Constipation
  5. Infections due to poor resistance
  6. Blotchy, sallow skin
  7. Lanugo (fine, downy hair seen on newborns
  8. Dryness and loss of hair
  9. Amenorrhea
  10. Loss of secondary sex characteristics; says "I used to wear a bra"
  11. Electrolyte imbalances, dehydration
  12. Girl is usually bright, ambitious, and obedient
  13. Low self-esteem
  14. Preoccupied with food
  15. Depression
  16. Manipulation
  17. Compulsive exerciser

D. Nursing diagnoses (see Table 17.10)

Table 17.9 Comparison of Anorexia and Bulimia

Anorexia	Bulimia
25% weight loss from original	Weight fluctuates 10 lbs
Amenorrhea	None
Starvation	Binge eating followed by purging: emetics, finger down throat, laxatives
Deny abnormal eating	Sees patterns and fears loss of control
Intense fear of becoming obese	Hide and hoard food
Prefer health foods	Prefer high-calorie food
Preoccupation with buying, planning, and preparing foods	Repeated cycle of crash diet, use of diuretics, laxatives, amphetamines
Rigorous exercise	Abuse of alcohol and/or drugs, petty crime

Table 17.10 Nursing Diagnoses Related to Eating Disorders

- Impaired nutrition: less than body requirements related to refusal to eat, exercise in excess of caloric intake, self-induced vomiting
- Risk for deficient fluid volume related to inadequate intake of food and liquids, excessive use of laxatives, diuretics, emetics, and self-induced vomiting
- Activity intolerance related to fatigue secondary to malnutrition
- Constipation related to insufficient food and fluid intake
- Ineffective individual coping related to self-induced vomiting, denial of hunger, and insufficient food intake secondary to feelings of loss of control and inaccurate perceptions of body states
- Disturbed self concept related to inaccurate perception of self as obese
- Disturbed thought processes related to severe electrolyte imbalance or psychological conflicts
- Disturbed body image related to altered perception of body
- Impaired social interactions related to inability to form relationships with others or fear of trusting relationships with others

E. Interventions:
  1. Correct fluid and electrolyte imbalance.
  2. Intake and output
  3. Observe for two hours after eating to prevent self-induced vomiting
  4. Positive reinforcement for weight gain rather than amount of food eaten
  5. Allow opportunities for some choices in ADL.
  6. Client needs to accept responsibility for self without guilt or ambivalence
  7. Set and maintain limits.
  8. Assess for suicide potential.
  9. Family education and therapy
  10. Self-help groups
  11. Tranquilizers (phenothiazines)
  12. Antidepressants (fluoxetine hydrochloride, imipramine) to treat depression that is often associated with anorexia
  13. Psychotherapy
  14. Behavior modification

Bulimia

A. Recurrent binge-eating behavior (eating huge amounts of food in one sitting) followed by purging (self-induced vomiting, emetics, laxatives, diuretics) or excessive exercising
B. Assessment findings (see Table 17.9):
1. Electrolyte imbalances
2. Dental caries
3. Erosion of tooth enamel due to acid on teeth from frequent vomiting
4. Gingival (gum) infections
5. Infections
6. Bingeing
7. Vomiting
8. Abuse of laxatives and diuretics
9. Excessive exercising
C. Nursing diagnoses (see Table 17.10)
D. Interventions (See anorexia interventions)

LOSS AND GRIEF

See Death and Dying

Loss

A. Loss is any situation in which a valued object is changed or is no longer accessible to the individual. Types of loss include:
1. Actual: death of a loved one; loss of a body part such as a breast or a limb
2. Perceived: occurs when a sense of loss is felt by the individual but is not tangible to others
3. Potential: anticipation of a loss as in the preoperative period before an amputation or mastectomy
4. Physical: loss of an extremity in an accident; scarring from burns; a permanent injury
5. Psychological: woman feels inadequate after menopause and is no longer able to bear children
B. Loss precipitates anxiety and a feeling of being vulnerable.

Grief

A. Grief is a series of intense physical and psychological responses that occur following a loss. It is a universal, normal response to loss.
B. Grief has several stages:
1. Stage I: Shock and Disbelief:
   a. Person feels disoriented and helpless
   b. Denial gives protection until the person is able to deal with reality; may last from minutes to days.
2. Stage II: Developing Awareness:
   a. Emotional pain occurs with increased reality of the loss.
   b. Recognition that one is powerless to change the situation
   c. Feelings of helplessness
   d. Anger and hostility; may be directed at others
   e. Guilt
   f. Sadness, isolation, loneliness
3. Stage III: Restitution and Resolution:
   a. Emergence of bodily symptoms
   b. May idealize the deceased
   c. Mourner starts to come to terms with the loss
   d. Establishment of new social patterns and relationships
C. Grief reactions affect all areas of functioning:
1. Physiological:
   a. Loss of appetite and weight loss
   b. Insomnia and fatigue
   c. Decreased libido
   d. Increased susceptibility to illness due to decreased functioning of immune system
   e. General somatic complaints: headache, backache, and so on
2. Emotional:
   a. Profound sadness
   b. Helplessness and hopelessness
   c. Denial
   d. Anger, hostility
   e. Guilt
   f. Nightmares
   g. Thinking constantly about what was lost
   h. Loneliness and emptiness
3. Cognitive:
   a. Inability to concentrate
   b. Forgetfulness
   c. Poor judgment
   d. Inability to solve problems
4. Behavioral:
   a. Impulsive
   b. Indecisive
   c. Social withdrawal
D. Nursing diagnoses:
1. Anticipatory grieving: grieving in response to an expected significant loss
2. Grieving: normal response to loss
3. Dysfunctional grieving:
   a. Prolonged unresolved grief
   b. Dysfunctional activities in response to grief
E. Interventions:
1. Encourage client to express feelings related to loss:
   a. Use listening and communication skills.
   b. Understand that the process takes time.
2. Assure privacy.
3. Encourage client to share grief with significant others
4. Explain process of grieving so client understands it is a normal, expected response to loss
5. Help client to utilize support systems; family, church, community resources

MOOD DISORDERS

Depression

A. Sadness that is out of proportion to real events
B. Assessment findings:
    1. Physical symptoms:
        a. Sleep disturbance
        b. Alteration in weight: may be up or down
        c. Psychomotor agitation or retardation
        d. Fatigue
    2. Psychological symptoms:
        a. Decreased communication
        b. Decreased self-esteem
        c. Social withdrawal
        d. Tearful, crying
        e. Loss of interest, pleasure
        f. Recurrent thought of suicide
C. Nursing diagnoses (see Table 17.11)
D. Interventions:
    1. Primary goal is to increase self esteem.
    2. Schedule activities of daily living (ADL); encourage attention to physical needs.
    3. Encourage appropriate amounts of sleep.
    4. Structured activities
    5. Structure activities for success: assign tasks that client can achieve successfully, and give praise and recognition for success.
    6. Group and family therapy
    7. Give unconditional acceptance of the person.
    8. Encourage expression of feelings
    9. Focus on the client's strengths.
    10. Focus on non-competitive, non-intellectual activities such as leather work, sanding
    11. Frequent contacts to decrease loneliness
    12. Psychotherapy
    13. Milieu therapy
E. Suicide assessment and precautions:
    1. Say, "Often when people feel low, they think about hurting themselves. Have you thought about harming yourself?"
    2. Ask, "Do you have a plan?"
    3. Danger signs:
        a. Plan
        b. Giving away personal items
        c. Change in behavior
        d. Previous suicide attempts
        e. Verbal statement
    4. Presence of danger signs must be reported to charge nurse or physician and charted
    5. Greatest risk is when depression is lifting and client has more energy
    6. Place on suicide precautions if danger signs present:
        a. Observation
        b. Remove harmful objects such as razors, scissors, and neckties.
        c. Supervision during use of sharp objects
F. Antidepressant medication (see Table 17.12):
    1. Tricyclics
    2. Selective Serotonin Reuptake Inhibitors (SSRIs)
    3. Monamine Oxidase Inhibitors (MAOIs)

Table 17.11 Nursing Diagnoses Related to Depressive Disorders

- Risk for self-directed violence related to depressed mood and feelings of worthlessness and hopelessness
- Anxiety related to psychological conflicts
- Disturbed sleep pattern related to decreased serotonin, unresolved fears and anxieties, and inactivity
- Social isolation related to alterations in mental status and decreased energy
- Interrupted family processes related to situational crises of illness of family member
- Risk for injury related to electroconvulsive therapy
- Dressing/grooming self-care deficit related to decreased interest in body, inability to make decisions, and feelings of worthlessness
- Ineffective individual coping related to internal conflicts or feelings of rejection
- Chronic low self-esteem related to feelings of worthlessness
- Powerlessness related to unrealistic negative beliefs about self worth or abilities
- Ineffective sexuality patterns related to decreased sex drive loss of interest and pleasure
- Deficient diversional activity related to a loss of interest or pleasure in usual activities and low energy levels
- Colonic constipation related to sedentary lifestyle, lack of exercise, or inadequate diet
- Risk for imbalanced nutrition: less than body requirements related to anorexia secondary to emotional stress
- Risk for ineffective management of therapeutic regimen related to insufficient knowledge of condition, treatment options, and community resources

---

Table 17.12 Antidepressant Medications

Type	Generic Name	Trade Name	Daily Dose
Tricyclics	amitriptyline	Elavil	50–300 mg
	nortriptyline	Pamelor	20–150 mg
	protriptyline	Vivactil	5–60 mg
	amoxapine	Asendin	50–600 mg
	doxapin	Sinequan	75–300 mg
	clomipramine	Anafranil	50–250 mg
	desipramin	Norpramin	50–300 mg
	imipramine	Tofranil	50–300 mg
Selective Serotonin Reuptake Inhibitors (SSRI)	fluosetine	Prozac	20–80 mg
	paroxetine	Paxil	20–50 mg
	sertraline	Zoloft	25–200 mg
Monamine Oxidase Inhibitors (MAOI)	isocarboxazid	Marplan	30–70 mg
	phenelzine	Nardil	45–90 mg
Other	bupropion	Wellbutrin	50–600 mg
	maprotiline	Ludiomil	75–300 mg
	trazodone	Desyrel	50–600 mg
	venlafaxine	Effexor	25–375 mg

Table 17.13 Antidepressant Medications: Side Effects and Nursing Interventions

Side Effect	Nursing Interventions
Non-MAOI Antidepressants	
Drowsiness	Teach safety
Tremors, twitching	Observe
Seizures	Assess, safety, report
Insomnia	Give meds in AM
Blurred vision	May improve with time
Agitation (especially Prozac)	Observe
Hypotension	Monitor BP, teach safety
Pulse rate changes	Monitor pulse
Thrombocytopenia	Check blood work; observe for bruising
Agranulocytosis	Check blood work; observe for infection
Photosensitivity	Avoid sun
Dry mouth	Fluids, hard candy
Nausea and vomiting	Give with meals
Constipation	High-fiber diet
Urinary retention	Intake and output, decrease dosage
Altered libido	Reassure
MAOI	
As above	As above
Headache	Symptomatic treatment
Hypertensive crisis	Prevent by avoiding tyramine containing foods, monitor BP; do not lay down during crisis

Table 17.14 Foods Containing Tyramine

Aged cheese
Soy sauce
Alcoholic beverages
Pickled, smoked fish
Chocolate
Chicken/beef liver
Canned figs
Sauerkraut
Coffee
Raisins
Licorice
Processed meats
Yogurt
Spoiled /overripe fruit
Fava beans

4. Side effects and nursing interventions (see Table 17.13):
    a. Side effects relate to central nervous system depression, anticholinergic effects, photosensitivity, and blood dyscrasias
    b. MAOIs have additional problem of hypertensive crisis when client eats foods containing tyramine
5. Teach client about medications:
    a. It takes 3–6 weeks for a therapeutic effect.
    b. Continue medication until told otherwise.
    c. Use caution while driving until adjusted to the medications.
    d. Avoid abrupt withdrawal.
    e. Avoid sun.
    f. Report symptoms of infection.
    g. Report changes in heart rate or difficulty urinating.
    h. Do not drink alcohol.
    i. Do not take non-MAOIs with MAOIs or other CNS depressants.
    j. Persons taking MAOIs should avoid foods containing tyramine for two days before starting medication and two weeks after stopping medication (see Table 17.14).
    k. Persons taking MAOIs should avoid drugs affecting the CNS.

G. Electroconvulsive therapy (ECT):
    1. A grand mal seizure is induced by passing an electrical current through electrodes applied to the temples. It is used primarily to treat depression but has been used to treat schizophrenia and acute mania. Persons who do not respond to antidepressants often have significant improvement with ECT.
    2. Prepare client as if going to surgery: sign permit, NPO.
    3. Anesthesia and muscle relaxants are administered.
    4. The patient has no memory of the treatment.
    5. After the procedure, expect transitory memory loss and confusion.
    6. Recent literature states that ECT is safer than medication as a treatment for depression.

Bipolar Disorder

A. Periods of elation alternating with depression with or without a period of normalcy
B. Elation:
    1. A seemingly pleasurable affect that is characterized by an air of happiness and self-confidence as well as extreme motor activity
    2. Caused by a real or threatened loss of self-esteem or massive denial of depression
    3. May also have biochemical basis
    4. Assessment findings:
        a. Mild:
            (1) Euphoric
            (2) Life of the party
            (3) Superficial relationships
        b. Acute: hypomania (moderate degree of mania):
            (1) Thought disorders
            (2) Flight of ideas
            (3) Delusions of grandeur

Table 17.15 Nursing Diagnoses Related to Mania

- Risk for violence directed at others related to irritability, impulsive behavior, and delusional thinking
- Imbalanced nutrition: less than body requirements related to inadequate intake in relation to metabolic expenditures
- Risk for poisoning, lithium toxicity, related to narrow therapeutic range of drug, patient's inability to follow through with medication regimen and monitoring
- Disturbed sleep pattern related to hyperactivity
- Disturbed sensory perception related to decrease in sensory threshold, chemical alteration, psychologic stress, and sleep deprivation
- Interrupted family processes related to situational crises
- Impaired social interaction related to overt hostility, overconfidence, or manipulation of others
- Disturbed thought processes related to flight of ideas, delusions, or hallucinations
- Impaired verbal communication related to pressured speech and hyperactivity
- Risk for deficient fluid volume related to altered sodium excretion secondary to lithium therapy.
- Noncompliance related to feelings of no longer requiring medication
- Risk for ineffective management of therapeutic regimen related to insufficient knowledge of condition, pharmacological therapy, and follow-up care

Table 17.16 Lithium

Class	Generic Name	Trade Name	Dose	Notes
Lithium	Lithium	Eskalith Lithonate Lithotabs Lithobid	600–1800 mg daily	Initially dose is regulated by daily monitoring of blood levels 12 hours after last dose; blood levels less frequently after regulation. Blood Levels: 0.5–1.4 mEq/l = therapeutic level > 2.0 mEq/l = toxic > 2.5 mEq/l = lethal

Table 17.17 Lithium: Side Effects and Nursing Interventions

Side Effects	Interventions
Fine tremors	Monitor
Fatigue, drowsiness	Short naps
Headache	Medication
Acne	Treat symptoms
Anorexia, nausea, vomiting, diarrhea	Frequent small meals, hydrate
Diarrhea	Take with meals.
Polyuria	Avoid excessive caffeine.
Polydipsia	Drink 6–8 glasses water
Toxic effects: coarse tremors, lethargy, seizures, vertigo, hypotension, irregular pulse, ataxia, slurred speech, coma	Hold lithium, obtain lithium level, monitor vital signs

(4) Short attention span
(5) Little sleep
(6) Uninhibited
(7) Psychomotor activity greatly exaggerated; may need hospitalization

5. Nursing diagnoses (see Table 17.15)
6. Interventions:
   a. Deal with physical problems resulting from manic state; finger foods, cleanliness, and sleep.
   b. Set limits.
   c. Decrease stimuli.
   d. Give simple directions.
   e. Redirect thoughts.
   f. Pace speech.
   g. Provide activities with movement.
   h. Avoid arguing.
   i. Sometimes ECT
   j. Psychotherapy
   k. Milieu therapy
   l. Chemotherapy: lithium (see Tables 17.16 and 17.17)
   m. Teach client about lithium:
      (1) Takes 1–4 weeks to reach therapeutic level
      (2) Avoid driving until lithium dose stable
      (3) Don't reduce sodium in diet: lithium is excreted in the urine as a sodium salt
      (4) Avoid caffeine, thiazide diuretics, and NSAIDs.
      (5) Regular blood tests for lithium levels are essential.
      (6) Weight gain is a normal response.
      (7) Notify physician if there are signs of toxicity.

SCHIZOPHRENIA

A. A condition of extreme anxiety manifested by psychotic behavior with disturbances of mood, thought, feelings, perceptions, behaviors, personality disintegration, difficulty in functioning, and impairment in reality testing
B. Several theories exist as to the cause of schizophrenia. It is probably at least in part related to neurochemical imbalances, especially dopamine. The tendency for schizophrenia seems to be inherited.
C. Major types:
   1. Catatonic: psychomotor:
      a. Stupor

b. Excitement; may run around in circles
c. Waxy flexibility, bizarre posturing; when positioned will stay in that position for hours at a time without moving
d. Negativism; does the opposite of what is asked
e. Mutism; says nothing

2. Paranoid:
   a. Hallucinations; may be grandiose or persecutory
   b. Delusions of persecution or grandeur
   c. Emotions; often angry, anxious, violent, suspicious

D. Assessment findings:
   1. Associative looseness; disorganized thinking
   2. Affect (external expression of emotion):
      a. Inappropriate to situation
      b. Exaggerated (flat or overexcited)
   3. Ambivalence (conflicting strong feelings; hates and loves the same thing)
   4. Autism: preoccupation with inner thoughts, little connection to the real world
      a. Delusions: fixed false belief; "I am the King of England."
      b. Hallucinations: sensory experience (visual, auditory, touch, taste, smell) for which there is no organic basis
      c. Ideas of reference: incorrect idea that another person's words or actions refer to one's self (when seeing a nurse talking on the telephone, believing the nurse is talking about him)
      d. Depersonalization: sense of one's reality is lost; a feeling that one does not control one's own actions and speech

E. Nursing diagnoses (see Table 17.18)
F. Interventions:
   1. Psychotherapy
   2. ECT (see electroconvulsive therapy)

3. Antipsychotic medication (see Tables 17.19 and 17.20)
4. Teach client regarding medications:
   a. Use caution in driving until adjusted to medications.
   b. Do not abruptly stop medication.
   c. Wear sunscreen and protective clothing when exposed to sun.
   d. Report sore throat, fever, malaise, unusual bleeding, easy bruising, nausea, rapid heart beat, difficulty urinating, tremors, dark urine, yellow skin or eyes, or rash.
   e. Pink to reddish-brown urine is normal.
   f. Drink no alcoholic beverages because of CNS effects.
   g. Drug interactions: antidepressants, MAOI, CNS depressants, anticonvulsants, lithium

5. Medications to control Parkinson's syndrome from antipsychotic medications (see Table 17.21)
6. Short-term nursing care:
   a. Encourage trust.
   b. Encourage participation in milieu therapy.
   c. Encourage personal hygiene.
   d. Encourage decrease of hallucinations:
      (1) Respond to anything real.
      (2) Focus on feelings.
      (3) Avoid direct confrontations.
      (4) Voice doubt (I don't hear the voices).
      (5) Allow short, frequent contacts.
   e. Encourage decrease of delusions:
      (1) Help to recognize misinterpretations.
      (2) Help to reality test
   f. Assist in feeling safe in one-to-one relationship:
      (1) Use activity as a medium.
      (2) Avoid making demands or competition.

Table 17.18 Nursing Diagnoses Related to Schizophrenia

- Disturbed thought processes related to disintegration of thinking processes, impaired judgment, psychological conflicts
- Social isolation related to alterations in mental status, mistrust of others/delusional thinking, unacceptable social behavior
- Ineffective health maintenance/home management program may be related to impaired cognitive/emotional functioning, altered communications
- Risk for violence directed at self and others related to delusional thinking or hallucinations
- Ineffective individual coping related to personal vulnerability, disintegration of thought
- Interrupted family processes related to ambivalent family system, change of roles and difficulty coping with client's maladaptive behavior
- Self-care deficit related to perceptual and cognitive impairment
- Impaired verbal communication related to incoherent/illogical speech pattern and side effects of medications

Table 17.19 Antipsychotic Medications

Generic Name	Trade Name	Daily Dose
Phenothiazines		
chlorpromazine	Thorazine	30–1200 mg
fluphenazine	Prolixin	5–20 mg
thioridazine	Mellaril	200–600 mg
Thioxanthene		
thioxene	Navane	6–60 mg
Butyrophanons		
haloperidol	Haldol	2–20 mg
Atypical Antipsychotics		
clozapine	Clozaril	300–900 mg
risperidone	Risperdal	1–6 mg
olanzapine	Zyprexa	10 mg

Table 17.20 Antipsychotic Medications: Side Effects and Interventions

Side Effect	Nursing Intervention
Central Nervous System	
Sedation	Safety, do not drive until adjusted to medication; usually decreased over time; give at bedtime
Extrapyramidal Symptoms (EPS)	Report to physician; dosage may be changed
Tremors	
Parkinson's Syndrome (tremors, rigid posture, mask-like face)	Antiparkinson agents may be given
Neuroleptic Malignant Syndrome (NMS) (rigidity, confusion, fever, coma, death)	Notify physician
Akathisia (motor restlessness, need to keep moving)	Notify physician; change of drug may be ordered
Tardive dyskinesia (irreversible involuntary movements of tongue, face, extremities)	Notify physician; drug holiday, supportive treatment
Dystonia (sudden spasm in the face and neck, eyes roll back in head)	Notify physician; drug holiday, supportive treatment
Anticholinergic	
Nausea	
Dry mouth	Candies, fluids
Constipation	High fiber diet, laxatives
Urinary retention	Intake and output
Blurred vision	Disappears in a week
Cardiovascular	
Hypotension	Monitor BP.
Tachycardia	Monitor
Agranulocytosis	Report any signs of infection such as sore throats that do not go away.
Other	
Photosensitivity	Wear sunscreen and protective clothing when exposed to the sun.
Amenorrhea	Reassure that menstrual changes are due to medication

Table 17.21 Drugs Used to Treat Extrapyramidal Symptoms

Generic Name	Trade Name	Daily Dose
Anticholinergics		
benztropine	Cogentin	1–6 mg
trihexyphenidyl	Artane	1–10 mg
biperiden	Akineton	2–6 mg

7. Long-term nursing care:
    a. Encourage use of supportive agencies, people.
    b. Encourage resumption of work and relationships.
    c. Encourage pattern of regular eating and sleeping.

SUSPICIOUS AND PARANOID BEHAVIORS

A. Paranoia is a syndrome in which there is a tight, systematic, delusional system of persecution; a delusion is a false, fixed belief.

B. Assessment findings:
    1. Projection of one's unacceptable feelings to others
    2. Delusions of grandeur and control
    3. Ideas of reference
    4. Noncompliance with medical regime
    5. Loneliness
    6. Distrust, suspicion
    7. Argumentative, hostile
C. Nursing diagnoses (see Table 17.22)
D. Interventions:
    1. Delusions:
        a. Do not argue or confront.
        b. Distract to reality.
        c. Get to feeling level.
        d. Use anything real to communicate.
    2. Aggression and hostility:
        a. Monitor
        b. Help client to express hostility verbally rather than acting out.
        c. Set limits and offer alternatives.
        d. Provide outlets for aggression, such as punching bags or physical activity.
        e. No competitive activities, such as basketball games.
        f. Remind client of consequences.

Table 17.22 Nursing Diagnoses Related to Suspicious and Paranoid Behaviors

- Risk for violence directed at self or others related to perceived threats of danger, paranoid delusions, and increased feelings of anxiety
- Severe anxiety related to inability to trust
- Powerlessness related to feelings of inadequacy, maladaptive interpersonal interactions
- Disturbed thought processes related to inability to evaluate reality secondary to feelings of mistrust
- Ineffective family coping related to family disorganization and role changes
- Impaired social interactions related to feelings of mistrust and suspicions of others
- Social isolation related to fear and mistrust of situations and of others
- Risk for imbalanced nutrition: less than body requirements related to reluctance to eat secondary to fear of poisoning

g. Keep a safe distance.
h. Have backup personnel.
i. Be calm, direct, and simple.
j. Time out seclusion to decrease stimulation.
k. Medication (see Table 17.19)
l. Safety
3. Fear of being poisoned:
a. Serve food in individual containers.
b. Medications should be wrapped or in containers; unit dose.
4. Attitude of superiority:
a. One to one; small groups
b. Activities that insure success
c. Set limits without judging.
d. Increase self esteem.
5. Antipsychotic medications (see Table 17.19)

PERSONALITY DISORDERS

A. Disorders in which persons have difficulty adjusting to life situations and experience inadequate interactions with society; the individual exhibits behavioral problems rather than symptoms.
B. Causes may be both genetic tendency and learned responses; individual has poor ego and superego development; may have had unresponsive or inappropriate mother-child relationship
C. Assessment findings:
1. Antisocial behavior:
a. Superficial charm, wit, intelligence, manipulative; often seductive behavior
b. Inability or refusal to accept responsibility for self-serving, destructive behavior
c. Failure at school and work, delinquency, rule violations, inability to keep a job

Table 17.23 Nursing Diagnoses Related to Personality Disorders

- Ineffective individual coping related to subordinating one's needs to decisions of others
- Ineffective individual coping: inappropriate intense anger, poor impulse control, marked mood shifts, habitual disregard for social norms related to altered inability to meet responsibilities
- Impaired social interaction related to inability to maintain enduring attachments
- Ineffective individual coping related to resistance (procrastination, stubbornness, intentional inefficiency) in responses to responsibilities

Borderline Personality Disorder, add the following:
- Risk for self-mutilation related to used of projection as a major defense mechanism, distorted sense of self, feelings of guilt, and need to punish self
- Severe anxiety related to unconscious conflicts, perceived threat to self concept, unmet needs
- Chronic low self-esteem related to lack of positive feedback, unmet dependency needs, retarded ego development
- Social isolation related to immature interests, unaccepted social behavior, inadequate personal resources, and inability to engage in satisfying personal relationships

d. Promiscuity, desertion, two or more divorces and separations
e. Repeated substance abuse
f. Thefts, vandalism, multiple arrests
g. Inability to function as a responsible parent
h. Fights, assaults, abuse of others
i. Impulsiveness, recklessness, inability to plan ahead
j. Inappropriate affect; not sorry for violating others
2. Borderline personality:
a. Impulsive and unpredictable behavior in self-damaging areas—spending, sex, gambling
b. Unstable and intense interpersonal relationships
c. Inappropriate, intense anger
d. Identity disturbance with uncertain self image and imitative behavior
e. Unstable affect with mood swings
f. Intolerance of being alone; chronic feelings of emptiness or boredom
g. Self-destructive behavior, suicidal gestures, self mutilation, frequent accidents and fights
3. Passive-Aggressive:
a. Intentional inefficiency
b. Chronic lateness, procrastination
c. Complaining and blaming behavior
d. Feelings of confusion and mistreatment
e. Fear of authority
D. Nursing diagnoses (see Table 17.23)
E. Interventions:
1. Be aware of own feelings
2. Patience, persistence, consistency

3. Direct approach; confrontation
4. Teach social skills.
5. Reinforce appropriate behavior.
6. Set limits, rules, and regulations; consequences should be clear.
7. Encourage responsibility and accountability.
8. Help delay gratification.
9. Protect other clients from verbal and physical abuse.
10. Contract for behavioral changes.

SUBSTANCE ABUSE

A. Any process by which a person ingests any mind-altering, non-prescribed chemical that produces physiological and psychological dependence; withdrawal symptoms are usually manifest when substance is not taken.
B. Related terms:
   1. Abuse: drug use leading to legal, social, and/or medical problems
   2. Addiction: physical dependence
   3. Dependence: a need resulting from continued use; results in mental or physical discomfort upon withdrawal of the substance
   4. Tolerance: need for increasing amounts to achieve the same effect
C. Contributing factors:
   1. Genetic predisposition
   2. Peer pressure and social approval
   3. Low self-esteem
   4. Low frustration tolerance
   5. Availability of substance

Alcohol Dependence/Abuse

A. Characteristics of alcohol abuse:
   1. Alcohol is a CNS depressant with progression from relaxation to slurred speech and impaired motor activities to stupor and anesthesia.
   2. Blood alcohol concentration (BAC):
      a. 10% (10 mg/100 ml blood or 0.10) is legal intoxication for driving in most states; some have lowered the level (3–5 cocktails, 6 beers, and 20 oz. wine).
      b. Death may occur at levels of .30 or higher; death is due to respiratory paralysis (10 cocktails)
      c. At .60, death is likely due to cardio-respiratory impairment (20 cocktails).
      d. The liver detoxifies alcohol at 3/4 oz./hr. (3/4 oz. = 12 oz. beer or 4 oz. wine or one shot whiskey).
B. Assessment findings:
   1. Person initially uses alcohol for relaxation and freedom from anxiety
   2. Tolerance develops after prolonged use: person can drink larger amounts of alcohol without being affected; needs more alcohol to have an effect
   3. Loss of control
   4. Blackouts: fugue-like state where alcoholic acts normally but remembers nothing for that period of time
   5. Progression of alcoholism continues as tolerance reverses and alcohol quickly affects person
   6. Physical effects are apparent in all body systems:
      a. Nervous system:
         (1) Psychosis
         (2) Dementia
         (3) Seizure
         (4) Wernicke-Korsakoff's syndrome (motor and sensory disturbances and loss of memory due to alcoholism and vitamin B_1, or thiamine, deficiency)
         (5) Peripheral neuropathy
         (6) Poor coordination
      b. Cardiovascular system:
         (1) Dysrhythmias
         (2) Hypertension
         (3) Myopathy
         (4) Easy bruising and bleeding
      c. Gastrointestinal system:
         (1) Gastritis and ulcers
         (2) Pancreatitis
         (3) Cirrhosis of the liver
         (4) Hypoglycemia
         (5) Esophageal varices
      d. Respiratory system:
         (1) COPD
         (2) Pneumonia
         (3) Cancer
      e. Genitourinary system:
         (1) Fetal alcohol syndrome in infants born to women who drink during pregnancy
         (2) Decreased libido
      f. Skin and skeletal systems:
         (1) Ulcers
         (2) Spider angiomas
         (3) Fractures
      g. Psychological and social effects:
         (1) Erratic, impulsive, abusive behavior
         (2) Poor judgment
         (3) Memory loss
         (4) Family problems
         (5) Depression
         (6) Suicide: up to 21% of alcoholics commit suicide
         (7) Loss of job
   7. Withdrawal:
      a. Physical symptoms developing 8–48 hours after abstinence from or sharp reduction in alcohol; lasting 5–7 days
         (1) Shakiness and tremors
         (2) Anxiety
         (3) Mood swings

(4) Insomnia
(5) Impaired appetite
(6) Confusion
(7) Elevated vital signs
(8) Diaphoresis
  b. Delirium tremens (DTs):
      (1) Acute medical condition occurring 2–4 days after abstinence lasting 48–72 hours
      (2) Symptoms:
          (a) Confusion and disorientation
          (b) Visual, auditory, tactile hallucinations
          (c) Convulsions
C. Nursing diagnoses (see Table 17.24)

Table 17.24 Nursing Diagnoses Related to Alcoholism/Substance Abuse

- Imbalanced nutrition: less than body requirement related to anorexia
- Risk for deficient fluid volume related to abnormal fluid loss secondary to vomiting and diarrhea
- Risk for injury related to disorientation, tremors, or impaired judgment
- Risk for self harm related to disorientation, tremors, or impaired judgment
- Risk for violence related to impulsive behavior, disorientation, tremors, or impaired judgment
- Disturbed sleep pattern related to irritability, tremors, and nightmares
- Anxiety related to loss of control, memory losses, and fear of withdrawal
- Ineffective individual coping: anger, dependence, or denial related to inability to manage stressors constructively without drugs/alcohol
- Social isolation related to loss of work or withdrawal from others
- Ineffective sexuality patterns related to impotence/loss of libido secondary to altered self-concept and substance abuse
- Ineffective family coping related to disruption in family relationship and inconsistent limit setting
- Risk for ineffective management of therapeutic regimen related to insufficient knowledge of condition, treatments available, high-risk situations, and community resources
- Interrupted family process related to abuse of alcohol, resistance to treatment.

D. Interventions:
  1. Detoxification; 3–5 days to prevent withdrawal and DTs:
      a. Antianxiety medications to reduce tremors and prevent seizures
      b. Fluids and vitamins, especially thiamine
      c. Antidiarrheal medicine
  2. Delirium tremens (DTs):
      a. Quiet, moderately lighted area; no shadows because client may misinterpret shadows (illusions)
      b. Decrease stimuli to reduce illusions and chance of seizures.
      c. Restraints if needed and seclusion if needed

  d. Client safety is a major concern because client is impulsive and not fully rational.
3. Set limits.
4. Nonjudgmental support
5. Avoid being manipulated; substance abusers are good at manipulating people.
6. Monitor visitors to prevent introduction of addictive substances.
7. Confrontation of denial
8. Encourage rehabilitation programs and after care (AA).
9. Educate and support family; Alanon, Alateen
10. Rehabilitation:
      a. 30-day program essential with family therapy
      b. AA: 12-step recovery program
      c. Antabuse to prevent use of alcohol (see Table 17.25)

Table 17.25 Antabuse

Action	Interferes with breakdown of alcohol
Effects when alcohol is present	Nausea and vomiting Hypotension, rapid pulse, chest pain Flushing Confusion Respiratory and circulatory collapse
Patient education	NO ALCOHOL in any form No: cough and cold medicine, rubbing alcohol, shaving lotion, mouthwash; abstain 12 hours before taking Antabuse; no alcohol for two weeks after last dose; carry ID re: Antabuse Side effects: headache, dry mouth, flushing

Drug Abuse/Dependence

A. Assessment findings:
  1. Physiological:
      a. Effects on the CNS depends on the substance
      b. Endocarditis related to use of dirty needles
      c. Hepatitis
      d. HIV infection and AIDS
      e. Pulmonary emboli
      f. Gangrene from infections and poor circulation
      g. Malnutrition
      h. Trauma
      i. Psychosis
  2. Psychological and social effects:
      a. Isolation and withdrawal
      b. Family and work problems
      c. Loss of property
      d. Incarceration
B. Nursing diagnoses (see Table 17.24)
C. Interventions:
  1. Detoxification (see Table 17.26)
  2. Care for coexisting problems such as hepatitis, endocarditis, malnutrition

Table 17.26 Drugs Abused and Treatment

Drug	Symptoms When Using	Withdrawal Symptoms	Detox Regime
Barbiturates, Tranquilizers, Librium, Valium, Chloral Hydrate	Irritable, labile, impaired judgment, attention, memory, uncoordinated, talkative	Hypersensitivity, elevated vital signs, anxiety, delirium tremors, convulsions, irritability	Use same or similar drug in decreasing amounts over 3–5 days to prevent seizures
Opiates: Heroin, Morphine, Methadone	Euphoria, apathy; impaired judgment, memory and attention; anxiety; pupils constricted	Lacrimation (tearing), rhinorrhea, dilated pupils, yawning; elevated vital signs, insomnia, diarrhea	Methadone in decreasing doses over three days to prevent seizures
Cocaine	Agitation, elation, elevated BP and P, dilated pupils, talkative, grandiose	Depression, anxiety, irritability, paranoia, sleeplessness, convulsions, may attempt suicide	No drugs used
Amphetamines: Speed, diet pills	Agitation, elation, elevated BP and P, dilated pupil, talkative	Delusions, depression, anxiety, insomnia, aggression, agitation	Symptomatic only
Hallucinogens: PCP, LSD	Elevated BP and P, labile, Perceptual changes (thinks he can fly), impaired judgment, ideas of reference, ataxia, dilated pupils	Psychosis, agitation, hallucinations, may attempt suicide	None; Haldol if psychosis or out of control

3. Rehabilitation
   a. 30 days to 2 years in treatment
   b. Lifelong AA or NA
   c. Will need support in the community
   d. Job skills training, other community resources

Impaired Nurses

A. Nurses who abuse substances such as narcotics or alcohol
B. Assessment findings—warning signs:
   1. Frequent absenteeism
   2. Overworking
   3. Mood changes
   4. Inappropriate affect
   5. Inconsistent nursing care
   6. Narcotic count not accurate
   7. Altered judgment
   8. Alcohol on breath
   9. Frequent visits to restroom
   10. Frequent night shifts
   11. Patients complain of poor pain relief
C. Interventions:
   1. Client safety is first concern; report to supervisor
   2. Document
   3. Verify information with others.
   4. Employer may confront and offer treatment.
   5. Rehabilitation
   6. AA, NA
   7. If the nurse denies or refuses treatment, he/she will be dismissed.
   8. Report to Board of Nursing (usually done by supervisor or employer).
   9. Report to law enforcement if drug theft (usually done by supervisor or employer).

FAMILY VIOLENCE

A. Abuse of a violent physical or verbal nature within a family; crosses socioeconomic, religious, racial, and cultural lines; the abused can be wife, husband, child, or the elderly
B. Types of abuse:
   1. Physical: pushing, hitting, throwing, and so on
   2. Psychological: verbal degrading
   3. Sexual: wife, child, friend, stranger
   4. Neglect: not providing needed medical, physical, psychological care
C. Characteristics of abuser:
   1. Low self-esteem
   2. Alcohol or drug user
   3. Projects
   4. Anxious
   5. Depressed
   6. History of abuse as a child
   7. Socially isolated
   8. Impulsive, immature
   9. Guilt
D. Characteristics of abused:
   1. May have many of the characteristics of the abuser
   2. Accepts responsibility for others; "It's my fault he hit me, dinner was five minutes late."
   3. Helpless
   4. Suicidal at times
   5. Submissive
   6. Frightened
E. Assessment findings in the abused:
   1. Sleep disorders
   2. Headaches
   3. Anxiety
   4. Suicidal ideation

5. Substance abuse
6. Disruptive behavior at home, school, work
7. Physical abuse:
   a. Multiple injuries in various stages of healing
   b. Unexplained bruised, burns, fractures, lacerations
   c. Incongruence between explanation of injury and injury
   d. Wary of strangers
   e. Labile behavior
   f. Frightened, stiff, rigid, distant
8. Physical neglect: child, elderly:
   a. Poor hygiene, dress
   b. Medical and physical problems not cared for
   c. Fatigue
   d. Withdrawal
   e. Substance abuse
9. Sexual abuse:
   a. Venereal disease
   b. Pregnancy
   c. Pain or itching in vaginal area
   d. Unusual sexual behavior or knowledge (in children)
   e. Poor peer relations
   f. Reports of sexual assault
10. Emotional abuse or neglect:
    a. Decreased self-esteem
    b. Hypochondriasis
    c. Developmental lag (in children)
    d. Sleep disorders
    e. Behavioral extremes
F. Nursing diagnoses (see Table 17.27)
G. Nursing interventions:
   1. Ask in detail about the symptoms.
   2. Build trust.

Table 17.27 Nursing Diagnoses Related to Abuse

- Risk for trauma related to history of previous abuse, dependence, lack of support systems by caregiver
- Impaired parenting related to poor role model, presence of stressors, lack of support
- Self-esteem disturbance related to deprivation and negative feedback of family members
- Post trauma response related to sustained/recurrent physical or emotional abuse
- Ineffective family coping related to situational or developmental crisis and family disorganization
- Ineffective individual coping (abuser) related to history of abuse by own parents, marked lack of self esteem with low tolerance for criticism, emotional immaturity
- Ineffective individual coping (nonabusing parent) related to passive and compliant response to abuse
- Fear related to possibility of placement in a shelter or foster home.
- Parental fear related to responses of others, possible loss of child, and criminal prosecution
- Risk for imbalanced nutrition: less than body requirements related to inadequate intake secondary to lack of knowledge or neglect
- Risk for ineffective management of therapeutic regimen related to insufficient knowledge of parenting skills, stress management.

3. Be nonjudgmental.
4. Do not give advice.
5. Determine seriousness of battering; if child, call proper authorities
6. Identify resources: housing, money, legal aid, vocational, crisis center

RAPE

A. Rape is a crime of violence (force, penetration, and lack of consent) not passion; the motives are power and anger.
B. Common misconceptions about rape:
   1. It is provoked by actions of the victim.
   2. The victim is promiscuous or wears too-revealing clothes.
   3. A woman cannot be raped against her will.
   4. Rape is an impulsive act.
   5. Women frequently get revenge by accusing men of rape.
C. Assessment findings:
   1. Reports or evidence of sexual assault
   2. Acute phase
      a. Physiological responses:
         (1) Gastrointestinal irritability (nausea, vomiting, anorexia)
         (2) Genitourinary discomfort (pain, pruritus)
         (3) Skeletal muscle tension (spasms, pain)
      b. Psychological responses:
         (1) Denial
         (2) Emotional shock
         (3) Anger
         (4) Fear of being alone or that the rapist will return; children fear punishment, abandonment
         (5) Guilt
         (6) Panic upon seeing assailant or the scene of the attack
      c. Sexual responses:
         (1) Mistrust of men
         (2) Change in sexual behavior
   3. Long-term phase:
      a. Any response of the acute phase may continue if resolution does not occur.
      b. Psychological responses such as phobias, nightmares, sleep disturbances, anxiety, depression
D. Nursing diagnoses (see Table 17.28)

Table 17.28 Nursing Diagnoses Related to Rape

- Rape trauma syndrome
- Risk for injury related to violent assault
- Risk for infection
- Ineffective family coping related to disruption in family functioning, attitude of spouse

E. Interventions:
1. Crisis intervention
2. Emergency action:
    a. Evidence collection (aspirate vagina for semen, comb pubic hair for hairs from assailant)
    b. Treat physical wounds if present.
    c. Assign female nurses or physician if possible.
    d. Documentation of events, injuries
    e. Comfort; make her feel safe; one staff member care for client
    f. Involve the rape response team if available.
    g. Arrange for follow-up; make client aware of support services.
3. Will want to shower to get clean
4. Long term:
    a. Support groups
    b. Help with disrupted relationships
    c. Treatment of phobias, nightmares, and so on if they develop
    d. Encourage talking and working through.

Age-Related Disorders

AUTISTIC DISORDER

A. A syndrome beginning in infancy characterized by extreme withdrawal and an obsessive desire to maintain the status quo
B. Assessment findings:
1. Lack of awareness of the existence or feelings of others
2. Does not seek comfort from others
3. No mode of communication
4. Stereotyped body movements
5. Impaired social play
C. Nursing diagnoses (see Table 17.29)
D. Interventions:
1. Assess social and physical aspects of client and family.
2. Establish verbal or nonverbal communication.
3. Help the child to the next developmental level.
4. Use story telling, painting, and poetry.
5. Priorities of care:
    a. Safety
    b. Communication
    c. Re-education

Table 17.29 Nursing Diagnoses Related to Autistic Disorder

- Impaired social interaction related to abnormal response to sensory input, organic brain dysfunction, lack of intuitive skills to comprehend and accurately respond to social cues
- Impaired verbal communication related to inability to trust others, withdrawal into self, organic brain dysfunction, abnormal interpretation/response sensory stimulation
- Risk for self-mutilation related to organic brain dysfunction, inability to trust others, disturbance in self-concept, inadequate sensory stimulation
- Compromised family coping related to family members unable to express feelings, excessive guilt, anger, or blaming among family members

CHRONIC ORGANIC BRAIN SYNDROMES

A. Characterized by irreversible brain damage and gradual destruction of neurons
B. General assessment findings:
1. Confabulations (making up stories to fill in gaps in memory)
2. Blocking
3. Motor impairment
4. Disintegrating personality
5. Disintegrating behavior
6. Short-term memory impairment
7. Judgment impairment
8. Abstract thinking impairment
9. Months to years
C. Types of organic brain disease and assessment findings:
1. Wernike's— Korsakoff's Syndrome (dementia associated with alcoholism and thiamine deficiency):
    a. Long- and short-term memory impairment
    b. Confabulation
    c. Polyneuritis
    d. Flat affect
    e. Ataxia
    f. Confusion
    g. Learning impaired
2. Alzheimer's Disease (primary degenerative dementia):
    a. Onset after age 45
    b. Progressive and chronic
    c. Decreased cognitive function
    d. Behavior changes
    e. Can live up to 15 years after onset
    f. First phase: forgetfulness:
        (1) Anxiety
        (2) Recent memory impaired
        (3) Shortened retention of information

g. Confusion phase:
    (1) Orientation disturbance
    (2) Concentration decreases
    (3) Forgets words
    (4) Denies there is a problem
h. Dementia phase:
    (1) Disorientation
    (2) Anxiety and denial
    (3) Delusions, hallucinations, paranoia
    (4) Agitation
    (5) Physical deterioration

D. Nursing diagnoses (see Table 17.30)
E. Interventions:
1. Allow as much independence as is safe.
2. Treat medical symptoms.
3. Nutrition; finger foods
4. Limit fluids at night to reduce nocturnal incontinence.
5. Suggest tool softeners; use toilet regularly
6. ROM, walk, keep awake during day
7. Monitor safety; client may wander
8. Eliminate multiple stimuli.
9. Make short, simple conversation.
10. Speak slowly and distinctly.
11. Ask client to make only small decisions.
12. Break tasks into small steps.
13. Provide consistency in care; routines, persons.
14. Orient to person, place, time.
15. Visual cues: pictures, labels
16. Provide human contact.
17. Help families to understand.

Table 17.30 Nursing Diagnoses Related to Organic Brain Disorders

- Risk for injury related to lack of awareness of surroundings, confusion
- Chronic confusion related to physiologic brain changes
- Impaired physical mobility related to gait instability
- Risk for interrupted family processes related to effects of condition on relationships, role responsibilities, and finances
- Impaired home maintenance management related to inability to care for self, home, or inadequate or unavailable caregiver
- Unilateral neglect related to neurological pathology
- Self-care deficit
- Decisional conflict related to placement of person in a care facility
- Caregiver role strain related to multiple care needs and insufficient resources
- Disturbed sensory perception related to neurological deficit
- Disturbed sleep pattern related to sensory impairment, changes in activity patterns, neurological impairment
- Ineffective health maintenance related to deterioration affecting ability in all areas including coordination, communication, and cognitive impairment
- Risk for relocation stress syndrome related to little preparation for transfer to a new setting, inability to understand changes in daily routine, separation from support systems

Legal Aspects of Psychiatric Nursing

TYPES OF ADMISSIONS

A. Voluntary:
1. Persons who admit themselves
2. Must give consent for all treatment
3. Can refuse treatment including medications unless they are a danger to self or others
B. Involuntary judicial process:
1. Initiated when someone files a petition
2. Certification by two physicians that person possesses the likelihood of serious harm to self or others
3. Under 18: parents can confine
4. Must be released at end of statutory time or put on voluntary status or have another hearing

RIGHTS OF PSYCHIATRIC CLIENTS

A. Unless declared incompetent they maintain all previous rights:
1. Stationary and postage
2. Unopened mail
3. Visits by physician, attorney, and clergy
4. Visits by other people
5. Keep personal possessions
6. Keep and spend money
7. Storage space for personal items
8. Telephone access
9. Hold property, vote, marry
10. Education
11. Challenge retention
B. Right to treatment:
1. Humane psychological and physical environment
2. Qualified personnel and adequate nursing
3. Individual treatment plan
C. Least restrictive alternative
D. Informed consent must be obtained for procedures such as ECT, medications, seclusion, and restraint.

Sample Questions

1. When the nurse detects that a client is using defense mechanisms, the nurse should make

which of these interpretations of the client's behavior?

1. The client is attempting to reestablish emotional equilibrium.
2. The client is using self-defeating measures.
3. The client is demonstrating illness.
4. The client is asking for support from significant others.

2. The treatment goal for a client with severe anxiety will have been achieved when the client demonstrates which of these behaviors?
   1. The client recognizes the source of the anxiety.
   2. The client is able to use the anxiety constructively.
   3. The client can function without any sense of anxiety.
   4. The client identifies the physical effects of the anxiety.

3. The nurse is assessing a 22-month-old child who is thought to be autistic. During an interview with the nurse, the child's mother makes all of the following statements about his behavior until he was one year old. Which statement most strongly suggests that the child may be autistic?
   1. "He was a good baby and rarely cried when I left the room."
   2. "He slept very well after each feeding."
   3. "He spit out every new food the first time I gave it to him."
   4. "He started to walk without learning to crawl first."

4. In attempting to establish a therapeutic relationship with a child who may be autistic, the nurse should expect to encounter which of these problems?
   1. Hallucinating
   2. Impaired hearing
   3. Bizarre behavior
   4. Clinging to others

5. To initiate a relationship with a child who may be autistic, the nurse would probably be most effective by using which of these approaches?
   1. Playing peek-a-boo
   2. Having him point to designated body parts
   3. Sitting with him
   4. Playing an action game like Ring Around the Rosy

6. The nurse is caring for a 75-year-old widow admitted to the psychiatric hospital by her daughter, who became concerned when her mother began to talk in a confused manner about her husband who has been dead for seven years. In the hospital, especially at night, the client wanders in the other clients' rooms looking for her husband. What is the most appropriate action for the nurse to take when this woman wanders in the rooms of the other clients?
   1. Lock the door to her room.
   2. Tell her to stay in her room except for meals.

3. Take her by the hand and guide her back to her room.
4. Tell her that she will be restrained if she continues to wander.

7. The nurse is caring for an elderly woman admitted with chronic organic brain disease. When her daughter visits, she asks, "Are you my maid?" How should the nurse describe the client's behavior?
   1. Impaired judgment
   2. Disorientation
   3. Impairment of abstract thinking
   4. Delusions

8. An elderly woman is hospitalized with chronic organic brain syndrome. When her daughter visits, she does not recognize her. The daughter begins to cry and shares her concerns with the nurse. Which statement by the nurse would demonstrate an empathetic response?
   1. "It must be difficult for you to visit your mother when she is confused about who you are."
   2. "If you are going to cry when you come to visit, maybe you should not visit."
   3. "It is not unusual for people in your mother's condition to forget who other people are."
   4. "If these visits upset you, maybe you should telephone your mother instead of visiting."

9. An elderly woman with chronic organic brain syndrome refuses to eat and begins to lose weight. Which approach by the nurse will likely be most effective in getting the client to eat?
   1. Explaining to her the necessity of eating three meals daily
   2. Asking the client what she thinks should be done about her lack of eating
   3. Telling the client that if she doesn't eat, she will be given tube feedings
   4. Accompanying her to meals and assisting her in eating

10. A 25-year-old woman has admitted herself to the psychiatric unit for treatment of Valium addiction. She is currently taking 150 mg p.o. of Valium per day, which she gets from various doctors or buys off the streets. The first night she is on the unit, she dresses in a short, see-through night gown and approaches the male nurse. She states she is "coming down" and just needs a little comforting and conversation. What is the best initial response by the nurse?
    1. "Please put on your bathrobe and then we can talk."
    2. "I'm very busy now. Maybe one of the other nurses can help you."
    3. "What seems to be the problem?"
    4. "What you are experiencing is very common. It should get better soon."

11. A young woman has admitted herself to the psychiatric unit for treatment of Valium addiction. A schedule of drug withdrawal is ordered by the doctor. Which of the following

may the nurse expect to see as the Valium dose is decreased?

1. Decreased blood pressure
2. Tremors and hyperactivity
3. Increase in appetite
4. Grandiosity

12. Three days after admission for treatment of Valium addiction, a young woman briefly left the hospital to talk to a visitor. Her psychiatrist has threatened to discharge her for noncompliance with the treatment program. The client seems very despondent, refusing to get out of bed. The evening nurse finds the client crying, "I've screwed everything up. It's hopeless. It's no use." In responding to the client, which of the following would be most appropriate?

1. "You've screwed everything up?"
2. "Why do you feel it's no use?"
3. "Sometimes we have to hit bottom before things get better."
4. "You sound like you're feeling very sad. Are you thinking about harming yourself?"

13. A woman is admitted to the detoxification unit. She admits to drinking increasingly larger amounts of alcohol for the past five years. What question is most important for the nurse to ask initially?

1. "How much alcohol do you drink daily?"
2. "When was your last drink?"
3. "When did you last eat?"
4. "What type of alcoholic beverages do you drink?"

14. The morning after admission for withdrawal from alcohol, a client is restless, tremulous, and somewhat agitated. The nurse should take which of these actions at this time?

1. Offer her medicinal whiskey.
2. Observe her behavior closely.
3. Darken the client's room.
4. Prepare to place her in restraints.

15. Two nights after admission for alcohol withdrawal, the client runs out of her room. She is confused and disoriented and says, "Let me out of here. Bugs are crawling all over that room." The nurse should take which of these actions?

1. Escort her back to her room and show her that there is nothing to fear.
2. Assist her back into bed and then search her room for alcohol.
3. Take her to a quiet area and ask her if she usually has nightmares.
4. Have a staff member stay with her and notify the physician.

16. An adult woman is admitted to the detox unit for alcohol withdrawal. Her husband tells the nurse that he is fed up. Either she gets treatment or he is leaving her. Two days later the woman develops delirium tremens. At this time, which of these nursing diagnoses should be given priority in caring for this client?

1. Potential for physical injury related to impulsiveness
2. Noncompliance with medical regimen related to denial of illness
3. Anticipatory grieving related to her husband's threat of abandoning her
4. Translocation syndrome related to transfer to a strange environment

17. Following withdrawal from alcohol, the client agrees to participate in group therapy sessions for a period before being discharged. Initially, group therapy may have which of these effects on the client?

1. She will develop insight into her reasons for needing alcohol.
2. She will experience periods of extreme anxiety.
3. She will be able to set realistic goals for herself.
4. She will be able to identify the personality traits she needs to change.

18. Following withdrawal from alcohol, a client is to receive disulfiram (Antabuse). The medication is prescribed for which of these purposes?

1. To minimize the effects of alcohol
2. To improve detoxification by the liver
3. To increase her utilization of vitamins
4. To help her refrain from drinking alcohol

19. A client asks the nurse about participation in Alcoholics Anonymous. In addition to arranging for a visit by someone from Alcoholics Anonymous, the nurse should explain that the primary purpose of the organization is to:

1. Explore the individual member's need for dependence on alcohol.
2. Help members abstain from alcohol.
3. Teach members how to manage social situations without the need for alcohol.
4. Increase public awareness of the results of alcoholism.

20. Chlorpromazine hydrochloride (Thorazine) is prescribed for a young adult with schizophrenia. For three days, the Thorazine is to be administered intramuscularly. Before administering Thorazine intramuscularly to the client, the nurse should make which of these assessments?

1. Checking his blood pressure
2. Testing his urine for glucose
3. Testing his patellar reflexes
4. Checking laboratory results for his serum potassium level

21. While a client is taking Thorazine, he should be observed for which of these symptoms?

1. Pseudoparkinsonism
2. Dehydration
3. Manic excitement
4. Urinary incontinence

22. A 23-year-old premedical student is admitted to a psychiatric hospital in a withdrawn, catatonic

state. For two days prior to admission, she remained in one position without moving or speaking. On the unit, she continues to exhibit waxy flexibility as she sits all day. What is the first priority for the nurse during the initial phase of hospitalization?
1. Watch for edema and cyanosis of the extremities.
2. Encourage the client to discuss her concerns, which may have led to the catatonic state.
3. Provide a warm, nurturing relationship with a therapeutic use of touch.
4. Identify the predisposing factors in her illness.

23. A woman has been having auditory hallucinations. When the nurse approaches her, she whispers, "Did you hear that terrible man? He is scary!" Which would be the best response for the nurse to take initially?
1. "Tell me everything the man is saying."
2. "I don't hear anything. What scary things is he saying?"
3. "Who is he? Do you know him?"
4. "I didn't hear a man's voice, but you look scared."

24. A man who is being treated for paranoia walks toward the nurse's desk and observes the nurse making a telephone call. A few minutes later, he accuses the nurse of having called the police. How should the nurse interpret his behavior?
1. Projection
2. Reaction formation
3. Transference
4. Ideas of reference

25. A woman is admitted to the hospital because of recent overactive behavior. She enters the dining room for lunch after everyone is seated and eating. She runs around telling everyone that she has just been invited to speak at an important political meeting. She then sits down and starts to eat. After taking a few bites, she gets up and walks quickly out of the dining room. What initial action should the nurse take to meet the client's nutritional needs?
1. Serve her meals in her room.
2. Give her finger foods to eat.
3. Sit with her while she eats.
4. Discuss with her the importance of eating.

26. Lithium carbonate is ordered for a client with overactive behavior. The nurse should observe her for which of these side effects?
1. Diarrhea
2. Rhinitis
3. Glycosuria
4. Rash

27. A man who is severely depressed following the death of his wife sits in the dayroom for hours at a time, not speaking to anyone and showing no interest in unit activities. He does not answer when spoken to. Which action should the nurse take to help him at this time?

1. Encourage him to talk about his children.
2. Start playing a game in which he can participate.
3. Turn on the television for him to watch.
4. Speak to him briefly from time to time without expecting an answer.

28. A woman is being treated for severe depression. During the acute phase of her illness, which of these measures should have priority in her care?
1. Keeping her in seclusion
2. Repeating unit routines to her in detail
3. Urging her social interaction with other clients
4. Providing her with physical care

29. A woman who is severely depressed begins to improve. Which of these behaviors may be indicative of an impending suicide attempt?
1. Responding sarcastically when asked about her family
2. Avoiding conversation with some clients on the unit
3. Identifying with problems expressed by other clients
4. Appearing detached when walking about the unit

30. A young woman was referred to the psychiatrist by her family physician because she is fearful of getting into elevators. During the course of therapy, it was discovered that her initial fear was of men and that it had changed to elevators. Which of the following mechanisms is demonstrated by this change?
1. Repression
2. Identification
3. Projection
4. Displacement

31. A young woman who is fearful of getting into elevators is admitted. Two days after admission, she is scheduled for group therapy sessions which meet on the sixth floor. Her room is on the second floor. The other clients and the nurse go to the sixth floor on the elevator. The client starts trembling and refuses to get on the elevator. Which action is most therapeutic for the nurse to take?
1. Firmly insist that she get on the elevator with the other clients.
2. Explain to her that the elevator is safe and take her on a separate elevator from the rest of the group.
3. Excuse her from group therapy until she will get on the elevator.
4. Assign someone to walk up the stairs with her.

32. A 40-year-old man is admitted to the psychiatric unit for treatment of anxiety neurosis. For several weeks, he has had increasingly frequent periods of palpitations, sweating, chest pain, and choking. His nursing diagnosis is "severe anxiety, stressor

unidentified." Which of these measures is appropriate during the client's attacks?
1. Supporting and protecting him
2. Engaging him in socially productive behavior
3. Having him review the circumstances that precipitated the symptoms
4. Ignoring him until the symptoms subside

33. Which nursing action would help to reduce stress and to aid an obsessive-compulsive client in using a less maladaptive means of handling stress?
1. Provide varied activities on the unit, because a change in routine can break a ritualistic pattern.
2. Give him unit assignments that do not require perfection.
3. Tell him of changes in routine at the last minute to avoid the buildup of anxiety.
4. Provide an activity in which positive accomplishment can occur so he can gain recognition.

34. After the nurse has had several brief conversations with a newly admitted client, she suddenly says, "I'm afraid to ride in an elevator, I know it's silly, but I can't help it." Which of these responses by the nurse would be the best example of acknowledgment?
1. "It's hard to manage without using elevators."
2. "Being afraid to ride in elevators seems unreasonable to you."
3. "Perhaps you should consider why you are afraid to ride in an elevator."
4. "The speed of elevators frightens you."

35. A client with severe anxiety manifested by many somatic complaints starts psychotherapy. She becomes increasingly anxious, and her physical symptoms intensify. The nurse should make which of these interpretations of her observations?
1. The client needs to be involved in modifying the goals of therapy.
2. The client may be developing a physical illness unrelated to her emotional problems.
3. The client is responding to therapy as expected at this time.
4. The client is probably beginning to have insight into her behavior.

36. A young man who is admitted with antisocial behavior seeks the attention of a young, attractive nurse, and he finds many excuses to involve the nurse in conversation. The nurse should have which of these understandings of this situation?
1. The nurse should help him in any way possible.
2. The nurse is responsible for maintaining a therapeutic relationship with him.
3. The nurse should prepare to act as an advocate for him.

4. The nurse is uniquely able to gain his confidence.

37. A client says to the nurse, "I have something to tell you because I know you can keep a secret." To respond to his statement, the nurse should make which of these remarks?
1. "It's nice that you trust me to keep a secret."
2. "I would like to hear your secret."
3. "I cannot promise that I can keep your secret."
4. "A secret is not a secret when it is repeated."

38. A 75-year-old woman has been widowed for 12 years. She was forced to vacate her apartment several months ago when fire destroyed the building. She has been wandering about the city, begging for money to buy food, and sleeping on park benches or in secluded areas of large buildings. She carries her personal belongings in three bundles. One day she enters the bus terminal and becomes very noisy and quarrelsome. The police are called, and she is brought to a psychiatric unit. To plan care for this woman, which of these actions should be taken first?
1. Determine her interests.
2. Obtain information about her family.
3. Identify her emotional needs.
4. Evaluate her physical condition.

39. A homeless woman is admitted to the hospital. When she is admitted, she is asked to keep her possessions in a locker that is in her room. She insists on removing several articles to carry around with her. Following nursing interventions, she continues to carry most of her possessions around with her. The nurse should make which of these interpretations of this behavior?
1. The client needs to keep busy.
2. The client needs to maintain her identity.
3. The client needs to be a focus of attention.
4. The client needs a means of becoming involved with others.

40. A young woman who has a washing ritual has been late for breakfast each of the three days since admission. What is the most appropriate nursing intervention?
1. Give her a choice of getting to breakfast on time or not eating breakfast.
2. Restrict her privileges if she is late again.
3. Get her up early so she can complete her washing ritual before breakfast.
4. Insist that she stop washing her hands and go to breakfast.

41. A 15-year-old girl is brought to the hospital by her parents. She is 5 feet, 7 inches tall and weighs 80 pounds. Her parents report she eats very little. This evening she is very difficult to arouse and had to be carried into the emergency room. A diagnosis of anorexia nervosa is made. Which of the following is the

nurse most likely to observe/measure when assessing this client?
1. Enlarged breasts
2. Scanty pubic hair
3. Decreased visual acuity
4. Tachycardia

42. An adolescent with a diagnosis of severe anorexia nervosa is now on the adolescent psychiatric unit after being in intensive care to achieve fluid and electrolyte balance. In developing the nursing care plan, which will be of highest priority?
1. Weighing her before and after each meal
2. Observing her for two hours after each meal
3. Teaching her the elements of good nutrition
4. Recording her food intake

43. A 52-year-old man is admitted to the psychiatric unit. He states he does not sleep well, has not been eating, and has no energy. He tells the admitting nurse, "I don't think you can make me feel better. There's no use in talking to me. Leave me alone." What is the most appropriate interpretation of his behavior? The client:
1. Needs solitude. The nurse should leave him alone.
2. Is depressed. The nurse should stay with him.
3. Needs encouragement. The nurse should assure him that he will get well soon.
4. Is in a bad mood. The nurse should tell him to cheer up.

44. An adult man is being treated for depression and has been taking amitriptyline (Elavil) for three days. His wife says to the nurse, "I don't think the medicine is doing anything for him. He is still depressed." What is the best response for the nurse to make?
1. "I will observe him carefully and make a full report to the physician."
2. "Depression takes a while to clear. We are seeing small behavior changes."
3. "The medicine takes two to three weeks to be effective. It is too soon to see behavior changes."
4. "His doctor is pleased with his progress. Have patience."

45. An adult male is being treated for depression. He has been in the hospital for three weeks. Which observation by the nurse is indicative of improvement in his condition?
1. He appears for breakfast unshaven.
2. He says, "I now have the answer to my problems."
3. He refuses to eat, saying, "I don't like hospital food."
4. He initiates a conversation with another client.

46. An adult is being treated for depression. One day he appears at the nursing station and gives one of the nurses his favorite book. He smiles happily and says, "I want you to have this." The nurse's response is based on which understanding?
1. Nurses should not accept gifts from clients.
2. His actions indicate an improvement in communication skills.
3. The nurse should support actions which bring the client obvious pleasure.
4. Giving away objects of personal importance is a suicidal warning sign.

47. A client with cancer states he has no reason to live anymore. What is the most therapeutic response for the nurse to give at this time?
1. "You feel as though you have no reason to live?"
2. "Your wife needs you and wants you to live."
3. "Your children care about you."
4. "I care about what happens to you."

48. A young woman is admitted for the first time with a diagnosis of catatonic schizophrenia and is receiving Thorazine daily. She is to go home for a weekend pass. What is the most important instruction to give her relative to her medications?
1. "Use a sunscreen lotion, and do not drink alcoholic beverages."
2. "Do not drink wine or beer or eat hard cheeses."
3. "Stay away from persons with colds and infections and report any rashes immediately."
4. "Drink plenty of orange juice, and take your pills with milk."

49. Mr. S. is a man who has not spoken for years. He is diagnosed as having paranoid schizophrenia. One day, when Ms. J., another client, was standing facing the elevator, the man approached her from behind and reached for her as if to strangle her. What is the most appropriate action for the nurse to take at this time?
1. Grab Mr. S. by the arm to stop him.
2. Ask other clients to assist her.
3. Say, "Mr. S., that is not appropriate behavior."
4. Get Mr. S.'s attention and call for help.

50. Thorazine is prescribed for a client. Which of the following, if observed in the client, would suggest Thorazine toxicity?
1. Tremors
2. Sore tongue
3. Rash
4. Hoarseness

Answers and Rationales

1. (1) Defense mechanisms are measures that the client uses to reestablish emotional equilibrium. Some are self-defeating, and some are good.

2. (2) Anxiety can be used constructively as a learning and motivating tool. The goal is not to eliminate anxiety but to have the client respond appropriately to it and not be overwhelmed by it.

3. (1) The child with autistic behavior reveals a disturbance in the development of social relationships. There is often an absence of responsive behavior toward the approach of the parents, and typically the child seems as content alone as in the presence of the parents.

4. (3) The child often demonstrates peculiar motor behavior in the form of spinning, rocking, head banging, and repetitive arm movements. Hallucinations are not evident in the autistic child. Failing to respond to parents' voices is not evidence of impaired hearing. Autistic children tend to respond well to music. The child with autism does not relate to others so will not be seen clinging to others.

5. (3) Because of the autistic child's avoidance of interpersonal contact and the disturbance in language development that typically occurs, a therapeutic approach to the child offers the nurse's presence without making demands for a response or imposing personal closeness.

6. (3) Gently providing guidance allows her to maintain her esteem and communicates supportive caring. Locking the door to her room is not safe for the client and interferes with her independence. Telling the client to stay in her room is ineffective because she has a memory impairment. Restraints increase feelings of helplessness, frustration, and inadequacy.

7. (2) The client is unable to recognize her daughter. The symptom of disorientation in organic mental disorders is characterized by the inability to recall day or time, place, who they are, or the person or position of the person to which they are relating. Impaired judgment and impaired abstract thinking may be seen in organic mental disorders, but it is not the behavior described. They are both examples of impaired intellectual functioning, characterized by the inability to recall and use general knowledge in decision making and problem solving. Perceptual impairments such as delusions may occur in organic mental disorders, manifested by a fixed idea for which there is no factual basis. This is not the behavior described.

8. (1) This is empathetic, because it lets the daughter know that the nurse has an understanding of what the daughter must be feeling. Answers 2 and 4 are incorrect, because the nurse is giving advice and neglects the daughter's feelings. Answer 3 is not correct because it generalizes and minimizes the daughter's feelings.

9. (4) This approach conveys caring, support, and helpfulness. It also assures that the patient knows where and when to eat. Impaired intellectual functioning that is evident in organic mental disorders interferes with the person's ability to reason or solve problems. Answer 3 will increase frustration and anger.

10. (1) The client's behavior suggests an attempt at manipulation. Manipulative behavior is best handled by setting limits. Asking her to put on a robe sets limits. Answers 2 and 3 are incorrect because they avoid the problem. Answer 4 does not address the problem behavior, which is manipulation.

11. (2) Tremors and hyperactivity are common symptoms of Valium detoxification. Although blood pressure should be monitored, it generally does not decrease. Increased appetite and grandiosity are not symptoms of detoxification.

12. (4) The nurse is identifying the overall feeling tone of the client's communication and is directly asking for feedback about her suicide potential. Most suicide clients will give truthful information when directly asked. Answer 1 is a reflective statement and can allow her to continue talking, but it is appropriate after her suicide potential is assessed. Answer 2 asks for an analysis and may be distracting to the theme. Answer 3 invalidates the client's thoughts and feelings.

13. (2) The nurse must determine when the client had her last drink to help anticipate when withdrawal symptoms will occur.

14. (2) Physiological dependence on alcohol is responsible for the syndrome that occurs when alcohol is withdrawn. The syndrome includes the symptoms of tachycardia, elevated blood pressure, nausea, restlessness, tremors, hallucinations, convulsions, and ultimately may progress to delirium tremens. The client who is being detoxified must be monitored carefully for the development of these symptoms so that adequate measures can be taken to prevent injury, to meet metabolic and nutritional needs, and to minimize anxiety. Medicinal whiskey is not used during detoxification. Although the client in withdrawal may become confused and agitated, the use of physical restraints should be avoided if possible because they tend to increase agitation. The room should not be darkened, this tends to promote shadows that may be misintrepeted (this client is prone to illusions).

15. (4) Visual and tactile hallucinations are indicative of the development of delirium tremens. The presence of a staff member offering reassurance and orientation may reduce the client's growing sense of panic and prevent self-injury. The physician should be informed of the client's condition so that the use of a tranquilizer may be considered. Showing her that there is nothing to fear is not appropriate when the confusion is due to

withdrawal. There is no need to search her room for alcohol. The behavior suggests withdrawal, not intoxication. The behavior suggests withdrawal symptoms, not nightmares.

16. (1) When a client is in delirium tremens, the potential for physical injury may be life-threatening. Protective measures are a priority. All of the other diagnoses could be appropriate at some point in the care, but not at this time.

17. (2) It is expected that any client beginning group therapy will experience a period of uncertainty, during which considerable anxiety will be felt. Only when the client has progressed through this phase, and through the phases of aggression and regression, will she arrive at the adaptation phase—during which she may develop insight into her behavior. It is important to understand the phases through which participants move in group therapy.

18. (4) The purpose of Antabuse is to help the client abstain from alcohol. The client who takes Antabuse regularly will experience symptoms of nausea, vomiting, and palpitations when even a small amount of alcohol is consumed. The drug is usually used for only a limited time in conjunction with other treatment methods.

19. (2) Self-help and peer support are offered by AA in an ongoing education program that assists the members to achieve abstinence from alcohol. The other purposes may be secondary, but the primary purpose is to help members abstain from alcohol.

20. (1) The hypotension caused by Thorazine is more severe when the drug is administered IM. The other choices do not relate to side effects of Thorazine.

21. (1) Pseudoparkinsonism is one of the extrapyramidal side effects that occur with phenothiazine drugs. If this is severe, an antiparkinsonian drug is prescribed. The other choices are not side effects of Thorazine. The client is more apt to experience urinary retention than incontinence.

22. (1) Circulation may be severely impaired in a client with a waxy flexibility who tends to remain motionless for hours unless moved. She does not speak and will not be able to discuss her concerns or identify predisposing factors during the initial stages. Touch is not used at this stage.

23. (4) This is a reality-based response as well as one that acknowledges the client's nonverbal reaction. The nurse should not focus on the "voice," because that reinforces the hallucination and does not place doubt. Answer 2 voices doubt but focuses on the voice, not the client's feelings.

24. (4) Ideas of reference are a common symptom in paranoid disorders. The person interprets an event occurring in the environment as having particular significance or reference to himself.

25. (2) The client is too active to eat and at the moment is unable to control this overactivity. Nursing actions to meet nutritional needs include giving her finger foods that she can eat while moving about.

26. (1) Diarrhea is a common side effect of lithium carbonate and may indicate toxicity. Rhinitis (runny nose), glycosuria (sugar in the urine), and rash are not side effects of lithium.

27. (4) This client is severely depressed and needs an environment which places few demands on him. His self-esteem will be raised by knowing that someone cares enough about him to speak to him. In time, he may respond. Note that the scenario states twice that he does not speak; therefore, encouraging him to talk about his children is not appropriate.

28. (4) During the acute phase of depression, the client is not meeting her physical needs. The nurse must meet these needs.

29. (4) As the depressed client begins to improve, the risk of suicide is increased because the person now has a greater amount of energy. Behaviors that may indicate that the client is planning a suicide attempt include a sudden lightening of mood, an air of relaxation, or the appearance of detachment.

30. (4) The original fear of men was displaced onto elevators, a safer object.

31. (4) Her anxiety is high when faced with the elevator. Forcing her to get on the elevator may precipitate an anxiety attack or panic reaction. Note that this is early in the course of her hospitalization. The nurse must not force her to get on the elevator.

32. (1) He needs support during this time. He will be unable to pay attention to details or to think clearly during an anxiety attack. Note that his symptoms include chest pain and choking.

33. (4) Positive accomplishment will help to boost self-concept and self-confidence. A client with ritualistic behavior will do best when routine activities are set up and anxiety-producing changes are avoided. Perfection-type activities bring satisfaction (cleaning and straightening a linen closet). He needs to know changes in routine in advance in order to cope with the anxiety produced by the changes.

34. (2) Acknowledgment is really restating what the client says. This answer is a restatement of "I'm afraid to ride in an elevator, I know it's silly, but I can't help it."

35. (3) In the initial stage of psychotherapy, as clients begin to confront the conflicts that are the source of their symptoms, it is common for them to experience an intensification of anxiety and defensive behavior. The nurse should anticipate this phenomenon.

36. (2) It is common for the client with an antisocial personality disorder to single out a staff

member whom he will attempt to manipulate for the gratification of his wishes. The nurse must be aware of the client's motivations and of the responses that he may be attempting to elicit from the nurse. The nurse may mistakenly interpret the client's desire to communicate as an expression of real interpersonal closeness, or the nurse may engage in fantasies about saving the client from his destructive behavior. The realistic assessment of the situation is based on the understanding that the nurse can establish guidelines of the plan of care.

37. (3) The nurse cannot promise not to tell a client's secret. The client may tell of a suicide plan or something else that must be shared with the physician or other staff members.

38. (4) Since, in some cases, the symptoms of organic mental disorder are attributable to systemic illness, nutritional disorders and effects of drugs, it is imperative that the client be given a thorough physical examination so that physiologic problems that may be causing her behavior or may simply coexist can be addressed.

39. (2) The nurse should understand that the client's possessions represent an extension of herself and an affirmation of her personal identity in an alien environment. It is most therapeutic to allow the client to use this coping behavior as long as she is not dangerous.

40. (3) In the early part of hospitalization, the nurse should allow the client to perform the ritual and still eat. Given a choice, the obsessive-compulsive client would choose the ritual. Restriction privileges this early in treatment is not reasonable. Insisting that she stop washing her hands could precipitate a panic attack.

41. (2) Secondary sex characteristics tend to disappear. Her breasts will get smaller. She will have bradycardia, not tachycardia.

42. (2) Observing her to be sure she does not induce vomiting is the highest priority.

43. (2) He is exhibiting the classic symptoms of depression, and the nurse should stay with him. He should be evaluated for suicide potential.

44. (3) Elavilisa tricyclic antidepressants take 2–3 weeks for therapeutic effects to be seen.

45. (4) This indicates that he is less withdrawn. Answer 1 indicates poor self esteem. Answer 2 may be a suicidal warning sign.

46. (4) Giving away items may be a sign he is going to commit suicide.

47. (1) This response opens communication and encourages him to express his feelings.

48. (1) Thorazine causes photosensitivity. Because it is a central nervous system drug, alcohol should not be taken.

49. (4) The nurse should get his attention so that he will release the other client. Help is needed.

50. (1) Tremors suggest Thorazine toxicity.

Chapter 18

Pharmacology

BASIC CONCEPTS
PREPARING THE MEDICATION

A. Nursing actions:
1. Check medication order and label.
2. Check expiration date of medication.
3. Wash hands.
4. Check client identity:
   a. Check identification band.
   b. Ask client to state his/her name; do not ask the client "Are you Ms. _____?"
   c. Check picture ID in long-term care facility if no other ID available.
B. Administer the right dose of the right drug via the right route to the right client at the right time (Five R's of Medication administration).
C. Teach client:
1. Purpose of drug
2. Expected effects
3. Any adverse effects to be reported
D. Stay with client while he takes the medication.
E. Give medication within 30 minutes of prescribed time.
F. Chart immediately.
G. Observe for reactions.

METHODS OF ADMINISTRATION

A. Intramuscular:
1. Needle size: 18–23 gauge, 1–2 inch needle
2. Hold the skin taut.
3. Administer at a 90-degree angle (see Figure 18.1).
4. Maximum volume:
   a. 4 ml into large muscle (gluteus medius) in adult
   b. 1 to 2 ml in children and older adults
   c. 0.5 to 1.0 ml for deltoid muscle
5. Sites (see Figure 18.2)
   a. Dorsogluteal into the gluteus maximus muscle; not suitable for infants and preschool children
   b. Ventrogluteal into the gluteus medius muscle; not suitable for infants and preschool children
   c. Anterolateral aspect of thigh into the vastus lateralis muscle; suitable for infants
   d. Upper arm into the deltoid muscle
6. Z track IM injection (see Figure 18.3):
   a. Used for iron (Imferon) injections and almost any IM given in the ventrogluteal or dorsogluteal sites

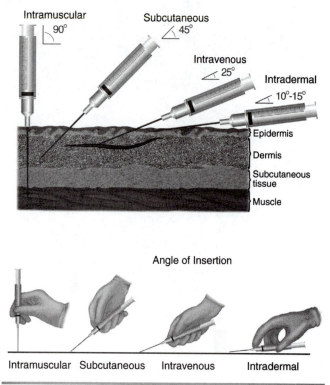

Angle of Insertion

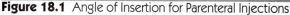

Intramuscular Subcutaneous   Intravenous   Intradermal

Figure 18.1 Angle of Insertion for Parenteral Injections

    b. With client in prone position pull the skin to one side and administer injection at a 90 degree angle into the muscle; wait 10 seconds and remove needle

    c. Do not massage

B. Subcutaneous:
1. Needle size: 25–27 gauge, 1/2–1 inch needle
2. Pinch skin
3. Administer at a 45 degree angle (see Figure 18.1)
4. Sites (see Figure 18.4):
   a. Abdomen: 1 inch away from umbilicus
   b. Lateral and anterior aspects of upper arm and thigh
   c. Scapular area on back
   d. Upper ventrodorsal gluteal area
5. Maximum volume should not exceed 1.5 ml.
6. Subcutaneous tissue sensitive to irritants; rotate sites if medication irritating

C. Intradermal:
1. Needle size: 25–27 gauge, 3/8- to 1/2-inch needle
2. Stretch skin taut.
3. Administer at 10- to 15-degree angle into the skin (see Figure 18.1).
4. Do not massage.
5. Sites (see Figure 18.5):
   a. Ventral forearm
   b. Upper chest
   c. Upper back (scapula)

6. Used for skin testing for disease (tuberculosis, histoplasmosis) and allergies and to administer local anesthetics

D. Rectal suppository (see Figure 18.6):
1. Have client void before inserting suppository.
2. Use rubber glove.
3. Moisten suppository and gloved finger with water-soluble lubricant.
4. Insert tapered end beyond anal sphincter: 4 inches for adult and 2 inches for child.
5. Do not insert suppository into feces.
6. Pinch buttocks until urge to defecate has passed.
7. Instruct client to retain for 15–20 minutes.

E. Vaginal suppository (see Figure 18.7):
1. Have client void before inserting suppository; a full bladder may cause discomfort and impede insertion.
2. Use nonsterile rubber glove.
3. Place client in dorsal recumbent position with knees bent or in Sim's position.
4. Assess perineum for odor and discharge; cleanse if necessary to prevent introduction of organisms into vagina.
5. Insert suppository into applicator's tip if applicator used.
6. Lubricate suppository and gloved finger if applicator not used.
7. Insert suppository at least 2 inches into vaginal canal or depress plunger of applicator.
8. Instruct client to remain in bed for 15 minutes to allow absorption of suppository.
9. Wash applicator under cold running water.

F. Eye (see Figure 18.8):
1. Position client supine with head turned to affected side.
2. Pull lower lid down, have client look up, and administer into conjunctival sac.
3. Apply pressure on inner canthus to prevent systemic absorption of medication and runny nose.
4. Terms:
   a. O.D. (right eye)
   b. O.S. (left eye)
   c. O.U. (both eyes)

G. Ear (see Figure 18.9):
1. Position client on unaffected side.
2. Clean outer ear.
3. Straighten ear canal:
   a. Up and back for adults
   b. Down and back for small children
4. Instill drops.
5. Instruct client to stay on side for 5–10 minutes for medication to be absorbed.
6. Insert cotton moistened with medication to prevent leaking of medication.

H. Intravenous:
1. LPN/LVN is not responsible for starting IVs and giving IV push medications.

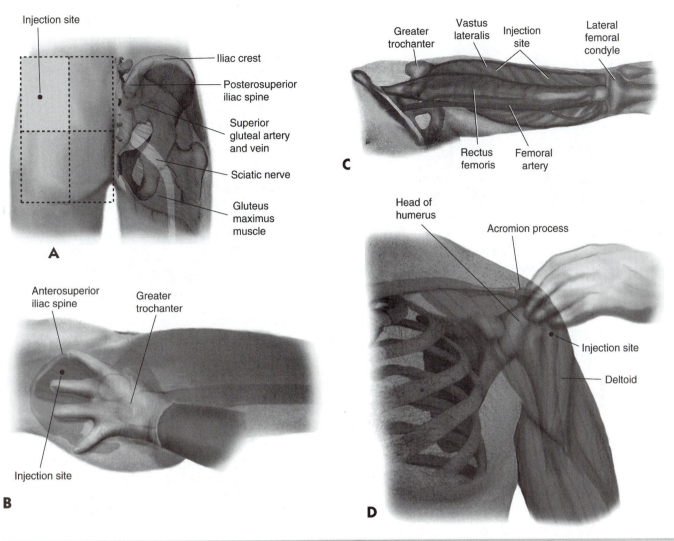

Figure 18.2 Intramuscular Injection Sites. A. Dorsogluteal, B. Ventrogluteal, C. Vestus Lateralis, D. Deltoid.

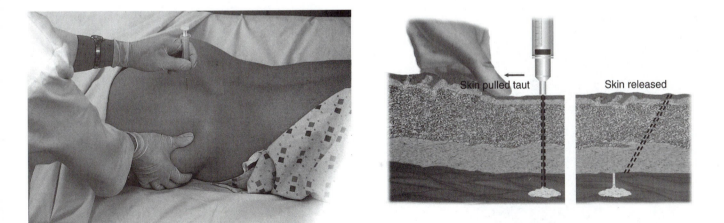

Figure 18.3 Z Track Technique for IM Injection.

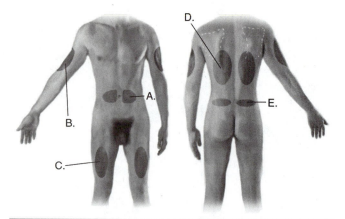

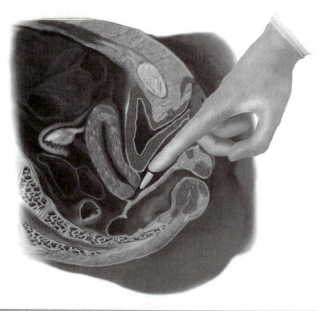

Figure 18.4 Subcutaneous Injection Sites. A. Abdomen, B. Lateral upper arm, C. Anterior upper thigh, D. Scapular area on back, E. Upper vertro dorsal gluteal area

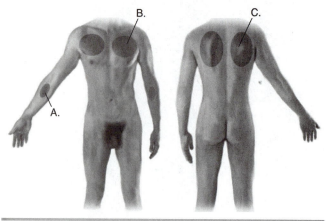

Figure 18.7 Inserting a Vaginal Suppository

Figure 18.5 Intradermal Injection Sites. A. Inner aspect of forearm, B. Upper chest, C. Upper back

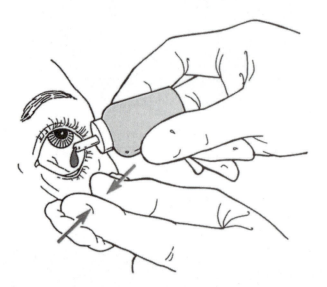

Figure 18.8 Administering Eye Medications

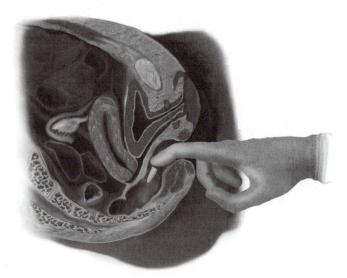

Figure 18.6 Inserting a Rectal Suppository

2. LPN/LVN should monitor clients with IV lines running.
3. Assess IV tubing for kinks.
4. Assess flow rate.
5. Assess infusion site:
   a. Redness and warmth may indicate phlebitis.
   b. Pallor and coolness may indicate infiltration.
6. Measure urine output.
7. Report any problems to the charge nurse.

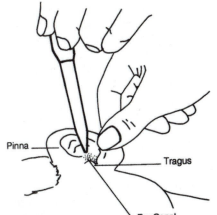

Pinna

Tragus

Ear Canal

(A) Child under 3 years

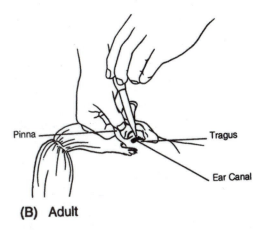

Pinna

Tragus

Ear Canal

(B) Adult

Figure 18.9 Administering Ear Medications

CALCULATING METHODS

A. General formula:

$$\frac{\text{Desire}}{\text{Have}} = \frac{X \text{ (unknown amount of drug)}}{\text{known amount of drug}}$$

Example:
Meperidine HCl (Demerol) 75 mg IM stat is ordered. The label on the available medication reads Meperidine HCl 50 mg/ml. How much should the nurse administer?

1. Set up formula

$$\frac{\text{Desire (75 mg)}}{\text{Have (50 mg)}} = \frac{X}{1 \text{ ml}}$$

2. Solve for X by cross-multiplying and then dividing

$50X = 75$

$X = \dfrac{75}{50}$

$X = 1.5$ ml

B. Conversion from pounds to kilograms
1. There are 2.2 pounds in 1 kilogram.
2. To convert pounds to kilograms, divide pounds by 2.2.
3. Example: Convert 165 pounds to kg.

165 divided by 2.2 lbs/kg = 75 kg.

C. Conversion from grams to milligrams
1. There is 1,000 mg in a gram.
2. Multiply number of grams by 1,000.
3. Example: Convert 2 grams into milligrams.

1,000 mg = 1 gram
1,000 mg × 2 grams = 2,000 mg

D. Conversion from ounces to milliliters
1. There is 30 ml in one ounce.
2. Multiply number of ounces by 30 ml per ounce.
3. Example: Convert 5 ounces to milliliters.

Multiply 5 ounces by 30 ml/ounce.
30 ml/ounce × 5 ounces = 150 ml.

E. Calculations requiring several steps
1. Do any conversion necessary.
   a. Convert pounds to kilograms if needed.
   b. Convert to like units if needed; i.e., grams to mg.
   c. Follow the steps one at a time.
2. Examples:
   a. A 132-pound adult is to receive Hyzyd 5 mg/kg PO divided into 3 equal doses. Each Hyzyd tablet contains 50 mg per dose. How many tablets would you administer per dose?
   (1) Convert pounds to kilograms.

   132 pounds divided by 2.2 pounds/kg = 60kg.

   (2) Calculate total dose.

   Multiply 60 kg by 3 mg/kg to determine the daily dose.
   60 kg × 5 mg/kg = 300 mg.

   (3) The medication is to be divided into three equal doses. 300 mg divided by 3 = 100 mg per dose.
   (4) Calculate the dose using the desired-over-have method.

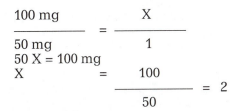

$$\frac{100 \text{ mg}}{50 \text{ mg}} = \frac{X}{1}$$
$50 X = 100$ mg
$X = \dfrac{100}{50} = 2$

   b. A client is to receive 1.5 gm of a drug. The tablets contain 500 mg per tablet. How many tablets should the nurse administer?
   (1) Convert to like units. Multiply 1.5 grams by 1,000 mg/gram.

(2) 1,000 mg × 1.5 gm = 1,500 mg.

(3) Calculate using the desire-over-have method.

$$\frac{1{,}500 \text{ mg}}{500 \text{ mg}} = \frac{X \text{ tablets}}{1{,}500 \text{ mg}}$$

500X = 1,500 mg

X = 3 tablets

c. A 22-pound child is to receive digozin (Lanoxin). The daily dosage is 0.012 mg/Kg daily in divided doses at 12 hour intervals. On hand is Lanoxin elixir 0.05 mg/ml.

(1) Convert pounds to kilograms. 22 lbs divided by 2.2 lbs/kg = 10 kg.

(2) Determine total daily dose by multiplying weight in kg by 0.012 mg/kg.

10 Kg × .012 mg/kg = .12 mg daily.

(3) Determine each dose. Given in 2 divided doses. Divide 0.12 mg by 2 = 0.06 mg/dose.

(4) Calculate ml/dose using desire-over-have method.

$$\frac{.06 \text{ mg}}{0.05 \text{ mg}} = \frac{X}{1 \text{ ml}}$$

0.05 X = 0.06 mg

Give 1.2 ml per dose.

F. Calculation of IV drip rates:

1. Drop factor must be known to calculate IV drip rate. Drop factors vary by manufacturer and may be 10,15, or 20 drops per ml.

2. A microdrip is 60 drops (gtts) per ml.

3. Calculation formula

$$\frac{\text{Amount of solution in ml}}{\text{Time}} \times \text{drop factor} = \text{drip rate in gtts/minute}$$

4. Example: A client is to receive 1,000 ml of Dextrose 5% in water over 8 hours. The drop factor is 12 gtts/ml. At what rate should the IV be running?

a. $\dfrac{1{,}000 \text{ ml}}{8 \text{ hours} \times 60 \text{ minutes (480 minutes)}} \times 12 \text{ gtts/ml}$

b. $\dfrac{1{,}000 \text{ ml}}{480 \text{ minutes}} \times 12 \text{ gtts/ml}$

c. Drip rate is 25 drops per minute.

Facts about Drug Action

A. Parenteral drugs go first to the systemic circulation, then to the liver—starting to work more quickly.

1. IM drugs are absorbed into the muscle before going into the blood stream.

2. IV drugs are absorbed directly into the blood stream and act the most quickly.

B. Oral drugs go first to the liver to be broken down, then to the systemic circulation; they are slower acting.

C. Dosage of parenteral drugs is less than oral drugs because they are not broken down before acting.

D. Parenteral drugs act more quickly than oral drugs.

E. Most drugs are broken down in the liver:

1. Liver disease affects the metabolism of drugs.

2. Most drugs have the potential for liver toxicity.

F. The principal route of excretion for most drugs is the kidney.

Pharmacologic Agents

Remember: Drugs in the same classification usually have similar generic names and similar actions and side effects.

ANTIMICROBIALS AND ANTIPARASITICS (SEE TABLES 18.1 AND 18.2)

Aminoglycosides (Mycins)

A. Used primarily for gram-negative organisms in serious infections
B. Examples:
   1. Gentamicin (Garamycin)
   2. Streptomycin

Table 18.1 General Rules for Administering Antimicrobials

- Culture before giving.
- Give at regular intervals.
- Check for superimposed infections.
- Can cause blood dyscrasias when given in high doses or for long periods of time.
- Most antibiotics can cause liver or renal damage when given in high doses for extended periods of time.
- Many antibiotics interfere with oral contraceptives.

   3. Tobramycin (Nebcin)
   4. Kanamycin (Kantrex)
   5. Neomycin
C. Method of administration:
   1. Given I.V. or I.M. for systemic action
   2. Oral administration for bowel disinfection only (neomycin and Kanamycin)
D. Adverse effects/nursing care:
   1. Eighth cranial (auditory) nerve damage: Tinnitus, hearing loss
   2. Nephrotoxicity: Monitor serum creatinine levels to assess possible kidney damage
   3. Neuromuscular blockade
   4. Monitor peaks and troughs:
      a. Peaks: Blood drawn one hour after I.M. and 30 minutes after IV administration
      b. Troughs: Blood drawn just before next dose
      c. Peaks above 12 mcg/ml and troughs above 2 mcg/ml are associated with higher toxicity.
   5. Contraindications: Clients in renal failure and those who are receiving other ototoxic (ear-damaging) drugs should receive a reduced dosage.

Table 18.2 Antimicrobial Summary

Drug Category	Major Uses	Major Side Effects	Major Nursing Interventions
Aminoglycosides (Mycins) **Vancomycin (Vancocin)**	Serious Gram (−) infections Methicillin-resistant infections, Penicillin-allergic	Nephrotoxicity, Ototoxicity Nephrotoxicity, Ototoxicity	Monitor peaks and troughs.
Penicillins (cillins)	Treponema (syphilis), Meningococcus, Pneumococcus Streptococcus, many others	Allergic reactions/ anaphylaxis, decrease effectiveness of oral contraceptives	Give oral forms 1–2 hours before or 2–3 hours after eating.
Cephalosporins "Cef-Kef" **Erythromycins**	Wide variety of organisms Persons who are allergic to penicillin, Legionnaire's Disease, Mycoplasma, Chlamydia, Lyme disease, H. influenzae, H. pylori (ulcers)	Penicillin cross allergy Low rate of side effects and toxicity	Check for a history of penicillin allergy. Do not give with meals or acids.
Tetracyclines (cyclines)	Rickettsial infections (Rocky Mountain Spotted Fever and Lyme Disease), Chlamydia, Mycoplasma, Helicobacter pylori, Acne	Gray tooth discoloration, photosensitivity, decreased effectiveness of oral contraceptives	Do not give with any product containing calcium, aluminum, iron, magnesium, or zinc.
Chloramphenicol	Infections that do not respond to other drugs: H. influenzae meningitis, Typhoid fever, Rickettsial infections such as Rocky Mountain Spotted Fever, Salmonella infections	Aplastic anemia, Granulocytopenia	Watch for signs of bone marrow depression: bleeding, infections.
Quinolones (oxacin)	Gram (−) bacteria, Pseudomonas, UTI	Hypersensitivity reactions	Food delays absorption. Milk and yogurt decrease absorption.
Sulfonamides "Sulfa," "Gant"	Urinary tract and genitourinary infections, Ulcerative colitis and Crohn's disease, bowel prep before colon surgery	Rash, Kidney stones, Fever, Photosensitivity, decreases effectiveness of oral contraceptives	Tell clients to avoid direct sunlight. I & O. Encourage fluids.
Urinary Anti-infectives	Urinary tract infections	Mandelamine is ineffective in alkaline urine.	Caution patient not to take alkalinizing agents such as antacid. I & O. Encourage fluids.

Vancomycin (Vancocin)

A. Unrelated to any other drug
B. Use reserved for severe infections because of its serious toxicity:
  1. Given IV for severe staphylococcal infections resistant to methicillin; may be given to penicillin-allergic clients
  2. Given PO for treatment of pseudomembranous colitis caused by antibiotics
C. Adverse effects/nursing care
  1. Adverse effects similar to aminoglycosides
  2. Ototoxicity
  3. Nephrotoxicity:
    a. Especially when given IV and to clients with reduced renal function or clients receiving high doses for prolonged periods
    b. Monitor BUN and creatinine levels to assess renal function.
  4. Monitor serum blood levels; concentrations usually under 40 mcg/ml
  5. Watch site of administration for tissue irritation.
  6. Never given by I.M. injection; very irritating to tissue; given by slow IV infusion

Penicillins (Cillins)

A. Used to treat treponema (syphilis), meningococcus, pneumococcus, streptococcus, and many others; penicillins are not used for viral, yeast, fungi, or rickettsial infections
B. Examples (note the cillin ending):
  1. Penicillin (Penicillin V Potassium—PenVee K)
  2. Amoxicillin trihydrate (Amoxil)
  3. Amoxicillin/clavelanate potassium (Augmentin)
  4. Ampicillin (Amcill)
  5. Methicillin (Staphcillin, Polycillin)
  6. Penicillin G (Pfizerpen-AS)
  7. Oxacillin (Bactocill)
  8. Ticarcillin (Ticar, Timentin)
C. Method of administration:
  1. Parenteral
  2. Oral
D. Adverse effects/nursing care:
  1. Allergic reactions/anaphylaxis
  2. Skin test when client has history of possible allergic reaction
  3. Gastrointestinal upset in orally administered drugs
  4. Give oral forms 1–2 hours before or 2–3 hours after eating.
  5. Probenicid (Benemid) may be given to increase blood levels of penicillins.
  6. Chemically incompatible with aminoglycosides (Neomycin, streptomycin); do not combine in an IV solution; if given concurrently, administer in separate sites at least one hour apart
  7. Penicillin V may decrease the effectiveness of oral contraceptives.
  8. Penicillins should be used cautiously in persons taking anticoagulants because they increase the potential for bleeding.
  9. Persons with allergies to cephalosporins may be allergic to penicillins.

Cephalosporins ("Cef-Kef")

A. Used to treat a wide variety of organisms; there are several generations of cephalosporins effective against different organisms
B. Examples (note that they have "cef" in the generic and often in the trade name):
  1. First Generation:
    a. Cephalexin (Keflex)
    b. Cefazolin (Ancef, Kefzol)
  2. Second Generation:
    a. Cefoxitin (Mefoxin)
    b. Cefaclor (Ceclor)
    c. Cefuroxime (Ceftin, Zinacef)
  3. Third Generation:
    a. Cefotaxime (Claforan)
    b. Ceftriaxone (Rocephin)
  4. Fourth Generation: Cefepime (Maxipime)
C. Method of administration:
  1. Oral
  2. Parenteral
D. Adverse effects/nursing care:
  1. Penicillin cross allergy; cephalosporins are similar in structure to penicillins and have similar side effects; be sure to assess for penicillin allergy.
  2. Nephrotoxicity may occur with high doses.

Erythromycins

A. Use to treat persons who are allergic to penicillin; Legionnaire's Disease; mycoplasma infections (mycoplasma are a cross between bacteria and a virus); chlamydia; Borrelia (carried by the deer tick, causes Lyme disease); Haemophilus influenzae
B. Biaxin is also used to treat Helicobacter pylori, associated with peptic ulcer disease, and Mycobacterium Avium (MAC) in AIDS.
C. Method of administration:
  1. Oral: Acidity decreases the activity of erythromycin; tablets are enteric-coated to prevent dissolving in the stomach; do not crush enteric-coated tablets
  2. Not usually given parenterally; I.M. is painful; I.V. is irritating
D. Adverse effects/nursing care:
  1. Erythromycin is noted for a low rate of side effects and toxicity.
  2. GI irritation (oral form)

3. Do not give with meals because food decreases absorption; take on an empty stomach with a full glass of water.
4. Do not give with acids such as fruit juices, because acidity decreases the activity of the drug.
5. Both partners are treated if given for a sexually transmitted disease.

Tetracyclines

A. Used to treat rickettsial infections (Rocky Mountain Spotted Fever and Lyme Disease); chlamydia infections; mycoplasma infections; and Helicobacter pylori; oral and topical preparations used in the treatment of acne vulgaris; rarely used in the treatment of common bacterial infections because of development of resistant organisms
B. Examples:
    1. Tetracycline
    2. Doxycycline (Vibramycin)
    3. Minocycline (Minocin)
C. Method of administration:
    1. Oral
    2. Parenteral possible but rare: I.M. very painful; IV has a high incidence of thrombophlebitis and local irritation
D. Adverse effects/nursing care:
    1. GI: Nausea, vomiting, diarrhea
    2. Do not give with any product containing calcium, aluminum, iron, magnesium, or zinc because these interfere with absorption. Tell the client not to take with milk or milk products and not to take with vitamins containing zinc or iron and not to take with antacids containing calcium or magnesium.
    3. Permanent gray tooth discoloration and enamel hypoplasia; do not give tetracycline during the last trimester of pregnancy, during lactation, or to children under 8 years of age
    4. Photosensitivity: Tell client to avoid direct exposure to sunlight or strong artificial light to prevent development of rash
    5. Decreased effectiveness of oral contraceptives

Chloramphenicol (Chloromycetin)

A. Because of its severe toxicity, chloramphenicol is used only for infections that do not respond to other drugs such as Hemophilus influenzae meningitis; typhoid fever; rickettsial infections such as Rocky Mountain Spotted Fever; and some types of salmonella infections.
B. Example of drug: Chloramphenicol (Chloromycetin)
C. Method of administration:
    1. Oral
    2. IV
    3. Ophthalmic

D. Adverse effects/nursing care:
    1. Aplastic anemia and granulocytopenia are most serious; monitor blood tests (CBC and platelets) baseline and every two days; do not give drug if signs of aplastic anemia are present: Low WBC, low RBC, decreased platelets, or signs of bleeding
    2. Penicillin antagonizes the antibacterial effect of chloramphenicol and should be given at least one hour before chloramphenicol.

Quinolones

A. Used against gram (–) bacteria including Pseudomonas and some gram (+) organisms
B. Examples (note the oxacin ending):
    1. Norfloxacin (Noroxin)
    2. Ciprofloxacin (Cipro)
C. Method of administration:
    1. Oral
    2. Usually given BID
D. Adverse effects/nursing care:
    1. GI disturbances: Nausea, abdominal pain, diarrhea
        a. Food delays absorption, so give on an empty stomach with a full glass of water.
        b. Milk and yogurt decrease the absorption of Cipro.
    2. CNS irritation: Dizziness, headache
    3. Hypersensitivity reactions, rash, pruritus, fever
    4. Encourage cranberry juice to acidify the urine.

Sulfonamides ("Sulfa," "Gant")

A. Used in the treatment of urinary tract and genitourinary infections; Sulfasalazine (Azulfidine) used in the treatment of mild to moderate ulcerative colitis and Crohn's disease; also used as a bowel prep before colon surgery to kill intestinal bacteria
B. Examples (note the "Sulfa" and "Gant"):
    1. Sulfisoxazole (Gantrisin)
    2. Sulfasalazine (Azulfidine; contains salicyclate)
    3. Sulfamethoxazole (Gantanol) is given primarily in combination with Trimethoprim (Proloprim) as Septra or Bactrim.
C. Method of administration:
    1. Oral
    2. Ophthalmic for eye infections
D. Adverse effects/nursing care
    1. Hypersensitivity reactions including rash
    2. Fever (7–10 days after starting therapy)
    3. Renal dysfunction caused by precipitation of sulfonamide crystals in the urinary tract; monitor intake and output; encourage fluids to avoid crystal formation and renal

dysfunction; check pH of urine; sodium bicarbonate may be given to make the urine more alkaline to decrease urine crystal formation
   4. Ecchymosis and hemorrhage caused by decreased synthesis of vitamin K by the intestinal bacteria
      a. Vitamin K is necessary for proper clotting and is made in the intestine by intestinal bacteria.
      b. Intestinal bacteria are very susceptible to sulfonamides; a decrease in intestinal bacteria means a decrease in vitamin K.
   5. GI reactions: nausea, vomiting, diarrhea
   6. Photosensitivity: Tell clients to avoid direct sunlight while taking sulfonamides
   7. Do not give to clients who have an allergy to other drugs containing sulfa, such as sulfonylureas (oral hypoglycemic agents—orinase) and thiazides.
   8. Do not give Sulfasalazine to clients who are allergic to salicylates.
   9. Decreases effectiveness of oral contraceptives

Urinary Anti-infectives

A. In acid urine, methenamine drugs are converted to ammonia and formaldehyde, which is antibacterial. Nitrofurantoin is bacteriostatic.
B. Used to treat urinary tract infections; they do not achieve blood levels high enough to treat systemic infections
C. Examples:
   1. Methenamine mandelate (Mandelamine)
   2. Methenamine hippurate (Hiprex)
   3. Nitrofurantoin (Macrodantin)
D. Method of administration: Oral
E. Adverse effects/nursing care:
   1. Nausea and vomiting
   2. Mandelamine is ineffective in alkaline urine.
      a. Caution client not to take alkalinizing agents such as antacids.
      b. Encourage cranberry juice or give ascorbic acid to maintain a pH of less than 5.5.
   3. Obtain a clean catch urine before starting therapy and prn thereafter.
   4. Intake and output; be sure there is adequate fluid intake.

Antitubercular Drugs

A. The mycobacterium tuberculosis has a tendency to develop resistant strains; therefore, two to four drugs are given for a period of 18–24 months.

B. Examples:
   1. Isoniazid (INH)
   2. Para amino salicylate sodium (PAS)
   3. Rifampin (Rimactane)
   4. Ethambutol (Myambutol)
   5. Also used but discussed earlier are streptomycin and kanamycin.
C. Method of administration:
   1. Usually given orally
   2. The mycins, as discussed earlier, are given I.M.
D. Adverse effects/nursing care:
   1. Isoniazid (INH):
      a. Peripheral neuritis:
         (1) Characterized by paresthesias of the hands and feet
         (2) Vitamin B_6 (pyridoxine) is given with INH to prevent peripheral neuritis.
      b. Elevated liver function tests; liver function tests should be done before and during INH therapy.
   2. PAS:
      a. GI disturbances; give with meals
      b. Liver toxicity
      c. Interferes with absorption of Rifampin; if Rifampin is being given in conjunction with PAS, the drugs should be given eight to 12 hours apart.
   3. Rifampin:
      a. Causes red-orange body secretions (remember, "Rifampin causes Red")
      b. Affects the actions of many drugs: Negates birth control pills; decreases the action of steroids, anticoagulants, and digitoxin
      c. GI disturbances and liver toxicity
      d. Give Rifampin on an empty stomach.
   4. Ethambutol:
      a. Optic neuritis:
         (1) Decreased visual acuity and loss of red-green color discrimination
         (2) Client should have visual testing before starting the medication and every two to four weeks while receiving it
      b. Elevated uric acid; monitor uric acid levels and watch for gout symptoms

Antiviral Agents

Viruses have no cell walls and are very difficult to destroy; antiviral drugs are moderately effective against certain viruses; most viruses such as influenza simply run their course; immunizations are used to prevent the spread of other viruses such as polio, measles, and small pox.

A. Antivirals used to treat herpes zoster and herpes simplex 1 and 2 (note the VIR in the

names of most antivirals): Acyclovir (Zovirax), famciclovir (Famvir)
1. Method of administration:
a. PO used to treat initial and recurrent genital herpes, cold sores, and shingles (herpes zoster)
b. At the first sign of an outbreak, the person should take several tablets (5–10) per day as ordered and continue until the lesions go away.
c. IV: Initial therapy for severe herpes
d. Topical:
(1) Systemic absorption is minimal.
(2) Topical application will reduce healing time and virus shedding time; topical use is less effective than oral.
2. Adverse effects:
a. Oral:
(1) GI symptoms
(2) Headache, can be severe
(3) Arthralgia
b. IV:
(1) Phlebitis and inflammation at injection site
(2) Should not be given as a large bolus
(3) Give over at least one hour.
(4) Hydrate well.
c. Topical: Transient burning, stinging, pain, rashes
B. Antivirals used to prevent and treat influenza type A
1. Examples:
a. Amantadine (Symmetrel); also used to treat Parkinson's Disease because it increases dopamine levels
b. Rimantadine (Flumadine)
2. Method of administration: PO as tablets or syrup
3. Adverse effects/nursing care:
a. Nausea, dizziness, insomnia, nervousness
b. Orthostatic hypotension: Take BP twice a day
c. Teach client to avoid aspirin and acetaminophen because these may decrease concentrations of rimantadine.
C. Antivirals to treat cytomegalovirus (CMV) infections in immunocompromised persons
1. Examples:
a. Ganciclovir (Cytovene)
b. Foscarnet (Foscavir)
c. Cidofovir (Vistide)
2. Method of administration: All given IV; ganciclovir also given po
3. Adverse effects/nursing care:
a. Bone marrow suppression; watch for infection and bleeding; check blood counts
b. Headache, seizures, neuropathy

c. Nausea, vomiting, abdominal pain
d. Eye problems
e. Renal damage; monitor creatinine clearance levels frequently during therapy

Antiretrovirals

Antiretrovirals are used to treat AIDS and HIV and are classified into three categories—nucleoside analogues, non-nucleoside analogues, and protease inhibitors. They all interfere with the replication of the virus but do it in different ways and in different stages of the virus life cycle.

A. Nucleoside analogues: Didanosine (Videx) (ddI), Lamivudine (3TC) (Epivir), Stavudine (d4T) (Zerit), Zidovudine (AZT) (Retrovir) inhibit the replication of HIV virus by inhibiting the transcription of RNA and DNA; AZT is used in persons who have been exposed to HIV as well as those who have AIDS
1. Method of administration: PO; all are given PO and zidovudine is also given IV
2. Adverse effects/nursing care:
a. Bone marrow suppression resulting in anemia and agranulocytosis and bleeding; seen especially with Didanosine and Zidovudine
(1) Epogen given to raise RBC count; transfusions may be needed during therapy
(2) Teach client to avoid exposure to infections.
(3) Assess blood counts every two weeks.
b. CNS: Headache, malaise, neuropathy
c. GI:
(1) Nausea and anorexia, pancreatitis
(2) Liver function tests should be done regularly.
d. Skin: Rash and itching
e. Use cautiously with other drugs because there are many drug incompatibilities.
f. Teach client and family:
(1) Drugs do not cure AIDS but will control symptoms.
(2) Call physician if signs of other infections such as sore throat or swollen lymph nodes
(3) Client is still infective and must use methods to prevent transmission of AIDS virus, including universal precautions and safer sex.
(4) Follow-up visits important to monitor for toxicity
(5) Avoid OTC products because of the many incompatibilities.

B. Non-nucleoside analogues: Delavirdine (DLV) (Rescriptor); Nevirapine (NVP) (Viramune)
   1. Method of administration: PO
   2. Adverse effects/nursing care:
      a. Monitor liver enzymes.
      b. Nevirapine decreases effectiveness of oral contraceptives.
      c. Nevirapine is always given with at least one other antiviral; resistance develops very quickly when given alone.
      d. Severe rash
C. Protease inhibitors: Indinavir (Crixivan); Nelfinavir (Viracept); Ritonavir (Norvir); Saquinavir (Invirase)
   1. Method of administration: PO
   2. Adverse effects/nursing care:
      a. Use cautiously with other drugs: Norvir may decrease effects of oral contraceptives and theophylline and may increase effects of antidepressants; Invirase has many interactions with drugs.
      b. Take with food.

Antifungals

A. Used to treat systemic fungi or yeast infections (histoplasmosis), vaginal fungal infections (candida), or skin fungal infections (tinea [ring worm])
B. Amphotericin B (Fungazone) used in the treatment of systemic fungal infections, such as histoplasmosis or coccidiomycosis
   1. Given IV
   2. Adverse reactions/nursing care:
      a. Very toxic
      b. Blood dyscrasias: CBC should be done weekly
      c. Give aspirin or acetaminophen, Benadryl, and steroids prior to infusion to prevent fever, chills, nausea, and vomiting
      d. Abnormal renal function with hypokalemia and azotemia
      e. Potassium supplements will be given to prevent hypokalemia.
      f. Monitor intake and output.
      g. Renal and liver function tests should be done weekly.
      h. IV infusion should be slow to prevent cardiovascular collapse, which may occur immediately after IV infusion.
      i. Don't mix antibiotics with Amphotericin B.
C. Griseofulvin (Grisastin):
   1. Treatment of ringworm infections of skin, hair, and nails
   2. Griseofulvin is a penicillin derivative; use with caution in persons with a penicillin allergy.

   3. Adverse effects/nursing care:
      a. Intense sunlight may cause redness and rash.
      b. Oral preparations are most effectively absorbed and cause the least GI distress when given with a high-fat meal.
D. Nystatin (Mycostatin):
   1. Used to treat gastrointestinal and vaginal candida (yeast) infections
   2. Can be given orally as tablets, oral suspension (for thrush), or as vaginal tablets
   3. Oral use is nontoxic.
   4. Tell client to take medication for two weeks after symptoms improve to prevent reinfection
   5. Teach client that antibiotics, birth control pills, steroids, diabetes, tight-fitting panty hose, and reinfection by the sexual partner are predisposing factors for vaginal infection
   6. Chlortrimazole (Gyne-Lotrimin) and miconazole (Monistat) vaginal suppositories are available without prescription for vaginal yeast infections.

Antihelminths

A. Rids the body of helminths (parasitic worms), including tapeworms, pinworms, hookworms, roundworms, and schistosomes
B. Examples:
   1. Quinacrine (Atabrine) treats giardiasis, malaria, and tapeworms; colors urine a deep yellow
   2. Mebendazole (Vermox) treats roundworm, whipworm, and hookworm.
C. Adverse effects/nursing care:
   1. Antihelmintics are relatively nontoxic.
   2. Teach clients and family about how the worm is spread; if one family member has parasites, all should be evaluated.

CENTRAL NERVOUS SYSTEM DRUGS
Local Anesthetics

A. Local anesthetics block nerve conduction, producing a temporary loss of sensation and motion in a limited area of the body; used for dental or minor surgical procedures such as suturing lacerations and for regional anesthesia.
B. Response to local anesthetic:
   1. Skin veins dilate because of vasomotor paralysis.

2. Temperature perception changes—sense of cold disappears, brief sense of warmth, absence of temperature.
3. Pain sensation blocked
4. Touch sensation lost
5. Motor function lost
6. Sensory functions return in reverse order.
7. Epinephrine may be given with local anesthetics to prolong action and to control bleeding; epinephrine is a peripheral vasoconstrictor; anesthetics are supplied in vials with and without epinephrine.
C. Examples (note the caine):
1. Benzocaine (Americaine)
2. Procaine (Novocaine)
3. Lidocaine (Xylocaine)
4. Mepivacaine (Carbocaine)
5. Tetracaine (Pontocaine)
6. Bupivacaine (Marcaine)
D. Regional anesthesia:
1. Spinal anesthesia:
   a. Needle is inserted into the spinal canal, and cerebrospinal fluid is lost.
   b. Client will be maintained in a flat position for eight hours to prevent headache.
   c. Epidural anesthesia:
      (1) Anesthesia is injected into the epidural space.
      (2) Because no cerebrospinal fluid is lost, the person is not likely to develop headaches and does not need to remain flat.
E. Adverse reactions/nursing care:
1. Skin irritation can occur.
2. Anaphylaxis, respiratory depression, dysrhythmias, and cardiac arrest can occur; serious reactions usually happen when the anesthetic is inadvertently injected into the vasculature and reaches high plasma concentrations.
3. Monitor vital signs.
4. Force fluids after spinal anesthesia to help the body quickly replace the CSF (cerebrospinal fluid) that was lost.

Non-narcotic Analgesics and Antipyretics

A. Salicylates:
1. Actions:
   a. Pain relief
   b. Anticoagulant effect in clients at risk for clotting, such as MI and TIA or CVA
2. Examples:
   a. Aspirin (acetyl salicylic acid)
   b. Methyl salicylate
   c. Sodium salicylate
   d. There are many trade names for aspirin and aspirin-containing products.

3. Actions (see Table 18.2):
   a. Analgesia: Produced by action on the hypothalamus and also by blocking the generation of pain impulses
   b. Antipyretic: Produced by acting on the hypothalamus (temperature regulating center) to produce peripheral vasodilation, which causes sweating and heat loss
   c. Anticoagulant: Produced by acting on prostaglandins, which inhibit platelet aggregation
   d. Anti-inflammatory: Produced by inhibition of prostaglandin synthesis, causing anti-inflammatory activity
B. Acetaminophen (Tylenol):
Acts similarly to salicylates in producing analgesia and reducing fever. It does not have anti-inflammatory properties and has a minimal anticoagulant effect (see Table 18.2).
C. Nonsteroidal Anti-inflammatory Drugs (NSAIDs):
1. Examples:
   a. Ibuprofen (Motrin, Datril)
   b. Naproxen (Naprosyn, Anaprox)
   c. Indomethacin (Indocin)
   d. Piroxicam (Feldene)
   e. Ketorolac tromethamine (Toradol); available PO, IM, IV and ophthalmic
2. Actions (see Table 18.2):
   a. NSAIDs are prostaglandin inhibitors that relieve pain and inflammation by blocking an early step in the inflammatory reaction; they are especially useful in the treatment of rheumatoid, osteo, and gouty arthritis; they help with pain but do not stop joint destruction.
   b. NSAIDs prolong clotting time and have some antipyretic action.
   c. It may take up to two weeks to see improvement.
   d. Ketorolac (Toradol) is used for short term relief of mild to moderate pain; the injection is not to be used more than five days.
D. Adverse reactions/nursing care (see Tables 18.3 and 18.4):
1. Bleeding:
   a. Seen primarily with salicylates and NSAIDs
   b. Acetaminophen can cause hemolytic anemia and thrombocytopenia.
   c. Assess the client for ecchymosis and other signs of bleeding.
   d. Salicylates may be prescribed therapeutically to prevent clot formation in clients on long-term bed rest with fractures or in the prevention of heart attacks.

e. Salicylates are contraindicated for clients with bleeding disorders.
f. Salicylates have an additive effect for persons receiving anticoagulants.

2. Gastrointestinal disturbances:
   a. Salicylates and NSAIDs can cause gastritis and GI bleeding.
   b. Contraindicated for persons with ulcer disease
   c. Give them with food.
3. Liver:
   a. Acetaminophen can cause liver toxicity, especially with an overdose or when alcohol is being consumed.
   b. NSAIDs can affect liver enzymes; monitor blood values.
4. Renal toxicity:
   a. High doses of salicylates can cause renal failure; monitor renal function tests in clients receiving high doses or those in salicylate toxicity.
   b. NSAIDs can cause hematuria and acute renal failure.
5. Hearing: Tinnitus (ringing in the ears) is the first sign of salicylate toxicity; hearing loss can occur
6. Rash can occur in all non-narcotic analgesics.
7. Reye's syndrome has been associated with the administration of salicylates to children who have viral infections; do not give salicylates to children with the chicken pox and influenza-like symptoms.
8. Allergic reaction: Allergies to salicylates are common; causes asthma symptoms (persons who are allergic to salicylates may also be allergic to Naprosyn)
9. Antidote for acetaminophen overdose is acetylcysteine (Mucomyst)

E. Antiheadache:
1. Sumatriptan (Imitrex)

2. Actions
   a. Classed as migraine agent
   b. Exerts antimigraine effect because it causes vasoconstriction in cerebral arteries
3. Adverse effects/nursing care:
   a. Feeling of pressure, dizziness, sedation, chest tightness
   b. Client instructed to give self a subcutaneous injection with a self-dose system
   c. Teach client to avoid tyramine foods because these may precipitate headache

Narcotic Analgesics

A. Narcotic analgesics alter the perception of and the emotional response to pain. Because of their addicting properties and abuse potential, they are controlled substances.
B. Uses:
1. Narcotic analgesics are used for the relief of severe pain and as a pre-operative medication.
2. Narcotics are not interchangeable; since potencies vary, use caution when switching from one drug to another or from one route to another.
3. Oral and parenteral dosages are not the same. Because oral forms go first to the liver to be metabolized, the oral doses are much higher than I.M. doses. Always be sure that the route is clearly indicated.
C. Examples:
1. Morphine
2. Codeine
3. Meperidine (Demerol)
4. Methadone (Dolophine)
5. Hydromorphone HCl (Dilaudid)
6. Pentazocine HCl (Talwin)

Table 18.3 Actions of Non-narcotic Analgesics

Drug Type	Analgesic	Antipyretic	Anti-inflammatory	Anticoagulant
Salicylates	X	X	X	X
NSAIDs	X	X	X	X
Acetaminophen	X	X	X	

Table 18.4 Adverse Effects of Non-narcotic Analgesics

Effect	Salicylates	NSAIDs	Acetaminophen
Bleeding	X	X	X
Gastrointestinal	X	X	
Liver		X	X
Renal	X	X	
Hearing	X		
Skin	X	X	X

7. Oxycodone HCl
8. Oxycodone and acetaminophen (Percocet)
9. Oxycodone and aspirin (Percodan)
10. Fentanyl (Duragesic) available in injection, transdermal patches, and lozenges; IM, IV, and lozenges used for pre-op and minor surgical or diagnostic procedures; transdermal patch used for chronic pain

D. Codeine is combined with empirin, fiorinal, or Tylenol.
E. Client-Controlled Analgesia (PCA)
   1. A type of intravenous pump that allows the client to administer his own narcotic analgesic (usually morphine) on demand within a preset dose and frequency limit
   2. Nurse must instruct the client in use of PCA pump and assess client for pain, pain relief, and signs of side effects frequently.
F. Adverse effects/nursing care:
   1. Respiratory depression:
      a. Monitor respirations.
      b. Do not give to clients with COPD or cor pulmonale.
      c. Pre-op narcotics should be given 1–2 hours before surgery so that the peak respiratory depressant effect will be over when anesthesia is administered.
   2. Drowsiness and sleep:
      a. Safety when ambulating
      b. Put up side rails.
   3. Mood changes
   4. Cough suppression; codeine may be used therapeutically as a cough suppressant
   5. Orthostatic hypotension:
      a. Monitor vital signs.
      b. Teach the client to get out of bed slowly.
   6. Decreased peristalsis:
      a. Observe for constipation.
      b. Administer stool softeners as ordered.
   7. Stimulates emetic chemo-receptors:
      a. Nausea and vomiting may occur.
      b. GI symptoms do not constitute an allergic reaction.
   8. Morphine increases intracranial pressure; do not give to clients with head injuries.
   9. Narcotics cross the placenta: Give at least two hours before delivery so that the fetus will not have respiratory depression
   10. May precipitate urinary retention; use with caution in clients with benign prostatic hypertrophy (BPH).
   11. Do not give to persons with convulsive disorders.
   12. Pupil constriction:
      a. Check pupils for reactivity.
      b. Chronic pupil constriction is a sign of addiction.
   13. Hypersensitivity reactions:
      a. Persons allergic to one drug may be able to tolerate another agent.
      b. Cross reactivity can occur.

   c. GI reactions are not allergic responses to the drug.
14. Alcohol potentiates CNS depressant effects of narcotics; teach client not to combine alcohol and narcotics.
15. Adjuvant drugs such as hydroxyzine (Viastaril, Atarax) and amytriptyline (Elavil) often given with narcotic analgesics for pre- and post-op sedation; because these drugs are also CNS depressants, be alert for drowsiness.

Narcotic Antagonists

A. Uses:
   1. Opiate-induced respiratory depression
   2. Acute opiate overdose
   3. Narcotic antagonists prevent or reverse many of the actions of morphine-type analgesics and meperidine by blocking opiate receptors in the central nervous system; will reverse opiate-induced respiratory depression within minutes.
B. Example of drug: Naloxone (Narcan)
C. Adverse effects/nursing care:
   1. Low incidence of toxicity
   2. Can cause nausea, vomiting, and elevated blood pressure
   3. Will cause acute withdrawal in clients who are addicted to opiates
   4. Frequently assess for recurrence of respiratory depression: The effects of the narcotic may last longer than the effects of the antagonist.
   5. Use with caution in clients with severe cardiovascular disease.

Sedatives and Hypnotics

A. Sedatives and hypnotics are thought to interfere with the transmission of impulses in various parts of the brain; they are used to provide sedation, treat insomnia, induce sleep before surgery and tests, and relieve anxiety.
B. Barbiturates:
   1. Barbiturates are readily absorbed after oral, rectal, and parenteral administration; they are distributed in all tissues, cross the placental barrier, and appear in breast milk.
   2. Actions and uses:
      a. CNS depression ranging from mild to death
      b. Sedation
      c. Pre-operative medications
      d. Anticonvulsants
   3. Examples (note that the barbiturates are barbitals)…
      a. Phenobarbital Sodium (Luminal)
      b. Amobarbital Sodium (Amytal)
      c. Butabarbital Sodium (Butisol)
      d. Pentobarbital Sodium (Nembutal)

e. Secobarbital Sodium (Seconal)
f. Thiopental Sodium (Pentothal Sodium)
B. Benzodiazepines (antianxiety agents):
  1. Actions and uses:
    a. Central nervous system depression
    b. Antianxiety
    c. Sedation
    d. Light anesthesia
    e. Skeletal muscle relaxation
    f. Anticonvulsant
  2. Examples:
    a. Diazepam (Valium)
    b. Alprazolam (Xanax)
    c. Midazolam (Versed)
    d. Oxazepam (Serax)
    e. Temazepan (Restoril)
    f. Alzapam (Ativan)
    g. Flurazepam (Dalmane)
    h. Triazolam (Halcion)
    i. Chlorazepate (Tranxene)
    j. Chlordiazepoxide (Librium)
C. Nonbenzodiazepines:
  1. Act similarly to other sedative hypnotics and have similar side effects
  2. Examples:
    a. Chloral hydrate
    b. Ethchlorvynol (Placidyl)
D. Adverse effects/nursing care:
  1. Addiction:
    a. Persons who are addicted to alcohol or any other CNS drug should not take any of the sedatives or hypnotics, because they are cross-addicting.
    b. Observe clients carefully for signs of addiction.
    c. When used as a hypnotic, do not give for more than 14–28 days.
  2. Drowsiness, lethargy, confusion, ataxia, vertigo, hallucinations
    a. Warn the client not to drive or operate dangerous machinery while taking barbiturates.
    b. Be alert for safety needs.
    c. Observe mental status of the client.
  3. Respiratory depression when given IV; monitor carefully.
  4. Blood disorders:
    a. Monitor blood counts.
    b. Report immediately signs of infection, such as sore throats and also bleeding and bruising.
  5. Renal and liver:
    a. Monitor kidney and liver function tests.
    b. Observe for urinary retention and jaundice.
  6. Do not use as an analgesic.
    a. Barbiturates do not control pain.
    b. They may cause a paradoxical excitement or may mask pain symptoms.
  7. Barbiturates and benzodiazepines should be tapered slowly when they are

discontinued; abrupt withdrawal can be life-threatening.
  8. Contraindications for benzodiazepines:
    a. Acute alcohol intoxication with respiratory depression
    b. Acute-angle glaucoma
    c. Suicidal persons
  9. When used to induce sleep, use nursing measures such as a back rub to enhance the effectiveness of the drug.
  10. Many interactions with other drugs
  11. Chlordiazepoxide (Librium) used in delirium tremens
  12. Midazolam (Versed) used for sedation and relief of anxiety as well as producing retrograde amnesia for short procedures (conscious sedation)

Benzodiazepine Receptor Antagonist: Flumazenil (Mazicon)

A. Antagonizes the actions of benzodiazepines on the central nervous system; used to reverse sedative effects of benzodiazepines and conscious sedation anesthesia
B. Adverse effects/nursing care:
  1. Hypertension
  2. Dysrhythmias; monitor cardiac status
  3. Convulsions, dizziness
  4. Nausea and vomiting; do not ingest food during IV infusion
  5. Monitor the client's airway.

Anticonvulsants

A. Anticonvulsants help to control seizures by preventing seizure activity in the brain or by preventing the spread of the seizure focus.
B. Categories of anticonvulsants:
  1. Barbiturates (Phenobarbital): Used for both generalized and absence seizures (petit mal)
  2. Benzodiazepines: Diazepam (Valium); drug of choice for status epilepticus; useful for absence seizures
  3. Hydantoins: Phenytoin (Dilantin): Used to treat grand mal seizures and status epilepticus
  4. Carbamazepine (Tegretol):
    a. Used for seizures that are unresponsive to other anticonvulsants
    b. Also used for neuropathies such as diabetic neuropathy and trigeminal neuralgia
C. Adverse reactions/nursing care:
  1. CNS effects: Drowsiness, ataxia, blurred vision; observe safety precautions
  2. GI effects: Nausea and vomiting
  3. Lowered blood counts: Monitor blood tests and watch for signs of abnormalities
  4. Renal and liver: Monitor renal and liver function tests

5. Dilantin may cause pink or red urine.
6. Hyperplasia of the gums with phenytoin (Dilantin); give good mouth care
7. Alcohol reduces the effectiveness of Dilantin.
8. Drug interactions:
   a. Check the client's medications.
   b. Anticonvulsants inhibit or potentiate many other drugs.
   c. Teach the client to let all physicians know what anticonvulsant is being taken.
9. Monitor serum hydantoin levels: Therapeutic level 10–20 mcg/ml.
10. Caution client not to suddenly stop taking anticonvulsants.
11. Do not mix Dilantin with dextrose; use normal saline.

Skeletal Muscle Relaxants

A. Uses:
   1. Skeletal muscle relaxants reduce the transmission of impulses from the spinal cord to the skeletal muscles.
   2. They are used to treat a wide range of skeletal muscle spasticity, from lower back pain to multiple sclerosis.
   3. Dantrolene is used to treat malignant hyperthermia and neuroleptic malignant syndrome.
B. Examples:
   1. Baclofen (Lioresal)
   2. Carisoprodol (Soma; Soma compound contains aspirin; available with codeine)
   3. Dantrolene (Dantrum)
   4. Cyclobenzaprine (Flexeril)
   5. Methocarbamol (Robaxin)
C. Adverse reactions/nursing care:
   1. CNS side effects: Drowsiness, dizziness as in all CNS drugs; safety is a nursing concern
   2. Dantrolene has serious side effects:
      a. Muscle weakness, neurologic symptoms
      b. GI and hepatic effects; monitor liver function tests; used cautiously in persons with liver dysfunction
   3. Used in combination with non-narcotic and narcotic analgesics
   4. Dantrolene (Dantrum) acts on skeletal muscles and relieves spasticity.

Anti-Parkinson Agents

A. Parkinson's disease is thought to result from a neurotransmitter imbalance in the central nervous system. There is too much acetylcholine and not enough dopamine; therefore, treatment consists of giving dopamine and blocking acetylcholine.

B. Cholinergic blocking agents:
   1. Examples:
      a. Benztropine Mesylate (Cogentin)
      b. Trihexyphenidyl HCl (Artane); relieves rigidity but has no effect on tremor
      c. Contraindicated in clients with glaucoma, tachycardia, duodenal ulcers, biliary obstruction, and prostatic hypertrophy
   2. Adverse reactions/nursing care:
      a. Constipation: Encourage fluids, activity, and stool softeners
      b. Dry mouth: Encourage cold beverages, hard candies, and gum
      c. Nausea: Give with food to decrease gastric symptoms
      d. Tachycardia, hypotension; monitor vital signs
      e. Dizziness, drowsiness; safety
      f. Decreased bronchial secretions
      g. Blurred vision, photophobia, acute glaucoma
      h. Suppression of sweating
      i. Loss of libido
      j. Urinary retention
      k. Do not withdraw drugs abruptly.
C. Dopamine agents:
   1. Carbidopa/Levodopa (Sinemet)
   2. Levodopa (Levopa)
   3. Amantadine (Symmetrel)
   4. Parlodel

Antipsychotic Agents

Note: When we look at drugs used to treat psychiatric disorders, we shall look only at the side effects in addition to the above. Remember, they can all cause anticholinergic side effects and hypotension.

A. Drugs used to treat psychiatric disorders have in common certain types of side effects (see Table 18.5).
   1. Anticholinergic effects:
      a. Red as a beet (vasodilation)
      b. Hot as a hare (tachycardia)
      c. Blind as a bat (mydriatic effect)
      d. Dry as a bone (drying of secretions)
      e. Mad as a hatter (nervousness and disorientation)
   2. Cardiovascular effects:
      a. Dysrhythmias
      b. Postural hypotension
   3. Hepatic effects
   4. Blood disorders
   5. Renal effects
   6. Central nervous system depression

Table 18.5 Major Side Effects of Antipsychotic Agents

Anticholinergic	Cardiovascular/ Hematologic
• "Red as a beet" (vasodilation) • "Hot as a hare" (tachycardia) • "Blind as a bat" (mydriatic effect) • "Dry as a bone" (drying of secretions)	• Postural hypotension • Agranulocytosis

Central Nervous System	
• "Mad as a hatter" (nervousness and disorientation)	• CNS depression; safety concerns

B. Phenothiazines:
   1. Actions and uses:
      a. It is thought that excess dopamine in certain parts of the brain may cause some psychoses. Phenothiazines block dopamine receptors in the brain and help to control psychoses, particularly schizophrenia.
      b. Antiemetic effects: Used in the control of nausea
      c. Phenothiazines can be given orally or by injection.
   2. Examples (zines):
      a. Chlorpromazine (Thorazine)
      b. Promethazine (Phenergan)
      c. Thiridazine (Mellaril)
      d. Fluphenazine (Prolixin)
      e. Promazine (Sparine)
   3. Adverse reactions/nursing care:
      a. In addition to the side effects discussed earlier, phenothiazines have many side effects involving most body systems.
      b. Extrapyramidal reactions ataxia and tremors; Cogentin is used to reduce or treat these symptoms.
      c. Dystonic reactions
      d. Drowsiness; particularly in the first few weeks of therapy
      e. Photosensitivity: Use sunscreen, wear long-sleeved shirts, avoid the sun
      f. Pink-colored urine
      g. Changes in libido and menses
      h. Agranulocytosis: Observe for a persistent sore throat; teach client to report persistent infections
      i. Potentiates CNS depressant effects of alcohol, narcotics, sedatives and hypnotics
      j. Neuroleptic malignant syndrome (NMS):
         (1) Observe for fever, tachycardia, tachypnea, diaphoresis, and rigidity.
         (2) NMS is rare but frequently fatal.
         (3) Withhold medication and notify the physician.
C. Other antipsychotic agents
   1. Examples:
      a. Haloperidol (Haldol): Used for psychoses and Tourette's syndrome

b. Clozapine (Clozaril): Used in treatment of schizophrenic persons who are unresponsive to or cannot tolerate other agents
   2. Adverse reactions/nursing care:
      a. Reactions are the same as for phenothiazines.
      b. Clozapine has fewer extrapyramidal side effects and more blood dyscrasias (agranulocytosis, leukopenia) than phenothiazines.
      c. Obtain a baseline CBC and then weekly a CBC while client is on clozapine and weekly for one month when the drug is discontinued.

Lithium

A. Lithium is thought to alter neurotransmitters in the central nervous system, reducing the characteristic highs and lows of bipolar disorder.
B. Examples (lith):
   1. Lithium Carbonate (Eskalith)
   2. Lithium Citrate (Cibalith-S)
C. Adverse reactions/nursing care:
   1. CNS and musculoskeletal effects (lethargy, fatigue, weakness, headache, hand tremors)
   2. GI effects (nausea, anorexia, dry mouth)
   3. Monitor serum lithium levels.
      a. Therapeutic levels are 0.4–1.6 mEq/l.
      b. Toxic level is 2 mEq/l.
   4. Give with meals.
   5. Maintain adequate sodium intake to reduce the danger of lithium intoxication.
   6. Avoid sodium-depleting diuretics (hydrochlorothiazidel to prevent under medication).
   7. Encourage fluid intake of 2.5–3 liters per day.
   8. Observe for lithium intoxication:
      a. Drowsiness, confusion, giddiness
      b. GI symptoms
      c. Muscle rigidity, fasiculations, ataxia
      d. Lithium intoxication is treated with IV normal saline and hemodialysis if levels > 3 mEq/l.

Antidepressants

A. Tricyclic antidepressants:
   1. Tricyclics block the reuptake of various neurotransmitters at the neuronal membrane, allowing for increased amounts of serotonin and norepinephrine. Tricyclics are used in the treatment of major depression.
   2. Examples:
      a. Amitriptyline (Elavil); remember Elavil elevates the mood
      b. Imipramine (Tofranil)
      c. Nortriptyline (Aventyl, Pamelor)
      d. Clomipramine (Anafranil)

3. Adverse reactions/nursing care: The following are in addition to the side effects common to all CNS drugs:
   a. Extrapyramidal effects: Tremor, rigidity; tricyclics are chemically related to the phenothiazines
   b. Blood disorders: Monitor CBC and differential for clients on long-term therapy.
   c. Takes 2–4 weeks for therapeutic effectiveness

B. Atypical antidepressants:
   1. Inhibit CNS neuronal uptake of serotonin and are used for short-term management of depression; Paxil and Zoloft also used for panic disorders
   2. Examples:
      a. Fluoxetine (Prozac)
      b. Paroxetine (Paxil)
      c. Sertraline (Zoloft)
   3. Adverse reactions/nursing care:
      a. CNS effects: Nervousness, insomnia, drowsiness
      b. Takes 2–4 weeks for therapeutic effectiveness
      c. Monitor liver enzymes with Zoloft.

C. MAO inhibitors:
   1. MAO inhibitors increase the concentration of amines in the CNS of the body. Amines are thought to elevate the mood. MAO inhibitors are used for the symptomatic management of clients with neurotic or atypical depression. Because of serious side effects, MAO inhibitors are not usually used unless other antidepressant drugs are ineffective.
   2. Examples:
      a. Phenylzine (Nardil)
      b. Tranylcypromine (Parnate)
      c. Selegiline (Eldepryl)
   3. Adverse reactions/nursing care:
      a. Hypertensive crisis: Severe headache, palpitation, stiff neck, nausea, vomiting, visual disturbances; monitor blood pressure
      b. Orthostatic hypotension (dose related); monitor blood pressure
      c. Persons taking MAO inhibitors should be taught to avoid food containing tyramine or tryptophan, including aged cheese, processed cheese, sour cream, wine, beer, chicken liver, raisins, bananas, avocados, chocolate, soy sauce, and caffeine, because these substances may precipitate hypertensive crises.
      d. MAO inhibitors have many drug interactions.
      e. Hepatic damage: Monitor liver function tests

Autonomic Nervous System

A. The autonomic nervous system regulates the basic physiologic functions of the body—respirations, blood pressure, heart rate, metabolism, digestion, bowel motility, salivation, perspiration, and pupil size.
   1. The autonomic nervous system is divided into two opposing systems: The sympathetic or "fight and flight" system and the parasympathetic or "feed and breed" system (see Table 18.6).
   2. The sympathetic system is the emergency response system; adrenalin is the hormone of the sympathetic nervous system.

Table 18.6 Autonomic Nervous System

	Sympathetic (Adrenergic)	Parasympathetic (Cholinergic)
Neurotransmitter	Adrenalin	Acetylcholine
Effects on		
Eye	Dilates pupil	Constricts pupil
Lacrimal gland	None	Stimulates secretion
Salivary	Thick, scanty, viscous secretions; dry mouth	Copious, thin, watery secretions
Heart	Increases rate and force of contraction	Decreases rate
Blood vessels	Constricts smooth muscles of skin, abdominal blood vessels, and cutaneous blood vessels	No effect
	Dilates smooth muscle of bronchioles, blood vessels of heart, and skeletal muscles	
Lungs	Dilates bronchi	Constricts bronchi
GI tract	Decreases motility	Increases motility
	Constricts sphincters	Relaxes sphincters
	Inhibits secretion	Stimulates secretion
	Inhibits gallbladder and ducts	Stimulates gallbladder and ducts
	Inhibits glycogenesis in liver	
Adrenal gland	Stimulates secretion of epinephrine and norepinephrine	No effects
Urinary tract	Relaxes detrusor muscle	Contracts detrusor muscle
	Contracts trigone sphincter (prevents voiding)	Relaxes trigone sphincter (allows voiding)

3. The parasympathetic system promotes storage and conservation of energy and the digestion and absorption of food; acetylcholine is the hormone of the parasympathetic nervous system.

B. Adrenergic drugs:
1. Treatment of shock:
   a. Examples:
      (1) Dopamine HCl (Intropin, Dopastat); dopamine is the immediate precursor to epinephrine in the body
      (2) Ephedrine Sulfate (Vatronol)
      (3) Epinephrine HCl (Adrenalin)
      (4) Levarterenol Bitartrate [Norepinephrine] (Levophed)
      (5) Metaraminol Bitartrate (Aramine)
   b. Adverse effects/nursing care:
      (1) Sympathetic effects such as hypertension, tachycardia, and dysrhythmias
      (2) Urinary retention
      (3) Nausea, vomiting
      (4) Aramine and Levophed are very potent; monitor BP frequently during administration.
      (5) Aramine and Levophed cause severe extravasation if they infiltrate.
      (6) When Levophed is being administered, have Regitine available to use at the site of extravasation to dilate local blood vessels.
2. Treatment of bronchospasm: (to be discussed under respiratory tract drugs)
   a. Examples:
      (1) Isoproterenol (Isuprel)
      (2) Metaproterenol (Alupent)
      (3) Theophylline
      (4) Terbutaline Sulfate (Brethine)
   b. Adverse effects/nursing care:
      (1) Rebound congestion can occur with prolonged use; caution the client to use only as often as directed.
      (2) Tachycardia, dysrhythmias, hypertension; should not be given to persons who are hypertensive
      (3) Persons with prostatic hypertrophy may develop urinary retention.

C. Adrenergic blockers:
1. Action and uses:
   a. Alpha adrenergic blocking agents reduce the tone of muscles around peripheral blood vessels, increasing peripheral circulation and lowering blood pressure.
   b. Beta adrenergic blockers work on the heart muscle and reduce muscle tone, also lowering blood pressure.

c. The beta blockers used primarily to lower blood pressure are discussed under antihypertensives.
2. Examples:
   a. Ergotamine Tartrate (Ergomar):
      (1) Decreases pulsations found in migraine headaches
      (2) Most effective when taken before the onset of an acute attack
      (3) Ergotamine has emetic and oxytocic effects.
      (4) Do not give in pregnancy, because it stimulates uterine contractions.
   b. Phentolamine Mesylate (Regitine):
      (1) Regitine is an alpha adrenergic blocking agent that produces vasodilation and cardiac stimulation.
      (2) Uses:
         (a) Treatment of hypertensive crises due to MAO inhibitors or sympathomimetic drugs
         (b) Treatment of pheochromocytoma (a secreting tumor of the adrenal medulla that causes serious hypertension)
         (c) Dermal necrosis following IV extravasation of levarterenol bitartrate (Levophed) or serotonin

D. Cholinergics:
1. Cholinergic drugs produce parasympathetic effects on the body. Acetylcholine is the neurohormone responsible for parasympathetic action. Cholinergic drugs are used to treat myasthenia gravis (a deficiency in acetylcholine); post-operative urinary retention, abdominal distention, and megacolon; and as an antidote in anticholinergic poisoning.
2. Treatment of Myasthenia Gravis:
   a. Ambenonium Chloride (Mytelase)
   b. Neostigmine (Prostigmin)
   c. Pyridostigmine (Mestinon)
   d. Edrophonium Chloride (Tensilon):
      (1) Used in diagnosis of myasthenia gravis to differentiate myasthenic from cholinergic crisis and as a curare antagonist
      (2) Tensilon acts rapidly but has the shortest duration, so it is not effective as a treatment for myasthenia gravis.
3. Bethanechol Chloride (Urecholine):
   a. Treatment of post-operative urinary retention and abdominal distention
   b. Urecholine is always given PO
4. Adverse effects/nursing care:

a. Cholinergic crisis:
  (1) Cholinergics are nonspecific and affect the whole parasympathetic nervous system.
  (2) Cholinergic crisis is characterized by nausea, vomiting, increased salivation, diarrhea, sweating, miosis (pupil constriction), and hypothermia.
  (3) Atropine is used to treat cholinergic overdose.
b. Monitor respirations, muscular weakness, temperature, urinary output, and GI function.
c. Do not give to clients with hyperthyroidism, peptic ulcer, active bronchial asthma, cardiac disease, or obstruction of the GI or urinary tract because parasympathetic effects will aggravate these conditions.

D. Anticholinergic:
  1. Anticholinergics block the effect of acetylcholine and inhibit parasympathetic actions. The effect is to increase the heart rate and decrease GI secretions. Anticholinergics are used as preanesthetic medications to decrease salivary and respiratory secretions and to treat Parkinson's Disease. Atropine can be used to treat poisoning due to organic phosphate insecticides.
  2. Uses:
    a. Preanesthetic medication:
      (1) Atropine sulfate
      (2) Scopolamine hydrobromide
      (3) Glycopyrrolate (Robinul)
    b. Parkinson's Disease:
      (1) Benztropine mesylate (Cogentin)
      (2) Trihexyphenidyl (Artane)
    c. Antiarrhythmic: Atropine sulfate
  3. Adverse effects/nursing care:
    a. Red, hot, dry, blind, mad
    b. Blurred vision, photophobia (pupils dilate); do not give to persons with chronic glaucoma
    c. Urinary hesitancy and retention; have client void before giving drug
    d. Tachycardia, palpitations; use with caution in clients with unstable cardiac conditions
    e. Dry mouth: Persons on long-term therapy may need saliva substitutes
    f. Do not give to persons with myasthenia gravis.

Central Nervous System Stimulant

A. Methylphenidate hydrochloride (Ritalin)
B. Action and uses:
  1. Blocks re-uptake of dopaminergic neurons.
  2. Used to treat attention deficit disorder.
C. Adverse effects/nursing actions:

1. Do not give in the afternoon or evening because it causes insomnia.
2. Suppresses weight gain
3. Tachycardia, palpitations, chest pain
4. Psychotic episode
5. Seizure
6. Coma
7. Monitor CBC.

DRUGS AFFECTING THE HEART AND CIRCULATORY SYSTEM
Cardiac Glycosides (Digoxin)

A. Action and uses:
  1. Cardiac glycosides are plant alkaloids.
  2. Cardiac glycosides act directly on the cardiac muscle to improve myocardial contraction, increasing blood flow to all organs including the kidneys (which causes diuresis), and also to decrease conduction through the AV node.
  3. Used to treat congestive heart failure and to slow ventricular rate in persons with atrial fibrillation or atrial flutter
B. Examples of drug: Digoxin (Lanoxin)
C. Method of administration/dose:
  1. When cardiac glycosides are started, a digitalizing dose is given to quickly raise the serum drug level to therapeutic levels.
  2. Cardiac glycosides stay in the body from two days to three weeks.
  3. Oral forms are usually used for maintenance doses and sometimes for digitalizing doses.
  4. Digoxin (Lanoxin):
    a. The digitalizing dose can be given IV or PO.
    b. Usual maintenance dose is 0.125 to 0.5 mg PO daily.
    c. Digoxin onsets in 1/2 to 2 hours and lasts 2–6 days.
D. Adverse effects/nursing care (see Table 18.7):
  1. Lab studies:
    a. Before administering a digitalizing dose, the client should have had hemoglobin, hematocrit, serum electrolytes, and liver and renal function studies.
    b. The dose must be reduced in persons with poor renal function because digoxin is excreted via the kidneys.
  2. ECG should be done before giving a digitalizing dose.
  3. Bradycardia and/or dysrhythmias:
    a. Do not administer digoxin preparations if the adult apical pulse is below 60 and the child apical pulse is below 90–110.
    b. The nurse should monitor the apical pulse for one minute, noting the rate, rhythm, and quality before administering digitalis preparations.

Table 18.7 Guidelines for Administering Digoxin

Digoxin

Action: Slows and strengthens heart; increases blood supply to organs
- Loading dose higher than maintenance dose
- Stays in system a week; risk for toxicity
- Assess for toxicity:
  - •• Check the apical pulse before giving.
  - •• Hold medication if pulse < 60 or > 100
  - •• Anorexia, nausea, and vomiting
  - •• Vision: Green and yellow halos
- Check K+ levels; report low levels.
- Check serum digoxin levels.
  - •• Withhold medication and report levels above 2.0 ng/ml.

4. GI symptoms: Assess client for anorexia, nausea, and vomiting
5. Central nervous system symptoms including headache, fatigue, and muscle weakness.
6. Visual disturbances: Green or yellow cast to vision
7. Digitalis toxicity:
   a. Monitor serum digoxin levels.
   b. Therapeutic levels 0.5–2.0 ng/ml
   c. Toxicity above 2.0 ng/ml
8. Monitor serum potassium:
   a. Normal 3.5–5.2 mEq/ml
   b. Digitalis toxicity occurs more quickly in the presence of a low serum potassium.
   c. Check potassium levels.
9. Watch for quinidine-digoxin reaction: When digoxin-stabilized clients are started on quinidine, the serum digoxin levels may double, which could lead to toxicity.
10. Increased digoxin levels are caused by anticholinergics, erythromycin, hydroxychloroquine (Plaquenil), tetracyclines, and verapamil (Calan).
11. Digoxin is not absorbed by fat; the dosage of an obese person should be based on ideal weight, not actual weight, to avoid overdose.
E. Digoxin immune FAB (Digibind) is the antidote used to treat life-threatening Digoxin (Lanoxin) intoxication.

Antianginal Drugs

A. Antianginal drugs are classified as coronary vasodilators and are used to reduce the pain of angina. All vasodilators dilate cerebral and peripheral arteries, as well as coronary arteries, causing headache and postural hypotension.
B. Nitrites and nitrates:
   1. Decrease myocardial oxygen needs
   2. Dilate large coronary arteries
   3. Examples:
      a. Isorbide dinitrate (Isordil)
      b. Nitroglycerin, Nitro-Bid, Nitro-Dur

   c. Transdermal Nitrodisc
   d. Topical: Nitrol
   e. Sustained-release Nitro-bid
   f. Sublingual: Nitrostat
   g. Sublingual or translingual aerosol to treat an acute anginal attack
   h. Sustained release capsule, ointment, transdermal patch to treat chronic angina
4. Adverse effects/nursing care (see Table 18.8):
   a. IV nitroglycerin should not be administered with any other medicines and is given in a glass bottle with manufacturer-supplied IV tubing.
   b. As with all vasodilators, side effects include headache and postural hypotension.
   c. Leave nitroglycerin tablets at the bedside of clients for whom they are prescribed; encourage clients to tell the nurse when they have anginal pain and when they take nitroglycerine and its effectiveness.
   d. Sublingual means under the tongue. Clients may repeat the dose every five minutes for a total of three doses if the pain is not relieved. If the pain is not relieved with this regimen of nitroglycerin and rest, the client may be having a myocardial infarction and should seek medical attention immediately.
   e. Nitroglycerin should be stored in a dark, glass container in a cool place; nitroglycerin is readily adsorbed into many plastics; nitroglycerin has a short shelf life—three to six months.
   f. Nitroglycerin ointment:
      (1) Apply ointment to a hairless area of the skin to promote uniform absorption.
      (2) Use a new site with each new dose.
      (3) Use the ruled applicator paper that comes with the ointment to measure the dose accurately.
      (4) Use the applicator paper to apply a thin, uniform layer of ointment.
      (5) Leave the applicator paper on the site.
      (6) Cover the applicator paper with plastic wrap, and secure it with tape.
   g. Tolerance may develop with regular, long-term use of nitrates.
B. Calcium channel blockers:
   1. Calcium channel blockers reduce oxygen demand by inhibiting the influx of calcium through the muscle cell, dilating the coronary arteries and reducing afterload (systemic vascular resistance).

Table 18.8 Nitroglycerine Highlights

Nitroglycerine

- Vasodilator
- Give sublingual q 5 min. × 3 doses
- Store in cool place in dark glass container
- Apply ointment and patches to hairless area; wash after removing
- Side effects: Headaches, hypotension

Table 18.9 Guidelines for Administering Antiarrhythmics

- All of the drugs except Bretylium can be given PO; most also given I.M. or I.V.
- Check apical pulse and ECG for bradycardia and dysrhythmias.
- Isuprel or atropine should be available.
- Give the drugs at equal intervals.
- Postural hypotension is a common side effect; check BP.

2. Examples (note "ipine" in the generic name):
   a. Given PO only:
      (1) Nifedipine (Procardia)
      (2) Felodipine (Plendil)
      (3) Amlodipine (Norvasc)
      (4) Nicardipine (Cardene)
      (5) Nimodipine (Nimotop)
      (6) Isradipine (DynaCirc)
   b. Given IV and PO
      (1) Verapamil (Calan, Isoptin)
      (2) Diltiazem (Cardizem)
3. Adverse effects/nursing care:
   a. Same as for all vasodilators
   b. A lower dose may be indicated when given with Beta blockers (Inderal), which also cause vasodilation.

PERIPHERAL VASODILATORS

A. Peripheral vasodilators act on the smooth muscle of blood vessels, causing peripheral vasodilation. They are used to treat peripheral vascular disorders such as Raynaud's disease, Buerger's disease, thromboangiitis obliterans, diabetic vascular disease, and varicose ulcers.
B. Examples (note the *spasm* and the *vaso* in some of the trade names):
   1. Cyclandelate (Cyclospasmol)
   2. Isoxsuprine HCl (Vasodilan)
   3. Papaverine HCl (Pavabid, Vasospan)
C. Adverse effects/nursing care:
   1. Headache, flushing, and GI symptoms are the primary adverse reactions.
   2. Vasodilators will dilate cerebral vessels and cause headache.
   3. Usually given orally

Antiarrhythmics

A. Drugs used to treat ventricular dysrhythmias:
   1. General guidelines for administering antiarrhythmics (see Table 18.9)
   2. Quinidine (Cardioquin, Quinaglute, Quinidex):
      a. Decreases the excitability of the heart
      b. Used for atrial fibrillation and ventricular dysrhythmias (it is also used to treat malaria)
      c. Has anticholinergic effects

   d. Adverse effects/nursing care:
      (1) Hearing loss, tinnitus
      (2) Blood dyscrasias
      (3) Diarrhea, nausea, vomiting
      (4) Monitor serum drug levels and blood counts.
3. Disopyramide (Norpace):
   a. Decreases the excitability of the heart
   b. Adverse effects/nursing care:
      (1) Congestive heart failure
      (2) Heart block: Monitor pulse rate before giving; do not give if pulse below 60 or above 120
4. Lidocaine (Xylocaine):
   a. Used to treat acute ventricular dysrhythmias
   b. Not effective for atrial dysrhythmias; does not affect blood pressure, cardiac output, or myocardial contractility
   c. Usually given IV bolus followed by IV drip for those with cardiovascular disease
   d. Adverse effects/nursing care:
      (1) Side effects of antiarrhythmics discussed above
      (2) CNS effects such as dizziness or stupor
      (3) Respiratory depression
5. Phenytoin Sodium (Dilantin):
   a. Used to treat ventricular and supraventricular dysrhythmias that are unresponsive to lidocaine or procainamide
   b. Adverse effects/nursing care:
      (1) Ataxia, lethargy
      (2) Give via slow IV push to prevent vascular collapse.
      (3) Nystagmus, diplopia
      (4) Gingival hyperplasia
      (5) Rash
      (6) Don't mix with dextrose 5% IV fluids; crystallization will occur; flush IV line with saline before and after administration.
6. Procainamide (Pronestyl):
   a. Used to treat PVCs, ventricular tachycardia, and some atrial dysrhythmias
   b. Adverse effects/nursing care:
      (1) Severe hypotension

(2) Keep the client supine during IV administration to decrease hypotension.
(3) Bradycardia
(4) Nausea, vomiting, anorexia, diarrhea, bitter taste

7. Bretylium (Bretylol):
    a. Used to treat ventricular fibrillation
    b. Adverse effects/nursing care:
        (1) Severe orthostatic hypotension
        (2) Keep the client supine until a tolerance to hypotension develops.
        (3) Monitor blood pressure and pulse.

8. Adenoside (Adenocard):
    a. Used in the treatment of supraventricular tachycardia
    b. Adverse effects/nursing care:
        (1) Monitor the heart rate and rhythm for dysrhythmias.
        (2) Monitor B.P.
        (3) Facial flushing and headache

9. Amiodarone (Cardarone):
    a. Used in the treatment of life-threatening, recurrent ventricular fibrillation and unstable ventricular tachycardia
    b. Adverse effects/nursing care
        (1) Do not give if pulse is less than 60/min. or systolic BP is less than 90 mm Hg.
        (2) Monitor liver function tests.

B. Beta blockers:
    1. Reduce cardiac oxygen demands by blocking adrenalin-related increases in heart rate, blood pressure, and force of myocardial contraction.
    2. Used to treat angina, hypertension, and ventricular and supraventricular dysrhythmias
    3. Examples (note the "olol" in the generic names):
        a. Nadolol (Corgard); PO
        b. Acebutolol (Sectral); PO
        c. Propranolol HCl (Inderal); PO and IV
        d. Metoprolol (Lopressor); PO and IV
        e. Atenolol (Tenormin); PO and IV
        f. Labetalol (Mormodyne, Trandate); PO and IV
    4. Adverse effects/nursing care:
        a. Severe bradycardia
        b. Heart block
        c. Severe hypotension
        d. Monitor BP
        e. Do not stop drugs suddenly
        f. Increased airway resistance; do not give to asthmatics
        g. Hypoglycemia

C. Cardiac stimulants:
    1. Cardiac stimulants are autonomic nervous system drugs that act to increase the heart rate either by enhancing cardiac

conduction (Isuprel) or by blocking vagal stimulation (atropine).

2. Atropine:
    a. Anticholinergic drug that blocks vagal stimulation increasing heart rate
    b. Acts throughout the body to block cholinergic activity causing side effects of dry mouth, dilated pupils, and blurred vision.

3. Isoproteronol (Isuprel):
    a. Enhances cardiac conduction, increasing the heart rate
    b. In contrast to the hypertensive action of most adrenergic drugs, Isuprel may cause a drop in diastolic blood pressure; the systolic pressure may rise slightly.
    c. Adverse reactions:
        (1) Headache
        (2) Palpitations
        (3) Dry mouth
        (4) Flushing, sweating
        (5) Bronchial edema

Anticoagulants (see Table 18.10)

A. Anticoagulants are given to clients who are at risk of developing clots or to prevent clot enlargement or fragmentation; anticoagulants do not dissolve clots.

B. Uses include persons with pulmonary embolus, myocardial infarction, CVA, deep vein thrombosis

C. Heparin:
    1. Heparin blocks the conversion of prothrombin to thrombin, thus prolonging clotting time.
    2. Heparin must be given parenterally (either IV or subcutaneous in the abdomen, at least one inch from the umbilicus), because Heparin is destroyed by gastric juices.
    3. The antidote for heparin is protamine sulfate.
    4. PTT (partial thromboplastin time) or aPTT (activated partial thromboplastin time) is done to monitor heparin administration.
    5. Platelet counts should be monitored every 2–3 days.
    6. Monitor hematocrit for evidence of bleeding.

D. Warfarin (Coumadin, Dicumarol):
    1. Warfarin blocks prothrombin synthesis.
    2. Given orally
    3. Antidote is vitamin K
    4. Prothrombin time should be monitored; when warfarin is being administered
        a. the PT should be 1 1/2 to 2 times the control.
        b. results may be reported in INR (international normalized ratio); goal is 2–3.

Table 18.10 Anticoagulants

Drug	Route	Action	Monitoring Tests	Normal Value	Value when on Medication	Antidote
Heparin	Parenteral; IV or SC (can't be given orally because it is destroyed by gastric juices)	Blocks the conversion of prothrombin to thrombin and prolongs clotting time	PTT (partial thromboplastin time aPTT (activated partial thromboplastin clotting time)	60–70 seconds 30–40 seconds	1 1/2 to 2 times normal 1 1/2 to 2 times normal	Protamine sulfate
Warfarin (Coumadin)	Oral	Blocks prothrombin synthesis	Prothrombin time (PT) INR	11–12.5 seconds	1 1/2 to 2 times normal 2–3 times normal	Vitamin K

E. Antiplatelets:
1. Antiplatelets prevent platelet aggregation and thus decrease clotting.
2. Abciximab (ReoPro): Used for cardiac ischemia and in clients who have had percutaneous transluminal coronary angioplasty (PTCA)
3. Dypyridamole (Persantine): Used in thromboembolic conditions
4. Ticlopidine (Ticlid): Used to decrease risk of stroke, in intermittent claudication, and in sickle cell

F. Adverse effects/nursing care for heparin, coumadin, and antiplatelets:
1. Bleeding is the primary adverse effect to watch for with all anticoagulants; assess client for bruising, hematuria, epistaxis, and bleeding from the gums.
2. Drug interactions:
    a. Do not give salicylates with anticoagulants unless ordered.
    b. Barbiturates, Rifampin, and Haldol decrease prothrombin time.
    c. Teach the client not to take any other drug without checking with the physician.
3. Avoid large quantities of vitamin K foods (spinach, broccoli, liver, and tomatoes), because these foods decrease effects of anticoagulants. Vitamin K is the antidote for warfarin.
4. Discontinue anticoagulants two weeks before surgery.
5. Monitor heart rate and BP.

Thrombolytic Drugs

A. Thrombolytic enzymes are used for lysis of thrombi, obstructing coronary arteries in acute myocardial infarction, lysis of pulmonary emboli, venous thrombosis, venous catheter occlusion, and stroke caused by thrombus or embolus.
B. Examples:
1. Alteplase (tissue plasminogen activator recombinant, tPA, Activase)
2. Streptokinase
3. Urokinase
C. Adverse effects/nursing care:
1. Bleeding
2. Heparin therapy may be started following thrombolytic treatment.
3. When given for myocardial infarction, should be given within six hours of episode
4. When given for cerebrovascular accident, should be given within 2–3 hours of episode

Antilipemic Agents

A. Antilipemic agents are used to treat atherosclerosis by lowering blood cholesterol, triglycerides, and low-density lipids (LDL).
B. Antilipemic drugs should always be used in conjunction with diet, weight control, and exercise to reduce atherosclerosis.
C. Examples (note the "fatty" sound to some of the drugs: Choley, clo, cole)
1. Cholestyramine (Questran):
    a. Binds bile acids in the intestine, causing increased fecal excretion, which causes increased production of bile acids from cholesterol
    b. Lowers LDL cholesterol
2. Gemfibrozil (Lopid): Acts by inhibiting lipolysis and triglyceride synthesis
3. Lovastatin (Mevacor), Atorvastin (Lipitor), Simvastin (Zocor); note the "astin" in the generic names and the "or" ending in the trade names
    a. Act by inhibiting HMG-CoA reductase, the enzyme that initiates cholesterol synthesis
    b. Lower LDL, VLDL, and triglycerides and raise HDL
D. Adverse effects/nursing care:
1. GI effects include nausea, vomiting and constipation; encourage fluids and high-fiber diet to combat constipation.
2. May need fat-soluble vitamins A, D, K, and folic acid in a water-soluble form so that deficiencies will not occur

3. Observe for bleeding tendencies due to decreased vitamin K.
4. Monitor cholesterol and serum triglyceride levels to measure effectiveness.
5. Teach the client to follow a diet low in cholesterol and saturated fats and high in fiber; weight loss and exercise are also a part of the therapeutic regimen.
6. Blurred vision: Encourage regular eye exams to detect possible cataracts
7. Myalgia in clients taking HMG CoA reductase inhibitors (Atorvastin, simvastin)
8. Monitor liver function tests.
9. Antilipemics should not be taken at the same time as other medications, because they may interfere with medication absorption; other medications should be taken one hour before or four hours after antilipemics.
10. Expect antilipemics to be administered for several months or years if they are effective.

Antihypertensives

A. Antihypertensive agents lower blood pressure by decreasing the constriction of blood vessels by various mechanisms.
B. Adverse effects/nursing care:
   1. Orthostatic hypotension and dizziness:
      a. Blood pressures should be taken both supine and upright.
      b. Teach clients to change positions slowly.
      c. Teach clients to avoid very hot baths and showers.
      d. Avoid alcohol.
   2. Rebound hypertension when discontinued abruptly
   3. Teach clients to report adverse reactions promptly.
   4. Do not take over the counter medications, especially cold medications, without the physician's approval.
C. Central acting drugs: Alpha agonists
   1. Clonidine (Catapres)
   2. Methyldopa (Aldomet)
   3. Catapres and Aldomet depress the activity of the sympathetic nervous system.
   4. Adverse effects include dry mouth and constipation.
D. Angiotensin Converting Enzyme (ACE) inhibitors:
   1. ACE inhibitors prevent the conversion of angiotensin I to angiotensin II, a potent vasoconstrictor, and also decrease aldosterone secretion.
   2. Examples:
      a. Captopril (Capoten)
      b. Enalapril, enalaprilat (Vasotec)
      c. Benazepril (Lotensin)
      d. Fosinopril (Monopril)
      e. Lisinopril (Prinivil, Zestril)
      f. Ramipril (Altace)
   3. Adverse effects:
      a. Blood dyscrasias
      b. Angioedema
      c. Renal failure, hyperkalemia
      d. Rash and fever
   4. Capoten should be taken one hour before meals, because food decreases absorption.
E. Vasodilators:
   1. Hydralazine (Apresoline):
      a. Hydralazine acts directly on the smooth muscle to lower blood pressure.
      b. Adverse effects of hydralazine include headache, tachycardia, angina, palpitations, and sodium retention.
      c. Hydralazine should be given with meals to increase absorption.
F. Alpha adrenergic blockers:
   1. Block alpha adrenergic receptors causing peripheral vasodilation, resulting in decrease in blood pressure and relaxation of muscles of bladder and prostate
   2. Examples (note that the generic names all end in "zosin"):
      a. Doxazosin (Cardura)
      b. Prazosin (Minipres)
      c. Terazosin (Hytrin)
   3. Adverse effects/nursing care:
      a. First dose is given at bedtime to decrease hypotension.
      b. Hytrin is frequently used in men who have benign prostatic hypertrophy to decrease urinary retention and difficulty urinating.
G. Beta blockers, discussed earlier, are also frequently used to lower blood pressure.

Diuretics

A. Diuretics reduce the body's total volume of salt and water by increasing their urinary excretion.
B. Uses:
   1. Mild hypertension
   2. Edema
   3. Congestive heart failure
C. Adverse effects/nursing care:
   1. All diuretics can cause orthostatic hypotension; clients should be taught to change positions slowly.
   2. Monitor output.
   3. Monitor weights.
   4. Monitor serum electrolytes.
D. Thiazide diuretics (note that thiazides have a zide in the generic name):
   1. Hydrochlorothiazide (Hydrodiuril, Esidrex)
   2. Thiazide diuretics increase the urinary excretion of sodium and water by inhibiting sodium reabsorption in the ascending loop of Henle; they also increase urinary excretion of chloride, potassium, and to some extent, bicarbonate.

3. Adverse effects/nursing care:
    a. Hypokalemia, hyperuricemia, hyperglycemia, and impairment of glucose tolerance occur.
    b. Monitor intake and output and weight.
    c. Monitor electrolytes, blood sugar, creatinine, and BUN.
    d. Teach client high-potassium foods.
    e. Thiazides are related chemically to the sulfonamides; they have no antimicrobial effect but do have cross allergies.
E. Loop diuretics:
  1. Examples:
    a. Furosemide (Lasix)
    b. Bumetanide (Bumex)
  2. Loop diuretics inhibit the reabsorption of sodium and chloride at the proximal portion of the ascending loop of Henle, increasing water excretion.
  3. Loop diuretics can be given PO or IV. IV acts within five minutes.
  4. Adverse effects/nursing care:
    a. Hypokalemia, hypochloremic alkalosis, hyperuricemia, fluid and electrolyte imbalances, hyponatremia, hypocalcemia, hypomagnesemia, hyperglycemia
    b. Agranulocytosis: Report a sore throat that persists
    c. Monitor electrolytes and blood values.
    d. Monitor blood pressure and pulse.
    e. Monitor for signs of hypokalemia.
    f. Monitor blood sugar levels in diabetics.
    g. Teach about high-potassium foods
    h. Give IM furosemide Z track to reduce pain.
    i. Sulfonamide-sensitive clients may have an allergic reaction to furosemide.
    j. Hearing impairment may follow rapid IV or IM administration.
F. Osmotic diuretics:
  1. Mannitol (Osmitrol)
  2. Osmotic diuretics increase the osmotic pressure of the glomerular filtrate inside the renal tubules; as a result, less fluid and electrolytes are reabsorbed by the tubules causing a greater loss of fluid, chloride, and sodium.
  3. Used to prevent acute renal failure, to reduce intraocular and intracranial pressure, and to promote diuresis in drug intoxication
  4. Adverse effects/nursing care:
    a. Solutions given IV only via an inline filter.
    b. Solutions above 15% have a tendency to crystallize; do not give solutions with undissolved crystals; give a warm solution to dissolve crystals.
    c. Monitor hourly vital signs, CVP, and I&O.

    d. Monitor daily weight, renal function tests, fluid balance, serum and urine potassium, and sodium levels.
G. Potassium-sparing diuretic:
  1. Examples:
    a. Spironolactone (Aldactone)
    b. Amiloride Hydrochloride (Midamor)
  2. These drugs block the sodium-retaining effects of aldosterone, causing increased elimination of sodium and fluid but not potassium.
  3. Useful in combination with other diuretics when it is important to avoid hypokalemia
  4. Adverse effects/nursing care:
    a. Hyperkalemia: Monitor potassium level
    b. The maximum hypotensive effect may not be seen for two weeks.
    c. Give with meals to improve absorption.
  5. Midamor: Monitor serum creatine kinase because Midamor may cause skeletal muscle myopathy
  6. Midamor: Watch for signs of hemorrhage

Potassium-Removing Resins

A. Sodium polystyrene sulfonate (Kayexalate):
  1. Kayexalate is a resin that exchanges sodium ions for potassium ions in the large intestine.
  2. Used in the treatment of hyperkalemia
B. Adverse effects/nursing care:
  1. Can be given orally or rectally via a high enema
  2. Needs to be in contact with GI tract for six hours to be the most effective
  3. Monitor for hypokalemia and loss of magnesium and calcium.
  4. Monitor for sodium overload: One-third of sodium is retained.
  5. Rectal administration helps to prevent constipation.
  6. Stop resin administration when serum potassium is 4–5 mEq.

HORMONAL AGENTS
Antidiabetic Agents

A. Insulin:
  1. Information:
    a. Normally produced by the beta cells of the islets of Langerhans in the pancreas
    b. Increases glucose transport across muscle and fat cell membranes
    c. Destroyed in the gastrointestinal tract
    d. Administered by subcutaneous injection
    e. Given to persons with diabetes mellitus to replace the insulin that they are not producing
    f. May also be added to IV hyperalimentation

2. Types of insulin (see Table 18.11):
  a. Rapid-acting insulins:
    (1) Regular
    (2) Humulin Regular
    (3) Onset in 1/2 to 1 hour
    (4) Peak in 2 to 4 hours
    (5) Duration is 6 to 8 hours.
    (6) Regular insulin will be given several times a day.
    (7) Regular insulin can be administered via IV.
  b. Intermediate-acting insulins:
    (1) NPH
    (2) Humulin NPH
    (3) Onset in 2 to 4 hours
    (4) Peak in 6 to 8 hours
    (5) Duration is 18 to 24 hours.
  c. Long-Acting Insulins:
    (1) Humulin U
    (2) Onset in 4 to 8 hours
    (3) Peak in 14 to 20 hours
    (4) Duration is 30 to 36 hours.
  d. Mixed:
    (1) Humulin 70/30
    (2) Novolin 70/30
    (3) Mixed insulins are manufactured to have a mixture of NPH (70%) and regular (30%).
  e. Regular insulin can be mixed with NPH.
  f. When mixing insulins, draw up regular insulin first and then NPH.
  g. Mixed insulins should be given immediately to avoid binding.
3. Adverse effects/nursing care:
  a. Hypoglycemia:
    (1) Hypoglycemia is manifested by behavior changes, irritability, pallor, cold sweats, a clammy appearance, and hunger.
    (2) Hypoglycemia onsets rapidly.
    (3) Treatment of hypoglycemia is the administration of glucose.
    (4) Glucagon raises blood glucose levels and may be given parenterally to reverse severe hypoglycemia.
    (5) Teach client not to skip meals and to follow diet.
  b. Atrophy or hypertrophy of subcutaneous fat tissue
    (1) Rotate injection sites.
    (2) Teach the client to keep a chart.
    (3) Sites on backs of upper arms, lower abdomen, and thighs may be used;

current recommendation is to rotate sites within the abdomen.
  c. Insulin administration:
    (1) Store extra insulin in a cool area.
    (2) Do not use insulin that has changed color.
    (3) Check the expiration date before using contents.
    (4) Always use the same type and brand of insulin unless prescribed otherwise.
    (5) When preparing insulin for injection, swirl the bottle gently or rotate between the palms; do not shake.
    (6) Inject at a 90-degree angle into the subcutaneous layer (use 45-degree angle if client emaciated); use a short needle.
    (7) Pat, don't rub, after an injection.
    (8) Teach the client to always wear diabetic identification.
    (9) Teach the client signs and symptoms of hypo- and hyperglycemia.
    (10) Monitor serum glucose levels, and teach the client how to do this.
  d. Insulin pumps (see Figure 18.10):
    (1) Small, externally worn devices that closely mimic normal pancreatic functioning
    (2) Insulin pumps contain a 3 ml syringe attached to a long (42-inch), narrow lumen tube with a needle or Teflon catheter at the end.
    (3) The needle or Teflon catheter is inserted into the subcutaneous tissue (usually on the abdomen) and secured with a tape or a transparent dressing.
    (4) The needle or catheter is changed at least every three days.
    (5) The pump is worn either on a belt or in a pocket.
    (6) The pump uses only regular insulin.
    (7) Insulin can be administered via the basal rate (usually 0.5–2.0 units/hr) and by a bolus dose (which is activated by a series of button pushes) prior to each meal.
  e. Drug interactions:
    (1) Cigarette smoking decreases the absorption of subcutaneously administered insulin; advise the

Table 18.11 Insulins

Insulin	Onset	Peak	Duration	Solution
Regular Humulin	1/2–1 hr	2–4 hrs	6–8 hrs	Clear
NPH Humulin	2–4 hrs	6–8 hrs	18–24 hrs	Cloudy

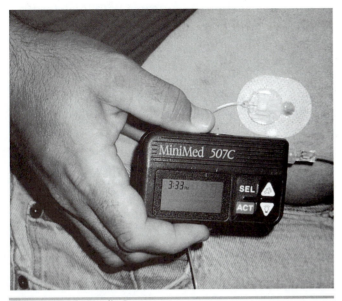

Figure 18.10 Insulin Pump

Table 18.12 Oral Hypoglycemic Agents

Drug	Onset	Peak	Duration
Sulfonylureas			
Chlorpropamide (Diabinase)	1 hour	2–4 hours	24 hours
Glipizide (Glucotrol)	15–30 minutes	1–3 hours	24 hours
Glyburide (Micronase, DiaBeta)	1–4 hours	2–4 hours	24 hours
Biguanide			
Metformin (Glucophage)	unknown	2–4 hours	unknown

client not to smoke for 30 minutes after insulin injection.

   (2) Marijuana use may increase insulin requirements.

   (3) Excessive alcohol intake may require a reduction in insulin dosage because alcohol potentiates the hypoglycemic effect of insulin; advise the client not to drink alcohol.

B. Oral hypoglycemic agents:

  1. Information:

    a. Oral hypoglycemic agents lower blood glucose concentrations by stimulating the secretion of endogenous insulin from beta cells of the pancreas, by reducing glucose output by the liver, and by enhancing peripheral sensitivity to insulin.

    b. Oral hypoglycemic agents are used in Type II diabetes (Non-Insulin-Dependent Diabetes).

  2. Examples of oral sulfonylurea hypoglycemic agents (see Table 18.12):

    a. Chlorpropamide (Diabinase):

     (1) Onsets in one hour

     (2) Peaks in 2 to 4 hours

     (3) Duration is 24 hours.

    b. Glipizide (Glucotrol):

     (1) Onsets in 15–30 minutes

     (2) Peaks in 1 to 3 hours

     (3) Duration is 24 hours.

    c. Glyburide (Micronase, DiaBeta):

     (1) Onsets in 1 to 4 hours

     (2) Peaks in 2 to 4 hours

     (3) Duration is 24 hours.

  2. Example of oral biguanide hypoglycemic agent:

    a. Metformin (Glucophage):

     (1) Onsets unknown

     (2) Peaks in 2 to 4 hours.

     (3) Duration is unknown.

     (4) Lowers basal and postprandial glucose by decreasing glucose production in the liver and decreasing intestinal absorption of glucose and improves insulin sensitivity

  3. Examples of oral alpha-glucosidose inhibitor hypoglycemic agent:

    a. Acarbose (Precose)

    b. Miglitol (Glyset)

    c. Delay glucose absorption and digestion of carbohydrates, resulting in smaller rise in blood glucose concentration after meals, lowering postprandial hyperglyclemia; does not enhance insulin secretion

  4. Adverse effects/nursing care:

    a. Hypoglycemia:

     (1) Seen particularly in older clients with renal disease

     (2) Monitor blood glucose levels.

     (3) Clients should monitor urine or blood glucose regularly.

    b. GI effects (nausea and anorexia)

    c. Pruritis, rash, jaundice; observe skin; monitor liver function tests

    d. Do not give sulfonylureas to clients who are allergic to sulfa drugs.

    e. During times of emotional or physical stress, many clients may need insulin instead of oral hypoglycemics.

    f. Diet, exercise, and weight reduction should be included in the treatment plan.

    g. Teach the client signs of hypoglycemia and how to treat it.

    h. Potentially fatal complication of Metformin is lactic acidosis; instruct client to report vomiting immediately

Pituitary Hormones

A. Corticotrophin (ACTH); Cosyntropin:

  1. Used primarily to diagnose adrenocortical insufficiency

2. Hypersensitivity reactions sometimes occur.
3. If corticotrophin is given over a period of time, Cushing syndrome may occur.

B. Desmopressin (DDAVP); Vasopressin (ADH, Pitressin); Lypressin spray:
  1. Used in the treatment of diabetes insipidus
  2. Sometimes used in the treatment of enuresis
  3. Adverse effects/nursing care:
    a. Water intoxication and hyponatremia
    b. Nausea, headache, and flushing
    c. Hypertension, arrhythmias, bradycardia

C. Use with caution in clients with seizure disorders, coronary artery disease, migraine headaches, and asthma.

Corticosteroids

A. Glucocorticoids (sugar) produce organic effects regulating carbohydrate, fat, and protein metabolism and are anti-inflammatory and immunosuppressant.
B. Mineralocorticoids (salt) produce inorganic effects regulating water and electrolyte metabolism.
C. Adrenal androgens and estrogens (sex) produce sex hormonal effects.
  1. Examples of corticosteroids (note the "sone" in the generic name):
    a. Prednisone (Deltasone)
    b. Prednisolone (Cortalone)
    c. Methylprednisolone (Solu Medrol)
    d. Cortisone (Cortone)
    e. Dexamethasone (Decadron)
    f. All of the above have glucocorticoid actions.
    g. Fludrocortisone (Florinef) has mineralocorticoid actions.
  2. Uses:
    a. Replacement for deficient hormone production
    b. Decrease inflammation
    c. Treat allergic conditions
    d. Reduce cerebral edema
    e. Respiratory disease/asthma
    f. With antineoplastics in the treatment of cancer
  3. Adverse effects/nursing care:
    a. Adrenocortical insufficiency
    b. Taper steroids when they are discontinued.
    c. Increased susceptibility to infections
    d. Fluid and electrolyte disturbances; monitor serum electrolytes; explain that edema is expected
    e. May cause ulcers; antacids may be prescribed to reduce ulcer formation; give oral doses with food to reduce gastric symptoms

f. Cushing's syndrome with long-term administration of steroids:
  (1) Moon face
  (2) Hirsutism
  (3) Buffalo hump
  (4) Protruding abdomen, purple striae, thinning of extremities
  (5) Glycosuria, elevated blood sugar
  (6) Edema, hypertension
  (7) Muscle weakness
  (8) Assure the client that these symptoms will disappear when the drug is discontinued.
g. Ocular effects
4. Steroid dosages are not interchangeable (see Table 18.13).

Table 18.13 Steroid Dosage Equivalents

Steroid	Dose in mg
Cortisone	25
Hydrocortisone	20
Prednisone	5
Prednisolone	5
Methylprednisolone	4
Dexamethasone	0.75
Betamethasone	0.6

D. Topical corticosteroids:
  1. Topical steroids reduce inflammatory and pruritic symptoms.
  2. The ointments are spread in a thin film 2–4 times daily.
  3. Never place an occlusive dressing over a topical steroid.
  4. The systemic effects of the drug are not seen at usual topical doses or if used for normal periods of time; caution clients to follow directions; do not use for longer than prescribed or on larger body surface areas.
E. Aerosol corticosteroids:
  1. Decrease number of inflammatory cells and inhibit bronchoconstriction
  2. Produce smooth muscle relaxation
  3. Decrease mucus secretion
  4. Used for allergic rhinitis and bronchial asthma
  5. Examples: Beclomethasone (Beclovent, Beconase, Vanceril, Vancenase)

Drugs Affecting the Thyroid Gland

A. Thyroid hormones:
  1. Examples:
    a. Dessicated thyroid
    b. Thyroglobulin (Proloid)
    c. Levothyroxine (Levothroid)
    d. Liothyronine sodium (Cytomel)
    e. Usually given PO once daily

2. Adverse effects/nursing care:
   a. Usually results from overdose
   b. Manifested as signs and symptoms of hyperthyroidism:
      (1) Weight loss
      (2) Palpitations, tachycardia, arrhythmias
      (3) Nervousness, tremors
      (4) Elevated blood pressure
      (5) Insomnia
   c. Angina
   d. The client will need periodic thyroid function tests.
B. Thyroid antagonists:
   1. Thyroid antagonists prevent the formation of thyroglobulin and iodothyronine.
   2. Thyroid antagonists are used in the treatment of hyperthyroidism and in preparation for thyroid surgery or radioactive iodine therapy to shrink the thyroid gland and make it less vascular and to make surgery safer.
   3. Examples:
      a. Methimazole (Tapazole)
      b. Propylthiouracil (PTU)
      c. These drugs are given orally.
   4. Adverse effects/nursing care:
      a. Very nontoxic
      b. Agranulocytosis very rare; observe for and report signs of agranulocytosis (fever, chills, sore throat)
      c. Monitor blood counts.
      d. Monitor thyroid function tests.
      e. Use with caution in clients older than 40 years.

Reproductive Hormones

A. Androgens (male hormones):
   1. Indications:
      a. Replacement therapy in androgen-deficient males
      b. Inoperable, advanced metastatic carcinoma of the breast in women
      c. Fibrocystic breast disease
      d. Endometriosis
   2. Examples (note the osterone in the generic names):
      a. Testosterone (Depo Testosterone)
      b. Fluoxymesterone (Halotestin)
      c. Danazol (Cyclomen); used to treat endometriosis and fibrocystic breast disease
   3. Adverse effects/nursing care:
      a. Acne, flushing of skin
      b. Gynecomastia
      c. Change in libido (increase or decrease)
      d. Edema
      e. Virilization in females
      f. Priapism (penis stays erect) in males

B. Estrogens (female hormones):
   1. Uses:
      a. Replacement therapy in menopause or when person is deficient in estrogens
      b. Postpartum breast engorgement
      c. Androgen dependent tumors (prostate cancer)
      d. Contraception (in combination with progestogen)
   2. Examples:
      a. Diethylstilbestrol (DES)
      b. Estradiol (Estrace)
      c. Conjugated estrogens (Premarin)
   3. Adverse effects/nursing care:
      a. Chloasma (mask of pregnancy)
      b. Nausea
      c. Elevated blood pressure
      d. Clotting problems: thrombophlebitis; pulmonary emboli; persons with a history of phlebitis or thromboembolic disorders should not take estrogens
      e. Gall stones; cholestatic jaundice
      f. Breakthrough bleeding
      g. Depression
      h. Estrogens are usually given cyclically if the woman has a uterus
C. Progestogens (progestins):
   1. Progestins transform a proliferative endometrium into a secretory one and stimulate the growth of mammary alveolar tissue; progesterone is the hormone of pregnancy.
   2. Uses:
      a. Amenorrhea
      b. Abnormal uterine bleeding caused by hormonal imbalance
      c. Endometrial cancer
      d. Combination estrogen-progestin birth control pills
   3. Examples:
      a. Hydroxyprogesterone (Duralutin)
      b. Medroxyprogesterone (Provera)
      c. Progesterone (Gestrol)
   4. Adverse effects/nursing care:
      a. Breakthrough bleeding
      b. Changes in menstrual flow
      c. Edema
      d. Thromboembolic disorders; do not give to persons with thromboembolic conditions
      e. Increased blood pressure
D. Oral contraceptives:
   1. Progestin only: Taken every day of the menstrual cycle
   2. Combination pill: Taken days 5–24 of menstrual cycle
   3. Adverse effects/nursing care:
      a. Same as for estrogens and progestins
      b. Discontinue one week before surgery to reduce risk of thromboembolism
      c. Advise the client to use an additional method of birth control for the first

week of administration in the initial cycle.

   d. Clients who smoke more than 15 cigarettes a day should not take oral contraceptives; this increases the risk of thromboembolic problems.

   e. Teach the client to have regular Pap smears.

   f. Teach the client that it may take longer to conceive after stopping birth control pills.

   g. If one menstrual period is missed and tablets have been taken on schedule, the woman should continue to take pills.

   h. If two periods are missed, the client should stop taking pills and have a pregnancy test.

E. Norplant system:
   1. Six capsules containing synthetic progestin are implanted subdermally in the midportion of the upper arm.
   2. Contraceptive efficacy lasts for five years.
   3. Side effects same as other progestins

F. Fertility agents:
   1. Stimulate ovulation
   2. Examples:
     a. Clomiphene (Clomid)
     b. Menotropin (Pergonal)
     c. Gonadorelin (Factrel)
     d. Bromcriptine (Parlodel): Inhibits prolactin; used to treat amenorrhea
   2. Adverse effects/nursing care:
     a. Drugs that stimulate ovulation (Clomid, Pergonal, Factrel) may cause multiple births.

G. Oxytocics:
   1. Oxytocics stimulate the smooth muscle of the uterus.
   2. Examples:
     a. Ergonovine (Ergotrate); Methylergonovine (Methergine):
       (1) Used to correct postpartum uterine atony and control postpartum uterine bleeding
       (2) Can be given PO, IM, or IV.
     b. Oxytocin (Pitocin, Syntocinon):
       (1) Induces labor or intensifies uterine contractions at term
       (2) May be used to control postpartum bleeding
       (3) IV administration allows the most control.
   3. Adverse effects/nursing care:
     a. Pitocin to induce or augment labor should only be given to women at term known to have an adequate pelvis.
     b. IV should be given by drip infusion only—never by bolus.
     c. Notify the physician and stop IV pitocin if contractions occur more frequently than every two minutes, last longer

than 60 seconds, or there is less than a 30-second rest period between contractions.

   d. Monitor the fetal heart rate during labor.

   e. Assess vital signs at least hourly.

   f. When given postpartum, monitor uterine fundus, amount of bleeding, and vital signs.

GASTROINTESTINAL DRUGS
Histamine (H₂) Antagonists

A. Histamine antagonists decrease the acidity of the stomach by blocking the action of histamine, which triggers gastric acid secretion; histamine antagonists are used to prevent and treat peptic ulcers.

B. Examples (note "itidine" in the generic name):
   1. Cimetidine (Tagamet)
   2. Ranitidine (Zantac)
   3. Famotidine (Pepcid)
   4. Roxotidine (Roxin)
   5. Nizatidine (Axid) (used for gastroesophageal reflux)

C. Adverse effects/nursing care:
   1. Diarrhea
   2. Dizziness, confusion, drowsiness, headache
   3. Elevated liver function tests
   4. Antacids decrease the absorption of cimetidine.
   5. Smoking decreases the effectiveness of histamine antagonists.
   6. Clients who are hypersensitive to one H₂ antagonist may not be allergic to another because they are structurally different.
   7. Oral histamine antagonists are available over the counter.
   8. Histamine antagonists may be given IV.

Omeprazole (Prilosec)

A. Blocks formation of gastric acid; not a histamine blocker

B. Used to treat esophagitis, gastroesophageal reflux disease, and duodenal ulcers

C. Adverse effects/nursing care:
   1. Abdominal pain
   2. Instruct the client to swallow capsules whole and not crush or open the capsule.

GI Anticholinergics

A. Gastrointestinal anticholinergics are used to relieve the pain of peptic ulcers by decreasing gastric secretions; they probably do not heal ulcers. Anticholinergics inhibit GI smooth muscle contraction and delay gastric emptying, so there is less time for gastric secretions to act on an empty stomach—enhancing the action of antacids. They can also be used to treat an irritable colon.

B. Examples:
1. Belladonna
2. Methaneline bromide (Banthine)
3. Propantheline bromide (Probanthine)
C. Adverse effects/nursing care (see anticholinergics section):
1. Dry mouth
2. Constipation
3. Blurred vision
4. Urinary retention
5. Confusion

Sucralfate (carafate)

A. Sucralfate forms a highly condensed, paste-like substance after reacting with gastric acid that binds to gastric and duodenal ulcers, forming a protective barrier to pepsin, acid, and bile—allowing ulcers to heal.
B. Method of administration: Oral 1 gm QID, one hour AC, and hour of sleep
C. Adverse effects/nursing care:
1. Minimal because it is not systemically absorbed
2. Binds with other medications; wait at least two hours after giving other medications before giving sucralfate
3. Constipation, diarrhea, nausea, indigestion, rash, and pruritus can occur.

Antacids

A. Antacids neutralize gastric acidity and help control ulcer pain.
B. Used as an adjunct to other therapy for peptic ulcer, heartburn, and esophageal reflux
C. Tablets should be chewed thoroughly before swallowing and followed by a glass of water; liquid antacids should be followed by a full glass of water to assure distribution throughout the stomach and to provide the necessary medium for the neutralizing reaction.
D. Magnesium-containing antacids:
1. Magnesium Hydroxide (Milk of Magnesia)
2. Magnesium-containing antacids may cause diarrhea and hypermagnesemia.
3. Do not give magnesium products to patients with renal failure.
E. Aluminum-containing antacids:
1. Aluminum hydroxide (Amphojel)
2. Aluminum-containing antacids may cause constipation and phosphorus depletion.
3. In renal failure, aluminum hydroxide is given to bind phosphates, reducing serum phosphate.
F. Calcium carbonate (Tums):
1. May cause hypercalcemia and hypophosphatemia
2. Should not be used in severe renal disease

3. Should not be administered with milk or other foods high in vitamin D
4. May cause milk alkali syndrome (headache, confusion, nausea and vomiting, hypercalcemia, hypercalcuria, and hypophosphatemia)
5. Can cause rebound hyperacidity
G. There are many aluminum and magnesium combinations:
1. Magaldrate (Riopan), Maalox, DiGel, Gelusil
2. Combinations reduce the diarrhea and constipation side effects.

Antidiarrheals

A. Antidiarrheals reduce the liquidity of stools and the frequency of defecation.
B. Bismuth subsalicylate (Pepto Bismol):
1. Bismuth has a water binding capacity and provides a protective coating for intestinal mucosa.
2. Contains a high quantity of salicylates.
3. May be used in the treatment of helicobacter pylori infection.
4. Bismuth is a heavy metal and should not be used in patients who are receiving radiation therapy, because heavy metals block radiation.
C. Kaolin-Pectate (Kaopectate):
1. Decreases the water loss in stools
2. May cause constipation
3. Should not be given if obstructive bowel lesions are suspected
D. Loperamide (Imodium):
1. Loperamide inhibits peristalsis, making intestinal contents take longer to pass through, allowing more water to be absorbed.
E. Diphenoxylate with atropine (Lomotil):
1. Increases smooth muscle tone in the GI tract, inhibits motility, and diminishes gastric secretions
2. Opium derivative
3. To decrease the risk of physical dependence, atropine is included in the drug.
4. Atropine side effects are unpleasant: Sedation, dizziness, dry mouth, and paralytic ileus.
F. Opium tincture (Paregoric):
1. Paregoric is a controlled substance.
2. Side effects:
a. Physical dependence in long-term use
b. Nausea and vomiting
c. Respiratory depression
G. General comments:
1. Antidiarrheals should not be used for more than two days.
2. They should not be used in acute diarrhea due to poisons until the toxic material is removed from the GI tract.

Laxatives

A. Laxatives may be given to relieve or prevent constipation or to prepare the bowel for surgery or diagnostic tests.
B. Hyperosmolar or saline cathartics:
   1. Increase the bulk of the stools by attracting and holding large amounts of fluids
   2. Should be given with enough fluid so that the patient will not become dehydrated
   3. Examples of saline cathartics:
      a. Magnesium citrate
      b. Milk of Magnesia
      c. Potassium citrate
      d. Glycerin
   4. Examples of bowel evacuant:
      a. Polyethylene glycol electrolyte solution (CoLyte, GoLytely, OCL, NuLytely, Colovage)
      b. Induce diarrhea and clean bowel in an electrolyte-sparing manner
      c. Used prior to surgery and diagnostic tests
      d. Clients must follow directions regarding fluid intake.
C. Bulk forming:
   1. Increase the bulk of the feces, stimulating peristalsis by mechanical means
   2. Safest of all laxatives
   3. Examples of bulk-forming laxatives:
      a. Methylcellulose (Cologel)
      b. Psyllium Hydrophilic Muciloid (Metamucil)
D. Lubricant (mineral oil):
   1. Coats the stool, creating a barrier between the feces and the colon wall—preventing the colon from reabsorbing water from the feces
   2. Do not take mineral oil with meals, because it will reduce the absorption of oil-soluble vitamins, particularly vitamins A and D.
E. Emollient (stool softener):
   1. Exert detergent activity and reduce the surface tension of feces and promote penetration by water and fat
   2. Used to prevent constipation, not to treat it
   3. Used when straining at stool is contraindicated: MI, rectal surgery, eye surgery, postpartum hemorrhage
   4. Examples of stool softeners: Docusate salts (Colace, Surfak)
F. Stimulant:
   1. Probably acts directly on the smooth muscle of the intestine, stimulating peristalsis.
   2. Examples of stimulant laxatives:
      a. Bisacodyl (Dulcolax)
      b. Cascara sagrada
      c. Castor oil
      d. Senna (Senokot)
G. Nursing care related to laxatives:
   1. Do not give laxatives when the client has:
      a. Abdominal pain, nausea, vomiting, or other symptoms of appendicitis
      b. Intestinal obstruction
   2. Avoid an over-administration of laxatives.
   3. Normal evacuation patterns may be as often as 1–2 times per day or as infrequent as 1–2 times per week.
   4. Laxatives should be used for a week or less to prevent the development of dependence.
   5. Encourage clients to eat a diet high in fiber and to have an adequate fluid intake to promote proper bowel function.

Antiemetics

A. Used to relieve nausea and vomiting
B. Antiemetics decrease stimulation of the chemoreceptor trigger zone (CTZ); phenothiazines and barbiturates have antiemetic effects (see section on phenothiazines)
C. Benzquinamide (Emete-Con):
   1. Used in the prevention and treatment of nausea and vomiting associated with anesthesia and surgery
   2. Adverse effects:
      a. Related to antihistamine and anticholinergic actions
      b. Central nervous system effects such as drowsiness and dizziness
      c. Anticholinergic effects such as dry mouth and blurred vision (because of mydriasis)
D. Dimenhydrinate (Dramamine):
   1. Antihistamine drug used to prevent motion sickness and also as an antihistamine to prevent allergic reactions
   2. Should be administered before nausea occurs
   3. Adverse effects:
      a. Drowsiness
      b. Dry mouth
E. Prochlorperazine (Compazine):
   1. Compazine is a phenothiazine and is used to treat nausea and vomiting.
   2. Adverse effects:
      a. Central nervous system depression: drowsiness and dizziness
      b. Hypotension
F. Metoclopramide HCl (Reglan):
   1. Stimulates motility of the upper GI tract by increasing lower esophageal sphincter tone
   2. Also blocks dopamine receptors at the chemoreceptor trigger zone
   3. Used to prevent or reduce nausea and vomiting induced by cisplatin and other chemotherapy

G. Ondansetron (Zofran):
   1. Prevention of nausea and vomiting associated with chemotherapy and surgery
   2. Adverse effects for Reglan and Zofran:
      a. Similar to other antiemetics
      b. Extrapyramidal symptoms
      c. Benadryl may be given to counteract extrapyramidal side effects with high doses.
H. Ganisetron (Kytril):
   1. Prevents nausea and vomiting associated with chemotherapy and radiation therapy
   2. Adverse effects/nursing care:
      a. May cause temporary taste disorder
      b. Administer 30 minutes before therapies.

Emetics

A. Emetics stimulate the vomiting center and induce vomiting; used to treat acute poisoning
B. Apomorphine:
   1. Given subcutaneously
   2. A controlled substance
   3. Emesis occurs 5 to 15 minutes after subcutaneous administration.
   4. Adverse effects/nursing care:
      a. Depression or euphoria
      b. Respiratory depression
      c. Orthostatic hypotension in large doses
      d. Do not give apomorphine to patients who are allergic to morphine or other opiates.
C. Ipecac syrup:
   1. Doses of 30 cc or less cause no systemic, adverse effects.
   2. Emesis occurs 20–30 minutes after administration of ipecac syrup.
   3. Contraindications for use:
      a. Semiconscious or unconscious patients
      b. Clients having seizures
      c. Clients who have ingested corrosives or caustic substances
      d. Clients who have ingested petroleum distillates
      e. 200–300 ml of water or clear liquid may facilitate the emetic action.

Pancreatic Enzymes

A. Pancreatic enzymes replace pancreatic enzymes and aid the digestion of starches, fats, and proteins.
B. Used in cystic fibrosis and when pancreatic secretion is insufficient
C. Examples (note the *ase* or *zyme* ending, indicating an enzyme):
   1. Pancreatin (Donnazyme)
   2. Pancrelipase (Pancrease, Viokase, Ilozyme)

D. Adverse effects/nursing care:
   1. Give with food; for infants, mix with applesauce.
   2. Do not give enteric-coated preparations with antacids; antacids may negate the pancreatin's effect.
   3. If enteric coated, do not crush or chew tablets.
   4. Use cautiously with patients who are hypersensitive to pork, because the product is pork based.

ARTHRITIS AND GOUT DRUGS

Gold Salts

A. Gold salts alter the immune response and are used to treat rheumatoid arthritis not responding to other therapy, as well as other autoimmune conditions.
B. Examples of gold salts:
   1. Auranofin (Ridaura)
   2. Aurothioglucose (Solganol)
   3. Gold sodium thiomalate (Myochrysine)
C. Adverse effects/nursing care:
   1. Given orally or deep IM, preferably in the gluteal muscle
   2. Oral compounds are less toxic than IM and are better tolerated.
   3. GI effects including loose stools, especially with auranofin; give with food to decrease GI effects.
   4. Check the mucus membranes for a rash; discontinue if rash or stomatitis develops.
   5. Glomerulonephritis: Monitor urine protein, BUN, creatinine
   6. Hematologic effects; monitor CBC
   7. Given under constant supervision of physicians; side effects can be reversed if the drug is stopped
   8. The client should use sunscreen.
   9. The client should not get pregnant.
   10. Therapeutic effects may not be seen for several months.

Antimalarials

A. Used to treat malaria; also useful in the treatment of rheumatoid arthritis that is unresponsive to NSAIDs
B. Examples:
   1. Chloroquine (Aralen)
   2. Hydroxychloroquine (Plaquenil)
C. Adverse effects:
   1. Visual disturbances such as retinopathy; ask client about changes in vision
   2. Epigastric discomfort; take with meals
   3. Rash
   4. Headache, fatigue

Gout Drugs

A. Allopurinol (Zyloprim):
1. Inhibits xanthine oxidase, which prevents the production of uric acid
2. Used in the treatment of primary and secondary gout
3. Used to prevent attacks; not useful for acute attacks
4. Adverse effects/nursing care:
   a. Agranulocytosis and aplastic anemia; monitor CBC
   b. GI effects such as nausea, vomiting, diarrhea, abdominal pain
   c. Minimize GI side effects by giving with meals or immediately after.
   d. The drug should be discontinued at the first sign of a skin rash.
   e. Drowsiness; advise client not to drive
   f. Push fluids to at least two liters per day.
B. Colchicine:
1. Reduces inflammatory response to deposition of monosodium urate crystals
2. Drug of choice in acute attacks of gout; also used in the prophylaxis of recurrent gouty arthritis
3. Adverse effects/nursing care:
   a. During acute attack colchicine is administered every hour until pain relief or toxicity (nausea and vomiting or diarrhea) occurs.
   b. GI effects: Nausea and vomiting
   c. Bone marrow depression; monitor CBC
   d. Rashes
   e. Extravasation if IV drug infiltrates; monitor IV carefully
   f. Do not give IM or SC; causes severe irritation
C. Probenecid (Benemid):
1. Used to prevent the recurrence of gouty arthritis and hyperuricemia secondary to thiazide therapy
2. Used to increase and prolong serum levels of penicillin
3. Adverse effects/nursing care:
   a. Administer with food or an antacid to minimize gastric irritation.
   b. Avoid aspirin, because salicylates decrease effectiveness.

DRUGS AFFECTING THE RESPIRATORY TRACT
Antiasthmatic Drugs

A. Drugs used to treat asthma are those which open blocked air passages and those which alter the characteristics of respiratory tract fluid; corticosteroids are used to decrease inflammation in the bronchi.

B. Respiratory smooth muscle relaxants (bronchodilators):
1. Theophylline derivatives:
   a. Relax the smooth muscles of the bronchial airways
   b. Used to treat asthma and reversible bronchospasm that may occur in association with chronic bronchitis or emphysema
2. Examples:
   a. Aminophylline
   b. Elixophylline
   c. Theo-Dur
   d. Somophyllin
   e. Slo-Bid Gyrocaps
3. Adverse effects/nursing care:
   a. Nausea and vomiting; oral preparations may be administered with antacids to reduce GI irritation
   b. Hypotension especially when administered IV; monitor blood pressure and heart rate often
   c. Palpitations and dysrhythmias
   d. Flushing
   e. Increased urinary frequency
   f. CNS stimulation; headache, irritability, dizziness, vertigo, and seizures
   g. Monitor serum levels of theophyllin:
      (1) Therapeutic levels are 10–20 micrograms per ml.
      (2) Levels above 20 micrograms require a change in dosage.
   h. Monitor the rate of IV infusion to be sure that it is not too rapid.
   i. Do not give to patients who are allergic to caffeine, because theophylline is a member of the xanthine (caffeine) family.
   j. Use with caution in patients who have peptic ulcer disease, hyperthyroidism, glaucoma, diabetes, hypertension, or severe cardiac conditions.
   k. Adverse effects occur more often in children than in adults.
   l. Do not give IM, because IM injections cause intense pain and sloughing of tissue; may be given subcutaneously.
C. Antihistamines:
1. Actions and uses:
   a. Effects of histamine on the body can be reversed by drugs that block histamine receptors (antihistamines) or by drugs that have effects opposite to histamine (epinephrine).
   b. Antihistamines do not prevent the release of histamine. They compete with histamine receptors, preventing or reversing the effects of histamines.
   c. There are several classes of drugs having antihistamine properties, including the phenothiazines.

2. Examples:
   a. Chlorpheniramine maleate (ChlorTrimeton)
   b. Dimenhydrinate (Dramamine)
   c. Diphenhydramine (Benadryl)
   d. Promethazine HCl (Phenergan)
   e. Clemastine (Tavist)
   f. Fexofenadine (Allegra)
   g. Loratadine (Claritin)
   h. Loratadine with pseudoephedrine (Claritin-D)
   i. Astemizole (Hismanal)
3. Adverse effects/nursing care:
   a. CNS sedation, which can range from mild sedation to deep sleep
   b. Children may develop paradoxical excitement including restlessness, insomnia, and even seizures.
   c. Use safety measures for the sedated patient:
      (1) Side rails
      (2) Support when out of bed
      (3) Tell patient not to drive or operate machinery.
   d. Antihistamines potentiate other CNS depressants; client should not drink alcohol or take any other CNS depressants while taking antihistamines.
   e. GI effects including epigastric distress and dryness of the nose, mouth, and throat
   f. Allergic reactions can occur.
D. Cromolyn Sodium (Intal, Nalcrom):
   1. Actions and uses:
      a. Respiratory inhalant used to treat bronchial asthma
      b. Acts on the lung mucosa to prevent the release of histamine
      c. Used prophylactically to reduce the number of asthmatic attacks and the intensity of the disease; not used in the treatment of acute asthmatic attacks
   2. Adverse effects/nursing care:
      a. Bronchospasm
      b. Teach client how to use inhaler.
      c. May take four weeks for asthma attacks to become less frequent

Mucolytics Acetylcysteine (Mucomyst)

A. Actions and uses:
   1. Reduces the viscosity of pulmonary secretions
   2. Used as adjunctive treatment of persons with abnormal mucus secretion in the treatment of acute and chronic bronchopulmonary disorders and pulmonary complications of cystic fibrosis
   3. Antidote for acute acetaminophen (Tylenol) overdose

B. Adverse effects/nursing care:
   1. Mucomyst has a wide margin of safety.
   2. Stomatitis or nausea and vomiting
   3. Bronchoconstriction and chest tightness; should be discontinued if bronchoconstriction progresses
   4. Be alert for problems when giving to elderly or debilitated patients with severe respiratory insufficiency.
   5. Drowsiness

Expectorants

A. Actions and uses:
   1. Given for the symptomatic management of cough associated with the common cold
   2. Treatment of bronchitis
B. Examples:
   1. Guaifenesin (Robitussin):
      a. Increases respiratory tract fluid, reducing the viscosity of secretions
      b. Nontoxic
      c. Often manufactured in combination with antitussives
   2. Terpin Hydrate Elixir:
      a. Directly stimulates the lower respiratory tract secretory glands
      b. Contains a high percentage of alcohol; do not use in children less than 12 years of age, and do not give to alcoholics

Antitussives

A. Antitussives suppress the cough reflex by direct effect on the cough center in the brain; given for the symptomatic relief of nonproductive cough.
B. Examples:
   1. Dextromethorphan (Benylin DM, Pertussin):
      a. Few adverse reactions
      b. May occasionally cause nausea and vomiting
      c. Should not be given to persons taking MAO inhibitors
   2. Codeine:
      a. Side effects include nausea, vomiting, and constipation.
      b. Teach patients who are taking codeine to drink plenty of fluids and to take a laxative if constipation occurs.
      c. Sedation; provide for safety
      d. More apt to have CNS effects if other CNS drugs are being given
      e. Respiratory depression at high doses; monitor respiratory rate
      f. Use with caution in patients with asthma or emphysema.
      g. Tolerance; codeine can be addicting; give in the smallest possible dose to reduce adverse effects and tolerance

EYE AND EAR MEDICATIONS
Eye Drugs

A. Mydriatics and cycloplegics:
   1. Actions and uses:
      a. Mydriatics dilate the pupil.
      b. Cycloplegics paralyze the sphincter muscle of the iris and the ciliary muscle of the lens.
      c. Mydriatics and cycloplegics are used to promote dilatation of the eye and paralysis of accommodation during opthalmoscopic examination and prior to eye surgery.
   2. Examples:
      a. Atropine (Isopto Atropine)
      b. Homatropine (Isopto Homatropine)
      c. Cyclopentolate (Cyclogel)
   3. Adverse effects/nursing care:
      a. May precipitate an acute crisis in patients with glaucoma.
      b. Tell clients vision will be temporarily impaired; do not drive until effects have worn off.
      c. May raise intraocular pressure.
B. Miotics:
   1. Actions and uses:
      a. Miotics lower intraocular pressure by increasing the cholinergic effect on the eye.
      b. Timolol is an beta adrenergic blocker that has essentially the same effects as cholinergic agents; the pupil is constricted, increasing the outflow of the aqueous humor.
      c. Miotics are used in the treatment of open-angle glaucoma and angle closure glaucoma.
   2. Examples:
      a. Carbachol (Isopto Carbachol)
      b. Echothiophate (Phospholine Iodide)
      c. Pilocarpine (Pilocar, Isopto Carpine)
      d. Betaxol (Betoptic)
      e. Levobunolol (Betagen)
      f. Timolol (Timoptic)
   3. Adverse effects/nursing care:
      a. Painful ciliary or accommodative spasm may occur.
      b. Blurred vision, poor vision in dim light may occur.
      c. A rebound increase in intraocular pressure can occur when medication is withdrawn.
      d. Use with extreme caution in patients with a history of retinal detachment.
C. Anti-glaucoma prostaglandin: Latanoprost:
   1. Increases outflow of aqueous humor, decreasing intraocular pressure.
   2. Adverse effects/nursing care:
      a. Transient blurred vision
      b. Burning, stinging

      c. May increase brown pigmentation of eye.
      d. Remove contact lenses prior to administration, and leave out for 15 minutes.
      e. Occasionally causes upper respiratory infection and rarely chest pain.
D. Carbonic anhydrase inhibitors:
   1. Action and uses:
      a. Carbonic anhydrase inhibitors promote the renal excretion of sodium, potassium, bicarbonate, and water. Bicarbonate ion excretion makes the urine alkaline. Serum bicarbonate falls, creating metabolic acidosis.
      b. Used to treat acute narrow-angle glaucoma.
   2. Examples:
      a. Acetazolamide (Diamox)
      b. Dorzolamide (Trusopt)
      c. Methazolamide (Neptazine)
   3. Adverse effects/nursing care:
      a. Hypokalemia, hyperchloremic acidosis
      b. Monitor lab values, I&O, and weight.
      c. Teach the client to eat high-potassium foods.

ANTINEOPLASTIC AND IMMUNOSUPPRESSIVE AGENTS
Antineoplastic Agents

A. Information:
   1. Anti-cancer drugs destroy cancer cells by interfering with their out-of-control cell division.
   2. Chemotherapy is most effective during the early stages of a tumor's growth, early in the disease.
   3. In the treatment of a solid tumor, chemotherapy is used in conjunction with surgery and/or radiation.
   4. Chemotherapy alone is the treatment of choice in blood-related malignancies, such as leukemias and lymphomas.
   5. Chemotherapy for cancer usually utilizes a combination of drugs.
B. Adverse effects/nursing care (see Table 18.14):
   1. Dosage calculations are based on body surface area.
   2. Cancer drugs affect not only rapidly dividing cancer cells, but also affect rapidly dividing normal cells.
   3. Adverse effects relate largely to the destruction of rapidly dividing normal cells: Bone marrow, skin, GI mucosa, hair follicles, and fetal tissue.
   4. Bone marrow depression is usually the dose-limiting adverse effect.
      a. Low white blood count:

Table 18.14 Major Side Effects of Cancer Chemotherapeutic Agents

Effect	Resulting Problems	Nursing Care
Bone marrow suppression		
Decreased RBC	Fatigue	Rest
Decreased WBC	Infection risk	Protective isolation
Decreased platelets	Bleeding risk	Bleeding precautions
Alopecia	Self-image problem	Support, scarves, wigs
Nausea, vomiting	Fluid electrolyte balance	Clear liquids
	Nutrition	TPN
Stomatitis	Pain, nutrition	Viscous Lidocaine mouth wash
Elevated uric acid	Kidney stones	Encourage fluids; allopurinol
Liver damage	Drug toxicity	Liver function tests

(1) Protect the client from infection; protective isolation.

(2) Teach the client to take his or her temperature and to be alert for signs of infection.

(3) Teach client to wash his or her hands frequently, avoid crowds and people with infectious diseases.

b. Low platelet count (thrombocytopenia):

(1) Protect the client from injury; avoid IM injections.

(2) Teach client to avoid aspirin and aspirin products.

(3) Assess the client for signs of bleeding, such as bleeding gums, hematuria, petechiae, and ecchymoses.

c. Low red count (anemia): Client will be fatigued and tire easily.

5. When administering IV chemotherapy, select a new peripheral vein.

6. Avoid extravasation: Antineoplastic drugs are very toxic; suspect extravasation if the patient complains of pain and burning.

7. If extravasation occurs, stop the IV; leave the needle in place. If hospital policy allows, place 10–15 ml of normal saline infused through tubing to dilute the drug's effects.

8. There is controversy about whether to apply cold compresses initially to localize the drug and slow cell metabolism or to apply warm compresses to increase the blood supply to the area and decrease local damage.

9. Nausea and vomiting and anorexia:

a. Monitor intake and output and fluid electrolyte balance.

b. Give antiemetics as ordered before antineoplastics are given.

10. Diarrhea and constipation; monitor stools and fluid, and electrolytes values.

11. Stomatitis:

a. Use a soft-bristled tooth brush.

b. Use hydrogen peroxide or viscous lidocaine mouth rinses; do not use alcohol-based mouth wash.

12. Hyperuricemia:

a. Massive cell destruction releases purines, which convert to uric acid; uric acid may precipitate crystals and lead to renal stones and failure.

b. Push fluids.

c. Give Allopurinol if ordered to encourage the excretion of uric acid.

13. Liver toxicity:

a. Most of the antineoplastic drugs are metabolized in the liver.

b. Advise the client not to drink alcohol, because this will increase liver damage.

c. Some drugs have an antabuse-like effect.

14. Alopecia—temporary hair loss often— occurs.

15. Handle chemotherapeutic agents very carefully:

a. Drugs should be prepared under a vertical laminar air flow hood.

b. The preparer should wear a gown and gloves for protection.

16. The above side effects pertain in general to all cancer chemotherapeutic agents, except for the hormonal agents.

C. Alkylating agents (see Table 18.15):

1. Mechanism of action:

a. Alkylating agents are derived from nitrogen mustard.

b. Agents settle in the cell nucleus and attack DNA, causing cross linking of strands of cellular DNA, causing an imbalance of growth that leads to cell death.

c. Agents act at all phases of the cell cycle (cell cycle nonspecific).

d. Alkylating agents are used to treat carcinomas, sarcomas, lymphomas, and leukemias.

e. Most of the alkylating agents cross the blood-brain barrier.

2. Examples of alkylating agents:

a. Cisplatin (Platinol)

b. Busulfan (Myleran)

c. Cyclophosphamide (Cytoxan)

d. Mechlorethamine HCl (Mustargen)

e. Thiotepa

Table 18.15 Cancer Chemotherapeutic Agents

Type	Action	Examples	Uses
Alkylating Agents	Produces breaks and cross linking in the DNA strands, interferring with cell reproduction	Cyclophosphamide (Cytoxan)	Cancer of ovary, breast, malignant lymphomas, retinoblastoma, multiple myeloma, leukemias, neuroblastoma
		Mechlorethamine (Mustargen)	Polycythemia vera, Hodgkin's Disease, Chronic leukemia, bronchogenic cancer
		Busulfan (Myleran)	Chronic myelogenous leukemia
Antimetabolites	Substances bearing close resemblance to one required for normal physiologic functioning; exerts effect by interfering with the utilization of the essential metabolite, causing cell death	Fluorouracil (Adrucil)	Cancer of colon, rectum, breast, stomach, and pancreas
		Methotrexate (Folex)	Acute lymphocytic leukemia
		Cytarabine (Cytosar-U or Ara-c)	Leukemias
Antitumor Antibiotics	Kill the host cell as well as organism	Doxorubicin (Adriamycin)	Leukemias, Wilm's tumor, neuroblastoma, sarcomas, lymphomas; brochogenic, gastric, thyroid, breast, ovarian cancers
		Bleomycin (Blenoxane)	Squamous cell carcinoma, lymphomas, testicular cancer
		Dactinomycin (Cosmegen)	Wilm's tumor, testicular cancer, Ewing's sarcoma
Vinca (plant) Alkaloids	Alkaloids extracted from the periwinkle plant; arrest cell division by disrupting the microtubules that form the spindle apparatus	Vincristine sulfate (Oncovin)	Leukemias, lymphomas, Wilm's tumor
		Vinblastine (Velban)	Leukemias, lymphomas, testicular cancer, Kaposi's sarcoma, breast cancer
		Etoposide (VP-16)	Testicular tumor, small cell lung cancer
Antihormonal Therapy	Inhibits natural hormones and stops growth of tumors dependent on that hormone	Tamoxifen (Nolvadex)	Breast cancer
		Flutamide (Eulexin)	Prostate cancer
		Goserelin acetate (Zoladex)	Prostate cancer
Hormonal Therapy	Manipulation of hormones to stop cancer cell growth	Estrogens (Diethylstilbestrol [DES])	Breast and prostate cancer
		Medroxyprogesterone (DepoProvera)	Endometrial and renal carcinoma
		Megastrol (Megase)	Breast and endometrial carcinoma
		Testolactone (Teslac)	Breast carcinoma
Miscellaneous	Work by different methods	L-asparaginase (Elspar)	Acute lymphotic leukemia
		Procarbazine hydrochloride (Matulane)	Hodgkin's Disease

3. Cytoxan is excreted through the urinary tract and can cause hemorrhagic cystitis; be sure that the patient drinks plenty of fluids and empties his or her bladder frequently.

D. Antimetabolites:
1. Antimetabolites interfere with protein synthesis and are classed as cell cycle specific.
2. Antimetabolites are divided into:
   a. Folic acid antagonists
   b. Purine antagonists
   c. Pyrimidine antagonists
3. Antimetabolites are very toxic.
4. Antimetabolites are used to treat carcinomas of the breast and GI tract; trophoblastic tumors such as choriocarcinomas and hydatidiform moles, medulloblastomas, and osteogenic sarcomas

5. Examples of antimetabolites (see Table 18.15):
   a. Methotrexate (Folex PFS)
   b. Cytarabine (Cytosine, Arabinoside)
   c. 5-Fluorouracil (5FU)
   d. Hydroxyurea (Hydrea)
   e. Mercaptopurine (Purinethol)
   f. 6-Mercaptopurine (6MP)
   g. Vidarabine (Vira-A)
   h. Thioguanine
E. Antibiotic antineoplastic agents:
   1. Mechanism of action:
      a. Isolated from naturally occurring microorganisms that inhibit bacterial growth
      b. Differ from the other aminoglycosides in that they disrupt the functioning of the host cells as well as the bacterial cells
   2. Examples of antibiotic antineoplastic agents:
      a. Bleomycin sulfate (Blenoxane)

b. Dactinomycin (Actinomycin D)
c. Daunorubicin HCl
d. Doxorubicin HCl (Adriamycin)
e. Mithramycin (Plicamycin)
f. Mitomycin (Mutamycin)
g. Procarbazine HCl (Matulane); procarbazine is technically not an antibiotic, but it acts like one and is usually placed in this group of antineoplastics.

F. Vinca alkaloids, asparaginase, and etoposide (see Table 18.15):
1. Derivatives of the periwinkle plant, a vine used to treat leukemias, lymphomas, sarcomas, and some carcinomas; Taxol is used for advanced ovarian cancer and small cell lung carcinoma.
2. Examples of Vinca alkaloids (note the *vin* or *vine* in the name):
   a. Vinblastine sulfate (Velban)
   b. Vincristine sulfate (Oncovin)
   c. Vindesine sulfate (Eldesine)
   d. Etoposide (VePesid)
   e. Paclitaxel (Taxol)
3. Adverse effects/nursing care:
   a. In addition to the usual side effects of chemotherapy, the vinca alkaloids cause neurological damage, numbness and tingling, foot drop, wrist drop, and slapping of the foot when walking.
   b. Constipation may be a sign of neurological damage.

G. Asparaginase:
1. Asparaginase or L-asparaginase is derived from Escherichia Coli and other sources.
2. Asparaginase is given in combination with other drugs in the treatment of acute lymphocytic leukemia.

H. Etoposide (VP-16): Prescribed primarily as a treatment for testicular cancer

I. Antineoplastics affecting hormonal balance:
1. Mechanism of action:
   a. Some are synthetic hormones.
   b. Others are hormone antagonists.
   c. Hormonal agents are valuable because they inhibit cancer growth in tissues, responding to hormones without directly causing cell toxicity.
2. Examples of antineoplastics affecting hormonal balance:
   a. Drugs used to treat breast cancer:
      (1) Tamoxifen (Nolvadex)
      (2) Dromostanolone
      (3) Megestrol
      (4) Aminoglutethimide (Cytadren)
   b. Drugs used to treat prostate carcinoma:
      (1) Estramustine phosphate sodium
      (2) Aminoglutethimide (Cytadren)
      (3) Flutamide (Eulexin)
   c. Drugs used to treat adrenal cancer:
      (1) Mitotane
      (2) Aminoglutethimide (Cytadren)

3. Adverse effects/nursing care:
   a. Adverse effects are related to the organ affected.
   b. Estrogen-dependent cancers are treated with antiestrogen drugs or male hormones. Cancers dependent on male hormones are given female hormones.
   c. A loss of libido may occur with drugs used to treat prostate cancer.

Immunosuppressants

A. Azathioprine (Imuran):
1. Imuran is an antimetabolite that is quickly split to mercaptopurine and is used for immunosuppression in organ transplants.
2. Causes immunosuppression and bone marrow suppression
3. Can cause severe liver damage

B. Cyclosporine (Sandimmune):
1. Cyclosporine inhibits the T-lymphocytes and is used in combination with corticosteroids to prevent rejection in kidney, liver, and heart transplants.
2. Cyclosporine causes bone marrow depression, nausea, and vomiting and liver and renal toxicity.
3. Since clients will be on long-term maintenance doses of this very toxic drug, teach the client and family about the side effects.
4. All the nursing care measures discussed earlier for bone marrow depression are applicable.
5. Mix oral solutions with milk or juice, and drink immediately after mixing.

IMMUNIZATIONS
Vaccines and Toxoids

A. Information:
1. Vaccines and toxoids initiate the formation of antibodies by stimulating the host's antigen-antibody mechanism.
2. Vaccines stimulate active immunity (see Table 18.16).
3. Active immunity is the manufacture of antibodies by the host in response to disease or by vaccination.
4. Passive immunity is the injection of antibodies formed some place other than the host (see Table 18.16).
5. Vaccines and toxoids should not be given to persons who are immunosuppressed, receiving corticosteroid therapy, or are pregnant.

B. Hepatitis B Vaccine (see Table 18.17):
1. The vaccine is given at birth, at one month, and at six months of age.
2. At-risk adults receive two doses a month apart followed by a third dose six months after the initial dose.

3. Vaccine is effective against all known types of hepatitis B
C. DTP (Diphtheria, Tetanus, Pertussis):
   1. Initial series of three shots at two-month intervals: 2, 4, 6, months
   2. Boosters: 18 months, 4–6 years
   3. DT (Diphtheria, tetanus) and IPV q 10 years starting age 14–16 years
D. IPV (inactivated polio vaccine):
   1. Vaccine is given at age two months and four months.

2. A booster is given at 15–18 months and again at 4–6 years.
E. Hib-Conjugate (haemophilus Influenza B):
   1. Given at 2, 4, and 6 months
   2. Given again at 12 months and 15 months
F. Pneumococcal conjugate vaccine
   1. Given at 2, 4, and 6 months
   2. Given again at 12–15 months
G. MMR (Measles, mumps, rubella):
   1. Vaccine is given at 15 months of age.
   2. Do not give within three months of a transfusion.
   3. Globulins inactivate the vaccine.
   4. DTP and OPV may be given simultaneously with MMR.
   5. Do not give the MMR if the child is allergic to eggs.
H. Tuberculin skin test:
   1. Done at 12–15 months, before starting school (4–6 years).
   2. May be done yearly.
   3. Repeated in adolescence (14–16 years) and when indicated.

Table 18.16 Active and Passive Immunity

Active Immunity	Passive Immunity
Takes time to develop	Immediate
Long lasting	Short lasting
Develops from immunization or disease	"Borrowed" from a donor
Toxoids, vaccines	Immunoglobulins

Table 18.17 Childhood Immunization Schedule

Vaccine		Age										
	Birth	1 mo	2 mo	4 mo	6 mo	12 mo	15 mo	18 mo	24 mo	4–6 mo	11–12 mo	14–18 mo
Hepatitis B	Hep B #1	Hep B #1	Hep B #2		Hep B #3	Hep B #3					Hep B	
Diphtheria tetanus toxids, and pertussis			DTaP	DTaP	DTaP		DTaP	DTaP		DTaP	Td	Td
H. influenzea type b			Hib	Hib	Hib	Hib	Hib					
Inactivated polio--			IPV	IPV	IPV	IPV	IPV			IPV		
Pneumococcal conjugate			PCV	PCV	PCV	PCV	PCV					
Measles-Mumps-Rubella						MMR	MMR			MMR	MMR	
Varicella						Var	Var				Var	
Hepatitis A	Hepatitis A									Hep A in selected area	Hep A in selected area	Hep A in selected area

 Range of recommended ages for vaccination.

 Vaccines to be given if previously recommended doses were missed or were given earlier than the recommended minimum age.

Recommended in selected states and/or regions.

I. BCG vaccine:
1. Vaccine is given to infants to prevent tuberculosis in countries where tuberculosis is endemic
2. It is not routinely used in the USA.
J. Influenza virus vaccine (see Table 18.18):
1. Annual vaccine recommended for people with cardiovascular or pulmonary disease, people over 65, nursing home residents, children with a chronic illness such as cardiopulmonary disorders, and health care providers.
2. Do not give to clients who are allergic to eggs.

Table 18.18 Adult Immunization Schedule

T(d)*	Every 10 yrs after 11–15 years of age
Tuberculin Test	Upon exposure; yearly for health care workers
Influenza Vaccine	Yearly after age 65; more often for people with chronic disease
Pneumococcal Vaccine	Once at 65 years

3. Do not administer during active infection or if the client is febrile.
K. Pneumococcal Vaccine: Given to persons at risk for pneumonia or persons who are immunocompromised, have cardiopulmonary disease, or are elderly.
L. Hepatitis A vaccine:
1. A single dose confers immunity in 15 days.
2. Booster dose is recommended 6 to 12 months later to ensure adequate antibody titers.
3. Recommended for nursing home residents, institutionalized clients, travelers to endemic areas, and persons engaging in high-risk sexual activity.

Immune Serums

Confer a passive immunity:

A. Hepatitis B Immune globulin, human:
1. Should be given within seven days after exposure
2. Repeated 28 days after exposure
B. Immune serum globulin (Immunoglobulin):
1. Given to nonimmunized individuals after exposure to measles, polio, or chicken pox.
2. Given as prophylaxis in primary immune deficiencies.
C. Tetanus immune globulin, human (Hyper-Tet):
1. Used only if wound is over 24 hours old or client has had less than two previous tetanus toxoid injections.
2. Lasts longer than antitoxin.

D. Immune serum globulin (Immunoglobulin): Given to nonimmunized individuals after exposure to measles, polio, chicken pox, and as a prophylaxis in primary immune deficiency disorders
E. RhoGam:
1. RhoGam is given to Rh negative mothers who have an Rh positive fetus and who have not developed antibodies to the Rh factor.
2. Also given to Rh negative women who have abortions or miscarriages even if the Rh factor of the fetus is not known
3. RhoGam prevents the development of maternal RH antibodies.
4. RhoGam must be given within 72 hours of delivery and should be given within three hours; sometimes given at 28 weeks gestation.

Sample Questions

1. The nurse is administering an IM injection to a client. When the nurse aspirates, there is a blood return. What is the most appropriate action for the nurse to take?
   1. Continue to administer the medication.
   2. Withdraw the needle and administer in another site.
   3. Withdraw the needle, discard the medication, and start over.
   4. Change the needle before administering the medication in another site.
2. The nurse is to administer a subcutaneous injection. Which technique is correct?
   1. Pull the skin taut. Insert a 21-gauge needle at a 90-degree angle.
   2. Pinch the skin. Insert a 25-gauge needle at a 45-degree angle.
   3. Stretch the skin taut. Insert a 27-gauge needle at a 10-degree angle.
   4. Pinch the skin. Insert a 21-gauge needle at a 60-degree angle.
3. The nurse is to administer an IM injection to a six-month-old. What is the most appropriate site to utilize?
   1. Vastus lateralis
   2. Dorsal gluteal
   3. Ventral gluteal
   4. Iliac crest
4. Ringers Lactate is running at 125 ml/hr. The administration set has 15 drops/ml. What should the drip rate be?
   1. 8 drops/min.
   2. 31 drops/min.
   3. 50 drops/min.
   4. 67 drops/min.

5. A two-year-old child who weighs 33 pounds is to receive a total daily dose of 25 mg/kg of a medication. It is to be administered in three evenly divided doses. The label reads 150 mg/ml. How many ml will be injected per dose?
   1. 0.5 ml
   2. 0.8 ml
   3. 3.75 ml
   4. 155 ml

6. An adult is receiving gentamicin IV q 8 h. Which laboratory tests does the nurse expect that the client will have done regularly?
   1. CBC and hemoglobin
   2. BUN and creatinine
   3. SGOT and SGPT
   4. Urine and blood cultures

7. Which observation, if reported by a client, is most suggestive of an adverse reaction to gentamicin?
   1. A WBC of 8000
   2. Ringing in the ears
   3. Itching
   4. Nasal stuffiness

8. Penicillin V Potassium (Pen-Vee-K) 500 mg PO qid is ordered for an adult client. He reports that he took penicillin for the first time two months ago. What should the nurse do?
   1. Be sure that skin testing for a penicillin allergy has been done.
   2. Observe for signs of an allergic response.
   3. Withhold the penicillin.
   4. Notify the physician.

9. The nurse in the physician's office is instructing an adult about taking penicillin V potassium (Pen-Vee-K) qid. When should the nurse tell him to take the medicine?
   1. With meals and at bedtime
   2. Once a day at 10 a.m.
   3. On an empty stomach at six-hour intervals
   4. With orange juice at four-hour intervals

10. A 10-month-old has been diagnosed as having acute otitis media. The pediatrician prescribed amoxicillin suspension. What instructions should the nurse give the child's mother?
    1. When your child's temperature has been normal for two days, discontinue the medicine.
    2. Discard any unused medication.
    3. If your child has symptoms of an ear infection again, start giving her the leftover medication.
    4. Give your child all of the medication in the bottle.

11. Keflex 250 mg PO q 6 h is ordered for an adult. The nurse notes that her history indicates that she has an allergy to penicillin. What is the most appropriate initial action for the nurse?
    1. Notify the physician.
    2. Observe the client carefully after giving the medication.
    3. Administer the Keflex IV instead of PO

4. Ask the client to describe the reaction that she had to penicillin.

12. Which of the following persons would be least likely to receive tetracycline?
    1. An adolescent with acne
    2. A woman with chlamydia who is seven months pregnant
    3. A 10-year-old with Rocky Mountain Spotted Fever
    4. A 32-year-old man with walking pneumonia

13. An adult is receiving Gantrisin 1 GM PO qid for a urinary tract infection. Which statement that she makes indicates a need for more teaching?
    1. "If I get a rash, I will apply calamine lotion."
    2. "I will take my pills with a full glass of water."
    3. "I will take all the pills even if I feel better."
    4. "I will stay out of the sun while I am taking the pills."

14. An adult client is seen in the clinic, and methenamine mandelate (Mandelamine) is prescribed. Which information is most appropriate for the nurse to include in the teaching?
    1. You should drink several glasses of cranberry juice each day.
    2. If it upsets your stomach, try taking it with an antacid.
    3. Avoid going out in the sun while taking Mandelamine.
    4. Take the tablets with orange juice or milk.

15. An adult client has pulmonary tuberculosis. He is receiving INH 300 mg PO and Ethambutol 1 GM PO daily and streptomycin 1 GM I.M. three times a week. When he comes in for a checkup, he tells the nurse that he hates getting shots and his ears ring most of the time. What is the best interpretation for the nurse to make regarding the client's complaints?
    1. He may be receiving too much Ethambutol.
    2. He should be evaluated for adverse reaction to streptomycin.
    3. Tuberculosis may have spread to the brain.
    4. He is experiencing a reaction commonly seen when INH and Streptomycin are given at the same time.

16. An adult client has pulmonary tuberculosis. He is receiving INH 300 mg PO and Ethambutol 1 GM PO daily and streptomycin 1 GM I.M. three times a week. When he comes in for a checkup, he tells the nurse that he hates getting shots and his ears ring most of the time. What advice does the nurse expect will be given to this client?
    1. Take pyridoxine daily.
    2. Expect red-colored urine and feces.
    3. Stop the medications when his cough is gone.
    4. Take streptomycin by mouth instead of by injection.

17. An adult client is being treated for genital herpes with acyclovir (Zovirax) tablets. Which statement she makes indicates that she understands her therapy?
    1. "It is safe now to have sexual relations."
    2. "I will stay home from work until the blisters are gone."
    3. "This medicine will cure the herpes infection."
    4. "If the blisters come back, I will start taking the pills immediately."

18. The clinic nurse is teaching an adult male who has AIDS. He is receiving zidovudine. Which statement he makes indicates that he understands the medication regimen?
    1. "If I get a sore throat and it is hard to swallow my capsules, I can empty the capsule into applesauce."
    2. "I am hopeful that this drug will get rid of this awful disease."
    3. "I understand I might need a transfusion."
    4. "I should take acetaminophen (Tylenol), not aspirin, if I get a fever."

19. An adult client has been diagnosed as having rheumatoid arthritis and is started on Piroxicam (Feldene) 20 mg daily. Two days later, the client calls the nurse and says that her joints still hurt. What is the best response for the nurse to make?
    1. "It may take up to two weeks before results are seen with Feldene."
    2. "Take aspirin with the Feldene. It has an additive effect."
    3. "Come in to see the physician. You should have pain relief by now."
    4. "You may need more medication. Take one additional pill each day."

20. A 13-month-old child is admitted to the emergency room with salicylate poisoning. Her mother found her beside the empty bottle of adult aspirin. She says there were "about 10" aspirin left in the bottle. What manifestations would the nurse most expect to see in the child?
    1. Bradypnea and pallor
    2. Hyperventilation and hyperpyrexia
    3. Subnormal temperature and bleeding
    4. Melena and bradycardia

21. A toddler who has swallowed several adult aspirin is admitted to the emergency room. When admitted, the child is breathing but is difficult to arouse. What is the immediate priority of care?
    1. Administration of syrup of ipecac
    2. Cardiopulmonary resuscitation
    3. Ventilatory support
    4. Gastric lavage

22. An adult client is on call for the operating room. The pre-op medication order is for meperidine HCl (Demerol) 100 mg IM and atropine 0.4 mg IM. The operating room calls at 11 A.M. and requests that the client be medicated. The nurse notes that the client last received meperidine for pain at 10 A.M. What is the most appropriate action for the nurse to take?
    1. Give the pre-op medication as ordered.
    2. Give half the dose of meperidine and all of the atropine.
    3. Check with the anesthesiologist before administering the medication.
    4. Withhold both the meperidine and the atropine.

23. An adult client had an abdominal hysterectomy this morning. Meperidine HCl (Demerol) 75 mg IM q 3–4 hrs prn for pain is ordered. At 9 P.M., she complains of lower abdominal pain. She was last medicated at 5:45 P.M. What is the most appropriate initial action for the nurse to take?
    1. Offer her a bed pan and a back rub.
    2. Reposition her.
    3. Administer meperidine HCl 75 mg IM.
    4. Encourage her to perform relaxation and breathing exercises.

24. An adult client has rheumatoid arthritis. Aspirin 975 mg q 4 hrs prn is ordered for pain. At 2 P.M. the client requests pain medication. Aspirin was last given at 9:30 A.M. What is the most appropriate initial action for the nurse to take?
    1. Give the aspirin as ordered.
    2. Question the order because it is a higher-than-normal dosage.
    3. Attempt to divert the client's attention from the pain.
    4. Assess the nature of the pain.

25. A 68-year-old man has been diagnosed as having Parkinson's Disease. He is started on Cogentin 0.5 mg PO daily. Which nursing action is most essential at this time?
    1. Monitor his blood pressure and pulse.
    2. Encourage cold beverages and hard candies.
    3. Observe for rashes.
    4. Monitor his stools for fluid loss.

26. A young adult, 20 years old, who is hospitalized for the first time with schizophrenia, is receiving chlorpromazine (Thorazine) 75 mg PO tid. The client is to go home for a weekend pass. Which statement that the client makes indicates a need for nursing intervention?
    1. "I won't drink any alcohol this weekend."
    2. "It will be good to taste home-cooked food again."
    3. "We plan to go dancing."
    4. "I'm looking forward to a relaxing weekend at the beach."

27. An adult client is receiving Lithium 600 mg PO tid for the treatment of bipolar disorder. The client should be taught that it is important to have adequate amounts of which substance?
    1. Potassium
    2. Sodium
    3. Calcium

4. Magnesium

28. An elderly adult is scheduled for repair of a fractured femur this morning. The nurse goes in to administer pre-op medication of Demerol 75 mg and Atropine 0.4 mg I.M. The client asks the nurse if he should take his eye drops before surgery. What is the best initial response for the nurse to make?
   1. "You can take them when you get back from surgery."
   2. "I'll give them to you now."
   3. "Let me check with your physician."
   4. "What kind of eye drops are you taking?"

29. A 68-year-old client was admitted with congestive heart failure, has been digitalized, and is now taking a maintenance dose of Digoxin 0.25 mg PO daily. The client is to be discharged soon. Which assessment is of most immediate concern to the nurse?
   1. The client's apical pulse is 66.
   2. The client says that he is nauseous and has no appetite.
   3. The client says that he will take his pill every morning.
   4. The client has lost eight pounds since his admission one week ago.

30. An adult has angina and is to be discharged on transdermal nitroglycerin. Which statement by the client indicates that the client needs additional teaching?
   1. "I am glad that I can continue walking."
   2. "I will change the site each day."
   3. "I will be able to continue to drink alcoholic beverages."
   4. "I will need to get up slowly."

31. A 48-year-old man is in the emergency room. He has crushing substernal pain, is diaphoretic, apprehensive, and ashen gray in color. The cardiac monitor shows runs of premature ventricular contractions. Which drug is most likely to be given to this client?
   1. Lidocaine
   2. Verapamil
   3. Digitalis
   4. Nitroglycerine

32. A 60-year-old client has been hospitalized for deep vein thrombosis. The client is to be discharged on coumadin 5 mg PO daily. Which statement that the client makes indicates the best understanding of the medication routine?
   1. "I will take aspirin for my arthritis."
   2. "I love to eat spinach salads."
   3. "I will get a blood test next week."
   4. "I made an appointment to have my teeth pulled."

33. A 67-year-old client is to be discharged from the hospital. The client is taking digoxin and furosemide daily. Which instruction is most essential for the nurse to give this client?
   1. Take your medicine early in the day.
   2. Be sure to drink orange juice and eat bananas or melons every day.

3. Avoid foods that are high in sodium.
4. Drink plenty of milk.

34. An adult client who has been taking furosemide (Lasix) 40 mg PO every day for several weeks is complaining of muscle weakness and lethargy. Which test will be of greatest value in assessing the client's condition?
   1. Serum electrolytes
   2. Urinalysis
   3. Serum creatinine
   4. Five-hour glucose tolerance test

35. An adult receives NPH insulin at 7 A.M. When is a hypoglycemic reaction most apt to develop?
   1. Mid morning
   2. Mid afternoon
   3. During the evening
   4. During the night

36. A 17-year-old, has been recently diagnosed as having diabetes mellitus Type I. Insulin is prescribed. The client asks why insulin can't be taken by mouth. What is the best answer for the nurse to give?
   1. "Insulin is irritating to the stomach."
   2. "Oral insulin is too rapidly absorbed."
   3. "Gastric juices destroy insulin."
   4. "You can take it by mouth when the acute phase is over."

37. An adult received regular insulin at 7 A.M. At 10 A.M., she is irritable and sweaty, but her skin is cool. What is the most appropriate action for the nurse to take?
   1. Have her lie down for a rest.
   2. Give her a cola drink.
   3. Give ordered insulin.
   4. Encourage exercise.

38. A woman who is taking cortisone for an acute exacerbation of rheumatoid arthritis is upset about the fat face she has developed. She says to the nurse, "I'm going to quit taking that cortisone." The nurse's response should be based on which understanding?
   1. Cortisone does not cause a fat face.
   2. The symptoms will lessen as her body adjusts to the medication.
   3. The drug should be immediately discontinued when adverse effects occur.
   4. Cortisone should never be abruptly discontinued.

39. An adult woman has been diagnosed as having hypothryoidism. She is taking Cytomel (liothyronine sodium) 50 mcg daily. Which of the following side effects should the nurse be especially alert for?
   1. Angina
   2. Fatigue
   3. Rash
   4. Gastritis

40. A 19-year-old, has just started taking birth control pills. She calls the clinic nurse to say that her breasts are tender and she is nauseous.

The nurse's response is based on which understanding?

1. These are serious side effects.
2. These effects usually decrease after three to six cycles.
3. Taking the pill in the morning reduces its side effects.
4. Taking the pills every other day reduces its side effects.

41. A young woman delivered a 7 lb., 8 oz. baby boy spontaneously. Ergotrate 0.4 mg q 6 hr for five days is ordered. A half hour after the nurse administers the first dose she complains of abdominal cramping. The nurse's best response is based on which understanding?
    1. Cramping indicates a serious adverse reaction.
    2. Cramping can be reduced by abdominal breathing.
    3. The medication is having the desired effect.
    4. The dosage needs to be reduced.

42. Aluminum hydroxide gel (Amphojel) is ordered for an adult who has acute renal failure. What is the primary reason for administering this drug to this client?
    1. To prevent the development of Curling's ulcers
    2. To bind phosphates
    3. To maintain normal pH
    4. To prevent diarrhea

43. An adult is hospitalized for an acute attack of gout. Which medication should the nurse expect to administer?
    1. Morphine
    2. Colchicine
    3. Allopurinol
    4. Acetaminophen

44. An adult is scheduled for a left cataract extraction. Homatropine and Cyclogel eye drops are ordered. What is the expected action of these drops?
    1. Mydriasis
    2. Miotic effects
    3. Relaxation of eye muscles
    4. Prevention of infection

45. When administering eye drops, the nurse should administer the drops into which place?
    1. The pupil
    2. The conjunctival sac
    3. The inner canthus
    4. The cornea

46. Ear drops have been ordered for a 10-month-old. How should the nurse teach the mother to pull the baby's ear to straighten the ear canal?
    1. Down and back
    2. Down and forward
    3. Up and forward
    4. Up and back

47. A client who has Hodgkin's Disease receives a weekly IV dose of nitrogen mustard. Which nursing order is most appropriate?

1. Encourage mouth care with an astringent mouth wash and dental floss after every meal.
2. Encourage organ meats and dried beans and peas.
3. Monitor vital signs daily.
4. Encourage fluid intake to 3,000 cc.

48. A woman who is receiving cancer chemotherapy exhibits all of the following. Which is most indicative of bone marrow depression?
    1. Alopecia
    2. Petechiae
    3. Stomatitis
    4. Constipation

49. A six-year-old is seen in the emergency room after stepping on a rusty nail. He has received no immunizations. What should the nurse expect to give him immediately to prevent a tetanus infection?
    1. Tetanus toxoid
    2. DPT
    3. Immune serum globulin
    4. Penicillin

50. A woman is two months pregnant when her five-year-old child develops rubella. What is most likely to be given to her?
    1. Immune serum globulin
    2. MMR
    3. RhoGam
    4. Rubella antitoxin

Answers and Rationales

1. (3) The nurse should not inject medication that has blood in it. Blood may interact with the medication and cause an adverse response.
2. (2) The skin should be pinched, and a 25-gauge needle should be inserted at a 45-degree angle. Answer 1 describes an IM injection. Answer 3 describes an intradermal injection.
3. (1) Infants and small children do not have enough muscle in the gluteal area to use that site. The iliac crest is a site used for subcutaneous injections, not IM.
4. (2) Divide 125 ml/hr by 60 min./hr and multiply by 15 drops/ml.
5. (2) Break the problem down into steps. First, determine the child's weight in kilograms. Divide the number of pounds by 2.2 obtaining 15 kg. Then, multiply 15 kg by 25 mg/kg and obtain 375 mg. Next, divide 375 mg by three daily doses, coming up with 125 mg/dose. The last step is to perform a desired over have calculation to determine the dose. Divide the desired dose (125 mg) by the have-on-hand amount (150 mg), obtaining .83 ml.
6. (2) BUN and creatinine are tests of renal function. Gentamicin is nephrotoxic. All persons receiving gentamicin should have these tests done regularly to assess for toxicity. Elevated levels indicate toxicity. CBC and

hemoglobin tests are done to indicate anemia or bone marrow suppression. SGOT and SGPT are liver function tests. Cultures are done before and after antibiotic treatments, not during treatment.

7. (2) Gentamicin is ototoxic (ears). Ringing in the ears suggests possible damage to the eighth cranial nerve, the auditory nerve. A WBC of 8,000 is normal.

8. (2) The client does not have a history of allergic response to penicillin, so there is no need to skin test or withhold the medication. However, the nurse knows that allergic responses rarely occur with the first administration of a medication. Most allergic responses occur following the second or later dose. In the United States, routine skin testing for penicillin allergy is not done. Skin testing is done when there is a question about whether the person has really had an allergic response.

9. (3) Penicillin V potassium (Pen-Vee-K) should be taken on an empty stomach at six-hour intervals.

10. (4) The nurse should tell the mother to give the child all of the medication in the bottle. The bottle contains the prescribed amount. Stopping the medication when the child begins to feel better is likely to cause antibiotic resistant strains of the microorganism to develop. There should be no unused medication. The amoxicillin suspension is only good for two weeks.

11. (4) The nurse knows that there is often a cross allergy between penicillin and the cephalosporins, like Keflex. The initial response by the nurse should be to determine what type of reaction the client had. The nurse should then notify the physician and describe the reaction. Reactions such as nausea or diarrhea are not allergic responses. A reaction such as hives or anaphylaxis would prevent giving Keflex.

12. (2) Tetracycline causes gray tooth syndrome in children under eight years of age. Tooth buds are developing during the third trimester of pregnancy and can be damaged if the mother takes tetracycline then. Tetracycline is effective for chlamydia but should not be given because the woman is pregnant. Tetracycline is often given to adolescents with acne. Tetracycline is effective against Rocky Mountain Spotted Fever. Note that the child is older than eight. Walking pneumonia is probably a mycoplasma infection; tetracycline is effective against mycoplasma.

13. (1) The client should be taught that a rash might be an adverse reaction to Gantrisin, and it should be reported to the physician, not self medicated. Gantrisin is a sulfa medication and should be taken with a full glass of water. Photosensitivity is common; the client should stay out of the sun. All antimicrobials should be taken for the full course of treatment even if the person feels better.

14. (1) Mandelamine is used to treat urinary tract infections. It works most effectively in an acid environment. The urine should be acidified by drinking cranberry juice. Antacids should not be taken with mandelamine; neither should orange juice and milk, which leave an alkaline urine. Photosensitivity is not a concern with mandelamine.

15. (2) A major toxic response to streptomycin is damage to the eighth cranial nerve, the auditory nerve. Ringing in the ears suggests streptomycin toxicity. Ethambutol might cause color blindness.

16. (1) Persons who are taking INH should also be taking pyridoxine (vitamin B_6) daily to prevent peripheral neuritis. Rifampin causes red-colored urine and feces. This client is not on Rifampin. A person with active tuberculosis will be on medication for a year or more. Streptomycin is not available in an oral form because it is not systemically absorbed when given orally.

17. (4) Persons with recurrent genital herpes should start taking their prescription acyclovir tablets at the first sign of an infection. This shortens the outbreak and makes it less severe. The client should avoid sexual relations whenever lesions are present. There is no need to stay home from work with genital herpes. The medicine shortens the outbreaks and makes them less severe but does not cure herpes infections.

18. (3) Zidovudine causes such a decrease in red blood cell count that transfusions are often necessary. The capsules should not be opened. Zidovudine does not cure AIDS. The client should not take over-the-counter medications such as acetaminophen when taking zidovudine.

19. (1) It takes up to two weeks for Feldene to reach therapeutic levels. The other options are not appropriate nursing interventions.

20. (2) Aspirin overdose causes an increase in metabolic rate and metabolic acidosis. The child will have an increased temperature (hyperpyrexia) from the increased metabolic rate. The pulse will be up. Compensation for metabolic acidosis is hyperventilation to blow off the acid. The child will be warm, flushed, tachycardic, and hyperventilating. The child is at risk for bleeding. Melena (blood in the stools) is unlikely at this time. Enough time has not elapsed for a GI bleed and hidden blood in the stool.

21. (4) The child is breathing, so CPR and ventilatory support are not needed. Once the child is breathing, the first priority is to remove the poison. The child is difficult to arouse, so gastric lavage is used, not syrup of ipecac, which induce vomiting.

22. (3) The client was medicated one hour ago. It is too soon to give meperidine again. The nurse should call the physician for instructions.

23. (3) The client has pain in the operative area and the time interval is appropriate, so medicate her. A back rub, repositioning, and relaxation and breathing exercises are not likely to relieve pain on the day of surgery.

24. (4) The client asked for pain medication, but there is no indication of where the client hurts. The nurse cannot assume that the pain is arthritis pain without asking. The aspirin dose is not high for someone with rheumatoid arthritis. The nurse should not divert attention from pain without first assessing.

25. (1) Cogentin can affect the blood pressure and pulse. The nurse must monitor vital signs. The client probably will also have a dry mouth as a result of taking Cogentin, and cold beverages and hard candies are also indicated. However, they are not the priority intervention. Rashes are not common side effect of Cogentin. He is likely to be constipated.

26. (4) Photosensitivity is a common side effect of Thorazine. The client should not drink alcohol. It is MAOIs that have food contraindications. There is no contraindication to dancing.

27. (2) Lithium is excreted from the body as a sodium salt. The client should be taught to have adequate amounts of sodium and water so that lithium can be excreted in the urine and not cause toxicity.

28. (4) The nurse knows that atropine is contraindicated in persons who have glaucoma. The client is elderly and takes eye drops. The nurse should determine the type of eye drops and the reasons for them before administering the preoperative medication.

29. (2) Anorexia and nausea are signs of digoxin toxicity. A pulse of less than 60 indicates toxicity. The client should take his pill every morning. Digoxin is not a diuretic effect, but the increase in pumping effectiveness of the heart will help to pump the accumulated fluid from congestive heart failure to the kidneys for excretion. A weight loss is normal when starting on digitalis.

30. (3) The client who is taking nitroglycerin should not drink alcohol. He should be able to walk. The site should be changed daily. He will need to get up slowly, because orthostatic hypotension is a common reaction to the vasodilating effects of nitroglycerin.

31. (1) The client is having premature ventricular contractions. Lidocaine is the drug of choice for frequent PVCs. Verapamil is a calcium channel blocker and is not the drug of choice for PVCs during an MI. Digitalis is used for CHF and atrial dysrhythmias. Nitroglycerine is used to treat angina. This client more likely has a myocardial infarction.

32. (3) Persons who are taking coumadin must have prothrombin times done on a regular basis. This indicates understanding. Aspirin is an anticoagulant and should not be taken by the person who is taking coumadin unless specifically ordered as part of the anticoagulant regimen. Spinach is high in vitamin K, a coagulant and the antidote for coumadin. Spinach should not be eaten in large amounts. The person who is taking anticoagulants should not have any teeth removed because of the possibility of hemorrhage.

33. (2) Furosemide (Lasix) is a potassium-depleting diuretic. The client who is also taking digoxin is at greater risk for digoxin toxicity when the serum potassium is low. The person must replace the potassium lost by eating foods high in potassium and possibly by taking a potassium supplement. The client should also be told to take the diuretic early in the day to prevent diuresing during the night and interfering with sleep. However, potassium replacement is of greater importance and takes priority. The client will also probably be told to avoid high-sodium foods, but that is not the highest priority. There is no need to tell the client to drink milk.

34. (1) The symptoms suggest hypokalemia. The client is at risk for hypokalemia because he is taking furosemide, a potassium-depleting diuretic. A urinalysis is used for many things, including picking up urinary tract infections. There is no indication of that in this client. Serum creatinine is the blood test for renal failure. There is no indication for that test. A five-hour glucose tolerance test is the definitive test for diagnosing diabetes. There is no indication for that in this question.

35. (2) Hypoglycemic reactions are most likely to occur at peak action times, when the insulin is taking the glucose out of the blood stream into the cells. Peak action time of NPH is 6–8 hours after the dose. That would be 1–3 P.M. Mid afternoon is the best answer. Regular insulin would be mid morning.

36. (3) Gastric juices break down insulin, which is a protein.

37. (2) The symptoms suggest hypoglycemia. The peak action of regular insulin is 2–4 hours after administration and the client took regular insulin three hours ago. The treatment for hypoglycemia is to administer sugar in some form—fruit juice, milk, cola drinks. Insulin would make her worse.

38. (4) When high doses of cortisone are taken, the body decreases its own production. If the client abruptly stopped the cortisone, she would develop Addisonian crisis. Cortisone does cause a moon face. The symptoms will not disappear until she stops the medication. Cortisone should never be abruptly discontinued.

39. (1) Angina is a frequent side effect when thyroid medication is started. Thyroid increases the metabolic rate and the heart rate. Persons with hypothyroidism are also likely to have atherosclerosis. When the heart rate increases, angina may result. Clients starting on thyroid medication should be instructed to call the physician if they develop chest pain or dysrhythmias.

40. (2) Breast tenderness and nausea are common side effects of the progesterone in birth control pills. These effects usually decrease after three to six cycles. Taking the pill at night reduces the nausea. If the client is sleeping, she is not aware of it. The pill must be taken to be effective. Skipping doses renders the regimen ineffective.

41. (3) Ergotrate is an oxytocic and is given to cause uterine contractions or cramping and prevent postpartum bleeding.

42. (2) Aluminum hydroxide gel binds phosphates when given to a client in renal failure. It can also help prevent the development of Curling's (stress) ulcers and is used as an antacid. Constipation is a side effect. It can be used as an antacid.

43. (2) Colchicine is given for acute gout. Allopurinol is given to prevent recurring attacks of gout. Morphine and acetaminophen are not indicated.

44. (1) Homatropine and Cyclogel are mydriatic drugs; that is, they dilate the pupil. Cyclogel paralyzes the ciliary muscles so that the pupil cannot constrict.

45. (2) Eye drops should be placed into the conjunctival sac.

46. (1) For infants and small children, the ear should be pulled down and back to straighten the ear canal. For older children and adults, the ear should be pulled up and back.

47. (4) The client should drink plenty of fluids and empty her bladder frequently to prevent hemorrhagic cystitis. Mouth care with an astringent mouth wash and dental floss are contraindicated because of mouth sores and the risk of bleeding with cancer chemotherapeutic agents. Organ meats and dried peas and beans are high in folic acid. The drug antagonizes folic acid. Daily vital signs are not often enough.

48. (2) Bone depression causes a decrease of white cells, red cells, and platelets. Petechiae (small, pinpoint bruises) are indications of bleeding and a decrease in platelets.

49. (3) A person who has stepped on a rusty nail is at risk for tetanus infection. He has received no immunizations. He needs immune serum globulin to give him an immediate, passive immunity. Later, he will receive tetanus toxoid to help him develop antibodies for future needs. Penicillin will not prevent tetanus.

50. (1) Immune serum globulin will give her a passive immunity and help keep her from developing rubella, which can have devastating effects on the unborn child. MMR is a live virus and is not given to pregnant women. RhoGam prevents anti Rh antibody development. There is no such thing as rubella antitoxin.

Chapter 19

Nutrition and Special Diets

CARBOHYDRATES, PROTEINS, AND FATS

CARBOHYDRATES (CHO)

A. Characteristics:
  1. Composed of carbon, hydrogen, and oxygen
  2. Sugars, starches, and cellulose
B. Functions:
  1. Energy: 4 calories/gram
     a. Glucose is a quick source of energy.
     b. Glucose is the only energy source for the central nervous system.
     c. Glucose exerts protein sparing and fat-sparing action.
  2. Regulatory function:
     a. Cellulose provides bulk, preventing constipation.
     b. Lactose ferments to lactic acid and encourages the growth of normal bacterial flora and discourages undesirable flora.
  3. Carry essential nutrients:
     a. Most carbohydrates contain other nutrients.
     b. Concentrated sweets (sugar, syrup) do not carry nutrients and should be limited in diet.
C. Sources:
  1. Milk group supplies lactose.
  2. Legumes and nuts supply cellulose and starch.
  3. Vegetables and fruits:
     a. Root and seed vegetables such as beets, turnips, squash, and peas contain starch.
     b. Raw, leafy vegetables (lettuce, spinach) and fruits contain cellulose.
     c. Some vegetables and most fruits contain sugars.
D. Nutritional problems related to CHO:
  1. Excessive CHO consumption
     a. Provides empty calories and reduces appetite for other foods
     b. Increases dental caries
     c. Causes increase in blood cholesterol and triglycerides
  2. Diabetes mellitus: lack of adequate amounts of insulin, which transports glucose across cell membranes
  3. Galactosemia:
     a. Lack of liver enzyme that converts galactose to glucose
     b. Milk must be restricted if mental retardation is to be prevented.

4. Lactase deficiency:
   a. Lack of lactase (the enzyme that breaks down lactose [milk sugar])
   b. Manifested by gas, cramps, and diarrhea after ingesting sweet milk
   c. Higher incidence in nonwhites; occurs in all races
   d. Treated by giving lactase in tablet form or drops to put in milk or using lactose-free milk
   e. Milk in fermented form (yogurt, cheese) is usually tolerated.
   f. Encourage client to get calcium from other sources if milk is not included in his/her diet.

PROTEINS

A. Characteristics:
   1. Made up of chains of amino acids; there are 20 different amino acids
   2. Intact proteins do not diffuse through capillary or cell membranes and play a role in fluid balance.
   3. When protein is dissolved in water, it forms a colloidal solution which attracts water; it acts like a sponge to pull up water, helping to regulate fluid balance.
   4. The eight essential amino acids cannot be made by the body and must be supplied in the diet.
   5. Nonessential amino acids are supplied by diet and can be made by the body.
   6. Complete protein foods supply all of the essential amino acids and come from animal sources (meat, milk, fish, and eggs), plus wheat germ and dried yeast.
   7. Incomplete protein foods supply some but not all of the essential amino acids and come from plants.
B. Functions:
   1. Provides structural components of all cells and regulatory compounds, including hormones and enzymes
   2. Regulates water balance
   3. Regulates acid-base balance
   4. Provides resistance to disease (antibodies)
   5. Can be used for energy as a last resort
C. Recommended daily amounts:
   1. Infant: 2.2 gm/Kg body weight
   2. Adult: 0.8 gm/Kg body weight
D. Protein deficiency:
   1. Persons at greatest risk include the chronically ill, elderly on fixed incomes, low-income groups, and strict vegetarians.
   2. Manifestations:
      a. Generalized weakness
      b. Weight loss
      c. Lowered resistance to infection
      d. Slow wound healing; prolonged recovery from illness

   e. Growth failure
   f. Brain damage to fetus or infant
   g. Edema due to decreased albumin in blood
   h. Anemia in severe deficiency
   i. Fatty infiltration of liver and liver damage
E. Indications for high-protein diet:
   1. Burns, massive wounds when tissue building is desired
   2. Mild to moderate liver disease
   3. Malabsorption syndromes
   4. Undernutrition
   5. Pregnancy to meet needs of mother and developing fetus
   6. Preeclampsia to replace protein lost in the urine
   7. Nephrosis to replace protein lost in the urine
F. Sources of protein:
   1. Animal sources: meats, fowl (chicken, turkey, duck), milk and cheese, egg whites
   2. Plant sources: legumes (soybeans, lentils, peanuts, and peanut butter)
G. Indications for low-protein diets:
   1. Liver failure (liver does not metabolize protein, causing nitrogen toxicity to brain)
   2. Kidney failure (kidneys can no longer excrete protein, and toxic nitrogen levels build in the brain)
H. Low-protein diets:
   1. Increase CHO so energy needs will be met by CHO, not protein breakdown.
   2. Small protein intake that is allowed will be complete proteins (animal sources).

FATS

A. Characteristics:
   1. Made up of carbon, hydrogen, and oxygen
   2. Insoluble in water
   3. 9 Cal/gm
B. Functions:
   1. Provide energy
   2. Carriers for fat-soluble vitamins
C. Sources:
   1. Saturated fats come from animal sources: meat, milk, and eggs.
   2. Unsaturated fats come from vegetables, nuts, or seed sources: corn oil, safflower oil, sunflower oil (liquids), olive oil, and canola oil.
   3. Palm oil and coconut oil are vegetable oils that are highly saturated.
   4. Nuts and salmon contain omega 3 fatty acids, which help to lower bad cholesterol (LDL) and increase good cholesterol (HDL).
D. Indications for low-fat diet:
   1. Cardiovascular disease
   2. Gallbladder disease
   3. Malabsorption syndromes, cystic fibrosis, pancreatitis
   4. Obesity
E. Advise clients not to fry foods but to bake or broil without butter to reduce fat content.

Vitamins

Vitamins are organic food substances and are essential in small amounts for growth, maintenance, and the functioning of body processes.

A. Water-Soluble Vitamins:
1. Water-soluble vitamins are the B vitamins and vitamin C (see Table 19.1)

Table 19.1 Vitamins

Vitamin	Functions	Deficiency Symptoms	Food Sources	Comments
Water-soluble vitamins				
B₁ Thiamin	Release energy from carbohydrates; nervous system functioning	Mental depression, neuritis, heart failure, beriberi	Whole grain and enriched breads and cereals; dried peas and beans	Prolonged high alcohol intake causes symptoms; not well stored in body
B₂ Riboflavin	Helps transform CHO, fats, and protein into energy	Sensitivity to light, itching, burning eyes, sore tongue and mouth, dry cracked lips and mouth	Milk, yogurt, cheese, dark green vegetables, meat, poultry, eggs, whole grain and enriched cereals and breads	Not well stored in body
Niacin	Helps transform CHO, protein, and fat into energy	Pellagra, inflammation of the tongue, diarrhea, nerve degeneration, dermatitis	Meat, poultry, fish, whole grain and enriched cereals and breads, nuts, dried beans and peas	Used to reduce serum cholesterol levels
B₆ Pyridoxine	Aids in the use of amino acids and formation of certain proteins; aids in the use of fats	Dermatitis, nervous irritability, convulsions	Meat, poultry, fish, dried beans and peas, whole grain breads, and cereals	Given with Isoniazid (INH) to prevent side effect of peripheral neuritis, converts glycogen to glucose
Folic Acid (Folacin, Folate)	Formation of hemoglobin and genetic material		Dark-green leafy vegetables, whole grain breads and cereals, dried beans and peas, fruits, especially orange juice	
Vitamin B₁₂ Cobalamin	Promotes nervous system functioning, helps to form red blood cells, synthesis of DNA and RNA	Pernicious anemia, neuropathy	Meat, milk, fish, eggs	Intrinsic factor is necessary for absorption.
C Ascorbic Acid	Helps to make collagen; production of steroid hormones; resistance to infection; converts folic acid to folinic acid; enhances iron absorption	Scurvy, bleeding gums, easy bruising, poor wound healing	Citrus fruits, tomatoes, melons, broccoli, raw cabbage	Known as a healing vitamin, not well stored in body, easily destroyed by cooking
Fat-soluble vitamins				
Vitamin A Retinol	Formation and maintenance of healthy skin, hair and mucous membranes; improves night vision; bone growth; tooth development; reproduction	Night blindness, poor bone and tooth development	Animal sources: liver, egg yolk, cheese, whole milk, butter, fish liver oils, deep yellow/orange and dark green vegetables: carrots, broccoli, spinach, sweet potatoes, pumpkin, winter squash, cantaloupe, peaches, apricots	Large amounts can be toxic, bile necessary for absorption
D Calciferol	Formation and maintenance of bones and teeth; absorption and use of calcium and phosphorus	Rickets, bowed legs, muscle spasms, delayed eruption of teeth	Milk fortified with Vitamin D, egg yolk, tuna, salmon, cod liver oil	Known as the sunshine vitamin because it is made in the skin when it is exposed to sunlight
E Tocopherol	Antioxidant; protects Vitamin A and essential fatty acids from oxidation; prevents cell membrane damage	Breakdown of red cells	Vegetable oils and margarines; nuts; wheat germ and whole grain breads and cereals; green leafy vegetables	Has anticoagulant effect; should not take extra amounts for one week before surgery, deficiency not likely
K Mephyton	Blood clotting; bone metabolism	Prolonged clotting time	Green leafy vegetables; cabbage and cauliflower, liver	Made by bacteria in intestines; newborns can't make Vitamin K until they are receiving milk feedings

2. Characteristics:
   a. Soluble in water; insoluble in fat
   b. Dissolves in cooking water
   c. Dietary excesses excreted in urine; lessens danger of overdose
   d. Minimal storage of dietary excesses; need daily intake
3. Deficiency symptoms develop quickly.

B. Fat-Soluble Vitamins (see Table 19.1):
   1. Fat-soluble vitamins are vitamin A (Retinol), vitamin D (Calciferol), vitamin E (tocopherol), and vitamin K (mephyton) (see Table 19.1).
   2. Characteristics:
      a. Soluble in fat; insoluble in water
      b. Follow absorption and circulation pathway of fats
      c. Dietary excesses stored in body; increases risk of overdose
      d. Dietary excesses not excreted in urine
      e. Deficiency symptoms develop slowly.
      f. Do not dissolve in cooking water

Minerals

Minerals are inorganic substances and essential for metabolic processes. See Table 19.2.

Nursing Care

Assessment:
   1. Obtain objective measurements:
      a. Weight in relation to height
      b. Recent gain or loss in weight
      c. Ask client to recall foods consumed in the last three days.
   2. Determine client's understanding of purpose of diet

B. Interventions:
   1. Discuss dietary instructions and answer questions.
   2. Provide written guidelines and lists of foods.
C. Evaluation:
   1. Have client describe diet and select menu choices
   2. Assess weight and related lab values.

Nutritional Guidelines

FOOD PYRAMID

A. Foods are grouped according to composition and nutrient value (see Figure 19.1).
   1. Bread, cereal rice, pasta group: 6–11 servings, fruit group: 2–4 servings
   2. Vegetable group: 3–5 servings
3. Meat, poultry, fish, beans, eggs, and nuts group: 2–3 servings
4. Milk, yogurt, cheese group: 2–3 servings
5. Use fats, oil, and sweets sparingly.

Table 19.2 Minerals

Mineral	Functions	Deficiency Symptoms	Food Sources	Indications for Increasing Mineral	Indications for Decreasing Mineral	Notes
Calcium: 1,000–1,200 mg/day	Building bones and teeth, muscle contraction, blood clotting; may help lower blood pressure, antacid	Tetany, hyperactive reflexes, bleeding	Milk, yogurt, and cheese; sardines; canned salmon eaten with bones; dark, green leafy vegetables; dried beans and peas	Children and adolescent age groups. Pregnanct and lactating, postmenopausal women to prevent osteoporosis	Calcium-based kidney stones	Vitamin D enhances the absorption of calcium
Phosphorus: 700 mg/day	Building bones and teeth; releases energy from CHO, proteins and fats; helps form genetic material and enzymes	Fragile bones and teeth, fatigue, joint pain and stiffness	Meat, poultry, fish, eggs, dried beans and peas, milk and milk products; soft drinks are high in phosphorus	High serum calcium	Renal failure causes high serum phosphorus levels	Aluminum hydroxide antacids such as Gelusil and Amphogel deplete phosphorus and cause bones to be fragile
Sodium	Regulates body fluid volume, regulates blood acidity, transmission of nerve impulses	Nausea and vomiting, cramps, confusion, convulsions; seldom seen due to nutritional deficiency, can occur with Addison's Disease or excessive loss of body fluids	Table salt, commercially processed foods, milk, cheese, canned soups, canned vegetables, canned tomato product (paste, puree, catsup), frozen peas, carrots, celery, spinach, baked goods (biscuits, muffins, cakes, cookies) contain baking powder or soda, some cereals (corn flakes); seafoods (lobster, clams, scallops, tuna, ocean perch, halibut and crab); beef, processed meats, ham and bacon, olives, pickles, soy sauce, steak sauce, salad dressings, onion salt, celery salt, potato chips, pretzels. *Foods low in sodium:* chicken, fresh fruits and vegetables (except carrots, celery, and spinach)	Persons taking lithium carbonate should have steady intake of sodium because lithium is excreted from the body as a sodium salt. Sodium loss is increased with cystic fibrosis, requiring additional intake especially in hot weather	Cardiovascular conditions including hypertension, CHF, and MI; renal failure; cirrhosis of the liver	Diet of 1,000 mg Na or less requires specially prepared foods

(continues)

Table 19.2 Continued

Mineral	Functions	Deficiency Symptoms	Food Sources	Indications for Increasing Mineral	Indications for Decreasing Mineral	Notes
Potassium: No RDA 2,000–3,000 mg usual recommendation	Muscle contraction including heart muscle; fluid and electrolyte balance in cells; transmission of nerve impulses; release of energy from CHO, proteins and fats; may help in blood pressure control	Muscle weakness, cardiac dysrhythmias, *Hyperkalemia* can occur in renal failure; symptoms include muscle weakness and cardiac dysrhythmias	Citrus fruits (oranges, grapefruit, melons, apricots), dried peas, soy beans, lima beans, kidney beans, meat, baked potatoes, squash, milk; *Foods low in potassium:* Breads and cereals, white sugar, fats, cranberry and grape juice, potassium is soluble in water (soaking vegetables in water before cooking reduces potassium content)	Thiazide diuretics and furosemide (Lasix); Cushing's syndrome; vomiting; diarrhea; NG tube	Kidney failure; burns (first 2–3 days)	Monitor output when potassium is being administered. Client must have adequate output to prevent hyperkalemia
Magnesium: Men: 350 mg; Women 280 mg	Builds bones, makes proteins, releases energy from muscle glycogen, regulates body temperature, helps to prevent irregular heartbeat, eases PMS and menstrual cramps	Alcoholics may have deficiencies (deficiency signs similar to delirium tremens) heart dysrhythmias; irritability; muscle spasms; confusion. Excess can cause diarrhea.	Leafy green vegetables, nuts and seeds, whole grains, dried beans and peas, shellfish	Alcoholism, cardiac dysrhthmias, constipation	Overdose unlikely	Give supplements with food to prevent GI irritation
Iron: Premenopausal women: 15 mg/ day; Pregnant women: 30 mg; Older women and men: 10 mg	Makes hemoglobin, which carries oxygen to cells; makes myoglobin in muscle; part of several enzymes and proteins	Iron-deficiency anemia (toddlers, adolescents, and pregnant women are especially vulnerable)	Red meats, liver, kidney, poultry, fish, egg yolks, green leafy vegetables, dried beans and peas, whole grain products, fortified breads and cereals	Iron-deficiency anemia, blood loss, pregnancy	Persons who have hemosiderosis (accumulation of iron in the tissues) should not take iron supplements	Vitamin C enhances absorption of iron; iron food sources should be given with a vitamin C source
Zinc: Men: 15 mg; Women: 12 mg	Formation of protein, wound healing, prevention of anemia, growth of genital organs, fights colds and flu; taste and smell	Loss of taste and smell, depressed immune system	Meat, poultry, shellfish, cheese, whole grain cereals, dried beans and peas, nuts and cereals	Older men to promote healthy prostrate	None	Doses over 100 mg/day can impair immunity. Zinc necessary to maintain proper amount of Vitamin E in the blood
Iodine	Major ingredient of thyroid hormones, reproduction	Endemic goiter	Iodized salt, seafood, shrimp, lobster, crab, seaweed	Iodine deficient goiter	Before iodine uptake studies	

(continues)

Mineral	Functions	Deficiency Symptoms	Food Sources	Indications for Increasing Mineral	Indications for Decreasing Mineral	Notes
Chlorine	Part of HCl in gastric juice, helps regulate blood acidity	Not common	Chief food source is salt—sodium chloride	None	None	
Flourine	Strong, decay-resistant teeth, bone strength	Poor teeth	Flouridated water, water naturally containing flouride, small ocean fish with bones, fluoride mouthwash and toothpaste	To promote strong teeth	None	
Selenium	Works with Vitamin E to help prevent cancer and heart disease; protects against cataracts and macular degeneration; fights viral infections, promotes pancreatic function	Muscle breakdown, cancer, heart disease	Meat, whole grains, Brazil nuts, broccoli, yeasts, onions, salmon	Intake usually adequate	No side effects known	

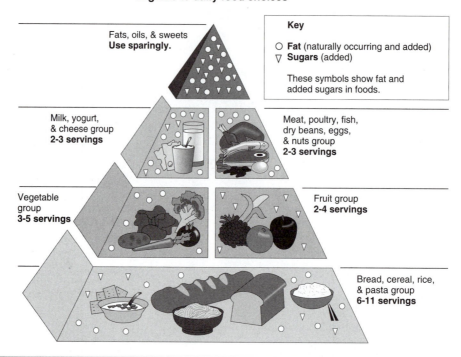

The Food Guide Pyramid
A guide to daily food choices

Fats, oils, & sweets
Use sparingly.

Key
○ **Fat** (naturally occurring and added)
▽ **Sugars** (added)

These symbols show fat and added sugars in foods.

Milk, yogurt, & cheese group
2-3 servings

Meat, poultry, fish, dry beans, eggs, & nuts group
2-3 servings

Vegetable group
3-5 servings

Fruit group
2-4 servings

Bread, cereal, rice, & pasta group
6-11 servings

Figure 19.1 Food Guide Pyramid (Courtesy of the U.S. Department of Agriculture and Health and Human Services, revised 1996)

Special Diets

CONSISTENCY MODIFICATIONS

A. Clear, liquid Diet:
  1. Purpose is to rest GI tract and maintain fluid balance
  2. Indications:
    a. Immediate post-operative period until bowel sounds have returned and nausea and vomiting ceased
    b. Diarrhea
    c. Nausea and vomiting
    d. Bowel preps before bowel X-rays or bowel surgery
  3. Foods allowed: "see-through foods"
    a. Water
    b. Tea
    c. Broth
    d. Jello
    e. Apple juice
  4. Not nutritionally adequate
B. Full, liquid Diet:
  1. Clear liquids

  2. Milk and milk products:
    a. Puddings
    b. Custards
    c. Cream soups
    d. Ice cream
    e. Sherbert
    f. All fruit juices
  3. Can be nutritionally adequate
C. Soft Diet:
  1. Full, liquid diet
  2. Pureed vegetables
  3. Eggs cooked any way except fried
  4. Tender meat
  5. Potatoes
  6. Cooked fruit
D. Bland Diet:
  1. Promotes healing of the gastric mucosa
  2. Chemically and mechanically nonstimulating
  3. Given in small, frequent feedings to assist in diluting or neutralizing stomach acid

(protein foods are good at neutralizing acid)
4. Spices such as pepper and chili are eliminated.
5. A soft diet without spices
E. Low-residue Diet:
1. Residue is the indigestible material left in digestive tract after food has been digested. It is not the same as fiber. High-fiber foods are high in residue. Other foods such as milk and milk products also leave a residue.
2. Indications:
a. Following colon, rectal, or perineal surgery to reduce pressure on the operative site
b. Prior to examination of the lower bowel to enhance visualization
c. Internal radiation for cancer of the cervix
d. Crohn's Disease or regional enteritis, ulcerative colitis to reduce irritation of the large bowel
e. Diarrhea to rest the bowel
3. Foods which should be avoided:
a. High fiber foods: fruits and vegetables
b. Milk and milk products
c. Whole grain breads and cereals
4. Foods allowed:
a. Clear liquids
b. Sugar, salt
c. Meats, eggs
d. Limited amounts of milk
e. Refined cereals
f. White breads
g. Peeled white potatoes
F. High-residue diet
1. Indications:
a. Constipation
b. Hemorrhoids
2. Foods to include are high-fiber foods
a. Fresh fruits and vegetables
b. Whole grain products

GLUTEN-FREE DIET

A. Purpose is to eliminate gluten (a protein) from the diet
B. Indicated in malabsorption syndromes such as sprue and celiac disease
C. Eliminate all barley, rye, oats, and wheat.
D. Avoid:
1. Cream sauces
2. Breaded foods
3. Cakes
4. Breads
5. Muffins
E. Allow corn, rice, and soy flour.

F. Teach client to read the labels of prepared foods.

PHENYLKETONURIA (PKU) DIET

A. Purpose is to control intake of phenylalanine, an amino acid that cannot be metabolized
B. Diet will be prescribed until age six or longer to prevent brain damage and mental retardation.
C. Avoid:
1. Breads
2. Meats
3. Fish
4. Poultry
5. Cheeses
6. Legumes
7. Nuts
8. Eggs
E. Give Lofenalac formula as ordered.
F. Teach the family to use low-protein flour for baking.
G. Sugar substitutes such as Nutrasweet contain phenylalanine and must not be used.

LOW-PURINE DIET

A. Indicated for gout, uric acid kidney stones, and uric acid retention
B. Purpose is to decrease the amount of purine, a precursor to uric acid
C. Foods containing purines should be avoided.
1. Organ meats
2. Other meats
3. Fowl
4. Fish and lobster
5. Lentils, dried peas and beans
6. Nuts
7. Oatmeal
8. Whole wheat

DIETS TO ALTER ACIDITY OF BLOOD

A. Acid Ash Diet:
1. Used to prevent alkaline kidney stones
2. Avoid most fruits and vegetables and milk.
3. Cranberries, plums, and prunes leave an acid ash and are encouraged.
4. Meats and breads are allowed.
B. Alkaline Ash Diet:
1. Used to prevent acid kidney stones
2. Avoid proteins, cereals, meats, fish, eggs, bread, cranberries, prunes, and plums.
3. Cranberries, prunes, and plums are not allowed.

DIETS FOR TREATMENT OF DIABETES

A. Exchange list (see Table 19.3)
  1. Purpose:
    a. Attain or maintain ideal body weight while ensuring normal growth.
    b. Maintain plasma glucose levels as close to normal as possible.
  2. Distribution of Calories:
    a. Protein 12–20%
    b. Carbohydrates 55–60%
    c. Fats 20–30%; fats should be unsaturated
  3. Daily distribution of calories:
    a. Breakfast   1/4
    b. Lunch   1/4
    c. Supper   1/4
    d. Snacks   1/4 divided among morning, afternoon, and evening snacks with the evening snack being the biggest
  4. Use foods high in fiber and complex carbohydrates.
  5. Avoid simple sugars, jams, honey, syrup, and frosting.
B. Glycemic index:
  1. Glycemic index refers to how fast and how much the food raises the blood sugar level.
  2. Persons with diabetes should eat foods with moderate- to low-glycemic index and have minimal amounts of high-glycemic index foods (see Table 19.4).

Table 19.3 Exchange Groups for Diabetic Diet

Milk	Vegetable	Fruit	Bread	Meat	Fat
Equivalent to 1 cup skim milk; most milk products also contain fat: whole milk is 1 milk and 2 fat exchanges	Equivalent to 1/2 cup of non-starchy, low-calorie vegetables: broccoli, carrots, string beans, tomatoes; lettuce and radishes can be eaten as desired	Contains more sugar and more calories than vegetable exchanges. Amount of fruit in an exchange varies with the sugar content of each fruit; 1 small apple, 1/2 cup orange juice, 1/3 cup pineapple juice, 1/4 cup raisins.	Contains about 70 calories. 1 slice bread, 1/2 hamburger roll, 1 tortilla, 1/2 cup bran flakes, 1/2 cup cooked cereal. Starchy vegetables: corn, potato, sweet potato, peas, lentils, dried peas and beans. Pasta such as macaroni and spaghetti. Biscuits, muffins, and pancakes are breads but also contain fat.	1 oz lean meat. Meat that is not lean also contains fat exchanges. An egg is 1 meat and 1 fat. 2 tablespoons of peanut butter equals 1 meat and 2 fat exchanges. 1/4 cup regular cottage cheese equals 1 meat and 1/2 fat exchange.	1 tablespoon butter or margarine is 1 exchange. Salad dressing, nuts, 1 slice bacon

Table 19.4 Glycemic Index

High	Moderate-High	Moderate-Low	Low
White bread	Pita bread	Apples	Broccoli
Bagels	Oat bran bread	Garbanzo beans	Plums
White rice	Brown rice	Navy beans	Leafy vegetables
Corn flakes	All-Bran	Pinto beans	Cherries
Pretzels	Oat bran	Potato chips	Squash
Cheerios	Rolled oats	Oranges	Peaches
Puffed rice/wheat	Carrots	Raisins	Tomatoes
Graham crackers	Parsnips	Dried fruits	Peanuts
Pasta (white)	Banana	Grapes	Yogurt
Grape Nuts	Kidney beans	Peas	Ice cream
Glucose	Potato	Mars bars	
	Honey	Sucrose	

Sample Questions

1. The nurse knows that the client understands a low-sodium diet when the client selects which of the following menus?
   1. Lobster salad, corn bread, and milk
   2. Hot roast beef sandwich, celery sticks, and coffee
   3. Sliced chicken, fresh tomatoes, and beets
   4. Liver and onions, creamed carrots, and a biscuit

2. An adult has chronic renal failure and asks why sodium must be limited. What is the best answer for the nurse to make?
   1. "Sodium causes high blood pressure, which is not good for your kidneys."
   2. "Kidneys normally help the body eliminate sodium. Your kidneys are not doing that now."
   3. "Sodium tends to increase the workload of the kidneys. Your kidneys need rest."
   4. "Sodium causes hypotension, which is dangerous when your kidneys don't work."

3. A low-sodium, low-fat diet has been prescribed for a client who recently had a myocardial infarction. Which of the following menu selections would be most appropriate for this client?
   1. Hot dog and roll, tossed salad with blue cheese dressing, and chocolate chip cookies
   2. Roast beef with gravy, baked potato, and sliced carrots
   3. Cream of mushroom soup, tuna sandwich, and sliced tomatoes
   4. Baked chicken, green beans, and mashed potatoes

4. Digoxin and furosemide (Lasix) have been prescribed for a client who is in congestive heart failure. Which snack would be best for the client?
   1. Crackers
   2. Honeydew melon
   3. Apple
   4. Carrots

5. Which foods should be omitted from the diet of a client who has gout?
   1. Eggs and cheese
   2. Lobster and liver
   3. Bread and peanut butter
   4. Apricots and melons

6. A client who is on a special diet for the treatment of gout asks the nurse why a special diet is prescribed. What is the best answer for the nurse to give?
   1. "When purines are used by the body, they break down into uric acid that deposits in your joints and causes pain."
   2. "Proteins make your lungs work harder and cause you pain."
   3. "Your heart cannot handle extra fluids."
   4. "Fats cause oxalates to deposit in your toes and legs, decreasing circulation."

7. A 10-year-old has a lactose intolerance. The child's mother asks the nurse for assistance in meeting calcium needs. What is the best nursing response?
   1. "Serve broccoli and other dark green vegetables frequently."
   2. "Give her ice cream."
   3. "Have Susan drink skim milk."
   4. "Serve carrots and other yellow vegetables frequently."

8. The wife of a man who has coronary artery disease asks the nurse how she can prepare foods that will be good for her husband. What should the nurse include when talking with this woman?
   1. Encourage her to use cream sauces to enhance the flavor of foods.
   2. Tell her to shop exclusively at health food stores.
   3. Suggest she substitute salmon or other fish for meat several times a week.
   4. Encourage her to use onion salt and celery salt to foods.

9. A client who has hypertension makes all of the following statements. Which statement indicates a need for more teaching?
   1. "I eat fresh fruit every day."
   2. "I just love dill pickles with my sandwich at lunch."
   3. "I prefer broiled meats to fried food."
   4. "I enjoy one cup of decaffeinated coffee at lunch."

10. An adult who has hypertension is taking furosemide (Lasix). The client has been placed on a low-sodium, high-potassium diet. What is the reason for the potassium alteration?
    1. To prevent sodium loss from the renal tubules
    2. To replace potassium lost from the kidneys
    3. To prevent osteoporosis secondary to diuresis
    4. To maintain an acid-base balance

11. Ferrous sulfate has been prescribed for a woman who is pregnant. The nurse should advise her to take the medication at which time?
    1. Upon arising
    2. With meals
    3. Immediately following meals
    4. At bedtime

12. A pregnant woman asks why iron has been prescribed for her. How should the nurse reply?
    1. "Iron helps to prevent sickle cell anemia in your baby."
    2. "Iron will help your baby to develop more intelligence."
    3. "Your body needs a lot of iron to make red blood cells for you and your baby."
    4. "Your morning sickness will be less if you have plenty of iron."

13. A pregnant woman asks the nurse for help in planning her diet to include iron sources. Which suggestion would be best?
    1. Be sure to eat at least one egg white a day.
    2. Drink orange juice with your morning egg.
    3. Drink milk with every meal.
    4. A peanut butter sandwich is a good snack.

14. A young mother is concerned about providing an adequate diet for her children and asks the nurse how to be sure they get enough B vitamins. Which response is best?
    1. Provide a glass of milk with every meal.
    2. Offer whole grains and cereals.
    3. Give citrus fruits as snacks.
    4. Offer carrots and melons.

15. An adult says to the nurse, "The doctor told me that I should have plenty of the healing vitamin to help my operation heal." What foods would best meet this prescription?
    1. Apple juice
    2. Strawberries
    3. Hamburger
    4. Peanut butter

16. An adult is on a low-sodium, low-fat diet for hypertension. What question is most important for the nurse to ask when starting to teach the client?
    1. "How do you prepare your foods?"
    2. "When do you eat your meals?"
    3. "Who eats with you?"
    4. "When do you sleep?"

17. Which of these meals would the nurse recommend to provide the highest amount of protein and calories?
    1. Vegetable soup, cottage cheese on crackers, applesauce, and a hot chocolate
    2. Cheeseburger, French-fried potatoes, carrot sticks, cantaloupe balls, and milk
    3. Fresh fruit plate with sherbert, buttered muffin, slice of watermelon, and a fruit-flavored milk drink
    4. Chicken noodle soup, cream cheese and jelly sandwich, buttered whole kernel corn, orange sherbert, and a cola drink

18. Mothers should be instructed that diets for infants and toddlers who drink a lot of milk and few other foods will most likely result in the development of a deficiency in which of these nutrients?
    1. Iron
    2. Carbohydrate
    3. Vitamin D
    4. Vitamin K

19. Following surgery, a clear liquid diet is ordered. Which of these foods would be contraindicated for this person?
    1. Tea with lemon
    2. Ginger ale
    3. Milk
    4. Gelatin desert

20. A 4-year-old child has phenylketonuria and must follow a special diet. Which food is allowed on this diet?
    1. Bread and butter
    2. Strawberries
    3. Peanut butter sandwich
    4. Hamburger

21. A low-residue diet is ordered for a man who has ulcerative colitis. The nurse knows that he understands his diet when he selects which foods?
    1. Spinach salad and roast beef
    2. Mashed potato and chicken
    3. Green beans and pork chop
    4. Lettuce salad and spaghetti

22. The nurse is to teach a client about a low-purine diet. What should the nurse do initially?
    1. Provide a list of foods to be avoided.
    2. Ask the client what he has eaten for the last three days.
    3. Obtain baseline weight and height measurements.
    4. Explain why he must follow this diet.

23. A woman who is in the seventh month of pregnancy has symptoms of preeclampsia. When discussing diet, the nurse instructs the client to eat a high-protein diet and to avoid foods that have a high sodium content. Which of these foods, if selected by the client, would be correct?
    1. Creamed chipped beef on dry toast
    2. Cheese sandwich on whole-wheat toast
    3. Frankfurter on a roll
    4. Tomato stuffed with diced chicken

24. An adolescent has been recently diagnosed as having type I insulin-dependent diabetes. She asks the nurse if she will ever be able to go out with her friends for pizza or ice cream. Which of these responses by the nurse would give accurate information?
    1. "You can go with the group, but you cannot eat pizza or ice cream."
    2. "You can have pizza but not ice cream."
    3. "If you eat when out with your friends, you will have to skip the next meal."
    4. "It is important for you to be with your friends. We will help you learn how to choose foods."

25. A pregnant woman tells the nurse she is constipated. What suggestion is best for the nurse to give the woman?
    1. Reduce your fluid intake.
    2. Reduce your intake of fruits.
    3. Increase your intake of raw vegetables.
    4. Increase your intake of rice.

Answers and Rationales

1. The correct answer is 3. Chicken is lower in sodium than seafood and beef. Fresh tomatoes are low in sodium. Canned tomato products are

not. Beets are not high in sodium. Seafood is high in sodium. Foods containing baking soda, such as corn bread and biscuits, are high in sodium. Milk and milk products are high in sodium. Creamed foods are high in sodium. Celery sticks and carrots are naturally high in sodium.

2. The correct answer is 2. This best explains the reason for reducing sodium in the diet of someone who has chronic renal failure. There is some truth to answer 1. Sodium is probably related to hypertension in some individuals, and hypertension is not good for the kidneys. However, answer 2 is better. Answer 3 is not correct. Answer 4 is not correct. Sodium causes hypertension, not hypotension.

3. The correct answer is 4. Chicken is lower in sodium and fat than beef and other meats. Green beans and mashed potatoes are low in sodium. Hot dogs are high in sodium and fat. Blue cheese dressing is high in sodium and fat. Chocolate chip cookies are high in sodium and fat. Roast beef and gravy are both high in sodium and fat. Carrots are naturally high in sodium. Creamed products are high in sodium and fat. Soups have about 1,000 mg of sodium per serving. Tuna is high in sodium. Bread contains about 200 mg of sodium per slice.

4. The correct answer is 2. Furosemide is a potassium-depleting diuretic. Melons are high in potassium. Crackers have very little potassium. An apple is not high in potassium. Carrots are high in sodium.

5. The correct answer is 2. Lobster and liver are high in purines. The other foods are not particularly high in purines.

6. The correct answer is 1. The prescribed diet for gout is a low-purine diet. Purines break down into uric acid. Persons who have gout do not excrete the uric acid normally, and it deposits in joints and causes severe pain. Answer 2 makes no sense. Extra fluid volume is not the problem in gout. Gout is faulty purine metabolism, not faulty oxalate metabolism.

7. The correct answer is 1. Broccoli and other dark green vegetables are high in calcium. The person who has lactose intolerance usually cannot eat ice cream or skim milk, both of which contain lactose (milk sugar). Carrots and yellow vegetables are high in vitamin A but are not high in calcium.

8. The correct answer is 3. Salmon and fish contain omega 3 fatty acids, which are "heart healthy" and help to increase HDL and lower LDL. Meat is high in omega 6 fatty acids, which raise the bad cholesterol (LDL). Cream sauces are high in fat and should be avoided if a person has coronary artery disease. There is no need to shop exclusively at health food stores. Onion salt and celery salt contain salt and are usually limited for a person who has coronary artery disease.

9. The correct answer is 2. The person who has hypertension should have a diet low in sodium and fat and avoid caffeine. Dill pickles are extremely high in sodium. Each slice of bread has about 200 mg of sodium. Sandwiches should be avoided on a low-sodium diet. Fresh fruit is low in sodium. Meats, when eaten, should be broiled, not fried. Decaffeinated coffee is recommended for persons who have hypertension.

10. The correct answer is 2. Furosemide (Lasix) is a potassium-depleting diuretic. Persons taking furosemide should increase their intake of potassium to replace the potassium lost in the urine. A high-potassium diet does not prevent sodium loss from the renal tubules. Sodium loss from the renal tubules is the mechanism by which furosemide works. Potassium in the diet does not prevent osteoporosis secondary to diuresis. Dietary potassium is not increased to maintain acid-base balance.

11. The correct answer is 2. Taking ferrous sulfate (iron) with meals helps to reduce nausea associated with the medicine. Absorption is best on an empty stomach. However, many people experience nausea when taking iron.

12. The correct answer is 3. The mother has to supply the iron needed for her increase in blood volume during pregnancy, for the baby's blood, and a six-month supply of iron for the newborn. Iron does not prevent sickle cell anemia. Iron does not increase intelligence. Iron does not reduce morning sickness. In fact, iron can cause nausea if it is taken on an empty stomach.

13. The correct answer is 2. Egg yolk contains iron. Iron is best absorbed when taken with a vitamin C source, such as orange juice. Egg white contains no iron. Milk contains no iron. A peanut butter sandwich is not a good source of iron.

14. The correct answer is 2. The best sources of B vitamins are whole grains and cereals. Milk contains good amounts of calcium. Citrus fruits are good sources of vitamin C and potassium. Carrots and melons are good sources of vitamin A.

15. The correct answer is 2. Strawberries are high in vitamin C. The other choices are not high in vitamin C. Vitamin C is called "the healing vitamin."

16. The correct answer is 1. A high-fat, low-sodium diet involves low salt and baking or broiling, not frying. The other questions are not particularly relevant to a low-sodium, low-fat diet.

17. The correct answer is 2. Protein is in the cheeseburger and the milk. The calorie load is high. The other choices have less protein and fewer calories.

18. The correct answer is 1. Milk contains no iron.

19. The correct answer is 3. Milk is not a clear liquid. All of the other choices are clear liquids.
20. The correct answer is 2. The PKU diet eliminates phenylalanine. Phenylalanine is a protein. The person should avoid all meats and protein foods. Bread contains small amounts of protein and should be avoided on a PKU diet.
21. The correct answer is 2. Mashed potatoes and chicken are low in residue. Residue sources have skins, seeds, and leaves. Spinach, green beans, and lettuce are all high in residue.
22. The correct answer is 2. Nutrition teaching should start with a diet history.
23. The correct answer is 4. Chicken contains protein and is relatively low in sodium. Fresh tomatoes are low in sodium. Creamed chipped beef on toast, a cheese sandwich, and a hot dog all contain protein but are also very high in sodium.
24. The correct answer is 4. This answer recognizes the adolescent's need to be with her friends and explains that she will learn how to choose foods. The answers do not give accurate information.
25. The correct answer is 3. Constipation is best prevented by increasing fiber intake. Fresh vegetables and fruits are good sources of fiber. Fluid intake should be increased, not reduced. Rice tends to cause constipation.

Appendices

Appendix A

Symbols and Abbreviations

Symbol	Meaning
~	similar
≅	approximately
@	at
√	check
Δ	change
↑	increased
↓	decreased
=	equals
#	pounds
>	greater than
<	less than
%	percent
+	positive
−	negative
♀	female
♂	male
△₁ △₂ △₃	trimester of pregnancy (one triangle for each trimester)

Abbreviation	Meaning
a.c.	before meals
ad lib	freely, as desired
b.i.d.	two times a day
c̄	with
cap	capsule
DC	discontinue
elix	elixir
h	hour
hrly	hourly
h.s.	at bedtime
ID	intradermal
IM	intramuscular
IV	intravenous
IVPB	intravenous piggyback

Abbreviation	Meaning
OD	right eye
od	every day
OS	left eye
OU	each eye
p.c.	after meals
po	by mouth
per	by
PRN	as needed
q	every
qd	every day
q2h	every 2 hours
q.i.d.	four times a day
qod	every other day
qs	sufficient quantity
SC	subcutaneous
Stat	immediately
supp	suppository
susp	suspension
tab	tablet
t.i.d.	three times a day
Tr or tinct	tincture

Metric System Equivalents

Liquid Measure (Volume)

Metric		Apothecary		Household
5 ml	=	1 fluid dram	=	1 teaspoonful
10 ml	=	2 fluid drams	=	1 dessertspoonful
15 ml	=	4 fluid drams	=	1 tablespoonful
30 ml	=	1 fluid ounce	=	1 ounce
60 ml	=	2 fluid ounces	=	1 wineglassful
120 ml	=	4 fluid ounces	=	1 teacupful
240 ml	=	8 fluid ounces	=	1 tumblerful
500 ml	=	1 pint	=	1 pint
1000 ml	=	1 quart	=	1 quart
4000 ml	=	1 gallon	=	1 gallon

Weight

Metric		Apothecary
1 mg	=	1/60 grain
4 mg	=	1/15 grain
10 mg	=	1/6 grain
15 mg	=	1/4 grain
30 mg	=	1/2 grain
60 mg	=	1 grain
1 g	=	15 grains
4 g	=	1 dram
30 g	=	1 ounce
500 g	=	1.1 pound
1000 g (1 kg)	=	2.2 pounds

Appendix C

Temperature Conversions

Fahrenheit to Celsius
C = (F − 32) × 5/9

97	36.1
98	36.6
98.6	37.0
99	37.2
100	37.7
101	38.3
102	38.8
103	39.4
104	40.0
105	40.5
106	41.1

Appendix D

Medical Prefixes and Suffixes

a-, an-	negative, without	cerebro-	brain
ab-	away from	cervico-	neck
acou-	hear	cheilo-	lips
ad-	to, toward	cholecyst-	gallbladder
adeno-	gland	chondro-	cartilage
alb-	white	chrom-	color
-algia	pain	cili-	eyelid
alve-	channel, cavity	circum-	around
ambi-	both	-cis-	incision
amphi-	both	-clasia	breaking
amyl-	starch	colo-	large intestine
andr-	man	colp-	hollow, vagina
angio-	vessel	corpora-	body
ankyl-	crooked, growing together	cortico-	bark, rind (outside covering)
ante-, anti-	before	costo-	rib
antr-	chamber	cranio-	skull
apo-	detached	cry-	cold
arachn-	spider	crypt-	hide, conceal
arthro-	joint	cune-	wedge
articul-	joint	cut-	skin
auri-	ear	cyan-	blue
		cyc-	circle
bi-	two	cysto-, vesico-	bladder
blasto-	bud, embryonic form	cyto-	cell
brachi-	arm		
brachy-	short	dactyl-	finger, toe
brady-	slow	de-	down from
broncho-	windpipe	dec-	ten
bucca-	cheek	dent-	tooth
		derm-	skin
capit-	head	dextr-	right-handed
carcin-	cancer	di-	two
cardi-, cordi-	heart	diplo-	double
cata-	down, negative	dis-	apart
caud-	tail	-docho-	common bile duct
cav-	hollow	dors-	back
cent-	hundred	-duct	lead, conduct
-centesis	puncture	duodeno-	duodenum
cephalo-	head	dys-	bad, painful

e-	apart, away from	kerato-	horny
ect-	outside	kil-	one thousand
-ectasis	dilation	kine-	move
-ectomy	excision		
ede-	swell	labi-	lip
-emia	blood	lact-	milk
endo-	inside	lapar-	flank
entero-	small intestine	laryngo-	throat
epi-	upon, after	later-	side
eso-	inside	-lep-	take, seize
estho-	perceive, feel	leuko-	white
en-	normal	lipo-	fat
eu-	normal	lithio-	stone or calculus
exo-	outside	lumb-	loin
		lute-	yellow
fasci-	band	-lysis	break down
fauci-	throat		
febr-	fever	macro-	long, large
ferr-	iron	mal-	abnormal
for-	door, opening	-malac-	soft
-form	shape	masto-	breast
fract-	break	mammo-	breast
		medi-	middle
galact-	milk	mega-	great, large
ganglio-	swelling, plexus	melan-	black
gastro-	stomach	men-	month
gingive-	gums	mening-	membrane
gloss-	tongue	ment-	mind
glott-	tongue, language	meso-	middle
glyc-	sweet	meta-	beyond, after
gno-	know, discern	metro-	uterus
gyn-	woman	micro-	small
gyr-	ring, circle	mill-	one thousand
		morph-	shape, form
hemi-	half	muco-	mucus
hemo-	blood	-myces	fungus
hemato-	blood	myco-	fungal
hepato-	liver	myelo-	bone marrow
histo-	tissue	myo-	muscle
hom-	same	myx-	mucus
hyper-	above, elevated	naso-	nose
hypo-	under, below	nephro-	kidney
hystero-	uterus	neuro-	nerve
		nod-	knot
-iasis	condition	nos-	disease
itro-	physician		
idio-	peculiar	ocul-	eye
ileo-	ileum	-odynia	pain
infra-	beneath	oligo-	few, little
inter-	between	-ology	study of
intra-	inside	-oma	tumor, swelling
is-	equal	onphal-	navel
-itis	inflammation	onych-	nail
		oophoro-	ovary
jejuno-	jejunum	ovari-	ovary
		optic, opth-	eye

orchi-	testicle	scop-	look at, observe
orth-	straight	-sect	cut
-osis	condition, state resulting	semi-	half
oss-, ost-	bone	sens-	perceive, feel
osteo-	bone	sep-	decay
-ostomy	new, opening	septo-	infection
-otomy	incision	sial-	saliva
oto-	ear	somat-	body
ov-	egg	-some	body
pancreato-	pancreas	spher-	ball
para-	beside	spirat-	breathe
-pathy	sickness, disease	spondyl-	vertebra
-pepsia	digestion	stear-	fat
ped-	child	sten-	narrow
pend-	hang down	-sthen-	strength
pept-	digest	stomato-	mouth
peri-	around, surrounding	splanchc-	entrails, viscera
pha-	say, speak	sub-	under
phag-	eat, swallow	super-, supra	above, extreme
pharyngo-	throat	syn-	together
phil-	affinity for		
phlebo-	vein	tact-	touch
phob-	fear, dread	tax-	arrange, order
phot-	light	tens-	stretch
-plasty	shape, repair	tetra-	four
pleuro-	membrane encasing lungs	thel-	nipple
pne-	breathing	thermo-	heat
pneumo-	lungs	thoraco-	chest
-pole-	made, produce	thromb-	clot, lump
poly-	much, many	-toc-	childbirth
procto-	anus and rectum	-tomy	cutting
pseudo-	false	tors-	twist
psych-	mind	tracheo-	windpipe
pto-	fall	tri-	three
-ptosis	prolapse	tricho-	hair
pulmo-	lungs	trop-	turn toward
pyelo-	kidney, pelvis	-trophy	nurture, nutrition
pyo-	pus	typ-	type
quadr-	four	un-	one
		uria-	urine
		uro-	urine
recto-	rectum	utero-	uterus
ren-	kidney		
retro-	backwards	vas-	vessel
rhino-	nose	vene-	vein
-rrhagia	break, burst	vesic-	bladder
-rrhaphy	suture, sew	vit-	life
-rrhea	flowing		
-rrhexia	break, rupture	xanth-	yellow, blond
salpingo-	fallopian tube	zo-	life
sanguin-	blood	zyg-	yoke, union
schis-	split	zym-	ferment
sclero-	hardening		

NANDA Nursing Diagnoses 2001–2002

Activity intolerance
Activity intolerance, Risk for
Adjustment, Impaired
Airway clearance, Ineffective
Allergy response, Risk for latex
Anxiety
Anxiety, Death
Aspiration, Risk for
Body image, Disturbed
Body temperature, Risk for imbalanced
Bowel incontinence
Breastfeeding, Effective
Breastfeeding, Ineffective
Breastfeeding, Interrupted
Breathing pattern, Ineffective
Cardiac output, Decreased
Caregiver role strain
Caregiver role strain, Risk for
Communication, Impaired verbal
Confusion, Acute
Confusion, Chronic
Constipation
Constipation, Perceived
Constipation, Risk for
Coping, Community, Ineffective
Coping, Community, Readiness for enhanced
Coping, Defensive
Coping, Family, Compromised
Coping, Family, Disabled
Coping, Family, Readiness for enhanced
Coping, Ineffective
Conflict, Decisional (specify)
Conflict, Parental role
Denial, Ineffective
Dentition, Impaired
Development, Risk for delayed
Diarrhea
Disuse syndrome, Risk for

Diversional activity, Deficient
Dysreflexia, Autonomic
Energy field, Disturbed
Environmental interpretation syndrome, Impaired
Failure to thrive, Adult
Falls, Risk for
Family processes, Dysfunctional: Alcoholism
Family processes, Interrupted
Fatigue
Fear
Fluid volume, Deficient
Fluid volume, Excess
Fluid volume, Risk for deficient
Fluid volume, Risk for imbalanced
Gas exchange, Impaired
Grieving, Anticipatory
Grieving, Dysfunctional
Growth and development, Delayed
Growth, Risk for disproportionate
Health Maintenance, Ineffective
Health-seeking behaviors (specify)
Home maintenance, Impaired
Hopelessness
Hyperthermia
Hypothermia
Identity, Disturbed personal
Incontinence, Functional urinary
Incontinence, Reflex urinary
Incontinence, Stress urinary
Incontinence, Total urinary
Incontinence, Urge urinary
Incontinence, Urge urinary, Risk for
Infant behavior, Disorganized
Infant behavior, Readiness for enhanced organized
Infant behavior, Risk for disorganized
Infant feeding pattern, Ineffective
Infection, Risk for
Injury, Perioperative positioning, Risk for

Injury, Risk for
Intracranial adaptive capacity, Decreased
Knowledge, Deficient
Loneliness, Risk for
Memory, Impaired
Mobility, Impaired bed
Mobility, Impaired physical
Mobility, Impaired wheelchair
Nausea
Noncompliance (specify)
Nutrition, Imbalanced: Less than body
    requirements
Nutrition, Imbalanced: More than body
    requirements
Nutrition, Imbalanced: More than body
    requirements, Risk for
Oral mucous membrane, Impaired
Pain, Acute
Pain, Chronic
Parent/infant/child attachment, Risk for impaired
Parenting, Impaired
Parenting, Impaired, Risk for
Peripheral neurovascular dysfunction, Risk for
Poisoning, Risk for
Post-trauma Syndrome
Post-trauma Syndrome, Risk for
Powerlessness
Powerlessness, Risk for
Protection, Ineffective
Rape-trauma Syndrome
Rape-trauma Syndrome, Compound reaction
Rape-trauma Syndrome, Silent reaction
Relocation stress Syndrome
Relocation stress Syndrome, Risk for
Role performance, Ineffective
Self-care deficit, Bathing/hygiene
Self-care deficit, Dressing/grooming
Self-care deficit, Feeding
Self-care deficit, Toileting
Self-esteem, Low, Chronic
Self-esteem, Low, Situational
Self-esteem, Low, Situational, Risk for
Self-mutilation

Self-mutilation, Risk for
Sensory perception, Disturbed (specify)
    (Visual, auditory, kinesthetic, gustatory, tactile,
    olfactory)
Sexual dysfunction
Sexuality patterns, Ineffective
Skin integrity, Impaired
Skin integrity, Impaired, Risk for
Sleep deprivation
Sleep pattern, Disturbed
Social interaction, Impaired
Social isolation
Sorrow, Chronic
Spiritual distress
Spiritual distress, Risk for
Spiritual well-being, Readiness for enhanced
Suffocation, Risk for
Suicide, Risk for
Surgical recovery, Delayed
Swallowing, Impaired
Therapeutic regimen management, Effective
Therapeutic regimen management, Ineffective
Therapeutic regimen management, Ineffective
    community
Therapeutic regimen management, Ineffective
    family
Thermoregulation, Ineffective
Thought process, Disturbed
Tissue integrity, Impaired
Tissue perfusion, Ineffective (specify type)
    (Renal, cerebral, cardiopulmonary,
    gastrointestinal, peripheral)
Transfer ability, Impaired
Trauma, Risk for
Neglect, unilateral
Urinary elimination, Impaired
Urinary retention
Ventilation, Impaired spontaneous
Ventilatory weaning response, Dysfunctional
Violence, Risk for other-directed
Violence, Risk for self-directed
Walking, Impaired
Wandering

Source: North American Nursing Diagnosis Association. (2001). *Nursing Diagnoses: Definitions and Classifications, 2001–2002*. Philadelphia, PA: Author.

Practice Tests

Comprehensive Practice Tests

This section contains five 100-question practice tests that are similiar in structure and concept to those you will find on the NCLEX-PN® examination. At the end of each test are the correct answers and rationales for the correct answers, as well as rationales explaining the incorrect answers. Also included are the identifiers for the clinical problems solving process, or nursing process (NP), the categories of client needs (CN), and the subject area (SA) for each question.

The following codes are used for the answers and rationales as identifiers to categorize the test items:

NP	=	CLINICAL PROBLEM SOLVING PROCESS (NURSING PROCESS)	Ps	=	Psychosocial Integrity
			Ps/5	=	Coping and Adaption
Dc	=	Data collection	Ps/6	=	Psychosocial Adaption
Pl	=	Planning	Ph	=	Physiological Integrity
Im	=	Implementation	Ph/7	=	Basic Care and Comfort
Ev	=	Evaluation	Ph/8	=	Pharmacological and Parental Therapies
CN	=	CLIENT NEED			
Sa	=	Safe Effective Care Environment	Ph/9	=	Reduction of Risk Potential
Sa/1	=	Management of Care	Ph/10	=	Physiological Adaption
Sa/2	=	Safety and Infection Control	SA	=	SUBJECT AREA
He	=	Health Promotion and Maintenance	1	=	Medical/Surgical
He/3	=	Growth and Development Through the Lifespan	2	=	Psych/Mental Health
			3	=	Female Reproductive
He/4	=	Prevention and Early Detection of Disease	4	=	Pediatrics
			5	=	Pharmacology
			6	=	Nutrition

The following sample answer should help you understand how to interpret these codes. The correct answer is listed first and is in bold type.

ANSWER	RATIONALE	NP	CN	SA
#1. **4.**	**Sterile gloves must be worn during the dressing change.**	lm	Sa/2	1
1.	This is not good practice. Sterile technique must be carried out during a dressing change.			
2.	Talking over a sterile field can cause bacteria to enter the wound.			
3.	This would be allowed if an irrigating solution were ordered by the physician. Do not irrigate any wound unless ordered by a physician.			

The elements of this previous example read as follows:
    Number 1 is the question of the item number in the test; Number 4 is the correct answer.
    The first rationale explains the correct rationale and appears in bold print.
    The remaining rationales explain the incorrect answers.
    The phase of the clinical problem solving process (nursing process) is implementation.
    The category of client need is Safe Effective Care Environment and Safety and Infection Control.
    The subject area is Medical/Surgical.

Practice Test One

1. The client is being admitted for surgery. During the admission assessment the client states she usually has 8–10 alcoholic drinks a day. How should the nurse reply?
   1. What type of alcohol do you drink?
   2. How long have you been drinking alcohol?
   3. When was your last drink?
   4. Why do you drink so much?

2. The nurse is caring for a woman who had a mastectomy following a diagnosis of breast cancer. When the nurse enters the room, the curtains are drawn and the client is lying with her body turned toward the wall away from the nurse. When the nurse approaches her, the client says, "Just leave me alone. I'm no use to anyone. I'm not even a real woman." How should the nurse respond?
   1. Leave the room.
   2. Open the curtains.
   3. Say, "You sound upset."
   4. Say, "Women are more than breasts."

3. The nurse is providing home care to a 78-year-old woman who has early dementia. The client tells the nurse, "My daughter is mean to me." What should the nurse do initially?
   1. Report suspected elder abuse to the supervisor.
   2. Report elder abuse to the authorities.
   3. Ask the daughter about the mother's comment.
   4. Ask the client to describe what the daughter does to be mean to her.

4. The nurse is inserting an indwelling catheter in a female. The nurse knows the urethral meatus is located where?
   1. Between the clitoris and the vagina
   2. Between the vagina and the rectum
   3. Above the clitoris
   4. Below the rectum

5. The nurse is caring for an adult male who is diagnosed with probable appendicitis. Which assessment finding is most consistent with the diagnosis?
   1. Pain in the right upper quadrant
   2. Decreased white blood count
   3. Nausea and vomiting
   4. High fever

6. How should the nurse position the client who has just had a liver biopsy?
   1. On the left side
   2. On the right side
   3. Semi-Fowler's
   4. Low Fowler's

7. An adult is to have a paracentesis performed today. What should the nurse do before the procedure?
   1. Encourage the client to drink large amounts of fluids.
   2. Ask the client to empty her bladder just before the test.
   3. Keep the client NPO until after the procedure.
   4. Premedicate the client as ordered.

8. The physician has ordered an oil retention enema and a cleansing enema for a client. How should the nurse plan to carry out these orders?
   1. Administer the cleansing enema first and several hours later give the oil retention enema.
   2. Administer the oil retention enema first and give the cleansing enema an hour later.
   3. Mix the oil and the cleansing enema and give together.
   4. Give the cleansing enema today and the oil retention enema tomorrow.

9. The nurse observes a certified nursing assistant (CNA) placing a hot water bottle directly on the skin of a 90-year-old client. What action should the nurse take initially?
   1. Report the act to the patient care supervisor.
   2. Interrupt the procedure.
   3. Talk to the CNA when the procedure is finished.
   4. Notify the physician.

10. The nurse is planning care for all of the following clients. Which client should be cared for first?
    1. A 60-year-old, who is three days post-op and needs a dressing change and ambulation.
    2. A 75-year-old, who had a suprapubic prostatectomy yesterday and says, "Take that tube out of me, I have to pee."
    3. A 90-year-old, who had a total hip replacement two days ago and is to get out of bed today.
    4. A 50-year-old, who had an abdominal cholecystectomy yesterday and is asking for pain medication.

11. An adult is admitted with advanced cancer of the GI tract. What question must be included in the admission assessment?
    1. "What foods do you like best?"
    2. "Do you have advance directives?"
    3. "Do you want CPR if you go into cardiac arrest?"
    4. "Do you understand the serious nature of your illness?"

12. The nurse is providing home care for an immobile client who has a stage IV decubitus ulcer that is not healing. Assuming all of the following are available, which person would be most appropriate to consult re: care of the wound?
    1. Physician
    2. Physical therapist
    3. IV therapist
    4. Enterostomal therapist
13. A woman reports to the physician's office complaining of urinary frequency and pain and burning on urination. The nurse expects which procedures will be ordered for this client?
    1. Urine for culture and sensitivity
    2. CBC, BUN
    3. Routine urinalysis
    4. BUN, creatinine
14. A 38-year-old who has mitral stenosis is hospitalized for a valve replacement. Which condition is the client most likely to report having had earlier in life?
    1. Meningitis
    2. Syphilis
    3. Rheumatic fever
    4. Rubella
15. Following cardiac surgery, a client's urine output for the last hour is 20 cc. The nurse understands this indicates which of the following?
    1. Possible hyperkalemia
    2. Insufficient cardiac output
    3. Inadequate fluid replacement
    4. Diuresis is occurring
16. A 20-year-old woman is admitted to the hospital following an accident. Her uncle, a physician from out of state, visits her and asks to see her chart. How should the nurse respond?
    1. Comply with the request and give the chart to the physician.
    2. Explain that written permission from his niece is needed first.
    3. Suggest that he discuss the case with the attending physician.
    4. Give him the chart but do not let him remove it from the nurse's station.
17. An adult is admitted for surgery today. Immediately after administering the pre-operative medication of meperidine and atropine, the nurse notes that the operative permit has not been signed. Which action should the nurse take?
    1. Have the client sign the operative permit immediately before the medication takes effect.
    2. Have the client's next of kin sign the permission form.
    3. Ask the client if he/she is willing to undergo surgery and sign the form for the

client and indicate your name as witness to the client's verbal consent.
    4. Report it to the physician so the surgery can be delayed until the client can legally sign a consent form.
18. The nurse is administering hygienic care to an elderly client in her home. What should the nurse wash first?
    1. Perineal area
    2. Face
    3. Upper torso
    4. Hands
19. The family of a 90-year-old resident in a long-term care facility asks the nurse why the client only gets a shower three times a week. What information is most important for the nurse to include when answering the question?
    1. The staff members have limited time and must schedule all the residents.
    2. The client's skin is dry; too many showers will dry the skin further.
    3. The client has limited energy and must conserve it.
    4. The client is not very active and doesn't get very dirty.
20. The nurse is giving home care to an elderly client with angina pectoris and Type II diabetes mellitus. Which observation is of most concern and should be reported immediately?
    1. The client reports chest discomfort yesterday while taking a walk.
    2. The nurse observes several brown spots on the client's arms and legs.
    3. The client reports an ingrown toenail that is getting more painful.
    4. The client reports shortness of breath when climbing stairs.
21. All the following clients assigned to LPN/LVN ring their call bells. Which client needs the most immediate attention?
    1. A 72-year-old diabetic who is blind says she has to go to the bathroom.
    2. A 75-year-old client who has rheumatoid arthritis asks for pain medication.
    3. A client who has a blood transfusion running says her chest hurts.
    4. A post-operative client who says he is in pain and wants a pain shot.
22. The nurse notes all of the following. Which should be attended to first?
    1. A blind client is calling out stating she cannot find the call bell.
    2. There is a water spill on the floor near the bed of an elderly client who ambulates regularly.
    3. A post-operative client is asking for pain medication.
    4. A diabetic client is asking for a glass of water.

23. The nurse is to insert an indwelling catheter in a male. Which action is appropriate?
    1. Cleanse the meatus before preparing the catheter for insertion.
    2. Wash hands before starting the procedure.
    3. Hold the penis at a 45-degree angle during insertion of the catheter.
    4. Inflate the balloon immediately before inserting the catheter.

24. A 75-year-old woman who is hospitalized with congestive heart failure falls out of bed. She has a bruise on her leg but X-rays reveal no fractures. How should the nurse record the incident in the client's chart?
    1. "Client fell out of bed at 10 a.m. Physician notified. Incident report completed."
    2. "Client found on floor beside bed at 10 a.m. Alert and oriented times 3. States she slipped as she was standing up. Bruise (3 inches by 2 inches) on left hip. Denies pain. Dr. _____ examined client. X-rays taken."
    3. "Client fell while getting out of bed. Seems okay. Charge nurse examined client. Doctor notified and incident report filed."
    4. "Found client on floor beside bed. Responds to questions. Red area on left hip. Notified charge nurse and physician."

25. The nurse is caring for a 78-year-old woman in a long-term care facility. The client is sitting in a geriatric chair with the attached tray in place. The client is agitated and appears to be sliding down in the chair. What is the best action for the nurse to take?
    1. Ask the supervisor for advice.
    2. Put a jacket restraint on the client.
    3. Tie a sheet around the client's waist.
    4. Use foam wedges beside the client.

26. The nurse is observing a Certified Nursing Assistant (CNA) caring for a client who has AIDS. Which action, if observed, is not correct?
    1. The CNA wears gloves when cleaning the client after an episode of fecal incontinence.
    2. The CNA uses chlorine bleach to wipe up blood after the client cut himself shaving.
    3. The CNA is observed giving the client a back rub without gloves on.
    4. The CNA wears a mask whenever entering the client's room.

27. An adult who has COPD is receiving oxygen at home via nasal cannula. In addition to instructing the client and his family about not smoking when oxygen is in use, what should the nurse plan to include in the teaching?
    1. If the prescribed liter flow does not relieve his difficulty breathing, increase the liter flow by up to 2 liters/minute every four hours.
    2. Try not to shuffle across the carpeted floor.

3. Clean the nasal cannula with alcohol several times a day.
4. Increase the oxygen flow rate if you develop shortness of breath.

28. An adult had major abdominal surgery this morning under general anesthesia. When the client arrives in the recovery room she is very lethargic and restless. Her BP is 150/98; pulse, 110 and irregular; respirations, 30 and shallow. Post-operative orders include meperidine (Demerol) 75 mg I.M. for operative site pain; reinforce dressings p.r.n.; O₂ at 6 liters/min p.r.n.; irrigate nasogastric tube q 2 hours and p.r.n.; IV 2500 cc D5W in 24 hours. What should the nurse do next?
    1. Carefully inspect the dressings for any drainage.
    2. Irrigate the nasogastric tube.
    3. Administer meperidine (Demerol) as ordered.
    4. Administer oxygen.

29. An adult client who had major abdominal surgery is returned to her room on the surgical nursing unit. The post-anesthesia nurse reports that the client is awake, and has stable vital signs. She has an NG tube in place that is attached to intermittent suction. How should the nurse position the client?
    1. Supine
    2. Semi-Fowler's
    3. Dorsal recumbent
    4. Prone

30. The nurse is to open a sterile package. How should the nurse plan to open the first flap?
    1. Toward the nurse
    2. Away from the nurse
    3. To the right side
    4. To the left side

31. A 66-year-old woman is being evaluated for pernicious anemia. Which assessment findings would be most apt to be present in a client with pernicious anemia?
    1. Easy bruising.
    2. Pain in the legs.
    3. Fine red rash on the extremities.
    4. Pruritus.

32. A Schilling test has been ordered for a client. What is the nurse's primary responsibility in relation to this test?
    1. Collect the blood samples.
    2. Collect a 24-hour urine sample.
    3. Assist the client to X-ray.
    4. Administer an enema.

33. A throat culture is positive for streptococcus. An antibiotic is prescribed. Which question is it essential for the nurse to ask the client before administering the medication?
    1. Has the client ever had an adverse reaction to sulfa drugs?
    2. Is the client currently taking vitamins?
    3. Does the client drink alcoholic beverages?

4. Is the client allergic to penicillin?

34. The nurse is caring for an adult who had a kidney transplant. He is taking maintenance doses of cyclosporine and prednisone. Which of the following is the greatest cause for concern to the nurse?
    1. Moon face
    2. Acne
    3. Sore throat
    4. Mood swings

35. During a home visit the nurse observes a man who is recovering from a left total hip replacement. Which observation indicates the client understands his care?
    1. He is sitting in a soft, overstuffed easy chair.
    2. He bends over to pat his cat.
    3. He crosses his legs when sitting.
    4. He holds the cane in his right hand when walking.

36. A 17-year-old client is admitted following a seizure. That evening the nurse goes into the room and notes that the client has obviously been crying. The client says to the nurse, "Now that I have epilepsy, I am a freak." What is the best initial response for the nurse to make?
    1. "It must be very difficult for you to realize you have epilepsy."
    2. "Don't say that. You might be having a few seizures now but I'm sure the doctor will be able to control them."
    3. "Don't think like that. You're still a bright, good-looking, young person."
    4. "Many famous athletes and actors have epilepsy and they can still do anything they used to do."

37. The physician orders phenytoin (Dilantin) and phenobarbital for a client admitted with a cerebrovascular accident. The nurse knows these drugs are administered for what purpose?
    1. To prevent seizures
    2. To promote sleep
    3. To stop clots from forming
    4. To stop bleeding

38. An adult who has cholecystitis reports clay-colored stools and moderate jaundice. The nurse knows that which is the best explanation for the presence of clay-colored stools and jaundice?
    1. There is an obstruction in the pancreatic duct.
    2. There are gallstones in the gallbladder.
    3. Bile is no longer produced by the gallbladder.
    4. There is an obstruction in the common bile duct.

39. Following a cholecystectomy, drainage from the T tube for the first 24 hours post-operative was 350 cc. What is the appropriate nursing action?
    1. Notify the physician.
    2. Raise the level of the drainage bag to decrease the rate of flow.
    3. Increase the IV flow rate to compensate for the loss.
    4. Continue to observe and measure drainage.

40. The nurse is caring for a client who had a total thyroidectomy. What should the nurse plan to observe the client for after his return to the nursing care unit?
    1. Hoarseness.
    2. Signs of hypercalcemia.
    3. Loss of reflexes.
    4. Mental confusion.

41. The nurse is caring for a woman who has diabetic neuropathy. The nurse knows the client needs more instruction when the client makes which statement?
    1. "I'll use a hot water bottle if my feet hurt."
    2. "I should dry my feet and toes carefully."
    3. "I go to the podiatrist to have my toenails cut."
    4. "The Tegretol seems to help my leg pain."

42. The nurse is auscultating an elderly bedridden client's breath sounds and hears crackles. What is the best interpretation of this finding?
    1. This is normal for the client's age.
    2. This is suggestive of an immediately life-threatening condition.
    3. This is an indication the client needs to take deep breaths.
    4. This is an indication the client may need nasal oxygen.

43. The nurse is providing home care to an elderly woman who had a cerebral vascular accident several weeks ago. All of the following need to be done. Which should the nurse plan to do first?
    1. Auscultate lung fields.
    2. Hygienic care.
    3. Assist with ambulation.
    4. ROM exercises.

44. An older adult is seen in clinic. During the assessment process all of the following are expressed or noted. Which is of most immediate concern to the nurse?
    1. The client's daughter says the client has become increasingly forgetful.
    2. The client has a productive cough.
    3. The client ambulates slowly.
    4. The client says "My arms aren't long enough for me to read the paper."

45. All of the following need to be done. Which should the nurse do first?
    1. A client who had surgery earlier today asks for pain medication.

2. A person who is two days post-operative needs a dressing change.
3. A client who had a cerebrovascular accident needs a bed bath.
4. A person scheduled for surgery tomorrow needs an enema.

46. The nurse is about to medicate a client who is to have surgery today. The client says, "I do not understand what the doctor is going to do," and asks the nurse to explain specific details of the surgery. The client has already signed an operative permit. What is the best action for the nurse to take at this time?
    1. Attempt to answer the client's questions.
    2. Notify the physician of the client's concerns prior to medicating the client.
    3. Reassure the client that the physician is well respected and very competent.
    4. Suggest that the client ask the physician her questions when in the operating room.

47. The nurse has completed teaching the client about his low-sodium, low-fat diet. Which menu, if selected by the client, would indicate to the nurse that the client understands his diet?
    1. Mashed potatoes, spinach, and meat loaf.
    2. Swordfish with Hollandaise sauce, carrots, and rice pilaf.
    3. Baked chicken, wild rice, and broccoli.
    4. Roast beef with gravy, baked potato with sour cream, and creamed peas.

48. The afternoon following a thyroidectomy, the client experiences all of the following. Which one indicates to the nurse the client is experiencing a serious complication?
    1. A sore throat
    2. Pain at the surgical site
    3. Temperature of 100.2°F
    4. Sudden hoarseness

49. The nurse is caring for a client who had a colostomy. Which comment by the client indicates that she is showing an interest in learning about her colostomy?
    1. "Why did this problem have to happen to me?"
    2. "What is the bag of water for?"
    3. "When will I get rid of this thing?"
    4. "The doctor didn't really do a colostomy."

50. The client is scheduled for a paracentesis. What should the nurse expect to do prior to the procedure?
    1. Insert an indwelling catheter.
    2. Have the client void.
    3. Keep the client NPO.
    4. Administer an enema.

51. The nurse is caring for a client who is to be on bed rest for two weeks. What should the nurse do to prevent atelectasis?
    1. Encourage the client to deep-breathe and cough every two hours.

2. Encourage the client to flex and extend her feet every two hours.
3. Apply antiembolism stockings as ordered.
4. Perform range-of-motion exercises several times a day.

52. The nurse is administering tuberculin skin tests. How should the nurse insert the needle when administering the skin test?
    1. At a ten-degree angle.
    2. At a thirty-degree angle.
    3. At a sixty-degree angle.
    4. At a ninety-degree angle.

53. The nurse is teaching a community group about healthy lifestyles to prevent cancer and heart disease. Which comment by a member of the group indicates a need for more teaching?
    1. "Smoking is not good for you."
    2. "Reducing fat intake helps reduce the risk of heart disease."
    3. "Walking every day puts a strain on your heart."
    4. "Eating lots of fruits and vegetables helps keep me healthy."

54. The parents of a child who is in for a one-year well-baby check ask what immunizations the child needs. The nurse checks the child's record and determines that the child has had immunizations as recommended during the first year. What should the nurse reply?
    1. MMR and DTP
    2. Hepatitis B and Polio
    3. Hemophilous and Chickenpox
    4. Pneumonia and Tetanus

55. The nurse is providing home care. Which assessment finding would suggest to the nurse that the elderly client should be evaluated for abuse?
    1. The client says, "My daughter takes some of my Social Security money. She says it's to pay for my food and medicine."
    2. The client has several bruises on her arms and legs.
    3. The client says her family is mean because they hire someone to stay with her when they go out.
    4. The client has several bruises and circular marks that look like cigarette burns on her back.

56. The nurse is assessing the client's abdomen. Which should the nurse do first?
    1. Auscultate
    2. Percuss
    3. Inspect
    4. Palpate

57. The nurse is teaching a young woman how to perform self breast examination. Which comment, if made by the client, indicates the teaching has been effective?
    1. "I should examine my breasts every year."

2. "I need to see the doctor every six months for a breast exam."

3. "I don't need to worry about breast cancer for a few years."

4. "I should examine all parts of my breasts both lying down and standing up."

58. The parents of an infant ask the nurse in the physician's office what diseases the DPT shot protects against. What should the nurse include when replying?
   1. Diarrhea, polio, and typhoid
   2. Diphtheria, whooping cough, and tetanus
   3. Diarrhea, pertussis, and typhus
   4. Diphtheria, paralysis, and tetany

59. The nurse is providing home care to a post-operative client who has a wound infection. What is essential to include when teaching the family about infection transmission?
   1. The client should stay isolated from the rest of the family.
   2. No one who is pregnant should care for the client.
   3. The family should wash hands before and after caring for the client.
   4. The client should not be allowed to have any visitors.

60. An adult is scheduled for surgery today and has signed an operative permit. As the nurse is about to administer the client's pre-operative medication, the client says that she has changed her mind and no longer wishes to have the surgery. How should the nurse respond?
   1. "Once you have signed the permit form you cannot change your mind."
   2. "I will give you the medication and call your doctor about your change of mind."
   3. "I will call your doctor so you can discuss it with her."
   4. "This is a safe procedure; you do not need to be afraid."

61. The nurse is providing home care to a confused client. The client's family is using a restraint to keep the client from pulling out her indwelling catheter. What should the nurse plan to include when teaching the family?
   1. Remove the restraints for one hour three times a day.
   2. Check the restrained extremities every two hours for circulation.
   3. Remove the restraints whenever someone is with the client.
   4. Do not remove the restraints unless the nurse is present.

62. A client who has Parkinson's disease is having difficulty ambulating. The nurse knows the client and his family understand safety issues when the client is seen wearing which type of shoe?

1. Rubber-soled shoe.
2. Smooth-soled shoes
3. Elevated shoes
4. Open-toed shoes.

63. The nurse administered an intramuscular injection to an adult. How should the nurse dispose of the needle and syringe?
   1. Immediately place syringe and needle in the disposal container.
   2. Recap the needle and place syringe and needle in the disposal container.
   3. Separate the syringe and the needle and place in the appropriate disposal containers.
   4. Recap the needle and cut the syringe before placing in disposal container.

64. The nurse is caring for a client who is receiving oxygen therapy. A visitor yells at the nurse saying there is a fire burning in the wastebasket on the other side of the room. What should the nurse do initially?
   1. Go for help.
   2. Ask the visitor to go for help while the nurse calms the client.
   3. Turn off the oxygen and remove the client from the room.
   4. Grab the nearest fire extinguisher and try to put out the fire.

65. A young woman comes to the physician's office seeking contraceptive advice. The client reports all of the following. Which contraindicates the use of oral contraceptives?
   1. A gonorrhea infection last year
   2. Thrombophlebitis in the legs six months ago
   3. A family history of diabetes
   4. A bladder infection last month

66. When planning care for a woman who is admitted in labor, it is most important for the nurse to obtain which of the following information about the client?
   1. Age of the client and due date
   2. Frequency and duration of contractions
   3. Whether the membranes have ruptured
   4. Who will be assisting the woman during labor

67. A woman who is 32 weeks gestation comes to her physician's office. Which finding is of most concern to the office nurse?
   1. Trace of glucose in the urine
   2. Weight gain of 4 pounds in one month
   3. Swelling around the client's eyes
   4. Ankle and foot edema

68. The nurse is planning care for a group of senior citizens. The nurse should plan activities that promote achievement of which developmental task?
   1. Identity
   2. Intimacy
   3. Generativity

4. Ego integrity

69. A young couple asks the nurse what method of contraception they should use. What information is most important for the nurse to have before giving an answer?
   1. The exact age of the couple
   2. The sexual history of both partners
   3. The method they find most acceptable
   4. How soon they want to start a family

70. The nurse is making a home visit to the mother of an eight-pound baby boy born five days ago. Which observation indicates the mother understands the care of the newborn?
   1. The mother is concerned about the fact the baby has a soft stool after every breast feeding.
   2. The mother cleans the cord stump with alcohol when changing the diaper.
   3. The mother cleans the circumcised penis with alcohol when changing the diaper.
   4. The mother nurses the baby hourly.

71. The nurse in a college health clinic is teaching the male students self testicular examination. Which statement made by one of the young men indicates a need for more teaching?
   1. "I should do a self testicular examination every month."
   2. "When I am taking a shower is a good time to do the self exam."
   3. "If I feel any lumps I should report it to the physician."
   4. "Testicular cancer is usually found in older men."

72. The nurse has been interacting for several weeks with a client on the psychiatric unit. The nurse is to be transferred to another unit. Which comment by the client indicates separation anxiety?
   1. "We had a good time at the party last night. You should have been here."
   2. "Some of us are going to the museum next week. Too bad you can't go."
   3. "I was thinking about my friend last night; the one who died in the car crash."
   4. "I was telling my wife what a good nurse you are."

73. The nurse is caring for a client who is very demanding. She frequently rings the bell and asks to have her pillow fluffed or the water glass filled. Which response by the nurse will likely be most effective?
   1. Answer the bell quickly each time she rings.
   2. Tell her you do not have time to be in her room constantly.
   3. Say, "Why are you so upset?"
   4. Say, "You seem concerned about something."

74. An elderly client is severely dehydrated. Which is the best way to assess the effectiveness of fluid restoration therapy?
   1. Assess the client's skin turgor every shift.

2. Record weights daily.
3. Ask the client if she is thirsty.
4. Record all intake.

75. The nurse is caring for a client who is recovering from a cerebrovascular accident and is partially paralyzed on the right side. How should the nurse position the chair when getting the client out of bed?
   1. On the right side of the bed facing the foot of the bed
   2. On the right side of the bed facing the head of the bed
   3. On the left side of the bed facing the foot of the bed
   4. On the left side of the bed facing the head of the bed

76. An adult woman who broke her right ankle is seen in the physician's office one week after the cast was applied. Which observation indicates to the office nurse that the client is using crutches correctly?
   1. The client moves the left crutch forward, then the right foot, then the right crutch, and finally the left foot.
   2. The client moves the left crutch and the right foot together, and then moves the right crutch and the left together.
   3. The client moves the left foot and the crutches forward while bearing weight on the right foot.
   4. The client bears weight on the left foot and moves the right foot and the crutches forward.

77. The nurse observes a certified nursing assistant (CNA) moving a client up in bed. Which action by the nursing assistant indicates a need for more instruction in how to move a client?
   1. Using a pull sheet
   2. Asking another nursing assistant to help
   3. Lowering the head of the bed
   4. Pulling the client by the shoulders

78. The client tells the nurse she is having trouble falling asleep. What initial nursing action is least appropriate?
   1. Asking the physician for a sleeping medication
   2. Offering the client a back rub
   3. Asking the client if she is concerned about something
   4. Repositioning the client

79. The nurse is caring for a client who is ordered to be on bed rest for a prolonged period of time. What should be included in the nursing care plan to prevent venous stasis?
   1. Deep-breathe and cough every two hours
   2. Range-of-motion exercises every shift
   3. Antiembolism stockings on legs
   4. Turn every two hours

80. The nurse is caring for a client who is receiving intravenous fluid therapy. Which

observation needs to be reported to the charge nurse?

1. The client says the IV fluid feels cool when it goes in.
2. The infusion site is covered with clear tape.
3. The client is ambulating while the IV infusion is running.
4. The area around the infusion site is cool and blanched.

81. The nurse is to administer the daily dose of digoxin to an adult client. What is it essential for the nurse to do before administering the medication?
    1. Check the client's temperature
    2. Check the client's blood pressure
    3. Check the client's respirations
    4. Check the client's apical pulse

82. An adult client who has a fractured tibia is ordered one baby aspirin a day. He says to the nurse, "I don't think the aspirin is doing any good. I still have pain." What should the nurse include when replying to this client?
    1. "The aspirin is given to prevent clots from forming."
    2. "The aspirin is given to keep your temperature normal."
    3. "The aspirin is given to control your pain and should be helping."
    4. "The aspirin is given to decrease inflammation at the fracture site."

83. A client who is about to be discharged from the acute care facility is receiving warfarin (Coumadin). The nurse should plan to teach the client which of the following?
    1. Take the medication on a full stomach.
    2. Do not take any over-the-counter medications without checking with your physician.
    3. Take aspirin if you need an analgesic.
    4. Avoid prolonged exposure to the sun while taking warfarin.

84. A spansule is ordered twice a day for a client in the outpatient clinic. What should the nurse teach the client about taking a spansule?
    1. Take the spansule before breakfast and dinner.
    2. If the spansule is difficult to swallow, open it up, and put the contents in food.
    3. Spansules should be taken at 12-hour intervals.
    4. Spansules can safely be cut for partial doses.

85. The client says to the nurse, "I don't see why I should live any longer." How should the nurse respond initially?
    1. Ask the client why she doesn't want to live any longer.
    2. Ask the client if she is considering suicide.
    3. Tell the client that life is precious and worth living.
    4. Help the client see the good things that she has in her life.

86. A client who has had a right below-the-knee amputation refers to himself as "a freak " and "old peg-leg." What initial response by the nurse is most therapeutic?
    1. "You are not a freak."
    2. "Lots of people have amputations and live a normal life."
    3. "You feel like a freak."
    4. "You shouldn't say that, you are very attractive."

87. The nurse is caring for a client who is suffering from severe anxiety. What must the client do first when learning to deal with his anxiety?
    1. Recognize that he is feeling anxious.
    2. Identify the situations that precipitated his anxiety.
    3. Understand the reason for his anxiety.
    4. Select a strategy to use to help him cope with his anxiety.

88. The nurse is caring for a client who had a right below-the-knee amputation three days ago. The client complains of pain in the right foot and asks for pain medication. What nursing action is appropriate initially?
    1. Elevate the stump.
    2. Administer a placebo.
    3. Administer ordered medications.
    4. Encourage the client to discuss his feelings.

89. An adult woman has obsessive-compulsive disorder. She continually washes her hands and misses meals because she has not completed her washing rituals. What should be in the nursing care plan for this woman?
    1. Interrupt the ritual and insist the woman go to meals.
    2. Bring meals to the client if she is unable to get to the dining room.
    3. Remind her an hour before meals so she can perform her washing ritual.
    4. Give her a choice of performing her washing ritual or going to meals.

90. An eight-month-old infant is admitted with head injuries and suspected child abuse. Which comment, if made by the mother, would be most suggestive of child abuse?
    1. "He always cries just to irritate me."
    2. "I get worried when he cries and I don't know what he wants."
    3. "When he cries I usually just feed him and hope that is what he wants."
    4. "I wish he could talk to me and tell me what he wants."

91. An 82-year-old woman who has Alzheimer's disease is admitted to the acute care unit. She frequently gets out of bed and wanders in the hall, unable to find her way back to her room. She even gets in the beds of other clients. What nursing action is most appropriate for this client?

1. Restrain her so she will not wander in the halls.
2. Ask her roommate to call the nurse whenever she leaves the room.
3. Punish her when she gets in a bed other than her own.
4. Put her favorite picture on the door to her room.

92. A 35-year-old woman with three children is seen in the emergency room for a broken arm and facial lacerations. This is the third emergency room visit in the last three months for injuries. Each time she tells the staff that she fell. This time she confides to the LPN/LVN that "my husband accidentally pushed me." What should the LPN/LVN do with this information?
    1. Ask the client why she stays with a man who has caused her to get hurt.
    2. Notify the charge nurse so the client can receive a referral.
    3. Ask the client if she wants a referral to a divorce lawyer.
    4. Tell the client that she has rights and does not have to put up with abuse.

93. An adult is receiving external radiation as part of her treatment for cancer. She asks what precautions are necessary for her to take because of the radiation therapy. The nurse replies that the client should not be around which of the following persons?
    1. Pregnant women
    2. People who are sick
    3. People who have pacemakers
    4. Elderly persons

94. An adult client is showing signs of developing hypovolemic shock. Which finding is most likely to be present?
    1. Elevated systolic and lowered diastolic blood pressure
    2. Decreased heart rate
    3. Decreased urine output
    4. Decreased respiratory rate

95. The nurse finds a person unresponsive on the floor. What is the initial nursing action?
    1. Start chest compressions.
    2. Assess respirations and pulse.
    3. Place on a hard surface.
    4. Start mouth-to-mouth breathing.

96. A home care client is scheduled for dialysis. He asks the nurse if he should take his antihypertensive medication before going for dialysis. How should the nurse respond?
    1. He should take all regularly scheduled medications.
    2. Antihypertensives should not be taken before dialysis because the blood pressure drops during dialysis.
    3. He should check with the physician because it varies from person to person.
    4. He should take it with him and take it if his blood pressure rises during the treatment.

97. During suctioning of the client's tracheostomy tube the catheter appears to attach to the tracheal wall and creates a pulling sensation. What is the best action for the nurse to take?
    1. Release the suction by opening the vent.
    2. Continue suctioning to remove the obstruction.
    3. Increase the pressure.
    4. Suction deeper.

98. The client has a chest tube attached to a Pleurovac® drainage system. Four hours after the chest tube is inserted the nurse notes there is no bubbling in the water seal compartment. What is the most likely explanation for this?
    1. The lung has reexpanded.
    2. There is an obstruction in the tubing coming from the pleural cavity.
    3. There is an air leak in the drainage system.
    4. The suction is not turned on.

99. An adult client was admitted for congestive heart failure today. An IV is running. The nurse enters the room and notes the client is having increased difficulty breathing. Before calling the physician, what action should the nurse take?
    1. Increase the IV drip rate.
    2. Place the client in a supine position.
    3. Ask the client if this has happened before.
    4. Raise the head of the bed.

100. An adult client is receiving oxygen at 6 liters/min. The client asks the nurse why the oxygen is running through bubbling water. What should be included in the nurse's reply?
    1. The water cools the oxygen and makes it more comfortable.
    2. Oxygen is very drying to tissues; the water humidifies it.
    3. The water prevents fires when oxygen is in use.
    4. The water helps to prevent infections from developing in the tubing.

Answers and Rationales for Practice Test One

Answer	Rationale	NP	CN	SA

#1. 3. Admitting to 8–10 alcoholic drinks a day is suggestive of alcoholism. It is important to know when the client last had a drink of alcohol in order to anticipate the onset of withdrawal symptoms.   Dc Ps/6 1

    1. The type of alcohol the client drinks is not the key issue. The key issue is when to anticipate withdrawal symptoms.

    2. The key issue is when to anticipate withdrawal symptoms, not how long the client has been drinking.

    4. The key issue is when to anticipate withdrawal symptoms, not why the client drinks so much. "Why" questions are usually not therapeutic because they make the client defensive.

#2. 3. Acknowledging the client's feelings is an appropriate response to this common grief reaction following the loss of a body part.   Im Ps/5 2

    1. Leaving the room would reinforce the client's perception that she is useless.

    2. Opening the curtains does not address the client's concerns; it merely forces the nurse's perception of appropriateness on the client.

    4. While this statement is true, it is not an appropriate response to the client. The nurse should recognize the client's feelings, not put them down.

#3. 4. The client's statement is very vague and needs to be clarified. Initially the nurse should ask the client what the daughter does that is mean to her. Examples of behavior are important in evaluating whether the client is the victim of abuse or whether the client's dementia is affecting her perceptions.   Dc Ps/6 2

    1. The nurse does not have enough data at this point to report the client's claim.

    2. The nurse does not have enough data at this point to report the client's claim.

    3. Initially the nurse should clarify the accusation with the client. After doing that, it would be appropriate to discuss the issue with the daughter.

#4. 1. The urethral opening is located between the clitoris and the vagina.   Dc Ph/7 1
    2. The urethral opening is located between the clitoris and the vagina.
    3. The urethral opening is located between the clitoris and the vagina.
    4. The urethral opening is located between the clitoris and the vagina.

#5. 3. Nausea and vomiting are typically seen in persons who have appendicitis.   Dc Ph/10 1

    1. The pain of appendicitis is in the right lower quadrant, not the right upper quadrant.

    2. The white blood count is elevated in the person with appendicitis.

    4. The temperature of a person with appendicitis is likely to be a low-grade fever, not a high fever.

#6. 2. The person who has had a liver biopsy should be positioned on the right side so that there is pressure on the liver to stop any potential bleeding. The liver is located on the right side.   Im Ph/9 1

    1. The person who has had a liver biopsy should be positioned on the right side so that there is pressure on the liver to stop any potential bleeding. The liver is located on the right side.

    3. The person who has had a liver biopsy should be positioned on the right side so that there is pressure on the liver to stop any potential bleeding. The liver is located on the right side.

    4. The person who has had a liver biopsy should be positioned on the right side so that there is pressure on the liver to stop any potential bleeding. The liver is located on the right side.

#7. 2. **The client should empty her bladder before a paracentesis so the bladder will not be in the abdominal cavity during the procedure. This reduces the risk of accidental puncture of the bladder.**   Im   Ph/9   1

    1. The bladder should be empty during a paracentesis to avoid accidental puncture.

    3. A paracentesis is usually done at the bedside with only a local anesthetic prior to insertion of the needle. There is no need to keep the client NPO.

    4. A paracentesis is usually done at the bedside with only a local anesthetic prior to insertion of the needle. There is no need to premedicate the client.

#8. 2. **The oil retention enema is given first to soften the feces. An hour later a cleansing enema is given to help remove the feces.**   Pl   Ph/7   1

    1. The oil retention enema is given first to soften the feces. An hour later a cleansing enema is given to help remove the feces.

    3. The oil retention enema is given first to soften the feces. An hour later a cleansing enema is given to help remove the feces.

    4. The oil retention enema is given first to soften the feces. An hour later a cleansing enema is given to help remove the feces.

#9. 2. **Applying heat directly to skin with no barrier is dangerous. The client, especially an elderly client, is at risk for skin burn. The nurse's first responsibility is for the safety of the client. The act must be stopped before the client is injured.**   Im   Sa/1   1

    1. The nurse should first stop the dangerous act, then discuss it with the CNA. If the problem cannot be resolved, the nurse should talk with the patient care supervisor.

    3. The nurse cannot wait until after the heat has been applied. Applying heat directly to skin with no barrier is dangerous. The client, especially an elderly client, is at risk for skin burn. The nurse's first responsibility is for the safety of the client. The act must be stopped before the client is injured.

    4. The nurse should first stop the dangerous act. There is no need to notify the physician unless the CNA carries out the improper procedure and the client's skin is damaged.

#10. 2. **An urgent feeling of having to urinate in a client who has a suprapubic tube or an indwelling catheter suggests the tube may be blocked. The nurse should further assess the client immediately and irrigate the catheter if ordered or notify the physician if no irrigation order is present.**   Pl   Sa/1   1

    1. This client's needs can wait for a few minutes.

    3. This client's needs can wait a few minutes.

    4. This client's needs can wait a few minutes. Caring for a blocked catheter is of higher priority than administering pain medication.

#11. 2. **All persons should be asked upon admission if they have advance directives.**   Dc   Sa/1   1

    1. All persons should be asked upon admission if they have advance directives. Asking about favorite foods might be appropriate in some situations but is not something that must be included in an initial assessment.

    3. All persons should be asked upon admission if they have advance directives. CPR is only one item that may be included in advance directives. Initiation of a feeding tube might be an issue with this client, for instance.

    4. All persons should be asked upon admission if they have advance directives. At some point in the course of caring for this client, it might be appropriate to ask if they understand the serious nature of the illness, but it is not something that must be done during the admission assessment.

#12. 4. **An enterostomal therapist is a Registered Nurse who is an expert in wound care, including stomas such as colostomies and decubitus ulcers.**   Im   Sa/1   1

     1. Most physicians are not expert on the care of decubitus ulcers. The enterostomal therapist is the expert in wound care.

     2. A physical therapist is not an expert in wound care. The enterostomal therapist is the expert in wound care.

     3. An IV therapist is not an expert in wound care. The enterostomal therapist is the expert in wound care.

#13. 1. **The symptoms suggest a urinary tract infection. A clean catch urine for culture and sensitivity will most likely be done to confirm the diagnosis.**   Pl   Ph/9   1

     2. CBC and BUN are not the tests most likely to be ordered for this client. An elevated BUN is a sign of renal failure. However, the client's signs and symptoms suggest urinary tract infection. An elevated WBC indicates infection. However, the diagnostic test for UTI is urine for C&S.

     3. The symptoms suggest a urinary tract infection. A clean catch urine for culture and sensitivity will most likely be done to confirm the diagnosis.

     4. The symptoms suggest a urinary tract infection. A clean catch urine for culture and sensitivity will most likely be done to confirm the diagnosis. BUN and serum creatinine are done to diagnose renal failure. The client's findings suggest urinary tract infection.

#14. 3. **The most common cause of mitral valve stenosis is rheumatic fever.**   Dc   Ph/9   1

     1. Meningitis is not a cause of mitral valve stenosis. Sequelae from meningitis would most likely be neurological problems.

     2. Tertiary syphilis can cause cardiovascular problems such as aortic aneurysm. However, this would be unlikely at age 38. The most common cause of mitral valve stenosis is rheumatic fever.

     4. Rubella in the mother can cause cardiac defects in the unborn child. While any viral infection has the potential to cause heart problems, mitral stenosis is not a common sequela of rubella.

#15. 2. **Urine output below 30 ml/hr indicates the onset of shock. Remember that urine is made from blood. If there is insufficient blood flow to the kidneys there will be a decrease in urine output.**   Dc   Ph/10   1

     1. Hyperkalemia is not characterized by decreased urine output. Renal failure could cause hyperkalemia.

     3. Inadequate fluid replacement could cause a decrease in urine output; however, there is not enough data to suggest that. More likely, the heart is not beating effectively.

     4. The urine output is less than normal. Diuresis would be characterized by an increase in urine output.

#16. 2. **The client's right to confidentiality requires that only persons with a need to know have access to her chart. If she wants her physician uncle to read the chart, she needs to sign written permission.**   Im   Sa/1   1

     1. The client's right to confidentiality requires that only persons with a need to know have access to her chart. The physician uncle who is from out of state is clearly not actively involved in the case. If she wants her physician uncle to read the chart, she needs to sign written permission.

     3. The client's right to confidentiality requires that only persons with a need to know have access to her chart. The physician uncle who is from out of state is clearly not actively involved in the case. If she wants her physician uncle to read the chart, she needs to sign written permission. The client needs to give permission for her physician to discuss the case with her physician uncle.

     4. The client's right to confidentiality requires that only persons with a need to know have access to her chart. The physician uncle who is

from out of state is clearly not actively involved in the case. If she wants her physician uncle to read the chart, she needs to sign written permission.

#17. 4. A consent form must be signed before surgery can be legally performed. A client who has been medicated may not sign the consent form. The surgery will be delayed or postponed until the client is free of the influence of mind-altering medications and can legally sign a consent form.   Im   Sa/1   1

   1. Even though the client has just received the medication, the client can not legally sign documents until free of the influence of mind-altering drugs.

   2. If the client is otherwise able to sign the consent form (the client is of age and alert and oriented before being medicated), the next of kin are not authorized to sign for her.

   3. If the client is not legally able to give written consent, the client is not legally able to give verbal consent for surgery.

#18. 2. The nurse should start the bath by washing the eyes and face first.   Im   Ph/7   1

   1. The perineal area is the last to be washed. The nurse should start the bath by washing the eyes and face first.

   3. The upper torso is washed after the face and hands and arms have been washed. The nurse should start the bath by washing the eyes and face first.

   4. The hands are washed after the face. The nurse should start the bath by washing the eyes and face first.

#19. 2. Elderly clients usually have dry skin. Bathing every day is not recommended for persons with very dry skin. Showers two or three times a week are usually recommended.   Im   Ph/7   1

   1. Elderly clients usually have dry skin. Bathing every day is not recommended for persons with very dry skin. Showers two or three times a week are usually recommended. The nurse should not tell family members that the staff does not have time to care for their loved one.

   3. Elderly clients usually have dry skin. Bathing every day is not recommended for persons with very dry skin. Showers two or three times a week are usually recommended. The client may have limited energy but from the data given, the primary reason for showering only three times a week is the client's dry skin due to aging.

   4. Elderly clients usually have dry skin. Bathing every day is not recommended for persons with very dry skin. Showers two or three times a week are usually recommended. It may also be true that the client does not get very dirty, but the primary reason for showering only three times a week is the client's dry skin due to aging.

#20. 3. An ingrown toenail in a person who has diabetes can be very serious. Diabetics have poor circulation and are prone to infection, especially in the feet and legs. An ingrown toenail should be reported immediately to the nurse supervisor so an appropriate referral can be made.   Dc   Ph/9   1

   1. Chest discomfort while exercising is a common occurrence in persons who have angina.

   2. Brown spots on the arms and legs are common in elderly persons; these are sometimes called age spots.

   4. Shortness of breath when climbing stairs occurs frequently in persons who are elderly and who have angina. The nurse should note this so comparisons can be made to see if the shortness of breath is getting worse. However, the greatest concern at the moment is the painful ingrown toenail.

#21. 3. Chest pain in a person receiving a transfusion may indicate a transfusion reaction that could be immediately life-threatening.   Im   Sa/1   1

The transfusion should be stopped immediately and the charge nurse notified.

1. Assisting a blind person to ambulate to the bathroom is important; however, a possible transfusion reaction could be immediately life-threatening and takes priority.

2. Administering pain medication is important; however, a possible transfusion reaction could be immediately life-threatening and takes priority.

4. Administering pain medication is important; however, a possible transfusion reaction could be immediately life-threatening and takes priority.

#22. 2. A water spill on the floor next to the bed of an elderly client who ambulates creates an immediate hazard and should be wiped up immediately. Wiping up the spill is not a time-consuming process and immediately assures the safety of the client. The other clients can safely wait until the immediate hazard has been dealt with.   Im   Sa/2   1

1. The blind client obviously can speak to get attention. The need for the call bell is not an immediate safety need. A water spill on the floor next to the bed of an elderly client who ambulates creates an immediate hazard and should be wiped up immediately.

3. A post-operative client who needs pain medication is not an immediate safety concern. A water spill on the floor next to the bed of an elderly client who ambulates creates an immediate hazard and should be wiped up immediately.

4. A diabetic client who asks for a glass of water is not an immediate safety need and can wait for a few minutes. A water spill on the floor next to the bed of an elderly client who ambulates creates an immediate hazard and should be wiped up immediately.

#23. 2. Hands should be washed before starting any procedure.   Im   Ph/7   1
1. The nurse should lubricate the catheter and test the balloon before touching the client. Once the nurse touches the client's penis to cleanse the area, that hand is contaminated.

3. The penis should be held at a 90-degree angle to insert the catheter.

4. The nurse may test the balloon before draping and cleansing the client. However, the balloon is not inflated during insertion of the catheter. It would be dangerous, if not impossible, to try to insert a catheter with an inflated balloon.

#24. 2. This answer is most complete. The client's mental status is described; the bruise is described; and the actions taken are described.   Im   Sa/1   1

1. The notes are too vague. The nurse should not make reference to an incident report in the written notes. However, an incident report should be completed. The purpose of the incident report is for the hospital to follow untoward events. The client's chart is a legal record.

3. The notes are too vague. The nurse should not make reference to an incident report in the written notes. However, an incident report should be completed. The purpose of the incident report is for the hospital to follow untoward events. The client's chart is a legal record.

4. The notes are too vague. Answer Number 2 gives more information.

#25. 4. The nurse should use only one form of restraint. The tray is considered a restraint. Foam wedges and pillows are not considered restraints.   Im   Sa/2   1

1. The nurse should be able to solve this problem without asking a supervisor.

2. The nurse should use only one form of restraint. The tray is considered a restraint. A jacket restraint is a second form of restraint.

3. The nurse should use only one form of restraint. The tray is considered a restraint. Tying a sheet around her waist is a second form of restraint.

#26. 4. There is no reason to wear a mask whenever entering the room of a person who has AIDS. A mask might be worn when suctioning if the client had a lot of secretions.   Ev   Sa/2   1

   1. This action is correct. Gloves should be worn when there is contact with any body fluids.
   2. This action is correct. Chlorine bleach 1:10 dilution should be used to clean up blood spills.
   3. This action is correct. There is no need to wear gloves when touching the client's intact skin such as when giving a backrub.

#27. 2. Shuffling across a carpet may create static electricity and the possibility of fire with oxygen running.   Pl   Sa/2   1

   1. Persons with COPD should not have oxygen at levels above 2–3 liters because their drive to breathe is a low oxygen level.
   3. The nasal cannula can be cleaned with soap and water but should not be cleaned with alcohol, which is flammable.
   4. Persons with COPD should not have oxygen at levels above 2–3 liters because their drive to breathe is a low oxygen level.

#28. 4. Most cases of restlessness in combination with lethargy are due to hypoxia. Hypoxia will cause an irregular pulse and rapid shallow respirations. The client may be in pain. However, the priority is to treat anoxia first and then reassess the client before giving analgesia.   Im   Ph/9   1

   1. The nurse will inspect the wounds for drainage on a regular basis. The data do not suggest an immediate need to inspect the wound. The data are more consistent with hypoxia.
   2. There is no data to suggest the nasogastric tube needs irrigating.
   3. The data are more consistent with hypoxia than pain. Airway takes precedent over pain.

#29. 2. Semi-Fowler's position will facilitate respirations, take pressure off the abdominal incision, and aid drainage if a drain is in place. Semi-Fowler's position is indicated when a client has a nasogastric tube in place to prevent backflow of gastric juices.   Im   Ph/9   1

   1. A person who has a nasogastric tube should not be placed in the supine position because of the risk of aspiration.
   3. A person who has a nasogastric tube should not be placed in the dorsal recumbent position because of the risk of aspiration.
   4. A person who has a nasogastric tube should not be placed in prone position because of the risk of aspiration.

#30. 2. The first flap is opened away from the nurse; then the side flaps and finally the last flap are opened toward the nurse. This way the nurse does not have to reach across a sterile field. Reaching across a sterile field contaminates the field and it is no longer considered sterile.   Pl   Sa/2   1

   1. If the first flap is opened toward the nurse, the last flap will be opened away from the nurse, causing the nurse to reach across the sterile field.
   3. The first flap is opened away from the nurse; then the side flaps and finally the last flap are opened toward the nurse. This way the nurse does not have to reach across a sterile field. Reaching across a sterile field contaminates the field and it is no longer considered sterile.
   4. The first flap is opened away from the nurse; then the side flaps and finally the last flap are opened toward the nurse. This way the nurse does not have to reach across a sterile field. Reaching across a sterile field contaminates the field and it is no longer considered sterile.

#31. 2. Neuropathy, as evidenced by pain in the legs, is characteristic of pernicious anemia. Vitamin B₁₂ is necessary for neurological function.   Dc   Ph/9   1

   1. Easy bruising would be seen in a clotting disorder such as hemophilia, in leukemia, or in bone marrow depression.
   3. Rash is not seen in pernicious anemia.

ANSWER	RATIONALE	NP	CN	SA

    4. Pruritus is characteristic of Hodgkin's disease.

#32. 2. The client is given radioactive Vitamin B$_{12}$ orally and a 24-hour urine is collected to see if Vitamin B$_{12}$ is absorbed from the GI tract into the blood stream and excreted in the urine. The nurse should collect a 24-hour urine.   Dc   Ph/9   1

    1. There are no blood samples to be collected in a Schilling test.

    3. The Schilling test does not involve X-rays.

    4. No enema is administered before or during a Schilling test.

#33. 4. Penicillin is usually prescribed for streptococcal infection. Penicillin allergy is fairly common. The nurse should ask the client about allergic reactions to penicillin.   Dc   Ph/8   5

    1. Sulfa drugs are not usually prescribed for streptococcal infections.

    2. Vitamins are not a contraindication for penicillin therapy.

    3. Alcoholic beverages do not cause adverse reactions when taken with penicillin. Alcohol will cause an Antabuse-like reaction when taken with metronidazole (Flagyl).

#34. 3. A sore throat is probably symptomatic of immunosuppression as a result of taking immunosuppressants.   Dc   Ph/8   5

    1. Moon face is an expected side effect of prednisone therapy.

    2. Acne is an expected side effect of prednisone therapy.

    4. Mood swings are an expected side effect of prednisone therapy.

#35. 4. When walking with a cane, the cane should be held in the nonaffected hand, which in this case is the right hand. This action indicates understanding of his care.   Ev   Ph/7   1

    1. The client who has had a total hip replacement should keep the hips in extension. Sitting in a soft, over-stuffed easy chair causes hip flexion and indicates the client does not understand his care.

    2. The client who has had a total hip replacement should keep the hips in extension. Bending over to pat his cat causes hip flexion and indicates the client does not understand his care.

    3. The client who has had a total hip replacement should keep the hips abducted. Crossing the legs causes adduction, which may cause the hip to move out of the socket. Crossing his legs indicates the client does not understand his care.

#36. 1. Initial responses should open communication and let him express his feelings.   Im   Ps/5   2

    2. This response is not therapeutic in that it argues with the client and encourages denial of illness.

    3. This response denies the client's feelings.

    4. This response is not an appropriate initial response. Telling the client about successful people who also share his condition may be appropriate later on.

#37. 1. Phenytoin and phenobarbital are prescribed to prevent seizures.   Dc   Ph/8   5

    2. These drugs do have a sedating effect. However, that is a side effect and not the purpose for which they are given to this client.

    3. These drugs do not prevent clotting. Heparin followed by coumadin might be given to stop clots from forming.

    4. These drugs do not stop bleeding.

#38. 4. Clay-colored stools mean bile is not getting through to the duodenum. The bile duct is obstructed so bile backs up into the bloodstream, causing jaundice.   Dc   Ph/10   1

    1. An obstruction in the pancreatic duct might cause fatty stools but would not block bile and therefore would not cause clay-colored stools and jaundice.

    2. Gallstones in the gallbladder would cause pain but would not cause clay-colored stools and jaundice unless they blocked the common bile duct.

    3. Bile is not produced in the gallbladder. The liver produces bile and the gallbladder stores it.

#39. 4. **350 ml in 24 hours after surgery is a normal amount of bile drainage.**   Im Ph/9 1

1. There is no need to notify the physician, because the normal T tube drainage in the immediate post-operative period is 350–500 ml.
2. Raising the level of the drainage bag might cause reflux of bile. There is no need to do anything, as this amount of drainage is normal.
3. The drainage is normal. The LPN/LVN should not readjust the IV drip rate unless there is an obvious problem or emergency.

#40. 1. **Hoarseness may occur after thyroidectomy if the laryngeal nerve is damaged.**   Pl Ph/9 1

2. The nurse should observe the post-thyroidectomy client for signs of hypocalcemia, which may occur if the parathyroids were damaged or removed. Signs of hypocalcemia are tetany and Trousseau's or Chvostek's sign.
3. The nurse should observe the post-thyroidectomy client for hyperreflexia, not loss of reflexes. Hyperreflexia can be determined by assessing for Trousseau's or Chvostek's sign.
4. Mental confusion is not a sign of the usual post-thyroidectomy complications.

#41. 1. **A person who has diabetic neuropathy has altered sensation in the extremities and should not use a hot water bottle. This answer indicates a need for further instruction.**   Ev Ph/9 1

2. A person who has diabetes needs meticulous foot care. This response indicates the client understands her care.
3. A person who has diabetes and especially one with diabetic neuropathy should have professional assistance with cutting toenails. This response indicates the client understands her care.
4. Tegretol is a drug frequently given to persons who have diabetic neuropathy. It is an anticonvulsant and blocks painful nerve impulses, reducing the pain of neuropathies.

#42. 3. **Crackles are an indication that fluid is beginning to collect in the alveoli and the client needs to take deep breaths to expand the alveoli.**   Dc Ph/9 1

1. Crackles in the lung fields are not normal findings.
2. Crackles are an early sign that the alveoli are not well-expanded and that fluid is collecting. Crackles are not suggestive of an immediately life-threatening condition.
4. Crackles are an early sign that the alveoli are not well-expanded and that fluid is collecting. The client who has crackles needs to take deep breaths and cough. Crackles do not indicate the client needs oxygen.

#43. 1. **The nurse should auscultate the lung fields before doing hygienic care. If the client should have crackles and need additional deep-breathing and coughing exercises, the nurse can incorporate these into the hygienic care.**   Pl Ph/7 1

2. Hygienic care should be done after assessing the client's breath sounds so corrective actions can be incorporated into the care if necessary.
3. Assessing lung fields should be done before ambulating.
4. Range-of-motion exercises can be incorporated into hygienic care.

#44. 2. **A productive cough could indicate an immediate infectious process and is of most immediate concern.**   Dc He/3 1

1. Forgetfulness could be a sign of chronic brain disease. It is not an inevitable sign of aging. However, it is not as immediate a concern as a productive cough.
3. Ambulating slowly can be a normal part of the aging process or could indicate a condition such as arthritis or even visual deficits. It is a concern, but not as immediate as a productive cough.
4. Difficulty reading at close range (presbyopia) is a normal part of aging. The nurse will want to recommend to the client that a

prescription for reading glasses may easily correct the problem. However, this is not as immediate a concern as a productive cough.

#45. 1. **The client who had surgery earlier today may be in acute pain and should be assessed immediately for pain and the administration of ordered pain medication.**   Pl Ph/9 1
2. Changing the dressing of a post-operative client can safely be delayed until the nurse has assessed the pain of the fresh post-op client.
3. Assisting a client with ambulation can safely be delayed until the nurse has assessed the client who is in pain.
4. Administering an enema can safely be delayed until the nurse has assessed the client who is in pain.

#46. 2. **The client should talk with the physician if the questions are about specific details regarding the surgery. The nurse might be able to answer general questions. The client should talk with the physician before being medicated.**   Im Sa/1 1
1. The question states that the client wants to know specific details of the surgery. These are questions the physician should answer, not the nurse. The nurse can answer general questions about pre-operative and post-operative care, etc.
3. The client has specific questions about the details of the surgery. The nurse should not ignore these questions by reassuring the client.
4. The nurse is about to medicate the client for surgery. The client will be under the influence of medications when she is in the operating room.

#47. 3. **Baked chicken is lower in both salt and fat than beef. Wild rice and broccoli are low in fat and sodium. This choice indicates understanding of his diet.**   Ev Ph/7 6
1. Spinach is high in sodium and meat loaf is high in sodium and fat. This choice indicates the client does not understand his diet.
2. Swordfish, like all ocean fish, is high in sodium. Hollandaise sauce is high in sodium and fat. Carrots are naturally high in sodium. This choice indicates the client does not understand his diet.
4. Roast beef is higher in sodium and fat than chicken. Gravy is high in sodium and fat. Sour cream is high in sodium and fat and creamed peas contain fat. This choice indicates the client does not understand his diet.

#48. 4. **Sudden hoarseness following a thyroidectomy may indicate damage to the laryngeal nerve. This should be reported to the charge nurse or physician immediately.**   Ev Ph/10 1
1. A sore throat is normal following a thyroidectomy. Most people who have a general anesthetic and are intubated complain of a sore throat.
2. Pain at the surgical site on the day of surgery is a normal finding.
3. A low-grade temperature on the day of surgery may well indicate mild dehydration and is quite normal.

#49. 2. **Asking questions about procedures indicates a readiness to learn more about it.**   Ev Ps/5 1
1. Asking "why" a problem happened indicates the client has not yet accepted the condition. It is typical of the anger stage of reaction to an illness or problem.
3. Asking, "When will I get rid of this thing?" in reference to a colostomy indicates the client has not accepted the condition and is probably not ready to learn more about it.
4. Saying, "The doctor didn't really do a colostomy" indicates the client is in denial and not ready to learn about her colostomy.

#50. 2. **The client should void prior to a paracentesis. If the client has a full bladder, the needle could puncture the bladder rather than remove fluid from the abdominal cavity.**   Pl Ph/9 1
1. There is no need to insert an indwelling catheter. Having the client void prior to the procedure will empty the bladder.
3. There is no need to keep the client NPO prior to a paracentesis. This is performed at the bedside with a local anesthetic in the skin.

ANSWER	RATIONALE	NP	CN	SA

4. There is no need to administer an enema prior to the procedure. During a paracentesis, fluid is removed from the peritoneal cavity.

#51. 1. Deep-breathing and coughing helps to prevent atelectasis.   Pl   Ph/9   1

2. Flexing and extending the feet will help to prevent thrombophlebitis and is appropriate for a client on bed rest, but does not prevent atelectasis.
3. Antiembolism stockings may be ordered for a client on bed rest. However, they help to prevent thrombophlebitis. They do not prevent atelectasis.
4. Range-of-motion exercises are appropriate for someone who is on prolonged bed rest, but they do not prevent atelectasis.

#52. 1. A tuberculin skin test is an intradermal test and is administered at a 10- to 15-degree angle.   Im   He/4   1

2. A tuberculin skin test is an intradermal test and is administered at a 10- to 15-degree angle.
3. A tuberculin skin test is an intradermal test and is administered at a 10- to 15-degree angle. A subcutaneous injection is administered at a 60-degree angle.
4. A tuberculin skin test is an intradermal test and is administered at a 10- to 15-degree angle. An intramuscular injection is administered at a 90-degree angle.

#53. 3. Walking is one of the best forms of exercise. Walking daily is good for the heart and helps keep weight under control. This statement indicates the client does not understand the teaching.   Ev   He/4   1

1. Smoking is thought to be a factor in the development of heart disease and several types of cancer. This statement indicates the client understands the teaching.
2. A high fat intake increases the risk of heart disease. This statement indicates the client understands the teaching.
4. A diet that is high in fruits and vegetables is thought to reduce the risk of heart disease and several types of cancer. This statement indicates the client understands the teaching.

#54. 3. The last Hemophilous (HIB) immunization is usually given at 12–15 months. Varicella or chickenpox vaccine is recommended at 12 months.   Im   He/4   4

1. Measles, Mumps, Rubella (MMR) is given at 15 months. The child does not develop adequate antibody levels when MMR is given before 15 months. Diphtheria, Tetanus, and Pertussis (DTP) is usually given at two, four, and six months with a booster at 18 months and another booster when the child starts school.
2. Hepatitis B is given at birth and at one month and six months. Polio vaccine is given at two months and four months and a booster at 18 months, with another booster when the child starts school.
4. Most well children do not receive pneumonia vaccine. Tetanus is part of the DTP and is usually given at two, four, and six months with boosters at 18 months and when the child starts school.

#55. 4. Bruises and areas that look like cigarette burns on the back are not likely to be due to bumping into things. These findings suggest abuse and should be reported so they can be investigated.   Dc   Ps/6   1

1. Taking some of the client's social security money for food and medicine does not indicate abuse.
2. Elderly clients bruise easily. While the nurse should carefully assess these bruises, they do not necessarily suggest abuse. Bruises on the back and those that look like cigarette burns are much more suggestive of abuse.
3. Hiring a sitter when the family is not at home is an indication of concern about the client's safety, not an indication of abuse.

#56. 3. The nurse should first inspect the abdomen. Then the abdomen can be auscultated, followed by percussion and palpation.   Dc   He/4   1

1. The nurse inspects the abdomen before auscultating.

    2. The nurse should first inspect the abdomen. Percussing may affect the bowel sounds so auscultation should be done prior to percussing.

    4. The nurse should first inspect the abdomen. Palpation may change the bowel sounds so auscultation should be done prior to palpation.

#57. 4. The woman should use either a circular or an up-and-down pattern to assess every part of both breasts in both an upright and a supine position. This statement indicates the client understands the teaching.   Ev   He/4   3

    1. The client should examine her breasts every month following her menstrual period. This statement indicates the client does not understand the teaching.

    2. The woman can do a self breast exam. There is no need to see a physician for a breast exam every six months. This statement indicates the client does not understand the teaching.

    3. While the incidence of breast cancer increases with age, breast cancer can occur at any age, even in teens. This statement indicates the client does not understand the teaching.

#58. 2. DPT stands for diphtheria, pertussis (whooping cough), and tetanus.   Im   He/4   4

    1. DPT stands for diphtheria, pertussis (whooping cough), and tetanus.

    3. DPT stands for diphtheria, pertussis (whooping cough), and tetanus.

    4. DPT stands for diphtheria, pertussis (whooping cough), and tetanus.

#59. 3. Hand-washing is the best way to prevent transmission of infection. The nurse should teach the family proper hand-washing technique.   Pl   Sa/2   1

    1. There is no need to isolate the client from the rest of the family. Good hand-washing technique should prevent the spread of infection.

    2. Good hand-washing technique should prevent transmission of infection.

    4. There is no need to restrict visitors. Good hand-washing technique should prevent the spread of infection.

#60. 3. Permission can be revoked. The client does have a right to change her mind. The nurse should call the physician and have her talk with the client.   Im   Sa/1   1

    1. Permission can be revoked. The client does have a right to change her mind.

    2. The nurse should not medicate the client for two reasons. First, the client said she did not want surgery. Second, the client should be alert when talking with the physician.

    4. This response does not address the client's statement that she had changed her mind about having the surgery. This is not the appropriate response at this time.

#61. 2. The nurse should teach the family to check the restrained extremities at least every two hours for circulation. The restraints should also be removed periodically, usually one at a time, to perform range-of-motion.   Pl   Sa/2   1

    1. The restraints should be removed periodically, usually every two hours, for range-of- motion exercises. They should be removed one at a time.

    3. Removing the restraints whenever someone is with the client may not be feasible. If the caregiver is busy, the client could remove the catheter.

    4. The restraints should be periodically removed, when it is safe to do so. The nurse does not need to be present when the restraints are removed.

#62. 2. The person who has Parkinson's Disease shuffles when he walks. Smooth-soled shoes allow him to walk without tripping and falling.   Ev   Sa/2   1

    1. The person who has Parkinson's Disease shuffles when he walks. Rubber-soled shoes do not allow the client to shuffle without tripping.

3. The person who has Parkinson's Disease shuffles when he walks. Elevated shoes would tend to make him unstable.

4. The person who has Parkinson's Disease shuffles when he walks. If the client wears open-toed shoes, he is likely to injure his toes when he shuffles.

#63. 1. **The nurse should immediately place the syringe with needle attached into the disposal container. The needle should not be recapped. Recapping needles is one of the most common types of injuries to nurses and a common way to spread HIV infection and hepatitis.** Im   Sa/2   1

2. The needle should not be recapped. Recapping needles is one of the most common types of injuries to nurses and a common way to spread HIV infection and hepatitis.

3. The needle and syringe should not be separated before placing in the disposal container. This increases the risk of nurse exposure to blood and to needle sticks.

4. The needle should not be recapped. Recapping needles is one of the most common types of injuries to nurses and a common way to spread HIV infection and hepatitis. There is no need to cut the syringe before placing in disposal container. This would increase the risk of nurse exposure to client's body fluids and needle sticks.

#64. 3. **Oxygen supports combustion so the nurse should immediately turn off the oxygen and then remove the client from the area. Remember RACE (Remove, Alarm, Contain, Evacuate).** Im   Sa/2   1

1. The nurse should assure the client's safety first, then sound the alarm. The nurse should not leave the client in danger.

2. Asking the visitor to tell someone else might be appropriate, but the nurse should turn off the oxygen and remove the client from danger immediately. If the nurse can also calm the client, that might be appropriate, but is not the initial action.

4. The client's safety is the nurse's first priority. Remember RACE (Remove, Alarm, Contain, Evacuate). Turning off the oxygen should be done immediately. Oxygen supports combustion.

#65. 2. **Clotting disorders such as thrombophlebitis contraindicate the use of oral contraceptives as they can cause clotting. Other vascular conditions such as migraine headaches and smoking more than half a pack of cigarettes a day also contraindicate the use of oral contraceptives.** Dc   He/3   5

1. A history of gonorrhea is not a contraindication for oral contraceptives. The client should be advised to use barriers such as condoms in addition to the oral contraceptive to prevent disease transmission.

3. A family history of diabetes does not contraindicate the use of oral contraceptives.

4. Bladder infection does not contraindicate the use of oral contraceptives.

#66. 2. **When a woman is admitted in labor, the nurse should assess the frequency and duration of contractions.** Dc   He/3   3

1. Age of the client is "nice-to-know information." It is most critical to know the frequency and duration of contractions. Due date is also important information.

3. Status of the membranes is important information, but not as critical as frequency and duration of contractions.

4. Who will be assisting the woman during labor is "nice-to-know" information, but not as important as frequency and duration of contractions.

#67. 3. **Swelling in the upper body is suggestive of pregnancy-induced hypertension. The woman is in the third trimester, when PIH is most apt to occur.** Dc   He/3   3

1. A trace of glucose in the urine is common in pregnant women. The woman will be followed carefully, but this should not cause great alarm.

2. During the third trimester, the client should gain about a pound a week. This is a normal finding.

4. Ankle and foot edema in the third trimester is a normal finding. The enlarging uterus decreases venous return from the lower extremities and causes foot and ankle edema.

#68. 4. Ego integrity is the developmental task of the older adult.   Pl   He/3   2

1. Identity is the developmental task of the adolescent.

2. Intimacy is the developmental task of the young adult.

3. Generativity is the developmental task of the middle adult.

#69. 3. The best method of contraception is usually the one the couple finds most acceptable. If a method is recommended that the couple will not use, the statistics are of little relevance.   Dc   He/3   1

1. The question states that it is a young couple. The exact age is not very important information.

2. The sexual history of both partners is less important information than the method of contraception they find most acceptable.

4. How soon they want to start a family may have some relevance. However, the method of contraception they find most acceptable is the most important information for the nurse to obtain.

#70. 2. The cord stump should be cleaned with alcohol at every diaper change. This finding indicates the mother understands the care.   Ev   He/3   4

1. A soft stool after every feeding is normal for a newborn. There is no need for the mother to be concerned.

3. The circumcised penis should not be cleaned with alcohol. Vaseline gauze may be on the penis, but not alcohol.

4. The baby should be nursed every 3–4 hours. It is not likely that an eight-pound baby needs to be nursed every hour.

#71. 4. Testicular cancer is primarily a young man's disease. It is highly curable when found early. This statement indicates the client does not understand the teaching and needs more instruction.   Ev   He/4   1

1. Self testicular examination should be done every month by every man from puberty onward. This answer indicates an understanding of the teaching.

2. The self testicular examination should be performed while the client is in the shower. This answer indicates an understanding of the teaching.

3. Lumps should be reported to the physician. This answer indicates an understanding of the teaching.

#72. 3. When people are facing a painful separation, they often think about prior painful separations. Thinking about his friend who died is evidence of separation anxiety.   Dc   Ps/5   2

1. This statement does not indicate separation anxiety.

2. This statement does not indicate separation anxiety.

4. This statement does not indicate separation anxiety.

#73. 4. The client's behavior indicates anxiety. This response will open communication and help the client to verbalize concerns.   Im   Ps/5   2

1. Answering the bell quickly is appropriate but is not likely to help control the behavior. A better response is to open communication.

2. This response is very nontherapeutic.

3. Asking a person "why" is not likely to be therapeutic because it puts the person on the defensive.

#74. 2. Daily weights are a good indication of fluid restoration. As the fluid is restored, the weight will increase.   Ev   Ph/10   1

1. Skin turgor assessment will give some idea of fluid balance, but daily weights are a better assessment. The client is elderly and most elderly clients have poor skin turgor.

3. Thirst is a late indicator of fluid loss. By the time a client complains of thirst, there is significant fluid loss. Daily weights give a better indication of the effectiveness of fluid restoration.

4. The nurse will record all intake. Recording intake shows what measures were taken to restore fluid balance but does not indicate if the measures were effective.

#75. 3. The chair should be on the client's unaffected side so the client can stand on the unaffected leg, pivot, and sit in the chair.   Im   Ph/7   1

1. The chair should be on the client's unaffected side so the client can stand on the unaffected leg, pivot, and sit in the chair. The client's affected side is the right.

2. The chair should be on the client's unaffected side so the client can stand on the unaffected leg, pivot, and sit in the chair. The chair should face the foot of the bed.

4. In this answer, the chair is on the correct side of the bed, but it should face the foot of the bed.

#76. 4. This correctly describes the three-point gait for someone who is unable to bear weight on the right foot. This gait is correct for this client.   Ev   Ph/7   1

1. This describes the four-point gait. The four-point gait is not appropriate for someone who has a broken right ankle and cannot bear weight on one foot. This gait is not correct for this client.

2. This response describes the two-point gait. The two-point gait is not appropriate for someone who has a broken ankle and cannot bear weight on both feet. This gait is not correct for this client.

3. This response describes the three-point gait for someone who cannot bear weight on the left foot. The client has a fractured right ankle. This gait is not correct for this client.

#77. 4. Pulling the client by the shoulders is not appropriate. A better approach would be to use a turning sheet or a pull sheet to pull the client up in bed. Pulling the client by the shoulders can damage the shoulders and also cause friction, which may lead to decubitus ulcer formation.   Ev   Ph/7   1

1. Using a pull sheet or a turning sheet is appropriate. This makes it easier for the nursing assistant and reduces skin breakdown in the client.

2. Asking another nursing assistant to help is appropriate. This makes it easier for both the nursing assistant and the client.

3. The head of the bed should be lowered before the client is pulled up in bed.

#78. 1. The nurse should try nonpharmacologic methods to help the client relax and go to sleep before asking for sleeping medication. This is not an appropriate initial action.   Im   Ph/7   1

2. A back rub often helps a person relax and makes it easier to go to sleep. This is an appropriate initial action.

3. Asking the client if she is concerned about something is an appropriate initial action. This opens communication and may reduce anxiety.

4. Repositioning the client who is having trouble sleeping may promote relaxation and is appropriate initially.

#79. 3. Antiembolism stockings will do most to help prevent venous stasis.   Pl   Ph/7   1

1. The immobilized client should deep-breathe and cough every two hours. However, this is done to prevent atelectasis, not thrombophlebitis.

2. Range-of-motion exercises are performed primarily to prevent joint contractures. They may be a little help in preventing thrombophlebitis. During range-of-motion exercises, the joint is moved. Exercises to prevent thrombophlebitis.

4. Turning every two hours is done primarily to prevent atelectasis and skin breakdown.

ANSWER	RATIONALE	NP	CN	SA

#80. 4. **A cool and blanched area around the infusion site suggests the IV may be infiltrated. This should be reported to the charge nurse immediately, because the IV must be discontinued.**   Dc   Ph/8   1

    1. Intravenous solutions are at room temperature and may feel cool to the client as they infuse. This is normal and does not need to be reported to the charge nurse.

    2. The infusion site is normally covered with clear tape. This does not need to be reported to the charge nurse.

    3. It is safe for clients to ambulate when an IV infusion is running. This does not need to be reported to the charge nurse.

#81. 4 **Before administering digoxin, the nurse should always check the client's apical pulse. If the adult client's pulse is below 60/min., the nurse should hold the medication and notify the physician.**   Im   Ph/8   5

    1. There is no need to check the client's temperature before administering digoxin. The nurse should check the client's apical pulse.

    2. There is no need to check the client's blood pressure when administering digoxin. The nurse should check the client's apical pulse.

    3. There is no need to check the client's respirations before administering digoxin. The nurse should check the client's apical pulse.

#82. 1. **Small doses of aspirin are frequently given to persons with long bone fractures to prevent clots from forming. A fat embolus is a potential complication of a long bone fracture. The tibia is a long bone in the lower leg.**   Im   Ph/8   5

    2. Small doses of aspirin are frequently given to persons with long bone fractures to prevent clots from forming. Baby aspirin is not given to an adult to lower body temperature.

    3. Baby aspirin is not given to an adult to control pain. Small doses of aspirin are frequently given to persons with long bone fractures to prevent clots from forming.

    4. Aspirin does have an anti-inflammatory effect. However, this is not the reason it is given to the client with a long bone fracture. Small doses of aspirin are frequently given to persons with long bone fractures to prevent clots from forming.

#83. 2. **Many drugs affect the action of warfarin. Both aspirin and acetaminophen potentiate the action of warfarin and could cause bleeding if taken when warfarin is being administered. Clients should be taught to avoid over-the-counter drugs without first checking with their physician.**   Pl   Ph/8   5

    1. There is no need to take warfarin on a full stomach.

    3. Aspirin is an anticoagulant and potentiates warfarin, which is also an anticoagulant. Taking aspirin with warfarin could cause the client to bleed.

    4. There is no need to avoid sun exposure when taking warfarin.

#84. 3. **Spansules are capsules with particles of medication that are coated so they will be absorbed at different times. Spansules should be given at 12-hour intervals.**   Pl   Ph/8   5

    1. Spansules should be taken at 12-hour intervals.

    2. A spansule should not be opened up. The little pellets are designed to be absorbed at different rates. The contents of the spansule should not be put in food.

    4. A spansule should not be cut.

#85. 2. **The client's remarks sound suicidal. The nurse should ask the client if she is considering hurting herself. This is a safety issue. The nurse should also record and report the client's remarks.**   Im   Ps/5   2

    1. Asking the client "why" questions puts her on the defensive. This is not therapeutic.

3.   The nurse should first assess suicide potential. Telling her that life is precious does not give recognition to what she is expressing. It is almost arguing with her and is not therapeutic.

4.   The nurse should first assess for suicide potential. Helping her see the good things in life does not give recognition to what she is expressing at the moment.

#86. 3.   Restating the client's remarks will open communication and allow the client to further express his feelings.   Im   Ps/5   2

1.   Saying "you are not a freak" is not therapeutic. This is arguing with the client and denying his feelings.

2.   Telling the client that lots of people have amputations and live a normal life is a true statement but is not the most therapeutic response. The nurse should initially let the client express his feelings.

4.   Responding by telling the client he shouldn't say what he said is very judgmental and will not open communication.

#87. 1.   In order to deal with his anxiety, the client must first recognize that he is anxious.   Dc   Ps/5   2

2.   Identifying the situations that precipitated his anxiety is a later step in the process. The client must first recognize that he is anxious.

3.   Understanding the reason for his anxiety is a later step in the process. The client must first recognize that he is anxious.

4.   Selecting a strategy to cope with his anxiety is a later step in the process. The client must first recognize that he is anxious.

#88. 3.   The client is experiencing phantom pain. This is real pain. The nurse should administer the ordered medications first. Later, the nurse can encourage the client to discuss his feelings.   Im   Ps/5   2

1.   Elevating the stump will not relieve the pain. The stump should only be elevated for the first 24–48 hours following an amputation.

2.   The client is experiencing phantom pain. This is real pain. The nurse should administer the ordered medications first.

4.   The client is experiencing phantom pain. This is real pain. The nurse should administer the ordered medications first. After medicating the client, the nurse can encourage the client to express his feelings.

#89. 3.   Reminding her an hour before meals that mealtime is coming up will allow her time to complete the washing ritual so she will be able to get to meals.   Pl   Ps/6   2

1.   Interrupting the ritual will increase the client's anxiety and may precipitate a panic attack.

2.   The client needs to learn to function. Bringing meals to her only encourages the ritualistic behavior.

4.   The rituals are so important to the obsessive-compulsive client that if given a choice between the rituals and meals, the rituals will seem more important and the client will not eat.

#90. 1.   This comment indicates the mother does not understand the developmental level of an eight-month-old. A child of eight months does not cry just to irritate his parents. Parents who abuse their children often have unrealistic expectations of the developmental level.   Dc   Ps/6   4

2.   This comment is one that most parents would make and indicates concern and a desire to understand what the infant needs. This is not suggestive of child abuse.

3.   This comment indicates the mother is trying to meet the infant's needs. It indicates a need for instruction about infants and needs other than feeding. However, it does not indicate possible child abuse.

4.   This comment indicates a desire to understand what the infant wants. It does not suggest child abuse.

#91. 4.   Putting her favorite picture on the door to her room should help her find her room.   Pl   Ps/6   1

1.   Wandering is not an indication for restraints.

ANSWER	RATIONALE	NP	CN	SA

2. Asking a roommate in an acute care setting to take responsibility for another client is not appropriate.

3. Punishing the client is not appropriate. She is not deliberately misbehaving. The disease process makes her confused.

#92. 2. The LPN/LVN should notify the charge nurse regarding this information. The client needs referral to a battered women's shelter. The psychiatric clinical specialist nurse may be called in to talk with this client. This situation needs referral; it is beyond the scope of the practical nurse. — Im — Ps/6 — 2

1. The woman who is abused often feels helpless and unable to get out of the situation. Asking the client why she stays with a man who has caused her to get hurt may give her more guilt.

3. Asking the client about divorce is premature at this time. The practical nurse should notify the charge nurse so appropriate referrals for the client's safety can be made is more appropriate. This situation is beyond the scope of the practical nurse.

4. Simply telling the client she has rights will not assure her safety. This situation is beyond the scope of the practical nurse and should be referred to the charge nurse.

#93. 2. The client should avoid persons who are sick because radiation therapy causes bone marrow depression making the client susceptible to infection. — Im — Ph/10 — 1

1. The person receiving external radiation is not a danger to others.

3. The person receiving external radiation is not a danger to others.

4. The person receiving external radiation is not a danger to others.

#94. 3. When a person is in shock and has a decreased circulating blood volume, the urine output decreases. — Dc — Ph/10 — 1

1. When a person is in shock, the systolic and diastolic blood pressure drop. The systolic pressure drops more than the diastolic so the pulse pressure narrows. Elevated systolic and lowered diastolic pressure is seen with increasing intracranial pressure.

2. When a person is in shock, the heart rate increases.

4. When a person is in shock, the respiratory rate increases.

#95. 2. When a person is unresponsive the nurse should initially assess respirations and pulse. — Dc — Ph/10 — 1

1. When a person is unresponsive the nurse should assess before starting chest compressions.

3. When a person is unresponsive the nurse should assess before starting CPR. If CPR is necessary, the client should be on a hard surface.

4. When a person is unresponsive the nurse should assess before starting mouth-to-mouth breathing.

#96. 2. Antihypertensives and vasodilators should not be given before dialysis because the blood pressure drops significantly during the procedure. — Im — Ph/10 — 5

1. Antihypertensives and vasodilators should not be given before dialysis because the blood pressure drops significantly during the procedure.

3. Antihypertensives and vasodilators should not be given before dialysis because the blood pressure drops significantly during the procedure.

4. Antihypertensives and vasodilators should not be given before dialysis because the blood pressure drops significantly during the procedure.

#97. 1. The nurse should release the suction by opening the vent to stop the pulling action of the suction (take your finger off the hole). — Im — Ph/10 — 1

2. If the suction is pulling the tracheal wall, the nurse should not continue to suction. This causes further damage to the tracheal wall.

3. The nurse should not increase pressure as this would cause further damage to the tracheal wall.

    4. When the catheter is attaching to the tracheal wall it will be nearly impossible to suction deeper. The nurse should release the suction by taking the finger off the hole.

#98. 2. When there is no bubbling in the water seal compartment it means either that the lung has reexpanded or that there is an obstruction in the tubing coming from the pleural cavity. It is not very likely that the lung has reexpanded in four hours. It is much more likely that there is an obstruction in the tubing.   Dc   Ph/9   1

    1. When there is no bubbling in the water seal compartment it means either that the lung has reexpanded or that there is an obstruction in the tubing coming from the pleural cavity. It is not very likely that the lung has reexpanded in four hours. It is much more likely that there is an obstruction in the tubing.

    3. An air leak would cause no bubbling in the suction control chamber.

    4. When the suction is not turned on there is no bubbling in the suction control chamber. There may still be bubbles in the water seal chamber as there will still be gravity drainage.

#99. 4. Increasing respiratory difficulty indicates the congestive heart failure is worsening. Before calling the physician, the nurse should raise the head of the bed to ease the client's breathing.   Im   Ph/10   1

    1. Increasing respiratory difficulty indicates the congestive heart failure is getting worse. Increasing the drip rate will further increase the overload situation and make the client worse. The nurse should decrease the IV drip rate and raise the head of the bed.

    2. Increasing respiratory difficulty indicates the congestive heart failure is getting worse. Placing the client in a supine position will make the symptoms worse. The client should be placed in a semi- to high Fowler's position to make breathing easier.

    3. Increasing respiratory difficulty indicates the congestive heart failure is getting worse. The nurse should take measures to make the client more comfortable. Asking questions that require him to talk waste energy without giving useful information.

#100. 2. Oxygen is very drying to tissues. Humidifying oxygen helps to prevent drying of tissues.   Im   Ph/10   1

    1. The water doesn't cool the oxygen; it humidifies the oxygen.

    3. The water humidifies the oxygen. The purpose of the water is not to prevent fires.

    4. The reason for humidifying oxygen is to keep the tissues from drying out. Humidifying oxygen does not prevent infections from developing in the tubing.

Practice Test Two

1. An adult client who had major abdominal surgery is returned to her room on the surgical nursing unit. The post-anesthesia nurse reports that the client is awake and has stable vital signs. She has a nasogastric tube in place that is attached to intermittent suction. The nurse should position the client in which of the following positions?
   1. Supine
   2. Semi-Fowler's
   3. Dorsal recumbent
   4. Prone

2. An adult post-operative client vomits and his abdominal wound eviscerates. What is the best initial action for the nurse to take?
   1. Cover the exposed coils of intestine with sterile moist towels or dressings.
   2. Pack the intestines back into the abdominal cavity.
   3. Irrigate the exposed coils of intestines with sterile water.
   4. Take the client's vital signs.

3. Thirty-six hours after major surgery a client has a temperature of 100°F. What is the most likely cause of the temperature elevation?
   1. Dehydration
   2. Atelectasis
   3. Wound infection
   4. Bladder infection
4. The nurse is preparing to administer pre-operative medication of meperidine and atropine to an elderly adult who is scheduled for surgery. The client tells the nurse he has glaucoma and wants to take his eye drops before going to the operating room. What is the best action for the nurse to take?
   1. Administer medication as ordered and encourage the client to take his eye drops.
   2. Check with the physician before administering pre-operative medication.
   3. Administer pre-operative medication as ordered and suggest the client not take his eye drops.
   4. Administer the meperidine; withhold atropine and suggest the client take his eye drops.
5. An adult client has been medicated for elective surgery. The operating room nurse discovers that the consent form for surgery has not been signed. What should the nurse do?
   1. Have the client sign the consent form.
   2. Tell the physician that the consent form has not been signed.
   3. Have the client's spouse sign the consent form.
   4. Continue preparation for surgery as the client has given implied consent.
6. An elderly man has just returned from the operating room where he spent several hours in lithotomy position during a perineal prostatectomy. Which assessment should the nurse make because the client was in lithotomy position during surgery?
   1. Lower extremity pulses, paresthesias, and pain
   2. The presence of bowel sounds
   3. Radial pulse, sensation, and movement of the arms
   4. Palpation of the bladder
7. An elderly client is admitted to a skilled nursing care facility. When doing a skin assessment the nurse notes a 3-cm round area of partial-thickness skin loss that looks like a blister on the client's sacrum. The nurse interprets this to be a
   1. stage I pressure ulcer.
   2. stage II pressure ulcer.
   3. stage III pressure ulcer.
   4. stage IV pressure ulcer.
8. The nurse is caring for a client who has been placed on a hypothermia blanket. What should the nurse include in the care plan?

1. Take frequent vital signs and perform frequent skin assessments.
2. Leave the hypothermia blanket on until the client's temperature reaches 98.6°F.
3. Place the client directly on the blanket.
4. Apply iced alcohol sponges to the part of the client's trunk not in contact with the blanket.
9. The physician's orders include warm compresses to the left leg three times a day for treatment of an open wound. Which action is appropriate when carrying out these orders?
   1. Use medical aseptic technique.
   2. Leave the wet compress open to the air.
   3. Place both a dry covering and waterproof material over the compress.
   4. Remove the compress after five minutes.
10. An adult is on a clear liquid diet. Which food should the nurse offer him?
    1. A milk shake
    2. Fruited gelatin
    3. Sherbet
    4. Apple juice
11. Four clients have signaled with their call bell for the nurse. Whom should the nurse observe first?
    1. An adult who needs assistance walking to the bathroom
    2. A postoperative client who is asking for pain medication
    3. An adult who has just been given penicillin
    4. An elderly client who is in a gerry chair with a restraint vest on
12. The nurse is caring for a client who was in a motor vehicle accident. His blood pressure is dropping rapidly. What should the nurse observe the client for before placing the client in shock position?
    1. Long bone fractures
    2. Air embolus
    3. Head injury
    4. Thrombophlebitis
13. The nurse is teaching family members how to correctly transfer a client who has right hemiplegia from the bed to a wheelchair. Which observation indicates the family understands how to transfer the client?
    1. The wheelchair is placed parallel to the bed on the affected side.
    2. The family members lift the client up by having her place her arms around their necks.
    3. The wheelchair is placed at a 45-degree angle to the bed on the client's unaffected side.
    4. The family members ask for a trapeze bar for the client to use in the transfer.
14. An adult is being discharged from the emergency room with instructions to apply a cold pack to his sprained ankle. The client

asks why it is necessary to use a cold pack. The nurse replies that the cold pack will do which of the following?
1. Keep the sprain from becoming a fracture
2. Prevent bruising and ecchymosis from occurring
3. Keep the client from developing a fever
4. Help reduce swelling and pain

15. An adult has received an injection of immunoglobulin. The client asks what this injection will do for him. The nurse's reply includes the information that he will develop which type of immunity as a result of this injection?
1. Active natural immunity
2. Active artificial immunity
3. Passive natural immunity
4. Passive artificial immunity

16. An adult is receiving total parenteral nutrition (TPN). Which assessment is essential for the nurse to make?
1. Number of bowel movements
2. Confirmation that the tube is in the stomach
3. Auscultation of bowel sounds
4. Daily weights

17. An adult is on long-term aspirin therapy and complains of tinnitus. Which interpretation by the nurse is accurate?
1. The aspirin is working as expected.
2. The client ingested more medication than was recommended.
3. The client has an upper GI bleed.
4. The client is experiencing a minor overdose.

18. An adult is to receive a narcotic analgesic via patient-controlled analgesia (PCA). Which statement by the client indicates that the client understands how the PCA works?
1. "When I press this button the machine will always give me more medicine."
2. "I will press the button whenever I begin to experience pain."
3. "I should press this button every hour so the pain doesn't come back."
4. "With this machine I will experience no more pain."

19. The nurse is caring for a client who had knee surgery this morning. Post-operative orders include a narcotic every 3–4 hours as needed for operative-site pain and an ice bag. At 7 p.m. the client asks for pain medication. He was last medicated at 3:30 p.m. What is the best initial nursing action?
1. Administer the prescribed analgesic.
2. Assess the location and nature of the pain.
3. Refill the ice bag as needed.
4. Reposition the client.

20. An adult is receiving external radiation therapy. What should the nurse include in the teaching plan about care of the skin at the radiation site?

1. Tape a loose dressing to the radiation site.
2. Shower each evening before therapy.
3. Apply ice compresses to the site to relieve pain.
4. Avoid washing the skin in the area being radiated.

21. A client is receiving chemotherapy for cancer and develops thrombocytopenia. What should the nurse include in the client's plan of care because of the thrombocytopenia?
1. Place the client in a semi-upright position.
2. Limit the client's intake of fluids.
3. Administer no injections.
4. Exercise the client's lower extremities.

22. An adult is admitted with a head injury following an accident. He has a severe headache and asks the nurse why he cannot have something for pain. The nurse understands that the client should not receive a narcotic analgesic for which reason? Narcotic analgesics
1. cause mydriasis, which will raise intracranial pressure.
2. are not effective for pain caused by brain trauma.
3. cause vomiting, which would mask a sign of increased intracranial pressure.
4. may depress respirations, which would cause acidosis and further brain damage.

23. A client is scheduled for a cataract extraction. Pre-operatively 1% atropine is instilled into the client's right eye. The nurse knows this drug would be contraindicated if she also had which of the following conditions?
1. Bradycardia
2. Hypothyroidism
3. Diabetes
4. Glaucoma

24. An adult is admitted with Guillain-Barré syndrome. On day three of hospitalization, the client's muscle weakness worsens and he is no longer able to stand with support. He is also having difficulty swallowing and talking. The priority in the nursing care plan at this time is to prevent which problem?
1. Aspiration pneumonia
2. Decubitus ulcers
3. Bladder distention
4. Hypertensive crisis

25. A young woman is admitted to the hospital complaining of severe fatigue and weakness of one week duration. Her physician suspects a diagnosis of myasthenia gravis. Which additional findings would the nurse expect the client to have?
1. Ataxia and poor coordination
2. Diplopia and ptosis of the eyelids
3. Slurred speech
4. Headaches and tinnitus

26. The nurse is caring for a client who has a C-6 spinal cord injury. He complains of blurred vision and a severe headache. His blood

pressure is 210/140. What action should the nurse take initially?
1. Check for bladder distention.
2. Place in Trendelenburg position.
3. Administer prn pain medication.
4. Continue to monitor blood pressure.

27. The charge nurse in a long-term care facility is making assignments. When assigning personnel to care for residents, which principle is important?
1. Assignments should be rotated on a daily basis.
2. Clients who are confused often do better with the same caregiver for several days.
3. Female caregivers should not care for male residents.
4. Caregivers should be allowed to select the residents they will care for.

28. The family of a young man who has been declared brain dead following an accident tells the nurse that the doctors said their son would be a good organ donor. They ask the nurse if donating his organs would mean that they could not have a regular funeral. Which response by the nurse is most accurate?
1. "Donating organs does deface the body, so a closed casket is necessary."
2. "Ask the physician which organs would be donated."
3. "Organ donation involves a surgical incision but should not interfere with any type of funeral."
4. "Donating organs is a wonderful service to humanity."

29. All of the following tasks need to be done. Which one can the LPN/LVN safely delegate to the certified nursing assistant (CNA)?
1. Tube feeding for a client with a nasogastric tube
2. Routine vital signs for a group of clients
3. Blood pressure monitoring for a client who is in congestive heart failure
4. Wound care for a client with a stage III decubitus ulcer

30. The nurse is new to the resident facility and is administering medications. One of the clients does not have a readable identification band in place. What should the nurse do?
1. Ask the client what his name is.
2. Ask the client if he is Mr. _____.
3. Ask the roommate if this is Mr. _____.
4. Check the bed tag for the name.

31. The nurse is caring for all of the following persons. Which one is most in need of restraints?
1. An elderly man who is sitting in a chair
2. A confused post-operative client who is picking at his nasal oxygen and NG tube
3. A confused woman who is in bed with the side rails up

4. An adult who has just returned to the surgical floor from a post-anesthesia care unit

32. The RN charge nurse hands the LPN/LVN a syringe filled with medication that the RN has just drawn and asks the LPN/LVN to administer this to a client. How should the LPN/LVN respond?
1. Do as requested by the charge nurse.
2. Ask the charge nurse what the medication is and then administer it.
3. Ask the charge nurse what the medication is, check the order and then administer it.
4. Refuse to administer the medication.

33. An adult client in an acute care facility says to the nurse, "I hope this hospital doesn't have student doctors and nurses. I do not want a student taking care of me." The nurse's response should be based on which of the following understandings?
1. When a client signs permission for treatment in a hospital, this includes treatment by medical and nursing students.
2. The client has the right to know if the hospital is affiliated with a medical school and to refuse care by students.
3. The client may sign a special form that says he refuses to be cared for by medical or nursing students.
4. The client should be informed if any caregivers are students but the client does not have the right to refuse to be cared for by students.

34. An adult client in an acute care setting asks the nurse to show him his hospital records. The nurse's response should reflect which understanding?
1. The client has no right to see his records without a court order.
2. The client must have the physician's approval before he can see his records.
3. The client has the right to see his records and to have information explained when necessary.
4. The client must ask permission to view his records from the medical records department and must appear before a special committee.

35. The LPN/LVN has delegated basic hygienic care of several clients to a certified nursing assistant. Which action by the nurse will assure that the clients receive the best care?
1. Observe the nursing assistant during the performance of all care.
2. Ask the nursing assistant if there were any problems.
3. Check the nursing assistant's charting.
4. Observe the clients following administration of care by the nursing assistants.

36. A client who is withdrawing from alcohol says to the nurse, "There are snakes on the wall." Which action should the nurse take initially?
   1. Reassure the client there are no snakes.
   2. Turn the lights on brighter.
   3. Tell the client that while he may see snakes there are really no snakes.
   4. Reassure the client the snakes will not hurt him.

37. The client is scheduled for a myelogram today. The permit has been signed. The client tells the nurse that she has changed her mind and does not want to have the procedure. What should the nurse do?
   1. Tell the client that once permission has been given the procedure has to be done.
   2. Tell the client that the physician will be very upset if she does not have it done.
   3. Suggest to the client that it is in her best interests to have the procedure as scheduled.
   4. Understand that the client has the right to change her mind about procedures.

38. The nurse is caring for a woman who is receiving internal radiation for cancer of the cervix. Which nursing action will do most to reduce the risk of radiation exposure to other clients?
   1. Keep the door to the client's room closed.
   2. Place the client in the bed closest to the outside window.
   3. Place the client in a room close to the nurse's station for continuous observation.
   4. Place a "do not enter" sign on the door to the client's room.

39. The nurse is caring for a 79-year-old client. Which observation is not normal and should be reported for follow-up?
   1. The client has several brown spots on her cheek and neck.
   2. The client says, "I move slower than I used to."
   3. The client is short of breath when walking down the hall.
   4. The client says, "I have trouble telling the colors of my socks."

40. The nurse is caring for an aging client. Which statement the client makes indicates he is having difficulty with the developmental tasks of aging?
   1. "I like to make toys for my grandchildren."
   2. "I used to be a farmer, now I can't do all that hard work."
   3. "I wish I had changed careers when I really wanted to; now it's too late."
   4. "We don't have as much money now as we did before I retired."

41. A young woman who is at 32 weeks gestation reports to the physician's office for a routine prenatal visit. Which comment by the woman must be reported to the physician?

   1. "I had to stop wearing my rings because my fingers are swollen."
   2. "I seem to be hotter than everyone else."
   3. "My feet tend to swell in the hot weather."
   4. "My breasts are so big and tender."

42. The nurse is caring for an older adult. Which statement made by the client is not typical of normal aging?
   1. "I seem to be more sensitive to the taste of salt than I used to be."
   2. "I have trouble reading the newspaper."
   3. "I don't drive at dusk any more."
   4. "Sometimes I have trouble matching my socks."

43. The nurse is to obtain pedal pulses on a client following a cardiac catheterization. Which is the proper procedure?
   1. Place the fingertips against the wrist bone.
   2. Place the stethoscope over the apex of the heart.
   3. Place the fingertips against the side of the neck.
   4. Place the fingertips on top of the foot.

44. The nurse is to obtain an apical-radial pulse on a client. Which statement is true regarding obtaining an apical-radial pulse?
   1. After taking the apical pulse the nurse immediately takes the radial pulse.
   2. The radial pulse is usually higher than the apical pulse.
   3. One person takes the apical pulse while the second person takes the radial pulse at the same time.
   4. The nurse should take the radial pulse while listening to the apical pulse.

45. The nurse is assessing the client's vital signs and notes that the client is breathing very noisily. The nurse describes this pattern of breathing as
   1. hyperpnea.
   2. Cheyne-Stokes.
   3. orthopnea.
   4. sterterous.

46. The nurse is obtaining a blood pressure on a client who weighs over 300 pounds. The nurse chooses to use a large cuff for which of the following reasons?
   1. A large cuff is more comfortable for the client.
   2. Using a cuff that is too small causes the blood pressure reading to be abnormally high.
   3. When a regular cuff is used on a large person it is difficult to hear the pulse.
   4. A small cuff on a large person causes the systolic pressure to read lower than normal and the diastolic pressure to read higher than normal.

47. A post-operative client is to be discharged today. She will need to change her dressing daily. Which statement she makes indicates she understands the process?

1. "I will wash my hands before and after I change the dressing."
2. "I can touch the dressings with my hands if I only touch the edges."
3. "I should clean the area around the incision by moving the swab toward it."
4. "I can put the old dressings directly in the waste basket."

48. The nurse is caring for a client who is on bed rest for an extended period of time. When planning care the nurse knows that which nursing action will do most to help prevent muscle atrophy?
    1. Perform passive range-of-motion exercises on the client.
    2. Turn the client at two-hour intervals.
    3. Encourage the client to change positions frequently.
    4. Assist the client in the performance of active exercises.

49. The nurse is caring for a client who has been on bed rest for several weeks. Which problem is least likely to be related to bed rest?
    1. Muscle atrophy
    2. Hypostatic pneumonia
    3. Varicose veins
    4. Thrombophlebitis

50. The nurse is planning care for a client who must remain in bed for several weeks. Which action will do most to prevent the development of pressure ulcers?
    1. Performing range-of-motion exercises
    2. Deep breathing and coughing
    3. Keeping the feet against a footboard
    4. Changing position in bed frequently

51. The nurse is observing a certified nursing assistant move a client. Which action, if observed, indicates that the nursing assistant needs more instruction?
    The assistant
    1. stands with feet spread apart.
    2. bends from the waist.
    3. turns her whole body.
    4. keeps her back straight.

52. An adult client who is ambulating in the corridor with the nurse becomes dizzy and faint. What should the nurse do at this time?
    1. Have her put her head between her legs.
    2. Quickly go to get help.
    3. Guide her to a chair in the corridor and ease her into it.
    4. Encourage the client to walk faster.

53. The nurse is caring for a client admitted with a sickle cell crisis. What assessment finding is not consistent with the diagnosis?
    1. Enlarged liver and spleen
    2. Jaundice and icterus
    3. Decreased white blood count
    4. Abdominal and joint pain

54. The wife of a man who is diagnosed with angina pectoris asks the nurse how she would know if her husband had a heart attack rather than angina. What should the nurse include in the reply?
    1. Crushing chest pain not relieved by nitroglycerine is likely to be a heart attack.
    2. Epigastric pain relieved by antacids is likely to be angina.
    3. Chest pain that does not go down the left arm is usually angina.
    4. Chest pain not associated with activity or excitement is probably angina.

55. The nurse is caring for a man who has recently been diagnosed with angina. Which statement he makes indicates understanding of his condition?
    1. "I should not exercise now that I have angina."
    2. "If I have chest pain I will take a nitroglycerine."
    3. "Sexual activity is likely to cause a heart attack."
    4. "If I have any chest pain, I should immediately call my doctor."

56. The mother of a boy who has recently been diagnosed with sickle cell anemia is pregnant and asks the nurse if her unborn baby will have sickle cell. What information should the nurse include in the answer?
    1. Sickle cell anemia is a contagious disease but your child should no longer be communicable by the time the baby is born.
    2. When both parents are carriers there is a 25% chance that each child will have sickle cell anemia.
    3. Your sons have a 50% chance of having sickle cell, but daughters can only be carriers.
    4. The next child should be disease-free, but additional children have a chance of being born with the disease.

57. What nursing action is essential when oxygen is ordered for a client who is living at home?
    1. Assist the client and family in checking all electrical appliances in the vicinity for frayed cords.
    2. Encourage the client and family to purchase fire extinguishers.
    3. Remove electrical devices from the room where oxygen is in use.
    4. Encourage the client and family to carpet the client's room.

58. An adult who has a tracheostomy needs to be suctioned. How should the nurse position the client for this procedure?
    1. Supine
    2. Semi-Fowler's
    3. Sim's
    4. Semi-lateral

59. The client is admitted for a bronchoscopy this morning. Which question is essential for the nurse to ask the client?
    1. "When did you last eat?"

2. "Did you take the laxative as ordered?"
3. "What has the doctor told you about your procedure?"
4. "Have you had conscious sedation before?"

60. The nurse is caring for a client who had thoracic surgery yesterday and has a chest tube attached to water seal drainage. The client's family asks why he has to have a chest tube. What should the nurse include in the response?
The chest tube
1. allows air to enter the thoracic cavity to equalize pressures in the lung.
2. removes air from the pleural cavity and promotes re-expansion of the lung.
3. increases the amount of oxygen available to the lungs.
4. will help the wound heal faster and reduce scarring.

61. The nurse is caring for a client who had a chest tube inserted and attached to Pleurovac® drainage two days ago. There is no bubbling in the water seal chamber. What should the nurse assess initially?
1. Observe the wound for excess drainage.
2. Check the system for air leaks.
3. Auscultate the lungs.
4. See if the suction is turned on.

62. The client is receiving a gentamicin IV. Which finding may indicate an adverse response to gentamicin?
1. Decreased urine output
2. Blurred vision
3. Orange sputum
4. Hypertension

63. The nurse is caring for a client who had a cystoscopy earlier in the day. Which data from the client is of greatest concern to the nurse?
1. Complaint of back pain
2. Tea-colored urine
3. Leg cramps
4. Pink-tinged urine

64. A client who is diagnosed with cystitis has been given a prescription for pyridium. She asks the nurse why she has been given this medication. What should the nurse reply?
1. "Pyridium is an antibiotic that will kill the bacteria causing your infection."
2. "Pyridium is an analgesic that will make you less aware of the pain and discomfort."
3. "Pyridium is a urinary tract anesthetic that will kill the pain until the antibiotics have had time to work."
4. "Pyridium will help to prevent kidney damage from the bladder infection."

65. An adult is admitted with suspected urolithiasis. Which nursing diagnosis is of highest priority when planning nursing care for this client immediately after admission?

1. Acute pain
2. Diarrhea
3. Risk of ineffective health maintenance
4. Risk of infection

66. When admitting a client who has acute glomerulonephritis the nurse expects the client will report which information?
1. Recent bladder infection
2. History of previous kidney infections
3. Pharyngitis three weeks ago
4. Multiple sexual partners

67. The nurse is caring for an adult who has kidney stones. Which action is essential for the nurse to take?
1. Take blood pressure frequently.
2. Keep the client on bed rest.
3. Position the client supine.
4. Strain all urine.

68. The client is to be discharged after passing a uric acid kidney stone. This is the third time the client has been hospitalized for kidney stones. The nurse should teach the client to do which of the following?
1. Eat generous amounts of chicken and organ meats.
2. Drink lots of water.
3. Avoid vigorous activity.
4. Take the ordered allopurinol (Zyloprim) if the symptoms recur.

69. The client has just had a basal cell carcinoma removed in the doctor's office. Which statement the client makes indicates understanding regarding prevention and early detection of basal cell carcinoma?
1. "Moles that are round and brown should be seen immediately by my doctor."
2. "I should wear long sleeves when I am out in the sun."
3. "I should avoid using lotions and powders on my skin."
4. "I can use a tanning booth to get a tan since I can't stay in the sun very long."

70. Which statement made by an adolescent indicates understanding of how to reduce risk of osteoporosis later in life?
1. "I will be careful not to sprain my ankle when I play sports."
2. "I drink a glass of milk with every meal."
3. "As I get older I will reduce the amount of weight-bearing exercise I do."
4. "My favorite beverages are cola drinks."

71. The nurse is caring for a client who has right-sided weakness and has been told to use a cane for walking. Which action by the client indicates he can use a cane correctly?
1. He moves the cane with the right leg when walking.
2. He moves the cane from hand to hand when walking.
3. He carries the cane on his left side and moves it at the same time he moves his right foot.

4. He puts the cane forward, then moves the left foot forward followed by the right foot.
72. An adult has low back pain. Which position is likely to be most comfortable for the client?
    1. Prone
    2. Supine
    3. Side-lying with knees flexed
    4. Semi-Fowler's with legs extended
73. One of the campers at summer camp sprains his ankle. What action can the nurse take to help reduce the pain?
    1. Encourage the camper to gently exercise the ankle several times every hour.
    2. Apply an ice pack to the ankle.
    3. Keep the leg down to encourage blood flow.
    4. Apply a topical steroid ointment.
74. A home care client says she is having difficulty getting to sleep at night. Which suggestion could the nurse make to help the client?
    1. Exercise shortly before going to bed.
    2. Drink a cola beverage during the evening.
    3. Watch television after going to bed.
    4. Drink warm milk before going to bed.
75. The client's blood gas values are:
    pH 7.35; CO_2 60; HCO_3 34; pO_2 60.
    The nurse correctly interprets these to indicate the client is in which state?
    1. Compensated respiratory acidosis
    2. Partly compensated metabolic alkalosis
    3. Metabolic alkalosis
    4. Metabolic acidosis
76. What question should the nurse ask the client who presents for an MRI test?
    1. "Are you allergic to iodine or shellfish?"
    2. "When did you last eat or drink anything?"
    3. "Do you have any metal in your body?"
    4. "Did you take the laxative prep?"
77. The nurse notes all of the following. Which situation needs immediate attention?
    1. Dirty linen has fallen on the floor beside the bed of a bedridden client.
    2. Breakfast dishes remain on the overbed table two hours after mealtime.
    3. An elderly ambulatory client drops a glass of water on the floor beside the bed.
    4. The client's hi-low bed cannot be moved to the high position.
78. While caring for a woman who delivered a healthy term infant six hours ago, the nurse notes the fundus is soft, 2 cm above the umbilicus and off to the left. The lochia is red. The nurse suspects that the client has which problem?
    1. Retained placental fragments
    2. Perineal laceration
    3. Urinary retention
    4. Normal involution
79. The mother of a week-old infant says to the nurse "When will that ugly black cord thing come off?" How should the nurse reply?

1. "Are you wiping it with alcohol each time you change the baby's diaper?"
2. "It usually comes off in ten days to three weeks."
3. "It sounds as if it bothers you. Would you like to talk about it?
4. "It should be off by now. I'll have the doctor check to be sure there is no problem."
80. A six-month-old infant is being seen in the doctor's office. Which observation by the nurse should be brought to the physician's attention?
    The baby
    1. sits up but needs slight support.
    2. was seven pounds at birth and now weighs ten pounds.
    3. frequently drops objects and looks for them.
    4. smacks her lips and drools.
81. The nurse is to administer a tube feeding to an adult. What action is essential before administering the feeding?
    1. Position the client in a supine position.
    2. Check the position of the feeding tube.
    3. Give the client something to suck on during the feeding.
    4. Check to see when the client last had a bowel movement.
82. An adult who had a mastectomy yesterday says to the nurse, "I guess I'm not a real woman anymore. How could my husband possibly love me now?" What is the best response for the nurse to make?
    1. "You don't feel like a woman now?"
    2. "Has your husband said anything to you?"
    3. "Of course your husband will love you."
    4. "True love is not dependent on breasts."
83. A client who has been waiting for several hours in the clinic waiting room suddenly begins to shout, "I need some attention and I need it now!" How should the nurse respond initially?
    1. Tell the client to be quiet and that she will be seen as soon as possible.
    2. Immediately call security and the police.
    3. Talk with the woman and determine her immediate needs.
    4. Explain to the woman how busy the doctors are and that she will be seen soon.
84. The mother of six-month-old twins is in the doctor's office because one of the infants has an ear infection. The mother says to the nurse, "I just don't know if I can handle another problem. It is all so overwhelming." How should the nurse respond initially?
    1. "You're their mother. I'm sure you know what's best for them."
    2. "Have you called social services to see if you qualify for assistance?"
    3. "My sister had twins and she survived. You will too."

4. "It must be tough to have two little ones. What seems to be the biggest problem?"

85. There have been several clients recently who have fallen in the long-term care facility. The nurse would like to reduce the number of falls. Which action is likely to do the most to help prevent falls?
    1. Ask the nursing assistants to watch the clients more carefully.
    2. Restrain clients who cannot walk independently.
    3. Provide call bells the clients can carry with them when they walk.
    4. Keep beds in the lowest position unless the nurse is performing care for the client.

86. The nurse is observing a nursing assistant providing care. Which action indicates that the nursing assistant understands universal precautions?
    The nursing assistant
    1. washes hands first thing in the morning before giving care to any client and again after all morning care is completed.
    2. wears gloves during all client contact.
    3. wears a gown when changing linen soiled with urine and feces.
    4. changes gloves between clients but does not wash hands if gloves have been worn.

87. The nurse is changing a dressing. Which event indicates a break in sterile technique?
    The nurse
    1. opens the sterile dressing set by opening the first flap away from the nurse.
    2. turns around when answering a question asked by the client in the other bed.
    3. opens the dressing set on the overbed table.
    4. pours sterile saline into the container in the dressing set.

88. The nurse is assisting at a disaster shelter set up following a devastating earthquake. What is the most common problem the nurse is likely to see in those who come to the shelter?
    1. Thirst
    2. Traumatic injuries
    3. Stress
    4. Exacerbation of medical problems

89. The nurse is caring for a frail elderly client in her home. Which behavior, if observed or reported, should the nurse report to the supervisor for further evaluation of possible abuse?
    1. The client's daughter is attempting to be declared her mother's legal guardian.
    2. The client is frequently left in bed alone in the house for several hours at a time.
    3. The client has brown spots on her arms.
    4. The client says "My daughter doesn't like me very much. She yells at me."

90. A woman is being seen in the physician's office for a medical complaint. When she is called to see the physician she goes to the restroom and washes her hands over and over, missing her allotted time with the physician. How should the nurse deal with this woman?
    1. Send her home without seeing the doctor if she is not available when called.
    2. Give her advance warning that she will be seeing the physician and tell her if she needs to wash her hands she should do so.
    3. Interrupt her washing ritual and insist she see the physician when it is her turn.
    4. Give her a choice of seeing the physician or washing her hands.

91. A woman who was recently widowed says to the nurse, "I just can't believe he's gone. Sometimes I even think I see him standing there." What does this comment indicate about the client?
    1. She is in an early stage of normal grief.
    2. She may be hallucinating.
    3. She is having illusions.
    4. She may be in a severe depression.

92. The pre-operative client is from a different country and tells the nurse that his family will be coming for a prayer service. Eighteen persons arrive and start chanting in the client's semi-private room. What is the best response for the nurse?
    1. Explain that visitors are limited to two per client.
    2. Ask the client's roommate if they object to so many persons in the room.
    3. Ignore the large number of people and the chanting.
    4. Arrange for the group to go to the conference room or the chapel.

93. An adolescent is to be admitted to the orthopedic floor with several fractures. The client has been taking hallucinogens this evening. What should the nurse expect on admission because the client is using hallucinogens?
    1. Severe depression
    2. Violent behavior
    3. Respiratory distress
    4. Convulsions

94. An adult has completed an alcohol detoxification program and is being discharged with disulfiram (Antabuse). Which statement the client makes indicates a need for more teaching?
    1. "I have learned my lesson. I won't drink more than two beers."
    2. "I will not use mouthwash while I am taking Antabuse."
    3. "I should take the Antabuse every day."
    4. "If I have to go to the emergency room for any reason I will tell them I take Antabuse."

95. The nurse is caring for a woman who is admitted following a beating by her husband. The woman says, "It wasn't really his fault.

Dinner was late." The husband arrives to visit his wife with a large bouquet of flowers and a box of chocolates. The woman later says to the nurse, "He feels so bad about what he did and says it will never happen again." What concept should guide the nurse when replying to the client?
1. Men who abuse their wives and then repent usually do not do it again.
2. The woman is quite perceptive and should be safe when she is discharged.
3. Abuse is often followed by repentance and then again by abuse.
4. Spousal abuse is usually a result of misbehavior on the part of the abused.

96. Which characteristic is most likely to be present in persons who abuse others?
1. Financial security
2. Positive self image
3. Substance abuse
4. Physical illness

97. An adult man believes that someone is poisoning his food. What is the best nursing action in response to this belief?
1. Explain to him that no one is poisoning his food.
2. Tell him that the food is prepared in the hospital under secure conditions.
3. Taste his food to assure him that it is not being poisoned.
4. Offer him food that is in individual containers.

98. A newly admitted client is exhibiting signs of severe anxiety. She is pacing back and forth and has difficulty concentrating on the nurse's questions. What nursing action is most appropriate at this time?
1. Tell the client to sit down and get control of herself.
2. Leave the room until she regains control.
3. Whisper to her that everything will be all right.
4. Attend to her behavior and direct her to a quiet area.

99. A two-year-old child is seen in the pediatrician's office. The child screams when the nurse approaches him to give him the ordered IM medication. How should the nurse approach the child?
1. Tell him to stop screaming and he can have a lollipop after he gets the shot.
2. Ask him to point to the leg he wants you to use.
3. Tell him he is a big boy and shots don't hurt big boys.
4. Explain to him that the shot is important for his health and ask him to watch you.

100. An adult who is admitted for surgery today says to the nurse "I'm so afraid. Do you think the doctor knows what he is doing? Does anyone ever survive this type of operation?" How should the nurse reply?
1. "People who have this type of surgery almost always survive and get better."
2. "Don't worry, your doctor is very skilled and has done many operations like yours."
3. "You seem concerned about the surgery."
4. "I cared for a woman last week who had the same type of surgery and she did very well."

Answers and Rationales for Practice Test Two

Answer	Rationale	NP	CN	SA
#1. 2.	**Semi-Fowler's position will facilitate respirations, take pressure off the abdominal incision, and aid drainage if a drain is in place. Semi-Fowler's position is indicated when a client has a nasogastric tube in place to prevent backflow of gastric juices.**	Im	Ph/9	1
1.	Supine position is lying flat on the back. This position is not recommended when a nasogastric tube is in place as supine position would promote leakage of gastric contents into the esophagus.			
3.	Dorsal recumbent is lying on the back and is not recommended when a nasogastric tube is in place as this position would promote leakage of gastric contents into the esophagus.			
4.	Prone position is lying on the abdomen and is not recommended when a nasogastric tube is in place. Prone position would promote leakage of gastric contents into the esophagus.			
#2. 1.	**The first action indicated is to cover the exposed intestines with a sterile towel to prevent infection and moisten it to prevent intestines from drying and sticking.**	Im	Ph/10	1

| | | NP | CN | SA |

ANSWER   RATIONALE

2. The intestines will be reinserted into the abdominal cavity by the surgeon under sterile operating room conditions.

3. The exposed coils of intestines should be covered with a sterile moist towel. Normal saline is the solution of choice. Sterile water might cause fluid and electrolyte imbalances.

4. Taking the client's vital signs is not the initial nursing action. The first action indicated is to cover the exposed intestines with a sterile towel to prevent infection and moisten it to prevent intestines from drying and sticking.

#3. 2. **Pulmonary complications such as atelectasis usually develop 24 to 48 hours post-operatively.**   Dc   Ph/9   1

1. A low-grade fever related to dehydration usually occurs in the first 24 hours.

3. It takes at least 72 hours and often longer for a wound infection to develop and cause a fever.

4. Fever due to bladder infection is most likely to occur 48 to 72 hours after surgery.

#4. 2. **Atropine is contraindicated for persons with glaucoma. The nurse should check with the prescribing physician, who may not know the client has glaucoma.**   Im   Ph/8   5

1. Atropine is contraindicated for persons with glaucoma. The nurse should check with the prescribing physician, who may not know the client has glaucoma.

3. Atropine is contraindicated for persons with glaucoma. The nurse should check with the prescribing physician, who may not know the client has glaucoma.

4. Atropine is contraindicated for persons with glaucoma. The nurse should check with the prescribing physician, who may not know the client has glaucoma. Meperidine and atropine were ordered as a pre-operative medication. The nurse should not decide to give one drug, but not the other. Meperidine is a central nervous system depressant and decreases vital signs. Atropine is anticholinergic and will increase the heart rate in addition to slowing peristalsis and drying secretions.

#5. 2. **The client must sign a consent form before surgery. After a person has been medicated for surgery they cannot legally sign a consent form because they have received mind-altering drugs. The physician must be notified and surgery will be postponed.**   Im   Sa/1   1

1. The client must sign a consent form before surgery. After a person has been medicated for surgery they cannot legally sign a consent form because they have received mind-altering drugs. The physician must be notified and surgery will be postponed.

3. The client must sign a consent form before surgery. After a person has been medicated for surgery they cannot legally sign a consent form because they have received mind-altering drugs. If the person would have been able to sign the consent form except for the medication, the spouse cannot sign for them. We must wait until the medication has worn off and the client can sign the form.

4. The client must sign a consent form before surgery. After a person has been medicated for surgery they cannot legally sign a consent form because they have received mind-altering drugs. Even though the client has presented for surgery there must be a signed consent form before surgery can be performed. The only exception to this is a life-threatening emergency.

#6. 1. **Prolonged lithotomy position may interfere with circulation to the lower extremities.**   Dc   Ph/9   1

2. Presence of bowel sounds is not related to lithotomy position.

3. Lithotomy position should not affect the upper extremities.

4. The nurse may palpate the client's bladder, but not because he was in lithotomy position.

ANSWER	RATIONALE	NP	CN	SA

#7. 2. **A stage II pressure ulcer may look like a blister, abrasion, or shallow crater and only involves a partial-thickness skin loss of the epidermis and/or dermis.**   Dc   Ph/10   1

  1. A stage I pressure ulcer is red and the skin is intact.

  3. A stage III pressure ulcer is a full-thickness skin loss involving damage to or necrosis of subcutaneous tissue that may extend down to, but not through, underlying fascia. It generally looks like a deep crater.

  4. A stage IV pressure ulcer is a full-thickness skin loss with extensive destruction, tissue necrosis, or damage to muscle, bone, or supporting structures.

#8. 1. **The nurse should take vital signs frequently and assess the skin for signs of frostbite or breakdown.**   Pl   Ph/10   1

  2. The hypothermia blanket is turned off when the client's temperature is one to two degrees above the target temperature. The client's temperature will usually drift downward after the blanket is turned off.

  3. There should be a sheet between the client and the cooling blanket.

  4. Direct application of ice is not used as it may stimulate shivering (the temperature-raising mechanism) and may cause skin breakdown.

#9. 3. **The layers act as insulators and prevent moisture loss. Some nurses place the waterproof layer next to the compress and then cover with a dry cover, whereas others reverse the order, putting the waterproof layer on the outside.**   Im   Ph/10   1

  1. Surgical asepsis (sterile technique) is indicated. Medical asepsis is clean technique.

  2. The wet compress should be covered with a dry cover and a waterproof material. A wet dressing that is left open to the air can conduct organisms into the wound. It will also lose heat very quickly.

  4. Compresses are generally applied for 20 to 30 minutes.

#10. 4. **Apple juice is a clear liquid.**   Im   Ph/7   6

  1. Milk is not a clear liquid.

  2. Fruited gelatin is not a clear liquid. Gelatin without fruit is allowed on a clear liquid diet.

  3. Sherbert contains milk and is not allowed on a clear liquid diet.

#11. 3. **The client who has just been given penicillin should be checked on first. An adverse drug reaction is possible and could be life-threatening. The other clients all need to be checked but are not in potentially life-threatening situations.**   Im   Sa/1   5

  1. This client needs assistance but the nurse should first observe the client who has been given penicillin and is at risk for a reaction.

  2. This client needs to be medicated but the nurse should first observe the client who has been given penicillin and is at risk for a reaction.

  4. This client needs assistance but the nurse should first observe the client who has been given penicillin and is at risk for a reaction. The client is restrained and not likely to be in immediate danger.

#12. 3. **A client who has a head injury should not be placed in shock position as this would increase intracranial pressure. The other conditions would not be contraindications for shock position.**   Dc   Ph/10   1

  1. Long bone fractures will put the client at risk for fat emboli, but this is not a contraindication for putting the client in shock position.

  2. Air embolus is a serious condition. The treatment for air embolus would be to place the client's head lower than his chest. The client's head is lowered in shock position.

  4. Thrombophlebitis is not a contraindication for shock position. In shock position the legs are elevated. The legs are elevated for a client who has thrombophlebitis.

#13. 3. **The wheelchair should be placed on the unaffected side at a 45-degree angle. This position best allows the client to stand on the unaffected leg and pivot before sitting in the wheelchair. A**   Ev   Ph/7   1 person who has hemiplegia will have difficulty placing her arms around someone's neck and will not be able to use a trapeze effectively.

1. The wheelchair should be placed on the unaffected side so the client can pivot on the unaffected foot and sit in the chair.
2. The client has hemiplegia and will not be able to put her arms around the neck of a family member.
4. The client has hemiplegia and will not be able to use a trapeze bar. A trapeze bar would be appropriate for a client who had paraplegia.

#14. 4. **Cold applied to a sprained ankle should help reduce bleeding and swelling in the area. Cold has an anesthetic effect and should reduce pain.**   Im   Ph/10   1

1. Ice will not keep a sprain from becoming a fracture. Sprains are damage to soft tissue rather than to bone. Sprains do not become fractures.
2. There will be some bruising and ecchymosis following a sprain. Ice may reduce the amount of bleeding under the skin but will not eliminate it.
3. Ice applied to a sprain is not given to lower body temperature or to keep fever from developing. Fever is not common following a sprain.

#15. 4. **Passive artificial immunity occurs when antibodies are produced by another person or animal and injected into the recipient. This gives a temporary immunity to protect against this exposure to an organism.**   Im   He/4   1

1. Active natural immunity occurs when the person's own body produces antibodies in response to an active infection. This takes time to develop and the person has the disease.
2. Active artificial immunity is developed when antigens, either vaccine or toxoids, are administered to stimulate antibody response. This takes time to develop.
3. Passive natural immunity occurs when antibodies are transferred from an immune mother to a baby through the placenta or colostrum. This is usually temporary.

#16. 4. **The nurse must assess daily weights for a client who is receiving total parenteral nutrition (TPN).**   Dc   Ph/8   1

1. The number of bowel movements should be observed for any client but is not the most essential observation for the client who is receiving TPN. Remember TPN is nutrition given via a central venous line directly into the right atrium. It is not given into the GI tract.
2. TPN is nutrition given via a central venous line directly into the right atrium. There is no tube in the stomach.
3. TPN is nutrition given via a central venous line directly into the right atrium. Bowel sounds are not an issue related to TPN.

#17. 4. **Tinnitus (ringing in the ears) is a sign of aspirin toxicity and is consistent with a minor overdose.**   Dc   Ph/8   5

1. Tinnitus (ringing in the ears) is a sign of aspirin toxicity and is consistent with a minor overdose.
2. Tinnitus (ringing in the ears) is a sign of aspirin toxicity. The client does not have to exceed the recommended dosage. Some clients will develop toxicity at the recommended dosage.
3. Tinnitus (ringing in the ears) is a sign of aspirin toxicity. There is no evidence of an upper GI bleed. An upper GI bleed could occur with aspirin toxicity.

#18. 2. **Patient controlled analgesia (PCA) allows the client to administer analgesic before the pain becomes severe, thus allowing better pain control.**   Ev   Ph/8   1

1. The machine will only give the analgesic after a preset time has elapsed. This is designed to prevent overdosing. The client can see this by the ready light on the machine and the beep that accompanies the delivery of the medicine.

3. The client should press the button only when experiencing pain.

4. The client may experience pain when using the PCA pump correctly. If this happens the client should notify the nurse.

#19. 2. **The medication is ordered for operative pain. The client asks for pain medication but does not indicate where the pain is. The nurse should *initially* assess the client. If the pain is in the operative area, then the nurse can administer the ordered medication.**   Dc   Ph/8   1

1. The medication is ordered for operative pain. The client asks for pain medication but does not indicate where the pain is. The nurse should *initially* assess the client. If the pain is in the operative area, then the nurse can administer the ordered medication.

3. An ice bag will not usually be effective by itself for the relief of pain on the day of surgery.

4. Repositioning the client will not likely remove pain on the day of surgery.

#20. 4. **The skin at the radiation site should not be washed. The client should not attempt to wash off the purple marks.**   Pl   Ph/10   1

1. The skin will be dry so there is no need for a dressing.

2. The client should avoid washing the skin at the radiation site so showering is not indicated.

3. Ice should not be applied following radiation therapy. The skin is very sensitive and might be damaged from an ice bag.

#21. 3. **Thrombocytopenia (low platelet count) makes the client at risk for bleeding. The client should not receive injections. The other choices are not related to thrombocytopenia.**   Pl   Ph/10   1

1. Thrombocytopenia is a low platelet count, which places the client at risk for bleeding. A semi-upright position will not reduce the risk of bleeding.

2. Thrombocytopenia is a low platelet count, which places the client at risk for bleeding. Limiting the client's intake of fluids will not reduce the risk of bleeding.

4. Thrombocytopenia is a low platelet count, which places the client at risk for bleeding. Exercising the client's lower extremities will not reduce the risk of bleeding. Exercising the lower extremities will help prevent thrombophlebitis.

#22. 4. **Narcotic analgesics are respiratory depressants. Rising intracranial pressure causes respiratory depression. Further respiratory depression would cause acidosis, causing more blood flow to the brain, resulting in more cerebral edema and a further increase in intracranial pressure.**   Dc   Ph/10   5

1. Narcotic analgesics cause miosis or constriction of the pupil.

2. Narcotic analgesics would be effective for the pain but would increase intracranial pressure and are thus contraindicated.

3. Narcotic analgesics may cause vomiting. Vomiting can be a sign of increased intracranial pressure. However, this is not the reason they are contraindicated in persons who have head injuries.

#23. 4. **The treatment of glaucoma includes constriction of the pupil so the aqueous humor can flow more easily. Atropine is an anticholinergic which causes mydriasis (dilation of pupils).**   Dc   Ph/8   5

1. Atropine is an anticholinergic, which causes increased heart rate. Bradycardia is not a contraindication for atropine.

2. Atropine is an anticholinergic, which causes increased heart rate. Hypothyroidism is not a contraindication for atropine.

3. Atropine is an anticholinerigic agent. It is not contraindicated in diabetes.

#24. 1. **The client is having difficulty swallowing. The highest priority is to prevent aspiration pneumonia. Decubitus ulcers may also be a concern, but are not a higher priority than preventing aspiration pneumonia.**   Pl   Ph/9   1

		NP	CN	SA

2. Preventing decubitus ulcers is a concern for this client, who is having difficulty moving. However, preventing aspiration pneumonia is a higher priority. Aspiration pneumonia is more immediately life-threatening than decubitus ulcers.

3. Bladder distention could be a concern for this client, who has Guillain-Barré syndrome. Aspiration pneumonia is more immediately life-threatening. If the client develops bladder distention, he is likely to become incontinent, which is not life-threatening.

4. Hypertensive crisis is not likely to occur in the client who has Guillain-Barré syndrome.

#25. 2. Diplopia and ptosis of the eyelids are characteristic of myasthenia gravis. Upper-body symptoms occur before lower-body symptoms. Symptoms are related to cranial nerves.   Dc   Ph/9   1

1. Ataxia and poor coordination are lower-body symptoms. Upper-body symptoms occur before lower body symptoms.

3. Slurred speech is not an early sign of myasthenia gravis. The client may have a weak voice, however.

4. Headaches and tinnitus are not characteristic of myasthenia gravis.

#26. 1. The symptoms suggest autonomic hyperreflexia, which is usually caused by bladder distention. The patient will need to be catheterized and the physician notified. Autonomic hyperreflexia is a medical emergency.   Im   Ph/10   1

2. The client should be put in semi-Fowler's position, not Trendlenburg.

3. Pain is neither a symptom nor a cause of autonomic hyperreflexia.

4. Autonomic hyperreflexia is a medical emergency. The nurse must notify the charge nurse or the physician immediately. The client is likely to need antihypertensive medication as well as catheterization if a distended bladder is the cause.

#27. 2. Confused persons will often be more oriented if the same caregiver is assigned for several days in a row.   Pl   Sa/1   1

1. While some rotation of assignments may be appropriate, residents will often be more oriented and do better if there is consistency in caregivers.

3. Female caregivers frequently will need to care for male residents.

4. It is important to consider any special requests from caregivers. However, the nurse making the assignments has the big picture and should make assignments according to the needs of the unit.

#28. 3. This answer is accurate. There is a surgical incision to retrieve the organs but it is no more defacing than abdominal surgery and should not interfere with an open casket.   Im   Sa/1   1

1. This statement is not true. Donating organs does not deface the body and does not make it necessary to have a closed casket.

2. This response does not answer the client's direct request. The nurse should be able to give the information.

4. This response is a true statement. However, this does not answer the direct question that was asked. The nurse should not avoid answering the questions.

#29. 2. The certified nursing assistant should be able to take routine vital signs.   Pl   Sa/1   1

1. Tube feeding is more appropriately performed by a LPN/LVN. It is beyond the scope of a nursing assistant.

3. A client who is in congestive heart failure has to be monitored very carefully. The nurse should take the blood pressure for this client, who is not stable.

4. Wound care is a sterile procedure and should be performed by the nurse.

#30. 1. The best choice is to ask the client what his name is.   Im   Sa/2   1

2. Persons who are confused may not answer accurately if asked "Are you Mr. _____?"

    3.   Asking the roommate if a client is Mr. _____ may not give accurate information.

    4.   Clients may get in the wrong bed. Checking the bed tag is not as accurate as asking the client for his name.

#31. 2. **The client who is confused and picking at his nasal cannula and NG tube is endangering himself and may need restraints.**   Dc   Sa/2   1

    1.   There is no data in this answer that suggests the client is putting himself at risk. Restraints are indicated for persons who are putting themselves or others at risk.

    3.   Side rails are usually sufficient protection for a confused client who is in bed. There is no data to suggest that this is not true.

    4.   An adult who has just returned from a post-anesthesia care unit is probably not very alert, but there is no data to suggest that the client is putting himself or others in danger.

#32. 4. **The nurse should not administer medication that has been drawn up by someone else, even if that someone else is the RN charge nurse.**   Im   Ph/8   1

    1.   The nurse should not administer medication that has been drawn up by someone else, even if that someone else is the RN charge nurse.

    2.   The nurse should not administer medication that has been drawn up by someone else, even if that someone else is the RN charge nurse. Asking what the medication is does not assure the nurse that the medication was drawn up accurately.

    3.   The nurse should not administer medication that has been drawn up by someone else, even if that someone else is the RN charge nurse. Asking what the medication is does not assure the nurse that the medication was drawn up accurately.

#33. 2. **According to the Patient's Bill of Rights, the patient has the right to know who is caring for him/her and to know if any persons caring for him/her are students or other trainees. The client has the right to refuse any treatment.**   Im   Sa/1   1

    1.   The client has the right to refuse treatment by students. Signing permission for care does not take away these rights.

    3.   It is not necessary to sign a special form to refuse care by medical and nursing students.

    4.   The client should be informed if caregivers are students. However, the client can refuse to have students caring for him/her.

#34. 3. **According to the Patient's Bill of Rights, the client has the right to see his records and to have information explained and interpreted when necessary.**   Im   Sa/1   1

    1.   According to the Patient's Bill of Rights, the client has the right to see his records and to have information explained and interpreted when necessary. There is no need to obtain a court order.

    2.   According to the Patient's Bill of Rights, the client has the right to see his records and to have information explained and interpreted when necessary. It is not necessary to have the physician's approval to see his records.

    4.   According to the Patient's Bill of Rights, the client has the right to see his records and to have information explained and interpreted when necessary. It is not necessary to appear before a committee. It is the client's right.

#35. 4. **The nurse should determine that care was administered as delegated. One of the best ways to do this is to observe the clients. The nurse must follow up when delegating to other personnel.**   Pl   Sa/1   1

    1.   The nurse does not have time to observe the nursing assistant during the administration of all care. It is not necessary to observe the nursing assistant during all care.

    2.   Asking the nursing assistant if there were any problems is all right, but not the best way to determine that care was given as delegated.

3. Checking the charting of the nursing assistant does not ensure that the clients received the care that was charted.

#36. **2.** **The client is having an illusion—a misinterpretation of reality. The nurse should turn the lights up brighter so there are no shadows to be misinterpreted as snakes.** | | Im | Ps/5 | 2

1. The client is having an illusion—a misinterpretation of reality. The client is not likely to believe the nurse who simply reassures him there are no snakes. When dealing with an illusion the nurse should change the conditions that support an illusion.

3. The client is having an illusion—a misinterpretation of reality. The nurse should turn the lights up brighter so there are no shadows to be misinterpreted as snakes. Telling him there are really no snakes is not likely to change his interpretation of the shadows he sees.

4. The client is having an illusion—a misinterpretation of reality. The nurse should turn the lights up brighter so there are no shadows to be misinterpreted as snakes. Reassuring him the snakes will not hurt him confirms for him that there are snakes on the wall.

#37. **4.** **Permission is revocable. Clients have the right to change their minds about treatments and procedures and to revoke consent.** | | Im | Sa/1 | 1

1. Clients have the right to change their minds about treatments and procedures and to revoke consent.

2. Trying to coerce the client by telling her the physician will be upset is not appropriate. Clients have the right to change their minds about treatments and procedures and to revoke consent.

3. Clients have the right to change their minds about treatments and procedures and to revoke consent. Trying to talk the client into the procedure is not appropriate.

#38. **2.** **Increasing the distance of persons from the client who has internal radiation reduces the amount of exposure to radiation.** | | Pl | Sa/2 | 1

1. Keeping the door to the room closed will reduce the exposure only very slightly. Wooden doors do not stop radiation. Heavy metal stops radiation.

3. Placing the client close to the nurse's station where the traffic is high increases the amount of exposure to other clients and personnel.

4. Placing a "Do not enter" sign might be done. However, usually clients do not enter other client's rooms.

#39. **3.** **An older client should not be short of breath walking down the hall. This is abnormal and should be reported.** | | Dc | He/3 | 1

1. Brown spots or age spots are normal in the older adult.

2. Older persons usually move more slowly than they did earlier in life.

4. It is common for older adults to have difficulty with color discrimination.

#40. **3.** **This answer has a sense of regret for actions not taken in the past. This suggests despair rather than ego integrity. According to Erickson, the developmental task for the aging client is ego integrity versus despair.** | | Ev | He/3 | 2

1. Making toys for his grandchildren suggests the client has an interest in life and meaning in life. This indicates ego integrity.

2. This statement gives facts, but does not carry regret, as is obvious in statement number 3.

4. Adjusting to less income is a normal part of aging. This statement does not carry the tone of regret as statement number 3 does.

#41. **1.** **Edema in the hands and face is suggestive of pregnancy-induced hypertension and should be reported to the physician.** | | Dc | He/3 | 1

2. Pregnant women have an increase in metabolic rate and usually feel warmer than those around them. This is a normal finding.

3. Swelling of the feet is normal in pregnant women. The enlarging fetus reduces the venous return and causes swelling of the feet and ankles in latter part of pregnancy. This is a normal finding.

4.   The pregnant woman will have enlarged and tender breasts as a result of progesterone stimulation and in preparation for lactation. This is a normal finding.

#42. 1.   Most persons lose the sense of salt and sweet as they age.   Dc   He/3   6

2.   Most persons develop presbyopia, the farsightedness of aging, as they age. They have trouble focusing on close work.

3.   As people age there are pupillary changes with loss of light responsiveness, so they adapt to darkness more slowly and have difficulty seeing in dim light.

4.   As people age they often develop decreased color discrimination.

#43. 4.   The pedal pulse is felt by placing the fingertips on the top of the foot and gently pressing the artery against the bone.   Dc   He/4   1

1.   The radial pulse is obtained by placing the fingertips against the wrist bone.

2.   The apical pulse is obtained by placing the stethoscope over the apex of the heart.

3.   The carotid pulse is obtained by placing the fingertips against the side of the neck.

#44. 3.   An apical-radial pulse is obtained by having one person take the apical pulse while the second person takes the radial pulse at the same time.   Dc   He/4   1

1.   An apical-radial pulse is obtained by having one person take the apical pulse while the second person takes the radial pulse at the same time.

2.   The radial pulse is never higher than the apical pulse. Ideally both pulses are the same. A pulse deficit exists when the radial pulse is less than the apical pulse.

4.   An apical-radial pulse is obtained by having one person take the apical pulse while the second person takes the radial pulse at the same time. It is impossible for the nurse to count two pulses at the same time.

#45. 4.   Noisy breathing is best described as sterterous.   Dc   He/4   1

1.   Deep respirations are described as hyperpnea.

2.   Cheyne-Stokes respirations are periods of apnea alternating with hyperpnea.

3.   A person who has orthopnea must sit up to breathe.

#46. 2.   Using a cuff that is too small causes the blood pressure reading to be abnormally high.   Dc   He/4   1

1.   A large cuff may be more comfortable for the client. However, the reason the nurse uses a large cuff for a large person is that using a cuff that is too small causes the blood pressure reading to be abnormally high.

3.   Using a cuff that is too small causes the blood pressure reading to be abnormally high. It does not make the pulse hard to hear.

4.   Using a cuff that is too small causes both the systolic and diastolic blood pressure readings to be abnormally high.

#47. 1.   Handwashing is the best way to prevent spread of infection. Hands should be washed before and after changing the dressing. This indicates the client understands the procedure.   Ev   Sa/2   1

2.   Touching the edges of the dressings with bare hands contaminates the dressings. This indicates the client does not understand the procedure.

3.   A wound is cleansed from the wound out. The client should not move a swab from the outside into the wound. This statement indicates the client does not understand the procedure.

4.   The dressings should not be put directly into the wastebasket. They should be placed in a waterproof bag and sealed before being disposed of. This statement indicates the client does not understand the procedure.

#48. 4. **Active exercises prevent muscle atrophy. The other activities do not prevent muscle atrophy.**   Pl   Ph/7   1
   1. Passive range-of-motion exercises help to prevent joint contractures, but do not prevent muscle atrophy. Active exercises are necessary to prevent muscle atrophy.
   2. Turning the client at two-hour intervals will help to prevent respiratory complications and skin breakdown but will not prevent muscle atrophy.
   3. Changing positions frequently will help to prevent skin breakdown and may help in preventing respiratory complications but is not likely to prevent muscle atrophy.

#49. 3. **Varicose veins are related to venous stasis, which may be caused by prolonged standing. They are not a result of prolonged bed rest.**   Dc   Ph/7   1
   1. Muscle atrophy is a complication of prolonged bed rest.
   2. Hypostatic pneumonia is a complication of prolonged bed rest.
   4. Thrombophlebitis is a complication of prolonged bed rest.

#50. 4. **Changing position in bed frequently, thus avoiding prolonged pressure on any one bony prominence, will help to prevent development of pressure ulcers.**   Pl   Ph/7   1
   1. Passive range-of-motion exercises help to prevent joint contractures and active range-of-motion exercises help to prevent muscle atrophy. They do not prevent pressure ulcers.
   2. Deep breathing and coughing help to prevent atelectasis and hypostatic pneumonia. Deep breathing and coughing does not prevent pressure ulcers.
   3. Keeping the feet against a footboard helps to prevent foot drop. It does not prevent development of pressure ulcers.

#51. 2. **Proper body mechanics involves bending from the hip and knees, not the waist. Bending from the waist indicates the nursing assistant needs more instruction.**   Ev   Ph/7   1
   1. The feet should be separated to provide a wide base of support. This action indicates the nursing assistant understands body mechanics.
   3. Turning the whole body rather than twisting the body indicates an understanding of body mechanics.
   4. Keeping the back straight indicates an understanding of proper body mechanics.

#52. 3. **Having the client sit down will help to prevent her from falling and keep her safe.**   Im   Ph/7   1
   1. Putting her head between her legs is not going to prevent her from falling. In fact, it may cause her to fall.
   2. The nurse should never leave a client who is dizzy and faint.
   4. Encouraging her to walk faster is likely to aggravate the client's dizziness and faintness.

#53. 3. **A decreased white blood cell count is not typical of sickle cell crisis. The client will have a decreased red blood cell count.**   Dc   Ph/10   1
   1. Enlarged liver and spleen are often seen in persons who are in sickle cell crisis. The red blood cells live only 1 to 3 weeks rather than the usual 4 months. The spleen and liver are involved with RBC breakdown.
   2. In sickle cell crisis RBCs live only 1 to 3 weeks and are rapidly broken down by the spleen. The liver normally converts bilirubin (produced when RBCs are broken down) into bile. The liver cannot keep up with the extra load and jaundice and icterus result.
   4. Abdominal and joint pain are common in persons with sickle cell crisis. RBCs are broken down too rapidly and agglutinate and cause clumping in the vessel, blocking the blood supply and causing pain distal to the agglutination.

#54. 1. **Crushing chest pain not relieved by nitroglycerine or rest is likely to be a heart attack. Chest pain that is relieved by nitroglycerine or rest is usually angina.**   Im   Ph/9   5

2. Epigastric pain relieved by antacids is likely to be gastric in origin and is probably not either angina or a heart attack.

3. Both anginal pain and the pain of a heart attack can radiate down the left arm. Anginal pain is relieved by rest or nitroglycerine; heart attack pain is not.

4. Chest pain due to angina is usually related to excitement, exercise, environment (hot or cold), or eating.

#55. 2. Persons who have angina should take nitroglycerine at five-minute intervals times three when they have chest pain. If not relieved after three doses of nitroglycerine, they should call the physician or go to the emergency room.   Ev   Ph/9   5

1. Persons who have angina should exercise within the limits recommended by the physician. They should not remain completely sedentary.

3. Persons who have angina may have some chest pain with sexual activity. Heart attacks can occur during sexual activity but are not likely. The physician may recommend taking nitroglycerine before sexual activity.

4. If the client with angina has chest pain he should take nitroglycerine at five-minute intervals times three. If the chest pain is not relieved he should immediately call his physician or go to the hospital, as he may be having a heart attack.

#56. 2   Sickle cell anemia is an inherited disease transmitted as a recessive gene. When both parents are carriers there is a 25% chance that each baby will be born with sickle cell, a 50% chance that each child will be born with the trait, and a 25% chance that each child will be disease- and carrier-free. It is possible to have two children in a row with the disease.   Im   Ph/10   1

1. Sickle cell anemia is not contagious. It is an inherited disease transmitted as a recessive gene. When both parents are carriers there is a 25% chance that each baby will be born with sickle cell, a 50% chance that each child will be born with the trait, and a 25% chance that each child will be disease- and carrier-free. It is possible to have two children in a row with the disease.

3. This answer describes the transmission of an x-linked disease such as hemophilia or Duchenne's muscular dystrophy. Sickle cell anemia is an inherited disease transmitted as a recessive gene. When both parents are carriers there is a 25% chance that each baby will be born with sickle cell, a 50% chance that each child will be born with the trait, and a 25% chance that each child will be disease- and carrier-free. It is possible to have two or more children in a row with the disease.

4. Statistically parents who are both carriers of the sickle cell gene have a 25% chance of having a child who is both disease- and carrier-free. However, there is no way of knowing which child that will be. It is possible to have two or more children in a row with the disease.

#57. 1. The home should be assessed for items that might cause an electrical spark such as frayed cords.   Im   Sa/2   1

2. It is more important to check for frayed cords than it is to purchase fire extinguishers. It is more important to prevent a fire than to treat a fire.

3. It is not necessary to remove electrical appliances from a room where oxygen is in use. It is more important to assess for frayed cords because these could start a fire. A well-grounded electrical device does not produce sparks.

4. The client's room should not be carpeted. Shuffling across a carpet can produce static electricity, which can start a fire.

#58. 2. The client should be positioned in semi-Fowler's position to promote thoracic expansion.   Im   Ph/10   1

   1. Supine position will make it more difficult for the client to breathe and for secretions to be removed.

   3. Sim's position (semi-lateral with the lower arm behind the client's back) will make it more difficult for the client to breathe and for secretions to be removed.

   4. Semi-lateral position will make it more difficult for the client to breathe and for secretions to be removed.

#59. 1. The client must remain NPO before a bronchoscopy.   Dc   Ph/9   1

   2. There is no need for the client to take a laxative prior to a bronchoscopy. A rigid tube (bronchoscope) will be passed down the throat into the bronchi. The client will probably have a lidocaine spray to deaden the gag reflex during the procedure.

   3. This is "nice-to-know" information, but is not essential information.

   4. This is "nice-to-know" information, but is not essential before the procedure.

#60. 2. Air is in the pleural cavity following thoracic surgery. A chest tube removes air from the pleural cavity thus re-establishing negative pressure and allowing the lung to re-expand.   Im   Ph/9   1

   1. Air in the thoracic cavity causes the lung to collapse. The chest tube removes air from the thoracic cavity so the lung can re-expand.

   3. A chest tube does not bring oxygen to the lungs. A chest tube removes air from the pleural cavity, thus re-establishing negative pressure and allowing the lung to re-expand.

   4. A chest tube does not help the wound heal faster and reduce scarring. A chest tube removes air from the pleural cavity, thus re-establishing negative pressure and allowing the lung to re-expand.

#61. 3 The most likely cause for no bubbling in the water seal chamber two days following insertion of a chest tube is re-expansion of the lung. The nurse should auscultate the chest to determine if there are bilateral breath sounds.   Dc   Ph/9   1

   1. Excessive wound drainage is not a likely cause of absence of bubbling in the water seal chamber when a three-chamber system such as Pleuravac® is being used. The most likely cause for no bubbling in the water seal chamber two days following insertion of a chest tube is re-expansion of the lung. The nurse should auscultate the chest to determine if there are bilateral breath sounds.

   2. Air leaks cause lack of bubbling in the suction control chamber. No bubbling in the water seal chamber is usually due either to obstructions in the tubing or re-expansion of the lungs. Two days following insertion of a chest tube the most likely reason for no bubbling in the water seal chamber is re-expansion of the lung. Tubing obstruction is more likely to occur in the first day or so.

   4. If the suction is not turned on there will be no bubbling in the suction control chamber. The water seal chamber may still bubble if air is leaving the thoracic cavity by gravity drainage even when the suction is not turned on.

#62. 1. A major toxicity of gentamicin is nephrotoxicity. Diminished urine output indicates damage to the kidneys.   Dc   Ph/8   5

   2. Blurred vision is not a common adverse response to gentamicin. The major adverse responses are nephrotoxicity (kidneys) and ototoxicity (ears).

   3. Orange sputum is not an adverse response to gentamicin. Orange-colored secretions may occur with rimactane (Rifampin). The major adverse responses to gentamicin are nephrotoxicity (kidneys) and ototoxicity (ears).

   4. Hypertension is not an adverse response to gentamicin. Sometimes it can cause hypotension. The major adverse responses are nephrotoxicity (kidneys) and ototoxicity (ears).

#63. 1. Back pain following a cystoscopy could indicate kidney damage and should be reported to the charge nurse or the physician.   Dc   Ph/9   1

2. Tea-colored urine is a normal finding following a cystoscopy.

3. Leg cramps are common following a cystoscopy because the client has been in lithotomy position.

4. Pink-tinged urine is a normal finding following a cystoscopy.

#64. 3. Pyridium is a urinary tract anesthetic which will kill the pain until the antibiotics have had time to work.   Im   Ph/8   5

1. Pyridium is not an antibiotic. Pyridium is a urinary tract anesthetic which will kill the pain until the antibiotics have had time to work.

2. Pyridium is not an analgesic. Pyridium is a urinary tract anesthetic which will kill the pain until the antibiotics have had time to work.

4. Pyridium does not prevent kidney damage. Pyridium is a urinary tract anesthetic which will kill the pain until the antibiotics have had time to work.

#65. 1. The client who has a stone in the urinary tract is in severe pain. Acute pain is the priority nursing diagnosis.   Pl   Ph/10   1

2. Diarrhea often occurs from the pain and irritation caused by the stones. However, the client who has a stone in the urinary tract is in severe pain. Acute pain is the priority nursing diagnosis.

3. Risk for altered health maintenance related to insufficient knowledge of prevention of recurrence, dietary restrictions, and fluid requirements is an appropriate nursing diagnosis. This diagnosis is most appropriate related to discharge planning. Upon admission the client who has a stone in the urinary tract is in severe pain. Acute pain is the priority nursing diagnosis.

4. Risk for infection is not likely to be a realistic nursing diagnosis for the client who has a stone in the urinary tract. This client will be in severe pain. Acute pain is the priority nursing diagnosis.

#66. 3. Pharyngitis or sore throat caused by the beta hemolytic strep organism usually precedes acute glomerulonephritis. Acute glomerulonephritis is an antigen-antibody response to beta hemolytic strep. The antibodies made to attack the microorganism also attack the basement membrane of the glomerulus.   Dc   Ph/10   1

1. Pyelonephritis is caused by an ascending bladder infection. Acute glomerulonephritis is an antigen-antibody response to beta hemolytic strep.

2. A person with chronic glomerulonephritis is likely to have a history of previous kidney infections.

4. Acute glomerulonephritis is not a sexually transmitted disease. Acute glomerulonephritis is an antigen-antibody response to beta hemolytic strep.

#67. 4. The nurse should strain all urine to detect any stones, which the client may pass. If a stone is passed it will be sent to the laboratory for analysis.   Im   Ph/10   1

1. There is no need to take frequent blood pressures for the client with a kidney stone. The nurse should strain all urine to detect any stones which the client may pass. If a stone is passed it will be sent to the laboratory for analysis.

2. Persons who have kidney stones often prefer to ambulate. Walking not only helps the pain but also may help the stone to pass through the ureter and urethra.

3. The client will be uncomfortable in the supine position. Persons who have kidney stones often prefer to ambulate. Walking not only helps the pain but also may help the stone to pass through the ureter and urethra.

#68. 2. The nurse should teach the client to drink generous amounts of fluids each day to help prevent formation of kidney stones.   Pl   Ph/9   1

1. The person who has a uric acid kidney stone should be on a low purine diet. Chicken and organ meats are high in purines. The client should be taught to avoid purine-containing foods.

3. There is no need for the person who has a history of kidney stones to avoid activity. In fact, immobility predisposes to the formation of the kidney stone. The client should be active.

4. Allopurinol (Zyloprim) should be taken daily as ordered. This drug is used to promote excretion of uric acid and thus prevent the formation of kidney stones.

#69. 2. Exposure to the ultraviolet rays of the sun can cause skin cancer. The client should wear a long-sleeved shirt and a hat when exposed to the sun.   Ev   He/4   1

1. Moles that are round and a single color are usually not malignant. Moles that have irregular borders and multiple colors are more apt to be malignant and should be seen by the physician.

3. Lotions and powders do not cause skin cancer. Exposure to the ultraviolet rays of the sun cause skin cancer.

4. Tanning booths expose the person to ultraviolet rays and are a significant risk for the development of skin cancer.

#70. 2. Calcium deposits are laid down early in life. The time to prevent osteoporosis is in adolescence.   Ev   He/4   1

1. Athletic injuries are not risk factors for osteoporosis. They are more apt to be related to osteoarthritis.

3. Physical activity should be continued throughout life. Weight-bearing exercises are important to prevent osteoporosis.

4. Carbonated beverages pull calcium from the bones and increase the risk of osteoporosis.

#71. 3. The cane should be held on the nonaffected side. When walking with a cane the client should move the cane and the affected foot at the same time.   Ev   Ph/7   1

1. The cane should be held on the nonaffected side. When walking with a cane the client should move the cane and the affected foot at the same time.

2. The cane should be held on the nonaffected side. When walking with a cane the client should move the cane and the affected foot at the same time. Moving the cane from side to side could increase the risk of tripping over the cane.

4. The cane should be held on the nonaffected side. When walking with a cane the client should move the cane and the affected foot at the same time.

#72. 3. The client with low back pain will be most comfortable in a position that opens the spaces between the vertebrae, such as side-lying with knees flexed or semi-Fowler's with knees bent.   Pl   Ph/7   1

1. The client with low back pain will be most comfortable in a position that opens the spaces between the vertebrae, such as side-lying with knees flexed or semi-Fowler's with knees bent.

2. The client with low back pain will be most comfortable in a position that opens the spaces between the vertebrae, such as side-lying with knees flexed or semi-Fowler's with knees bent.

4. The client with low back pain will be most comfortable in a position that opens the spaces between the vertebrae such as side-lying with knees flexed or semi-Fowler's with knees bent.

#73. 2. Ice works in two ways to reduce pain of a sprained ankle. First, it has an anesthetic effect. Second, it helps to prevent swelling.   Im   Ph/7   1

1. Exercising a sprained ankle several times an hour is likely to increase the pain. The ankle should not be stressed.

3. The leg and ankle should be elevated.

4. Topical steroids help to prevent itching and inflammation. They do not reduce pain.

#74. 4. Drinking warm milk helps to induce sleep in many people.   Im   Ph/7   1

1. Exercising increases body metabolism and makes it harder to go to sleep. Exercise should be done several hours before going to bed.

2. Cola beverages contain caffeine, which is a stimulant and keeps many people awake. Cola beverages have a diuretic effect. If the client did get to sleep she is likely to have to get up during the night to urinate.

3. The bed should be for sleeping. Reading and watching television in bed tend to aggravate sleep difficulties.

#75. 1. The blood gas values indicate compensated respiratory acidosis. The pH is normal on the low or acid side. All the other values are abnormal, so the nurse knows this is compensated. Because the pH is on the acid side, it is compensated acidosis. CO_2 is high. Because CO_2 is acid, it is causing the acid pH. CO_2 is respiratory. The HCO_3 is also high. However, it is alkaline and is not causing the acid pH. It is compensating for the high acid. — Dc Ph/9 1

2. The values are not consistent with alkalosis. The blood gas values indicate compensated respiratory acidosis. The pH is normal on the low or acid side. All the other values are abnormal, so the nurse knows this is compensated. Because the pH is on the acid side, it is compensated acidosis. CO_2 is high. Because CO_2 is acid, it is causing the acid pH. CO_2 is respiratory. The HCO_3 is also high. However, it is alkaline and is not causing the acid pH. It is compensating for the high acid.

3. The values are not consistent with alkalosis. The blood gas values indicate compensated respiratory acidosis. The pH is normal on the low or acid side. All the other values are abnormal, so the nurse knows this is compensated. Because the pH is on the acid side, it is compensated acidosis. CO_2 is high. Because CO_2 is acid, it is causing the acid pH. CO_2 is respiratory. The HCO_3 is also high. However, it is alkaline and is not causing the acid pH. It is compensating for the high acid.

4. The values are not consistent with metabolic acidosis. The blood gas values indicate compensated respiratory acidosis. The pH is normal on the low or acid side. All the other values are abnormal, so the nurse knows this is compensated. Because the pH is on the acid side, it is compensated acidosis. CO_2 is high. Because CO_2 is acid, it is causing the acid pH. CO_2 is respiratory. The HCO_3 is also high. However, it is alkaline and is not causing the acid pH. It is compensating for the high acid.

#76. 3. MRI or magnetic resonance imaging using magnetic fields. Persons who have metal in their bodies such as artificial knees, hips, plates in the skull, or metal fragments from previous injuries such as gunshot wounds should not have that part of the body imaged. — Dc Ph/9 1

1. No iodine dye is used during magnetic resonance imaging so there is no need to inquire about iodine allergies.

2. There is no need for the client to fast prior to magnetic resonance imaging.

4. A laxative prep is not used prior to magnetic resonance imaging.

#77. 3. A glass of water dropped on the floor beside the bed of an elderly ambulatory client is a serious safety hazard and needs immediate attention. The other options are not immediate safety hazards. — Im Sa/2 1

1. Dirty linen on the floor beside the bed of a non-ambulatory client is less of a safety hazard than a glass of water dropped on the floor beside the bed of an elderly ambulatory client.

2. Breakfast dishes on the overbed table two hours after mealtime is unsightly but does not pose a hazard and does not need immediate attention.

4. A bed that cannot go from the low to high position does need attention. This bed is stuck in the low position, which does not present an immediate hazard for the client.

#78. 3. When the fundus is soft, high above the umbilicus and deviated to the left, the most likely cause is urinary retention. The woman is — Dc He/3 3 six hours post-partum. **The nurse should encourage her to void and if she is unable to do so, catheterize her as ordered.**

1. Retained placental fragments may cause bleeding and a soft fundus but would not cause the fundus to rise and deviate to one side. These findings are more consistent with a full bladder.
2. A perineal laceration would cause bright red perineal bleeding but would not cause changes in consistency and location of the fundus.
4. At six hours post-partum the fundus should be near the umbilicus but should be firm and there should be no deviation to one side. Red lochia is normal at this time. The findings are not normal; they are consistent with urinary retention.

#79. 2. **The cord usually dries up and falls off in ten days to three weeks.** Im He/3 4
1. The cord should be wiped with alcohol with each diaper change. However, the client asked for specific information. The nurse should answer the client's question.
3. The client does sound a bit upset about the cord. However, the nurse should give the client the information she asked for.
4. This answer is not correct. It usually takes ten days to three weeks for the cord to dry up and fall off.

#80. 2. **The baby should double her birth weight by six months and should now weigh close to 14 pounds. This observation indicates the baby is not gaining weight as expected.** Dc He/3 4
1. Infants should sit up with slight support and may lean forward at six months. This is normal and does not need to be brought to the physician's attention.
3. Infants at six months of age often drop objects and will look for them. This is normal and does not need to be brought to the physician's attention.
4. An infant of six months will smack her lips and drool. The infant gets her first tooth around six months of age.

#81. 2. **The nurse should determine that the feeding tube is in the stomach. This is essential.** Im Ph/7 1
1. The client should be positioned upright in a semi-Fowler's position.
3. There is no need to give the client something to suck on during the feeding.
4. It is not essential to check when the client last had a bowel movement.

#82. 1. **Reflecting the client's feelings helps to create a rapport with the client and should open communication and allow the client to further express her feelings regarding the loss of her breast.** Im Ps/5 2
2. This response focuses on the husband and not on the woman. It is not therapeutic.
3. This response does not let the client express her feelings, focuses on the husband, and is a false reassurance. It is not therapeutic.
4. Responding with a cliché type answer is not therapeutic. It does not allow the client to express her feelings.

#83. 3. **The nurse should initially talk with the woman and determine what her immediate needs are.** Im Ps/5 2
1. Telling the client to be quiet is not the best approach. The nurse should determine if the client has any immediate needs.
2. The data given are not sufficient to warrant calling security and the police. After talking with the client the nurse might determine the client was potentially violent and call security.
4. Simply telling the woman everyone is busy is not attending to the client's needs. This response is not therapeutic.

#84. 4. **The nurse should initially empathize and clarify the problem.** Im Ps/5 2
1. This response is not therapeutic. It does not allow the mother to express her feelings and it will probably make her feel guilty that she doesn't feel as though she can cope.

2. The nurse should initially respond with empathy and help to clarify the problem. If the use of social services is indicated the nurse should suggest this after determining the mother's needs and coping skills.

3. This response will probably make the mother feel guilty about her feelings of frustration. The nurse should initially respond with empathy and help to clarify the problem.

#85. 4. Keeping the beds in the lowest position except when the nurse is performing care for the client is likely to reduce the number of falls. Many falls occur when persons are getting out of bed. — Pl — Sa/2 — 1

1. Asking nursing assistants to watch the clients more carefully is very nonspecific. The nurse should give more specific directions.

2. The nurse should not restrain persons just because they cannot walk well independently.

3. Providing traveling call bells might help the clients to call the nurse for help quickly if they did fall, but is not likely to prevent falls. It is also a costly choice. Keeping beds in the lowest position costs nothing and should reduce the number of falls.

#86. 3. If linens are soiled with urine and feces the nursing assistant should wear a gown to prevent soiling of uniform with body secretions. This behavior indicates understanding of universal precautions. — Ev — Sa/2 — 1

1. The nursing assistant should wash hands before and after each and every client contact. This behavior indicates the nursing assistant does not understand universal precautions.

2. Gloves should be worn when the client does not have intact skin or when mucous membranes are being touched. The nursing assistant does not need to wear gloves for all client contact. This action indicates the nursing assistant does not understand universal precautions.

4. Hands should be washed before and after each and every client contact even if gloves have been worn. This action indicates the nursing assistant does not understand universal precautions.

#87. 2. The nurse should never turn her back on a sterile field and all sterile objects should be within view. Turning around to answer a question does not maintain sterile technique. — Ev — Sa/2 — 1

1. The first flap of a sterile dressing set or package should be opened away from the nurse. This allows the last flap to be opened toward the nurse avoiding the need to reach across the sterile field. This behavior maintains sterile technique.

3. Sterile objects should sit about waist high. The overbed table is an appropriate place to open the dressing set. This behavior helps to maintain sterile technique.

4. Pouring sterile saline into a container in the dressing set is appropriate providing the nurse does not spill any liquid on the sterile field. The behavior as described is consistent with sterile technique.

#88. 3. Although all of the problems could be seen, the most common problem seen in a disaster shelter is stress. — Pl — Sa/2 — 2

1. Thirst can be a problem and the disaster shelter should have water available. The most common problem seen in a disaster shelter is stress.

2. Traumatic injuries may be present. The most common problem seen in a disaster shelter is stress.

4. There may be persons who have exacerbation of medical problems. The most common problem seen in a disaster shelter is stress.

#89. 2. Leaving a frail elderly client in bed alone in the house for several hours at a time may well constitute abuse. This should be reported to the supervisor for further evaluation. — Ev — Ps/6 — 1

1. Asking to be a legal guardian for a frail elderly mother is not in any way indicative of abuse and does not need to be reported to the supervisor.

	ANSWER	RATIONALE	NP	CN	SA

3. Brown spots or even petecchiae on the body of an elderly adult are normal and not suggestive of abuse.

4. Before reporting that the daughter yells at her mother the nurse should check out the complaint, checking especially for hearing loss in the mother.

#90. 2. The client appears to have an obsessive-compulsive disorder. The nurse should give her advance warning that her turn is coming so she can perform her washing ritual to reduce her anxiety level.   Im   Ps/6   2

1. Sending her home without seeing the doctor is a punitive response and not appropriate.

3. Persons with an obsessive-compulsive disorder perform rituals to decrease anxiety. If the nurse interrupts the ritual the client may develop severe anxiety.

4. Given a choice of performing the ritual or seeing the doctor, the obsessive-compulsive client will usually choose the ritual.

#91. 1. Saying, "I just can't believe he's gone" is indicative of the denial stage of grief. People who have lost someone close to them often think they see the person standing there.   Dc   Ps/5   2

2. It is common for a recently bereaved person to think they see the loved one. This does not indicate hallucinations.

3. Illusions are a misinterpretation of reality. Thinking you see a recently deceased loved one standing there is not an illusion. It is a common part of the grief process.

4. Her behavior is indicative of early grief, not severe depression.

#92. 4. The nurse should arrange for the group to meet in a conference room or the hospital chapel. The client has a right to practice his religion. The nurse also has the responsibility to protect the rights of the other clients in the hospital.   Im   Ps/5   2

1. Rather than simply explaining the rules, the nurse should attempt to help the client meet his spiritual needs.

2. The nurse should not put the roommate on the spot. The nurse knows that 18 people are too many in a semi-private room and should help the client make alternate arrangements.

3. The nurse has a responsibility to the rest of the clients in the unit to maintain a therapeutic environment and cannot ignore the large number of people and the chanting.

#93. 2. Persons who are taking hallucinogens are apt to be violent. They may think they can fly and react with violence when forced to remain in bed.   Pl   Ps/6   5

1. Severe depression is not a characteristic manifestation of hallucinogen use. The client who is withdrawing from cocaine will get severely depressed.

3. Respiratory distress is not characteristic of persons who are taking hallucinogens. Persons who are taking cocaine may develop sudden cardiac arrest.

4. Convulsions are not typical of hallucinogen use. Persons who are withdrawing from heroin may develop convulsions.

#94. 1. Drinking any alcohol when taking Antabuse will cause a severe gastrointestinal upset and severe headache. The client should take no alcohol in any form. This statement indicates the client does not understand his treatment.   Ev   Ps/6   5

2. Mouthwash contains alcohol and can cause an Antabuse reaction. The client should not have alcohol in any form when taking Antabuse. This statement indicates the client understands his therapy.

3. The client should take the Antabuse daily. It stays in the system for up to three weeks so the client cannot decide he wants to drink in the evening and skip a dose. This statement indicates the client understands his treatment.

4. The client should tell emergency room personnel he is taking Antabuse. Many drugs including preps for intravenous and

intramuscular injections contain alcohol. This statement indicates the client understands his treatment.

#95. 3. Abusers often feel remorse after the episode and seek forgiveness. However, the next time they are frustrated, tired, or angry they are likely to strike out again and repeat the cycle.   Pl   Ps/6   2

   1. Abusers often feel remorse after the episode and seek forgiveness. However, the next time they are frustrated, tired, or angry they are likely to strike out again and repeat the cycle.

   2. Abusers often feel remorse after the episode and seek forgiveness. However, the next time they are frustrated, tired, or angry they are likely to strike out again and repeat the cycle.

   4. Spousal abuse is not caused by misbehavior on the part of the victim. The abuser does not know how to deal with his feelings. The victim often takes the blame and has poor self-esteem.

#96. 3. Persons who are violent and abuse others frequently have a substance abuse problem, which contributes to the problem.   Dc   Ps/6   2

   1. Abuse often happens in times of financial distress.

   2. Abusers usually have a negative self-image.

   4. Physical illness is not associated with the abuser. The abused is apt to suffer from numerous physical illnesses related to the abuse.

#97. 4. A person who has the delusion that his food is being poisoned will not be talked out of it. The nurse should offer him food in individually wrapped containers.   Im   Ps/6   2

   1. Delusions come from the unconscious mind and cannot be reasoned with. Logic is useless when a person is delusional.

   2. Delusions come from the unconscious mind and cannot be reasoned with. Logic is useless when a person is delusional.

   3. The nurse should not serve as the client's taster. If the client should eat the food the nurse has tasted, what will he do when the nurse is off-duty?

#98. 4. By attending to the client's behavior the nurse is sending a message to the client that she is concerned and that she is in control. Having the client go to a quiet area will decrease environmental stimuli. Extremely anxious persons respond to environmental stimuli.   Im   Ps/5   2

   1. Telling the client to do something is apt to increase the client's anxiety. At this time the client is so anxious that she has minimal voluntary control over her behavior. She is not likely to be able to get control of herself.

   2. Leaving the room when the client is severely anxious is likely to increase the client's anxiety level.

   3. The client may well not hear a whisper. Telling the client at this point that everything is going to be all right is false reassurance and something the client is not likely to believe.

#99. 2. Giving the child some control over what is happening to him is likely to reduce his fear.   Im   Ps/5   4

   1. The nurse should not bribe the child with candy.

   3. Telling him that shots don't hurt big boys is not truthful. When the shot does hurt he will feel betrayed, lose trust in the nurse and believe that he is not a big boy.

   4. A two-year-old is not able to respond to reason. A two-year-old will probably not do well watching the nurse give him a shot.

#100. 3. The client is expressing rather severe anxiety and fear. The nurse should respond with empathy and encourage her to vocalize her concerns.   Im   Ps/5   2

   1. The nurse should respond to the client's anxious feeling rather than giving her facts. This statement implies that sometimes people do not get better. This response would likely increase the client's anxiety.

2. The nurse should respond to the client's anxious feelings rather than giving her reassurance about her doctor. The doctor's competence is not the real issue.

4. The nurse should respond to the client's anxious feelings rather than sharing the story of another patient with her.

Practice Test Three

1. A client has fludrocortisone acetate (Florinef) prescribed. What blood tests would the nurse monitor when administering this drug?
    1. Liver function tests
    2. Renal function tests
    3. Serum electrolytes
    4. Complete blood count

2. A 40-year-old woman is admitted in labor with high blood pressure, edema, and proteinuria. She is started on magnesium sulfate. The nurse caring for her should be sure to keep which drug at the bedside?
    1. Calcium gluconate
    2. Narcan
    3. Ritodrine
    4. Glucose

3. A woman who is in labor is being treated for pre-eclampsia. How will the nurse know if the client develops eclampsia?
    1. The client has albuminuria.
    2. The client has a seizure.
    3. The client's face and hands are edematous.
    4. There are no fetal heart tones.

4. A two-month-old infant is admitted with pyloric stenosis and will be going to surgery. What toy should the nurse provide for this infant?
    1. A stuffed teddy bear with a large colorful bow.
    2. A "busy box."
    3. A mobile with large shapes and a music box.
    4. Spoons for each hand so he can bang them together.

5. A four-year-old child with Down syndrome is admitted to the hospital with pneumonia. She has a heart murmur and appears to be in respiratory distress. Her mother asks why her child has a heart murmur. What is the best nursing response?
    1. "Because she has pneumonia, her heart is working harder and causes the murmur."
    2. "Heart murmurs come and go in children. It is not a great concern."
    3. "Because of the pneumonia, her ductus arteriosus is functioning again."

4. "Heart defects are common in children with Down syndrome. Her illness may make the murmur louder."

6. A seven-year-old boy is in the hospital with Reye's syndrome. He has been ill for two weeks with the flu. He ran high fevers and was treated with four baby aspirin alternating with 325 mg chewable Tylenol and sponge baths to control the fever. He also had a rash on his body that was itchy and his mother used lotion and Benadryl to control the itching. Which factors in his history are associated with development of Reye's syndrome? History of the flu and
    1. the use of Benadryl.
    2. the use of Tylenol.
    3. aspirin treatment.
    4. the presence of a rash.

7. A 15-month-old child with Hirschsprung's disease comes for a checkup. The mother reports all of the following. Which indicates a need for more instruction?
    1. The mother limits the child's physical activity to preserve calories.
    2. The child receives daily saline enemas.
    3. The child eats a low-residue diet.
    4. The mother gives the child daily stool softeners.

8. A mother noticed a large abdominal mass when helping her three-year-old child bathe. The child is taken to the physician and admitted to the hospital after an IVP confirms the diagnosis of Wilm's tumor. Which nursing action is essential to include in the nursing care plan?
    1. Strain all urine and save for analysis.
    2. Avoid palpating the abdomen.
    3. Prepare the child for permanent dialysis.
    4. Help the family understand the poor prognosis.

9. A woman who is pregnant for the first time asks the nurse when during pregnancy is the best time to take Lamaze classes. What should the nurse respond?
    1. During the first trimester
    2. During the second trimester

3. During the third trimester
4. Whatever fits into your schedule

10. A woman who comes in for prenatal care has a history of herpes with outbreaks that occur every six months to a year. She asks if this means she will have a cesarean delivery. How should the nurse respond?
    1. "If you have active lesions when you go into labor, you will need a cesarean section."
    2. "Cesarean delivery is the only way to protect your baby from herpes."
    3. "Cesarean delivery is no longer recommended for persons with herpes."
    4. "Your obstetrician will decide at the time of delivery which is best for you."

11. The nurse is discussing health concerns with a group of adolescent girls. When discussing genital warts caused by condyloma acuminata (HPV), the nurse should emphasize that the organism increases the risk of which condition?
    1. Infertility
    2. Congenital anomalies
    3. Cervical cancer
    4. Uterine prolapse

12. The nurse caring for newborns observes for jaundice. Which type of jaundice is likely to be most serious?
    1. Jaundice that occurs during the first day of life.
    2. Jaundice occurring after 48 hours of life.
    3. Jaundice occurring 7–10 days after birth.
    4. Any jaundice is potentially life-threatening.

13. The mother of a newborn asks why the nurse is checking the baby's nose. The nurse replies that it is important to check nasal patency because the newborn:
    1. Does not have the ability to sneeze.
    2. Must breathe through his nose.
    3. Is subject to periods of apnea.
    4. Has rapid respirations.

14. The nurse is caring for a 31-year old gravida 2, para 1 woman who is in labor. The woman calls the nurse and says "My water has broken and I feel something between my legs." The nurse looks and sees a loop of umbilical cord at the vaginal outlet. After signaling for help, what should the nurse do?
    1. Try to replace the cord with a sterile gloved hand.
    2. Place the mother in knee chest position.
    3. Quickly apply manual pressure on the fundus.
    4. Expect a rapid vaginal delivery.

15. A laboring woman prefers to lie in the supine position during labor. The nurse teaches her that this is not a good position for which reason?
    1. It will cause more back pressure.
    2. Her baby will not come down well into the pelvis.
    3. Her blood pressure may drop and cause the baby's heart rate to drop.
    4. Contractions will be too close together, not giving her a rest.

16. All of the following clients are on the unit. Which one is most likely to have an order for catheterization for residual?
    1. A woman who had a modified radical mastectomy yesterday.
    2. A man who had an abdominal cholecystectomy this morning.
    3. A woman who had an abdominal hysterectomy yesterday.
    4. A man who had surgery for a ruptured appendix.

17. A client who had a total knee replacement is to be discharged today. Which statement the client makes indicates a need for further instruction?
    1. "When I am walking, I will wear that ugly immobilizer."
    2. "I will sit with my leg elevated."
    3. "I think I understand how to use the continuous passive motion machine."
    4. "I won't put any weight at all on my affected leg."

18. An adult is receiving cancer chemotherapy. Metoclopramide (Reglan) is also prescribed. The client asks why she is getting Reglan. How should the nurse respond?
    1. "Reglan helps to prevent bleeding that may occur as a side effect of your other medications."
    2. "Reglan helps to prevent any nausea and vomiting that may occur as a side effect of your other medications."
    3. "Reglan increases the effectiveness of the cancer chemotherapeutic agents."
    4. "Reglan helps to control pain associated with your disease."

19. A very tall, heavy-set man is admitted. The nurse is taking vital signs. Which statement is correct about taking the blood pressure?
    1. 10 mm should be added to each reading to compensate for the cuff size.
    2. 15 mm should be subtracted from the systolic reading and 10 mm from the diastolic reading.
    3. An extra-large cuff is needed to obtain an accurate measurement.
    4. The client should lie down before the blood pressure is taken.

20. The nurse is auscultating the lungs in a post-operative client and hears something that sounds like a cellophane bag being wrinkled when the client takes in a breath. How should the nurse record this finding?
    1. Crackles
    2. Stridor
    3. Stertor
    4. Wheezes

21. The client who is scheduled for a knee replacement asks the nurse why she should donate her own blood before surgery. How should the nurse respond?
    1. "The blood bank is very short of blood."
    2. "Your own blood is the correct type for you."
    3. "It eliminates the chance of blood-borne diseases such as hepatitis and HIV."
    4. "Your own blood increases your energy level after surgery."

22. The client who is receiving hydantoin (Dilantin) tells the nurse his urine is pink-colored. What action should the nurse take?
    1. Report this serious side effect immediately to the physician.
    2. Reassure the client that this occurs often in persons taking Dilantin.
    3. Ask the client if he drank cranberry juice or ate red gelatin recently.
    4. Strain the client's urine for possible urinary tract stones.

23. A woman who was recently diagnosed with multiple myeloma says to the nurse, "Why did this happen to me? I've always been a good person. What did I do to deserve this?" What should the nurse do initially?
    1. Remind the client that she is not dying now and has some time left.
    2. Call the chaplain to discuss why it happened to her.
    3. Respond by recognizing how difficult this situation must be.
    4. Tell her she didn't do anything to deserve it.

24. A client asks the home care nurse to look at the bruises on her arms and legs. The woman also tells the nurse that her gums bleed when she uses dental floss or brushes her teeth. The client is taking all of the following medications. Which is most likely related to the client's symptoms?
    1. Metformin (Glucophage)
    2. Estrogen (Premarin)
    3. Atenolol (Tenormin)
    4. Ibuprofen (Motrin)

25. The client is taking streptomycin, isoniazid, and rimactane. Which data indicates toxicity to isoniazid?
    1. My ears ring all the time.
    2. I have sharp pains in my legs.
    3. My urine is orange-colored.
    4. I'm having trouble at traffic lights.

26. The nurse observes the certified nursing assistant doing all of the following. Which action needs correction?
    1. Changing the dressing of a client with an abdominal wound
    2. Asking a standing client to sit down while vital signs are taken
    3. Emptying a urine drainage bag from the tube at the bottom

    4. Changing water in the middle of a bed bath

27. A man who has diabetes complains of hunger and is pale, shaky, perspiring, and has cool skin. What is the most appropriate initial action for the nurse?
    1. Call the physician for orders.
    2. Give the client cola to drink.
    3. Have the client lie down.
    4. Administer the next dose of insulin.

28. A client who had a total thyroidectomy this morning returns to the nursing care unit. How should the nurse position the client?
    1. Semi-Fowler's
    2. Supine
    3. Prone
    4. Sims

29. All of the following clients need care. Whom should the nurse see first?
    1. A diabetic whose blood sugar is 40
    2. A post-operative client who is complaining of severe pain
    3. A person with terminal cancer who is complaining of pain
    4. A client with an indwelling catheter who is complaining of bladder pain

30. The nurse is working with a person who was just diagnosed with diabetes mellitus Type II. What should the nurse teach the client first?
    1. How to self-inject insulin
    2. How to follow a diabetic diet
    3. Signs and symptoms of insulin reaction
    4. Complications of diabetes

31. The nurse is caring for a person admitted with myasthenia gravis. What should be included in the nursing care plan for this person?
    1. Have the client bathe late in the day.
    2. Check swallowing reflexes before feeding.
    3. Have the client void every hour.
    4. Observe for signs of neuropathy.

32. Which of the following clients should be cared for first?
    1. An elderly woman who has been incontinent of urine in bed
    2. An elderly man who has had fecal incontinence
    3. A man who has been up in the chair for two hours and wants to go back to bed
    4. A woman who needs to be turned every two hours and was last turned two hours ago

33. The nurse is caring for a person who is admitted with progressive amyotrophic lateral sclerosis. What nursing care measures should the nurse expect to be ordered for this client?
    1. Change dressing daily.
    2. Monitor IV fluids.
    3. Insert indwelling catheter.
    4. Chest physical therapy qid

34. All of the following need to be done. Which should the nurse delegate to the certified nursing assistant?
    1. Administering prn acetaminophen to a person who has arthritis
    2. Hygienic care to a person who had a CVA
    3. Catheterizing a client who is scheduled for surgery today
    4. Changing the dressing on a client who has a Stage III decubitus ulcer

35. The nurse is assessing a 78-year-old woman. The woman says she has some bladder discomfort and urinary frequency. She also says "I mind the cold so, but I don't seem to shiver. I don't have much energy these days." Her temperature is 98.9°F, pulse is 76, respirations 20, and blood pressure is 140/88. Which findings are of most concern to the nurse and need to be further evaluated?
    1. Temperature, pulse, respirations
    2. Blood pressure and temperature
    3. Bladder symptoms and fatigue
    4. Inability to shiver and cold sensitivity

36. All of the following individuals live at home with their families. Which of the following persons is least at risk for abuse?
    1. An 82-year-old woman who is incontinent and bosses people around
    2. An 80-year-old man who is ambulatory with help following a brain attack
    3. A 78-year-old woman who asks for help with all of her activities of daily living
    4. A 75-year-old man who wanders at night and frequently yells out

37. Triazolam (Halcion) 0.25 mg is ordered for a client at h.s. When the nurse goes to give the medication, the client asks the nurse to leave it at the bedside because she wants to finish reading a book. What is the best action for the nurse to take?
    1. Leave the medication at the bedside as requested.
    2. Return in one hour and offer the medication again.
    3. Tell the client to call when she is ready for the medication.
    4. Explain to the client that this is the time medications are given and she should take it now.

38. The family of a frail elderly man who is bedridden asks the nurse what they can do to prevent bedsores. Which response by the nurse is best?
    1. "Get him out of bed at least once a day."
    2. "Turn him every two hours."
    3. "Rub his buttocks and apply lotion several times a day."
    4. "Change the sheets every day."

39. After returning from the post-anesthesia care unit, a man who had abdominal surgery is ordered to be in semi-Fowler's position. What is the primary reason for this position for this client?
    1. To prevent venous stasis
    2. To promote circulation
    3. To reduce tension on the incision
    4. To prevent respiratory distress

40. A woman who has been hospitalized for several days says she is having trouble getting to sleep. What is the best initial nursing intervention?
    1. Offer her a back rub.
    2. Ask her what she is worrying about.
    3. Give the ordered prn sedative.
    4. Notify the physician.

41. The nurse is observing a nursing assistant move a client from bed to chair. Which action by the nursing assistant indicates a lack of understanding about transfer techniques?
    1. Bending from the waist when moving the person
    2. Keeping the feet separated when lifting and moving the person
    3. Turning the whole body when moving the person to the chair
    4. Asking for help in moving the person from bed to chair

42. A woman is scheduled for an electromyography procedure (EMG) in the outpatient department. What should the nurse say to the woman?
    1. "Do not eat or drink anything after midnight the night before the procedure."
    2. "Are you allergic to shellfish or iodine?"
    3. "Do not eat or drink anything that contains caffeine for 2–3 days before the procedure."
    4. "There is no special preparation for this procedure."

43. The nurse checks the lab values of a newly admitted client.
    RBC 4.0 million/mm^3
    WBC 1500/mm^3
    Platelets 40,000/mm^3
    What nursing actions are indicated because of these lab values?
    1. Keep the client on bed rest and protective isolation.
    2. Plan for protective isolation and do not give injections.
    3. Keep the client on bed rest and avoid trauma.
    4. There are no special nursing actions indicated.

44. The nurse is caring for a client who is receiving an intravenous infusion. Which finding would indicate the client's IV has infiltrated?
    1. The client's arm is red and warm to the touch.
    2. The IV is running faster than the desired rate.

3. The area around the infusion site is pale and cool to the touch.
4. The client complains of severe pain up and down the arm.

45. The nurse has been teaching a woman who has iron deficiency anemia. Which menu, if selected, indicates the woman understands her dietary instructions?
   1. Applesauce, green beans, bread, and butter
   2. Peanut butter and jelly sandwich, carrots, and milk
   3. Broccoli, spinach salad with tomatoes, and orange juice
   4. Macaroni and cheese, pickles, and hot chocolate

46. A client is admitted with pernicious anemia. The client reports all of the following. Which is most likely related to the admitting diagnosis?
   1. "I often have diarrhea."
   2. "My tongue is more red and thick than usual."
   3. "I have little bruise-like spots on my arms and legs."
   4. "I have been running a fever for the last two days."

47. A man who had a right below-the-knee amputation is placed in the prone position for one hour three times a day. The nurse explains to the man that this is done to prevent which problem?
   1. Atelectasis
   2. Thrombophlebitis
   3. Hip flexion contractures
   4. Wound infection

48. The client has contact dermatitis from poison ivy. Which statement, if made by the client, indicates he understands how to care for his condition?
   1. "A hot bath should make the itching go away."
   2. "I will use a good strong soap when I wash the affected areas."
   3. "A cool wet cloth to the area should help."
   4. "Wearing wool socks will help my itchy feet."

49. The nurse is caring for a client who has psoriasis. Which observation by the nurse is most consistent with the diagnosis?
   1. The client has thick, yellow toenails.
   2. The client has open, weeping lesions.
   3. The skin lesions are multicolored.
   4. The pain follows a nerve root.

50. The nurse is caring for a man who has severe burns and had a skin graft. What nursing care measures are appropriate at the graft site the day of the graft?
   1. Leave the graft site open to the air.
   2. Elevate the recipient site.
   3. Encourage range-of-motion exercises.
   4. Change the dressing twice a day.

51. The nurse is to make several home visits today. All of the visits are within a five-mile radius. All of the following persons need to be seen. Which person should the nurse visit first?
   1. An older adult who has diabetes, peripheral vascular disease, and leg ulcers and needs hygienic care and wound care
   2. An adult who has multiple myeloma and needs her weekly injection of Interferon
   3. A woman with multiple sclerosis that needs hygienic care
   4. An elderly woman who is recovering from a cerebral vascular accident and needs hygienic care and ROM exercises

52. The nurse is caring for a client who was admitted following a motor vehicle accident. The client's blood pressure one hour ago was 118/76, pulse was 80; now the blood pressure is 90/60, pulse is 98. What action should the nurse take initially?
   1. Continue to monitor the blood pressure.
   2. Ask another nurse to check the blood pressure reading.
   3. Elevate the client's legs.
   4. Call the physician.

53. The nurse is caring for a person who has a nasogastric tube attached to drainage. Which complaint by the client needs to be reported to the charge nurse?
   1. Dry mouth.
   2. Weak muscles.
   3. Sore throat.
   4. Irritated nose.

54. A cooling blanket is ordered for an adult client who has a temperature of 106°F. What nursing action is essential because the client has a cooling blanket?
   1. Keep a padded tongue blade at the bedside.
   2. Turn every two hours.
   3. Apply ice to the groin area.
   4. Cover with a sheet and blanket.

55. The nurse is to suction a client. What action is essential prior to inserting the suction catheter?
   1. Clear the mouth and throat of secretions.
   2. Lower the head of the bed.
   3. Oxygenate the client.
   4. Check the suction pressure.

56. The nurse is caring for a man who has chronic emphysema and is receiving oxygen at 2 liters per minute. The nurse enters the room to find his wife has turned the oxygen up to 10 liters per minute because her husband is having increasing difficulty breathing. What is the best immediate action for the nurse?
   1. Explain to the wife that his oxygen was ordered at 2 liters per minute and it should stay there until the physician orders something else.

2. Turn the oxygen setting back to 2 liters per minute.
3. Tell the wife that 10 liters per minute is too high and turn it back to 5 liters per minute.
4. Assure her that 10 liters per minute will ease her husband's breathing.

57. The nurse discovers that a client is not breathing and has no pulse. After calling for help, what should the nurse do next?
1. Give the client two breaths.
2. Administer five chest compressions.
3. Go get the emergency cart.
4. Defibrillate the client.

58. The nurse is caring for a man who has radiation pellets in his mouth for mouth cancer. The nurse discovers one of the pellets in the sheets. What should the nurse do initially?
1. Check the client's mouth for other loose pellets.
2. Using long-handled forceps, put the pellet in a lead-lined container.
3. Ask the client to hold the pellet until the radiologist arrives.
4. Call the radiation safety officer.

59. The physician has ordered crutches and specified the client use a four-point gait. Which action by the client indicates an understanding of the four-point gait? The client moves:
1. The left foot, then the left crutch, followed by the right foot and the right crutch.
2. The left foot, then the right foot, followed by the left crutch and the right crutch.
3. The left foot and the right crutch together followed by the right foot and the left crutch.
4. The left foot, then the right crutch, followed by the right foot and the left crutch.

60. A man is a client in a semi-private room. When a new person is admitted to his room he says to the nurse, "What is wrong with the man in the other bed?" How should the nurse respond?
1. Tell the man he should ask him himself.
2. Tell the man in general terms the new client's diagnosis.
3. Ask the man why he wants to know.
4. Tell him that all clients' diagnoses are confidential.

61. An adult is to go to surgery this morning. When the nurse goes to medicate the client she notes that she has a ring with several shiny stones in it on her left ring finger. There are no relatives present. What is the best nursing action?
1. Tape the ring before medicating the client.
2. Ask the client to put the ring in the bedside drawer.
3. Label the ring and place in an envelope in the hospital safe.

4. Have the client sign a waiver regarding responsibility for the ring.

62. The nurse is providing home care for a client who has Parkinson's disease and is ambulatory. Which activity will help to prevent slipping and falling?
1. Encourage the client to wear smooth-soled shoes.
2. Leave the bed rails up at all times.
3. Have the client spend several hours daily sitting in a chair.
4. Place a scatter rug beside his bed.

63. The LPN/LVN in a long-term care facility sees and hears a nursing assistant give a resident a hard slap. What initial action should the LPN/LVN take?
1. Be alert to further incidences of a similar nature.
2. Report the incident to the supervisor.
3. Write an incident report.
4. Report the incident to the police.

64. The nurse is giving pre-operative medication to an adult who is scheduled for surgery. The client says to the nurse that she does not want to have a transfusion during surgery because it is against her religion. The client has signed a consent form for surgery. How should the nurse respond?
1. Explain that she has signed a consent form for surgery and that includes the use of transfusions if necessary.
2. Explain that the surgeon will probably not perform surgery if she won't have a transfusion.
3. Have the client sign an addendum to the operative permit excluding transfusions.
4. Withhold the medication and notify the physician.

65. The daughter of a 78-year-old woman asks the nurse why her mother is giving away some of her belongings to her children and grandchildren. What should the nurse include when responding?
1. Older adults usually become more generous.
2. It is normal for older adults to think about and prepare for their own death.
3. Her mother probably does not trust her children to divide her things appropriately.
4. Her mother is probably thinking about suicide.

66. The nurse in a residence facility for older adults is planning for the year. During which month should the influenza vaccine be offered to the residents?
1. May
2. July
3. September
4. November

67. The nurse is giving instructions to a group of women about self breast examination. Which

statement indicates the client needs more instruction about the procedure?
1. "I will perform the exam every month after my period."
2. "I should do the exam both standing and lying down."
3. "Some ridges are normal in my breast."
4. "I will do the self breast exam every month until menopause."

68. The nurse is teaching a group of women about health issues. Today's topic is food poisoning. Which statement indicates a need for further instruction?
1. "I always wash my hands after I put raw meat in to cook."
2. "I should put foods away in the refrigerator immediately after meals."
3. "I will wash my kitchen counters with a bleach solution after preparing raw meat."
4. "Rare meat is okay to eat as long as it is eaten immediately after cooking."

69. The nurse is to administer a tuberculin skin test. What is the correct procedure?
1. Give it subcutaneously in the inner aspect of the forearm.
2. Use a 21-gauge needle and administer in the forearm.
3. Give it at a 10-degree angle in the volar surface of the arm.
4. Administer intradermal in the upper arm.

70. The nurse is planning care for a client who has a hearing impairment. Which action will likely help the most with communication?
1. Repeat everything twice.
2. Speak loudly.
3. Speak slowly and clearly.
4. Use gestures.

71. An 80-year-old woman has been hospitalized for three days with pneumonia. She is now able to sit in a chair for the first time. How should the nurse plan care for today?
1. Give her a bed bath and then get her up and make her bed while she is in the chair.
2. Get her up in the chair and have her give herself a bath while the nurse makes the bed.
3. Give her a bed bath and come back later to get her up in the chair. Make the bed while she is up in the chair.
4. Give her a bed bath and immediately get her up in the chair so the bed can be made.

72. The nurse is to administer a tube feeding to a client. Before administering the feeding, what is essential for the nurse to do?
1. Ask the client if she feels full.
2. Aspirate the nasogastric tube and check for acid.
3. Change the tubing.
4. Feel over the end of the tube and do not administer if air is felt.

73. The nurse is planning an approach to decrease urinary incontinence in an elderly client. Which activity will do the most to help prevent incontinence?
1. Restrict fluids until continence has been achieved, then hydrate well.
2. Offer the bedpan at two-hour intervals during the day and every four hours at night.
3. Encourage the client to ambulate frequently and have the client do deep-breathing exercises.
4. Encourage fluids during the day and offer the bedpan every two hours.

74. A woman in a residence facility is having difficulty sleeping at night. Which action by the nurse is most appropriate initially?
1. Ask the physician for a sleeping medication.
2. Offer the woman a back rub and warm milk.
3. Suggest to the woman that she take a walk around the unit.
4. Offer the woman a cup of hot tea.

75. A post-operative client is having difficulty voiding. Palpation of the bladder indicates the bladder is full. What should the nurse do initially?
1. Ask the physician for a catheterization order.
2. Pour water over the client's perineum.
3. Encourage the client to take deep breaths.
4. Administer pain medication.

76. The physician has recommended that the client increase the amount of dietary iron. The nurse knows the client understands the recommendations when the client selects which foods?
1. Orange juice, scrambled eggs, and toast
2. Hot dog and roll, French fries, and cola
3. Roast beef, carrots, and rice
4. Baked chicken, peas, and noodles

77. The nurse is to start oxygen therapy via nasal cannula. Which action is correct?
1. Set the oxygen at 12 liters per minute.
2. Lubricate the cannula with petrolatum before inserting.
3. Give 100% oxygen by mask before inserting the cannula.
4. Insert the cannula 1 cm into the nostrils.

78. A woman calls the physician's office stating that her 16-year-old daughter took 20 or 30 sleeping pills. The mother tells the nurse that her daughter is awake and says, "Leave me alone. I just want to die." How should the nurse respond?
1. "Ask her why she wants to die."
2. "Try to convince her she wants to live."
3. "Give her a glass of milk to bind the medication."
4. "Do you have syrup of Ipecac in the house?"

79. A wet-to-dry dressing is ordered for a client who has a decubitus ulcer. Which technique is appropriate?
    1. Irrigate the wound, then apply a dry dressing and cover with a wet compress.
    2. Apply a wet dressing for two hours followed by a dry dressing for 2 hours.
    3. Apply a wet dressing and cover with a dry dressing.
    4. Apply a wet dressing above the wound and a dry dressing below the wound.

80. The nurse is providing home care to a confused older adult. The family members have tied the client in a chair with a large leather belt. They say the client wanders if he isn't restrained. What initial nursing action is most appropriate?
    1. Report the family to family protective services.
    2. Congratulate the family on solving the problem.
    3. Help the family think of ways to make the environment safer for the client.
    4. Tell the family that you are not allowed to restrain the client with a leather belt.

81. The nurse is assessing the nursing care unit in a long-term facility for fire hazards. Which finding is the greatest fire hazard?
    1. Some of the nurses and nursing assistants smoke in the restroom.
    2. There are several cardboard boxes and cleaning supplies stored in the room with the emergency oxygen supply.
    3. Several residents have dust under their beds.
    4. Two of the residents have closets that are stuffed full of photo albums and sewing supplies.

82. A woman who recently had a simple mastectomy is about to be discharged. She seems very concerned about such things as where to find the best prosthesis, suitable underwear, and swimsuits, and adjusting to life with only one breast. Which resource is appropriate for the nurse to recommend?
    1. A psychologist or psychiatrist
    2. Reach for Recovery
    3. Pastoral counseling
    4. Her physician

83. A man who had a cerebral vascular accident has expressive aphasia. Which approach will help communication the most?
    1. The nurse should write to the client and the client should write back.
    2. The nurse should anticipate the client's needs as much as possible.
    3. The nurse should encourage the client to speak as much as possible.
    4. A family member should stay with the client and express the client's needs to the nurse.

84. An upset client says to the nurse, "Where did you learn to be a nurse? You don't know anything." How should the nurse respond?
    1. "I'm sorry you feel that way."
    2. "I went to a fine nursing school."
    3. "You sound upset."
    4. "Please don't speak to me that way."

85. A terminally ill client says to the nurse, "Do you believe in heaven?" How should the nurse respond?
    1. "Yes, I believe in heaven and hell."
    2. "My personal belief is private."
    3. "Do you believe in heaven?"
    4. "Do you want to see your clergyman?"

86. The nurse is assessing a child admitted who has a fractured humerus. The family says the child fell. Which piece of data would cause the nurse to suspect child abuse?
    1. The child has been to the emergency room twice in the last month.
    2. The child also has several bruises on the arms and legs.
    3. The child has small round burned areas on the abdomen and back.
    4. The child is holding his mother's hand.

87. Which comment, if made by the client, indicates adjustment to the diagnosis of insulin-dependent diabetes mellitus?
    1. "Will it ever get easier to give myself a shot?"
    2. "This can't be happening to me?"
    3. "When I get over this, I'm going to eat chocolate cake every day."
    4. "At least no one at work will know what they say I have."

88. An adult who is admitted to the hospital for a colostomy says to the nurse, "I'm so scared. Do you think I'll make it?" What is the nurse's best initial response?
    1. "Of course you'll make it."
    2. "Why are you so scared?"
    3. "You're not likely to die."
    4. "You sound scared."

89. The wife of a man who is comatose following a head injury asks the nurse if she should visit since he is unresponsive. How should the nurse reply initially?
    1. Explain that since he is unresponsive there is no need for her to be here.
    2. Tell her that the nurse will call if there is any change.
    3. Suggest her presence is important even though he seems unaware.
    4. Recommend that she ask his coworkers to visit.

90. A 14-year-old girl is brought to the emergency room because she is difficult to arouse. She is 5 feet, 8 inches tall and weighs 80 pounds. What additional findings would the nurse expect to be present?
    1. Tachycardia
    2. Amenorrhea

3. Wheezing
4. Acne

91. An adult is admitted to a detoxification unit for withdrawal from alcohol. Which medication does the nurse expect will be ordered for the client upon admission?
    1. Thiamin
    2. Antabuse
    3. Ascorbic acid
    4. Dilantin

92. The nurse is discussing dementia with the families of older adults. All of the following behaviors are reported. Which behavior is most suggestive of dementia?
    1. The woman can't remember what year each of her six children was born.
    2. A woman walked to the store and got lost on the way home.
    3. A woman forgot where she put her purse.
    4. A man is wearing one green sock and one red sock and doesn't see the difference.

93. A behavior modification program is planned for an adolescent who exhibits disruptive behavior. Which action by the nurse is most consistent with a behavior modification program?
    1. Punish the client if she becomes disruptive.
    2. Give the client extra privileges when she is not disruptive for a day.
    3. Remind the client what she is supposed to do at regular intervals.
    4. Ask the client what she sees as good behavior.

94. A client on the psychiatric unit does not get to the dining room to eat because she is continually washing her hands and doesn't finish until after lunch. What should be included in the nursing care plan?
    1. Give the client a choice between eating lunch and performing her ritual.
    2. Tell the client an hour before lunch so she can perform her ritual before lunch.
    3. Discuss the problem with the client and ask her why she washes her hands so long.
    4. Tell the client she cannot wash her hands at all if she is going to be late for lunch.

95. The nurse has been assigned a client who is thought to be suicidal. All of the following are in the client's room. Which is safe to leave in the room?
    1. Paper cup
    2. Leather belt
    3. Razor
    4. Pillow

96. The nurse has just completed a dressing change on an elderly client who is allowed bathroom privileges. Which action is most essential for the nurse to take before leaving the client's bedside?
    1. Wash hands.
    2. Lower the bed.
    3. Toilet the client.
    4. Assess for pain.

97. The nurse is caring for a woman who has internal radiation for cancer of the cervix. Which of the following situations poses the greatest risk for others?
    1. The client's daughter spends several hours sitting next to the client's bed.
    2. The client's husband kisses her and visits for five minutes before leaving.
    3. The nurse brings the client her lunch tray and sets it up on the overbed table for her.
    4. The cleaning lady damp mops the room.

98. An infant is to be admitted with severe diarrhea. Which room assignment is best for this infant?
    1. A private room
    2. A room close to the nurse's station
    3. A room with a two-year-old child who has a broken leg
    4. A room with another infant with severe diarrhea

99. A client who is blind is admitted to the hospital for surgery tomorrow. The client is able to get out of bed and eat until midnight. Which nursing action is most appropriate?
    1. Describe the surroundings and the objects in the room to the client.
    2. Put up the siderails and have the client ask for help when getting out of bed for any reason.
    3. Describe the voices of the personnel to the client.
    4. Remove objects such as water pitchers and glasses from the immediate vicinity.

100. The nurse is providing care in the home to a person who has AIDS. Which behavior, if observed by the nurse, indicates a need for further instruction?
    1. The client uses the same dishes as the rest of the family.
    2. The client shares a bathroom with the rest of the family.
    3. The client and his brother use the same razor.
    4. The client often cooks for the family.

Answers and Rationales for Practice Test Three

Answer	Rationale	NP	CN	SA

#1. 3. **Florinef is given to clients whose adrenal cortex is not functioning adequately or to clients who have had an adrenalectomy. It acts like aldosterone to cause sodium and water retention and potassium excretion. Serum electrolytes are important to monitor to determine sodium and potassium levels. The client may need potassium supplements.**   Dc   Ph/8   5

    1. Fludrocortisone acetate does not primarily affect liver function. Liver toxicity is not a common side effect of this drug.

    2. Renal toxicity is not a common side effect of this drug.

    4. This drug does not commonly affect the blood count.

#2. 1. **Calcium gluconate is the antidote for magnesium toxicity and must be available immediately for the respiratory depression that occurs when magnesium levels are too high.**   Pl   Ph/8   5

    2. Narcan is a narcotic antagonist and is used to treat respiratory depression caused by narcotic overdose.

    3. Ritodrine is used to treat pre-term labor.

    4. Glucose is used to treat hypoglycemia.

#3. 2. **Eclampsia means that the client has seizures.**   Dc   Ph/10   3

    1. Albuminuria is a classic symptom of pre-eclampsia.

    3. Edema of the hands and face is a classic symptom of pre-eclampsia.

    4. Absence of fetal heart tones is suggestive of fetal death and could be associated with severe eclampsia but is not definitive of eclampsia. Eclampsia means the client has developed seizures.

#4. 3. **This choice is most age-appropriate. The infant can focus on the large shapes and listen to the music box.**   Im   He/3   4

    1. The teddy bear will not hold the attention of a two-month-old for long. The bow can present a choking hazard unless it is very well attached.

    2. A two-month-old infant does not have the dexterity to play with a "busy box."

    4. A two-month-old infant cannot bang spoons together.

#5. 4. **Heart disease is very common in children with Down syndrome. The strain on her system from pneumonia may increase blood flow through the defect making the murmur louder.**   Im   Ph/10   4

    1. It is true that pneumonia may make the heart work harder and may intensify a murmur. However, it does not cause the murmur. Heart defects are very common in children with Down syndrome.

    2. This is not correct information. Heart murmurs do not come and go in children.

    3. The ductus arteriosus should have closed at birth unless it was kept open by the defect. Pneumonia does not cause the ductus arteriosus to reopen.

#6. 3. **Reye's syndrome is associated with the use of aspirin in children who have a viral infection. Aspirin is not recommended for children.**   Dc   Ph/10   4

    1. Benadryl use is not associated with the incidence of Reye's syndrome.

    2. Reye's syndrome is not associated with the use of Tylenol.

    4. Reye's syndrome is not associated with a rash.

#7. 1. **There is no reason to limit activity in a child who has Hirschsprung's disease. This indicates the mother needs more teaching.**   Ev   Ph/9   4

    2. Daily saline enemas are part of the recommended treatment for a child with Hirschsprung's disease.

    3. A low-residue diet is part of the recommended treatment for a child with Hirschsprung's disease.

ANSWER	RATIONALE	NP	CN	SA

4. Stool softeners daily are part of the recommended treatment for a child with Hirschsprung's disease.

#8. 2. A Wilm's tumor is an encapsulated tumor. If palpated excessively it may rupture and spread cancer cells throughout the abdomen. It is essential that it not be palpated.   Pl   Ph/9   4

1. There is no need to strain and save urine. Straining urine is appropriate for kidney stones.
3. Following surgery the child will still have one kidney and will not need dialysis.
4. The prognosis for recovery from Wilm's tumor is good if it is caught early when it is confined to the kidney.

#9. 3. Taking Lamaze classes closer to delivery is ideal. The mother is thinking about labor and she is more likely to practice and keep up conditioning.   Im   He/3   3

1. Taking Lamaze classes closer to delivery is ideal. The mother is thinking about labor and she is more likely to practice and keep up conditioning.
2. Taking Lamaze classes closer to delivery is ideal. The mother is thinking about labor and she is more likely to practice and keep up conditioning.
4. Taking Lamaze classes closer to delivery is ideal. The mother is thinking about labor and she is more likely to practice and keep up conditioning.

#10. 1. Cesarean section delivery is only necessary if there are active lesions at the time of delivery. If active lesions are present at delivery, the baby could become severely ill or die.   Im   Ph/9   3

2. Cesarean section delivery is only necessary if there are active lesions at the time of delivery. If active lesions are present at delivery, the baby could become severely ill or die.
3. Cesarean section delivery is only necessary if there are active lesions at the time of delivery. If active lesions are present at delivery, the baby could become severely ill or die.
4. Cesarean section delivery is only necessary if there are active lesions at the time of delivery. If active lesions are present at delivery, the baby could become severely ill or die.

#11. 3. HPV infections are associated with an increased risk of cervical cancer.   Im   He/4   3

1. HPV infection is not associated with infertility. Pelvic inflammatory disease increases the risk of infertility.
2. Genital warts do not cause congenital anomalies. Diseases such as rubella and syphilis can cause congenital anomalies.
4. Uterine prolapse is not caused by genital warts.

#12. 1. Jaundice occurring in the first 24 hours of life is called pathological jaundice and is most serious because it is often related to blood incompatibilities.   Dc   Ph/9   4

2. Jaundice occurring after 48 hours is called physiologic jaundice and is related to an immature liver that can not keep up with the breakdown of red blood cells.
3. Jaundice that occurs 7–10 days after birth is usually breast milk jaundice and is usually of little concern.
4. Jaundice occurring after 48 hours and at 7–10 days is usually of little concern and is certainly not life-threatening.

#13. 2. The newborn is an obligate nose breather and can only breathe through his mouth when he is crying. When he becomes fatigued, he falls asleep and turns blue if he cannot breathe through his nose.   Dc   He/3   4

1. Newborns sneeze easily.
3. Newborns do have periods of apnea but this has nothing to do with being a nose breather.
4. Newborns have rapid respirations but this is not related to being a nose breather.

ANSWER	RATIONALE	NP	CN	SA

#14. 2. **The nurse should attempt to relieve pressure on the cord by putting the mother in knee-chest position. This lets gravity help to relieve pressure on the cord.**   Im   He/4   3

    1. The nurse should not attempt to replace the cord. If the nurse discovers a prolapsed cord during a sterile vaginal exam, the hand may be left in the vagina to help relieve pressure on the cord.

    3. The nurse should not apply manual pressure on the fundus.

    4. The baby will be delivered by c-section as rapidly as possible.

#15. 3. **Supine hypotension may occur as the weight of the uterus presses on the vena cava. This may cause the baby's heart rate to drop.**   Im   He/3   3

    1. The major problem with supine position is not back pressure but supine hypotension, which may occur as the weight of the uterus presses on the vena cava, causing the mother's blood pressure to drop and the baby's heart rate to drop.

    2. The supine position may or may not hinder descent. The major problem with supine position is supine hypotension, which may occur as the weight of the uterus presses on the vena cava, causing the mother's blood pressure to drop and the baby's heart rate to drop.

    4. Contractions usually slow down in the supine position.

#16. 3. **Catheterization for residual urine is usually done for persons who have been catheterized for a long period of time or persons who have had pelvic area surgery. It is frequently ordered for women who have had gynecological surgery. Surgery in the pelvic area often makes it difficult to regain bladder tone.**   Pl   Ph/7   1

    1. A mastectomy does not affect bladder tone. It would be unusual for the woman who had a modified radical mastectomy to have an order to be catheterized for residual urine.

    2. The client who had an abdominal cholecystectomy might or might not have an indwelling catheter for a few hours. A cholecystectomy does not affect bladder tone. It would be unusual for the client who had an abdominal cholecystectomy to have an order to be catheterized for residual urine.

    4. It would be unusual for the client who had surgery for a ruptured appendix to have an order to be catheterized for residual urine.

#17. 4. **The client should be gradually increasing weight-bearing on the affected leg. This answer indicates a need for further instruction.**   Ev   Ph/9   1

    1. The immobilizer should be worn when the client is walking. This answer indicates an understanding of instructions.

    2. The client should sit with leg elevated. This answer indicates an understanding of instructions.

    3. The client will use the continuous passive motion (CPM) machine at home. This answer indicates an understanding of instructions.

#18. 2. **Cancer chemotherapeutic agents frequently cause nausea and vomiting. Reglan is an antiemetic given to help control nausea and vomiting.**   Im   Ph/8   5

    1. Reglan does not control bleeding. Cancer chemotherapeutic agents frequently cause nausea and vomiting. Reglan is an antiemetic given to help control nausea and vomiting.

    3. Reglan does not increase the effectiveness of cancer chemotherapeutic agents. Cancer chemotherapeutic agents frequently cause nausea and vomiting. Reglan is an antiemetic given to help control nausea and vomiting.

    4. Reglan is not an analgesic. Cancer chemotherapeutic agents frequently cause nausea and vomiting. Reglan is an antiemetic given to help control nausea and vomiting.

#19. 3. **When the client's arm is long or larger around than average, a wide cuff should be used. If the regular cuff is used, the blood pressure reading will be higher than it actually is.**   Im   He/4   1

    1. When the client's arm is long or larger around than average, a wide cuff should be used. If the regular cuff is used, the blood pressure

    reading will be higher than it actually is. The nurse should not add numbers to the reading.

    2. When the client's arm is long or larger around than average, a wide cuff should be used. If the regular cuff is used, the blood pressure reading will be higher than it actually is. The nurse should use a larger cuff, not subtract numbers from the reading.

    4. When the client's arm is long or larger around than average, a wide cuff should be used. If the regular cuff is used, the blood pressure reading will be higher than it actually is. Lying down usually raises blood pressure.

#20. 1. The sounds described are crackles and are abnormal.   Dc   He/4 1

    2. Stridor is a shrill, harsh sound heard during inspiration in laryngeal obstruction.

    3. Stertor describes a breathing pattern that is noisy and caused by a partial obstruction of the upper airway.

    4. A wheeze is a high-pitched respiratory sound common in asthma.

#21. 3. The reason persons who are having elective surgery are often encouraged to donate their own blood is to reduce the risk of blood-borne diseases such as hepatitis and HIV, which can be contracted when donor blood is used. There is often significant blood loss with a knee replacement.   Im Ph/9 1

    1. It may well be true that the blood bank is short of blood. However, that is not the primary reason elective surgical clients are asked to donate their own blood.

    2. Donor blood of the correct type can be given to the client. This is not the reason clients who are scheduled for elective surgery are asked to donate their own blood.

    4. Blood transfusions are not given primarily to increase energy level following surgery, although that may be one effect. There would be no difference in effect on energy between donor blood and autologous transfusion.

#22. 2. Pink-colored urine occurs frequently in persons taking hydantoin (Dilantin).   Im Ph/8 5

    1. Pink-colored urine occurs frequently in persons taking hydantoin (Dilantin). It is not a serious side effect. The nurse should record the information.

    3. Cranberry juice and red gelatin do not turn the urine pink. Pink-colored urine occurs frequently in persons taking hydantoin (Dilantin).

    4. Pink-colored urine occurs frequently in persons taking hydantoin (Dilantin). It does not suggest kidney stones in this client.

#23. 3. The initial response should open communication. Responding with empathy or reflection is most appropriate.   Im Ps/5 2

    1. This response is not therapeutic and will only serve to close communication. The goal of initial communication is to open communication.

    2. Initially the nurse should open communication by responding with empathy or reflection. Later, the nurse might ask the client if she would like to talk with the chaplain. This is not appropriate initially.

    4. Telling the client she didn't do anything to deserve it may be appropriate at some point in the discussion, but is not appropriate initially. Initially the nurse should open communication and let the client express her feelings.

#24. 4. Ibuprofen is apt to cause bleeding as a side effect. None of the other drugs do.   Dc Ph/8 5

    1. Metformin is a drug used for Type II diabetics to lower blood sugar. Hypoglycemia and renal problems might be adverse effects. It does not cause bleeding as a side effect.

    2. Estrogen is a female hormone. It is more apt to cause clotting as an adverse effect. It does not cause bleeding as a side effect.

3. Atenolol is an antihypertensive. An adverse effect would be slow pulse or hypotension. It does not cause bleeding.

#25. 2. Peripheral neuropathy is a major side effect of isoniazid. Peripheral neuropathy is characterized by sharp pains in legs.   Dc   Ph/8   5

1. Ototoxicity is a toxicity of streptomycin.
3. Orange-colored urine is a side effect of rimactane.
4. Color blindness is a side effect of ethambutol.

#26. 1. A nursing assistant should not be changing a sterile dressing. That action is not within the scope of practice.   Dc   Sa/1   1

2. Asking a standing client to sit down while vital signs are being taken is an appropriate action and does not need correction.
3. Emptying a urine drainage bag from the tube at the bottom is an appropriate action and does not need correction.
4. Changing water in the middle of a bed bath is an appropriate action and does not need correction.

#27. 2. The diabetic client has the classic signs of hypoglycemia. The treatment is to administer sugar. Cola has sugar. The nurse could also do a glucose check but that is not one of the options.   Im   Ph/10   1

1. Initially the nurse should recognize the symptoms as those of hypoglycemia and give the client something with sugar in it to eat or drink. Calling the physician is not the initial action. The nurse should be able to handle the initial episode and then notify the physician if necessary.
3. Having the client lie down will not help with hypoglycemia. The client needs sugar.
4. The symptoms suggest hypoglycemia. Insulin is not what is needed for hypoglycemia. The client needs sugar in some form.

#28. 1. Semi-Fowler's position is the appropriate position to reduce edema and keep the airway clean.   Im   Ph/9   1

2. Supine is not the appropriate position. This position would promote edema and predispose to airway problems.
3. Prone is not the appropriate position. This position would promote edema and predispose to airway problems.
4. Sims is not the appropriate position. This position would promote edema and predispose to airway problems.

#29. 1. The nurse should attend to the client whose blood sugar is dangerously low. This client will soon lose consciousness. The nurse should give the person sugar in some form.   Pl   Sa/1   1

2. The post-operative client who is in pain needs pain medication but the pain is probably not life-threatening.
3. The person with cancer needs pain medication but the pain is probably not life-threatening.
4. The person with an indwelling catheter who is complaining of bladder pain should be seen soon, but the potential problem is not as immediately serious as the hypoglycemic client.

#30. 2. The key to controlling Type II diabetes mellitus is usually following a diet and losing weight. The client might also be on oral medication.   Pl   Ph/9   1

1. Most Type II diabetics do not need to self-inject insulin. Most Type II diabetics are controlled with diet and oral hypoglycemic agents.
3. Most Type II diabetics do not receive insulin on a regular basis and do not need to know the signs and symptoms of insulin reaction. They might need to know about hypoglycemia if they are taking oral hypoglycemic agents, but it would not be referred to as an insulin reaction.
4. The nurse will teach the client about the complications of diabetes, but not initially. First the nurse should teach the client what they need to know to help control the disease. Later, the nurse can teach about the complications.

#31. 2. **The person with myasthenia gravis has upper body weakness. The major symptoms include difficulty swallowing, double vision, and ptosis of the eyes. The nurse should check the swallowing and gag reflexes before feeding the person.**   Pl   Ph/9   1

    1. The client is usually strongest early in the day with the weakness getting worse as the day progresses. The client should bathe early in the day.

    3. There is no need for the person with myasthenia gravis to void every hour.

    4. Myasthenia gravis is not a neuropathy. There is no need to observe for this.

#32. 4. **The person who needs turning should be attended to first. This will help to prevent skin breakdown and respiratory complications. Turning usually can be done fairly quickly and the nurse can get on to the others who need attention.**   Pl   Sa/1   1

    1. This person needs attention but not first. It will probably take longer to change this person's bed than it will to turn the other client.

    2. This person needs attention but not first. The person who only needs turning can be done quickly and then this client can be cleaned and changed. This client will take several minutes to clean up.

    3. This person should be tended to but not first. There is nothing in the data that suggests that this client is in any immediate need to go back to bed.

#33. 4. **The person who has ALS will need chest PT at least qid. ALS is a motor neuron disease that results in progressive loss of function. Respiratory congestion is usually what kills persons with ALS.**   Pl   Ph/9   1

    1. The person with ALS is not likely to have dressings that need changing unless they develop a decubitus ulcer, which is possible. This question does not give that data.

    2. The person who has ALS is not likely to have an IV running unless there is an additional problem such as an infection requiring IV antibiotics. The question does not give that information.

    3. The person who has ALS might possibly need an indwelling catheter. That information is not given in the question.

#34. 2. **A nursing assistant is well qualified to give hygienic care. This act can safely be delegated.**   Pl   Sa/1   1

    1. The nurse should not delegate administration of medications to a nursing assistant. It doesn't matter what type of medication.

    3. A nursing assistant is not qualified to perform a catheterization.

    4. Changing the dressing on a Stage III decubitus ulcer is a sterile procedure. The nurse should not delegate this to the nursing assistant.

#35. 3. **The bladder symptoms suggest a bladder infection. In older people, temperature is not a very reliable indicator of infection. Other symptoms should be evaluated.**   Dc   He/3   1

    1. The vital signs are essentially normal.

    2. The blood pressure is borderline but not a cause for alarm in a 78-year-old.

    4. As people age they usually become more sensitive to the cold and often are less able to shiver. These are normal findings in a 78-year-old.

#36. 2. **This client has few risk factors for abuse.**   Dc   Ps/6   2

    1. Incontinence and being bossy are risk factors for elder abuse.

    3. Dependence is a risk factor for elder abuse.

    4. Wandering and yelling out are risk factors for elder abuse.

#37. 3. **Triazolam (Halcion) is a sleeping medication. If the client is not ready to go to sleep the nurse should have her call when she is ready for the medication.**   Im   Ph/8   1

    1. The nurse should not leave medication (with the exception of nitroglycerine) at the bedside. Leaving sedatives at the bedside

creates a risk of the client hoarding the medication and making a suicide attempt.

2. It is better for the client to call the nurse. The client may not be ready for the medication in one hour.

4. This response is very rigid. The nurse should be more flexible and give the client the medication at the client's hour of sleep.

#38. 2. The best way to prevent decubitus ulcers (bedsores) is to take the pressure off the pressure points by turning every two hours.   Pl   Ph/7   1

1. Getting him out of bed each day may well be a good thing. However, it is not the best way to prevent decubitus ulcers (bedsores).

3. Rubbing the skin on his buttocks may wear away the delicate skin and actually predispose him to skin breakdown. Sometimes gentle massage near the area is recommended to improve circulation.

4. Changing the sheets several times a day will not prevent pressure ulcers (bedsores). Straightening out the sheets to remove wrinkles is more important than changing the sheets each day, unless they are soiled or wet.

#39. 3. The primary reason for placing a client who has had abdominal surgery in semi-Fowler's position is to reduce tension on the suture line.   Dc   Ph/7   1

1. Elevating the legs and leg exercises are done to help prevent venous stasis. Semi-Fowler's position does not help to prevent venous stasis.

2. Semi-Fowler's position does not particularly promote circulation.

4. Semi-Fowler's position does help to promote thoracic expansion. It does not prevent respiratory distress. However, that is not the primary reason the client who has had abdominal surgery is placed in semi-Fowler's position.

#40. 1. The nurse should first try nonpharmacologic methods to induce sleep.   Im   Ph/7   1

2. The nurse could open communication, but asking her what she is worrying about is making an assumption that worry is the cause of her sleeplessness.

3. Before giving the ordered prn sedative, the nurse should try nonpharmacologic methods.

4. There is no need to notify the physician initially. The nurse should try nonpharmacologic methods to induce sleep and, if these are not successful, give the ordered sedative. If these efforts fail, the nurse should notify the physician.

#41. 1. The nursing assistant should keep the back straight when lifting and moving clients. This action indicates a lack of understanding about transfer techniques and body mechanics.   Ev   Ph/7   1

2. The nursing assistant should keep the feet separated when moving and lifting persons. This action indicates understanding of transfer techniques.

3. The nursing assistant should turn the whole body when moving the person from bed to the chair. This action indicates understanding of transfer techniques.

4. The nursing assistant should ask for help when necessary. This indicates an understanding of principles related to transfer techniques.

#42. 4. There is no special preparation for an electromyography procedure (EMG). There is no anesthesia given and no dyes are used. Needle electrodes are inserted into the muscle and the nerve conduction to the muscles is measured.   Im   Ph/9   1

1. No anesthesia is used during an EMG, and no dyes are used so there is no need for the client to be NPO.

2. No dyes are used during an EMG, so there is no need to ask the question about iodine allergy.

3. There is no need to limit caffeine before an EMG. Caffeine is restricted before an electroencephalogram (EEG).

#43. 2. **The WBC and platelet counts are low. The client should be on protective isolation because of the low white blood cell count and the resulting inability to fight infection. The client should also not receive any injections because of the low platelet count and the resulting inability to clot.**   Pl   Ph/9   1

    1. The client's RBC count is normal so there is no need to keep the client on bed rest. The client should be on protective isolation because of the low white blood cell count and the resulting inability to fight infection.

    3. The client's RBC count is normal so there is no need to keep the client on bed rest. The client should not receive any injections because of the low platelet count and the resulting inability to clot.

    4. This answer is not correct. There are special nursing actions indicated. The WBC and platelet counts are low. The client should be on protective isolation because of the low white blood cell count and the resulting inability to fight infection. The client should also not receive any injections, because of the low platelet count and the resulting inability to clot.

#44. 3. **When an IV infiltrates it means the IV needle is out of the vein and the IV fluid goes into the tissue outside the vein. This makes the area cool and pale.**   Dc   Ph/8   1

    1. A red and warm arm when an IV is infusing suggests phlebitis—inflammation of the vein.

    2. An infiltrated IV runs slower than the desired rate.

    4. Usually the discomfort is localized with an infiltration. There would not be pain up and down the entire arm.

#45. 3. **Broccoli and spinach both contain iron. Tomatoes and orange juice are vitamin C sources. When a person eats iron sources, they should also have a vitamin C source to increase absorption of iron.**   Ev   Ph/7   6

    1. None of these food choices contains a significant amount of iron.

    2. None of these food sources contains a significant amount of iron. Milk has protein but no iron.

    4. None of these food sources contains a significant amount of iron. Milk and milk products contain no iron.

#46. 2. **A beefy red tongue is usually seen in pernicious anemia.**   Dc   Ph/9   1

    1. Diarrhea is not a symptom of pernicious anemia.

    3. Ecchymotic areas are not usually seen in pernicious anemia.

    4. A fever is not usually seen in pernicious anemia.

#47. 3 **Prone position puts the hip in extension and helps to prevent the development of hip flexion contractures, which is a common complication following lower extremity amputation.**   Im   Ph/9   1

    1. Atelectasis is prevented by deep-breathing and coughing.

    2. Leg exercises and antiembolism stockings prevent thrombophlebitis.

    4. Hand washing and good technique will help to prevent wound infection.

#48. 3. **Cool moist compresses help with the itching of contact dermatitis.**   Ev   Ph/10   1

    1. A hot bath will most likely make the itching worse.

    2. The client with contact dermatitis should avoid strong soaps and detergents. They usually make the itching worse.

    4. Wool, nylon, and fur clothing should be avoided, as they tend to make the itching worse.

#49. 1 **The person who has psoriasis usually has thick, yellow toenails. Psoriasis is a chronic type of dermatitis that involves a turnover rate of the epidermal cells that is seven times the normal rate.**   Dc   Ph/10   1

    2. Psoriasis is not characterized by open, weeping lesions. Contact dermatitis caused by poison ivy would have open, weeping lesions. Psoriasis is characterized by sharply circumscribed bright red macules, papules, or patches covered with silvery scales.

ANSWER	RATIONALE	NP	CN	SA

3. Psoriasis is characterized by sharply circumscribed bright red macules, papules, or patches covered with silvery scales. Multicolored skin lesions are typical of skin cancer.

4. Skin eruptions and pain along a nerve root suggest herpes zoster, which is also called shingles.

#50. 2. Whenever possible the recipient site should be elevated to prevent edema formation.   Im   Ph/10 1

1. Warm compresses will probably be applied to the graft site.

3. The client should not do range-of-motion exercises as this might separate the graft from the area.

4. The nurse will not change the dressing twice a day. The nurse should apply sterile warm compresses if ordered.

#51. 2. The person who has multiple myeloma is immunocompromised. Multiple myeloma is cancer of the bone marrow and the bone. Interferon is an immunosuppressant. This person should be cared for before the client who has an open wound. This is also a short visit.   Pl   Sa/1 1

1. The client with leg ulcers has an open wound. The person who is immunocompromised should be cared for first.

3. This visit will take a long time. There is no reason to care for this person first.

4. This visit is also a lengthy one. There is no reason to care for this person first.

#52. 3. The vital signs suggest the client is in shock. The client's legs should first be elevated and then the nurse should notify the charge nurse or the physician.   Im   Ph 10 1

1. The blood pressure change is so significant that continuing to monitor the blood pressure is not sufficient.

2. The nurse should have confidence in his/her own actions and act on the basis of the results obtained.

4. The nurse will call the physician after elevating the client's legs. The question asked for the initial action.

#53. 2. Weak muscles may indicate hypokalemia. A nasogastric tube attached to drainage depletes potassium and sodium.   Dc   Ph/10 1

1. Most people who have a nasogastric tube in place complain of a dry mouth. This is not a serious problem.

3. Most people who have a nasogastric tube in place complain of a sore throat.

4. Most people who have a nasogastric tube in place complain of an irritated nose.

#54. 2. A person who is on a cooling blanket should be turned every two hours to prevent skin breakdown and to promote effective cooling.   Im   Ph/10 1

1. It is possible that the client who has a high fever might have seizures. However, a padded tongue blade is not used during a seizure.

3. A cool compress may be applied to the groin area and to the axilla. Ice is not used because it may stimulate shivering, which raises body temperature.

4. The client should be covered with a sheet but not with a blanket. A blanket will promote temperature increase.

#55. 3. Before inserting the suction catheter the nurse should oxygenate the client.   Im   Ph/10 1

1. The purpose of the suction catheter is to clear the mouth and throat of secretions.

2. The head of the bed should be raised, not lowered.

4. The wall suction is usually not regulated.

#56. 2. The stimulus to breathe in a person who has chronic emphysema is a low oxygen level. Ten liters of oxygen per minute will depress the respiratory drive and the person will die. The nurse must immediately put the oxygen level back to two liters per minute.   Im   Ph/10 1

1. After turning the oxygen back to a safe level the nurse can discuss the reason with the woman. This explanation is not sufficient. Simply stating it is the doctor's order is not adequate. The implication in this response is that the physician might order higher concentrations of oxygen. This is highly unlikely. The nurse should explain the reason to the woman so she does not try to do it again.
3. Five liters is too high. The nurse should immediately turn the oxygen flow rate back to two liters per minute.
4. The woman's actions are not appropriate and are putting her husband's life in danger.

#57. 1. The nurse should initially administer two breaths.   Im Ph/10 1
2. The nurse should first give two breaths when starting CPR.
3. The nurse should stay with the client, not leave the client to get the emergency cart.
4. The LPN should not initially defibrillate the client.

#58. 2. The nurse should use long-handled forceps to pick up the pellet and place it in a lead-lined container.   Im Ph/10 1
1. The initial action is to prevent radiation damage to the client, the nurse, and others. Checking the client's mouth for other loose pellets would be a later action.
3. The client should not hold the pellet. The pellet will cause radiation burns.
4. The nurse should call the radiation safety officer after safely putting the pellet in a lead-lined container.

#59. 4. This describes a four-point gait. In a four-point gait, the client moves one foot and then the opposite crutch, followed by the other foot and the opposite crutch.   Ev Ph/7 1
1. This is not the four-point gait. Walking as described in this response would be very hazardous.
2. This is not the four-point gait. This gait would be very difficult to do and very hazardous.
3. This is not the four-point gait. The gait described is the two-point gait.

#60. 4. The nurse should not discuss one client's diagnosis with another client.   Im Sa/1 1
1. This answer sounds rude. There is some truth to the fact that if one client wishes to discuss his illness with another he may do so.
2. This response might violate the client's right to confidentiality.
3. This answer is poor communication.

#61. 3 The nurse should identify the ring and place it in an envelope in the hospital safe.   Im Sa/1 1
1. The nurse may tape a ring without a stone. Taping a ring with a stone may cause the stone to become loose and even dislodge.
2. The ring needs to be placed in a secure place.
4. The client should not be asked to sign a waiver.

#62. 1. The client should wear smooth-soled shoes. Persons with Parkinson's disease shuffle when they walk. Smooth-soled shoes allow him to shuffle.   Pl Sa/2 1
2. Leaving the bedrails up at all times may make it more hazardous for the client to get out of bed. It is better to put the bed in the low position.
3. A person who has Parkinson's disease will get very stiff while sitting in a chair for hours at a time. He should ambulate several times. "The longer he sits, the stiffer he gets."
4. Scatter rugs would increase the likelihood of falling.

#63. 2. The LPN/LVN should report the incident to the supervisor.   Im Sa/1 1
1. The nurse will continue to be alert to other incidents. However, the nurse should initially report this incident.
3. This is not the type of event for which an incident report is made.

4. The LPN/LVN should first report the incident to the supervisor. The supervisor will make the determination as to any other action to be taken.

#64. 4.   The nurse should not medicate the client because the client will need to talk with the physician. The client has the right to refuse a transfusion. However, the surgeon may feel that surgery is not safe if a blood transfusion cannot be given if needed.   Im   Sa/1   1

1. The client has the right to refuse a transfusion and the right to rescind permission. The nurse must notify the physician immediately because the client is scheduled for immediate surgery.

2. This may be a true statement. However, answer #4 is a better response. This response sounds as if the nurse is trying to talk the client into having a transfusion. The nurse should not do that.

3. This is not the best response. The nurse should withhold pre-operative medication and notify the surgeon.

#65. 2.   It is a normal part of aging to think about one's own death and to prepare for it. This often includes giving belongings to the persons they want to have them. Unless this behavior becomes obsessive, it is normal.   Im   He/3   2

1. The basic personality type usually continues into older adulthood.

3. There is no data to suggest this response.

4. There is no data to suggest this response. If a younger person started giving away personal items it might be a sign of suicide. It could be a sign of suicide in the older adult if it is accompanied by other suicidal behavior.

#66. 4.   The best time to give influenza vaccine is November. This allows the antibody levels to rise for protection during the winter months when the incidence of influenza is highest.   Pl   He/4   5

1. The best time to give influenza vaccine is November.

2. The best time to give influenza vaccine is November.

3. The best time to give influenza vaccine is November.

#67. 4.   The woman should continue to do self-breast exams on a monthly basis as long as she is able. The incidence of breast cancer increases with age. This statement indicates the client does not understand and needs more instruction.   Ev   He/4   3

1. This statement is correct and indicates the client understands the teaching.

2. This statement is correct and indicates the client understands the teaching.

3. This statement is correct and indicates the client understands the teaching.

#68. 4.   Meat should be cooked to 160° Fahrenheit. Rare meat can cause food poisoning. This answer indicates the person does not understand how to prevent food poisoning and needs more instruction.   Ev   He/4   6

1. Hands should be washed after handling raw meat. This answer indicates the person understands how to prevent food poisoning.

2. Food should be placed in the refrigerator as soon as possible after eating to prevent the growth of microorganisms. This answer indicates the person understands how to prevent food poisoning.

3. Kitchen counters should be washed with bleach after raw meat has been handled on them. This answer indicates the person understands how to prevent food poisoning.

#69. 3.   A tuberculin skin test is given intradermal in the volar surface of the forearm. This answer is the correct procedure.   Im   He/4   5

1. This is not the correct procedure. A tuberculin skin test is given intradermal in the volar surface of the forearm.

2. This is not the correct procedure. A tuberculin skin test is given intradermal in the volar surface of the forearm.

			NP	**CN**	**SA**

4. This is not the correct procedure. A tuberculin skin test is given intradermal in the volar surface of the forearm.

#70. 3. Speaking slowly and distinctly will do the most to help with communication.   Pl   Ps/5   1

  1. Speaking slowly and distinctly is better than repeating everything twice.
  2. Speaking loudly is usually not as effective as speaking slowly and clearly. When speaking loudly the individual usually raises the pitch of the voice and makes it even harder to hear.
  4. Speaking slowly and distinctly is better than using gestures.

#71. 3. This is the approach that will allow the client to rest between activities.   Pl   Ph/7   1

  1. This approach does not allow the client to rest between activities.
  2. This approach does not allow the client to rest between activities.
  4. This approach does not allow the client to rest between activities.

#72. 2. The nurse should always check for residual and check to be sure that the aspirate is acid, which indicates that it is in the stomach.   Im   Ph/7   1

  1. It is essential to test for placement of the tube. Asking the client if she feels full is not the best way to assess that the tube is in the proper place.
  3. It is not necessary to change the tubing before giving a tube feeding. It is essential to test for placement of the tube.
  4. It is essential to test for placement of the tube. Feeling over the end of the tube for air is not an appropriate or accurate way to test that the tube is in the stomach.

#73. 4. The best way to achieve urinary continence is to encourage fluids during the day and offer the bedpan every two hours.   Pl   Ph/7   1

  1. This approach will not help to achieve urinary continence. You cannot bladder train an empty bladder.
  2. Offering the bedpan at two-hour intervals during the day is appropriate. The nurse should restrict fluids after 6 P.M. so the client does not need to use the bedpan during the night.
  3. Ambulation and deep-breathing exercises are not the protocol for promoting urinary continence.

#74. 2. The nurse should try nonpharmacologic methods first. A back rub should help the woman relax and encourages sleep. Warm milk has a sleep-inducing effect.   Im   Ph/7   1

  1. The nurse should try nonpharmacologic methods of inducing sleep before asking for sleeping medication.
  3. Exercise usually wakes people up. It does not induce sleep.
  4. Tea contains caffeine, which is a stimulant. Caffeine sources should not be consumed late in the day if the client has trouble sleeping.

#75. 2. The nurse should try a noninvasive method to encourage voiding such as running water or pouring water over the client's perineum.   Im   Ph/7   1

  1. The nurse might have to do this eventually. The nurse should try noninvasive methods first, such as running water or pouring water over the client's perineum.
  3. Taking deep breaths does not promote voiding.
  4. Narcotic pain medication makes it harder for the client to open the urinary sphincter.

#76. 1. The best food choices when an increase in iron is recommended contain iron (eggs) and vitamin C (orange juice) to increase the absorption of iron.   Ev   Ph/7   6

  2. There is very little iron and very little vitamin C in this choice.
  3. Roast beef has iron, but there is not vitamin C in this choice. Vitamin C increases absorption of iron.
  4. Baked chicken contains some iron, but there is no vitamin C in this selection. Vitamin C increases the absorption of iron.

#77. 4. The cannula should be inserted 1 cm into the nostrils. The other responses are incorrect.   Im   Ph/10   1

1. Twelve liters per minute is too high a setting for oxygen.
2. The cannula does not need to be lubricated. The nurse should not use petrolatum substances near oxygen.
3. The nurse does not give 100% oxygen before inserting the cannula.

#78. 4. Syrup of Ipecac should be given to induce vomiting, since the child is awake and talking.   Im   Ph/10 1

1. This answer is not correct for two reasons. First, this is not the time to talk. After the sleeping pills are removed from her system and she is physiologically stable, then the nurse may do further inquiry as to what happened. Second, asking a person why they want to kill themselves is poor communication.
2. There is a physiologic emergency. Until the client is stable physiologically, neither the nurse nor the parent should start trying to convince her she wants to live. It would be poor communication technique to try to convince her she wants to live initially. Initially the nurse and the parent should recognize the client's distress.
3. Milk is not the antidote for sleeping pills. Milk is given in acute lead poisoning.

#79. 3. When a wet to dry dressing is applied, the nurse first applies a wet dressing to the wound and then covers with a dry dressing.   Im   Ph/10 1

1. This is not the appropriate technique.
2. This is not the appropriate technique.
4. This is not the appropriate technique.

#80. 3. This approach helps the family to solve the problem and use a better, less restrictive way to keep the client safe.   Im   Sa/2   2

1. The nurse should work with the family to provide for the safety of the client. If the family refuses to work with the nurse, there might be a reason for notifying family protective services.
2. Restraining the client with a leather belt is not appropriate. The nurse should not congratulate the family.
4. This answer does not help the family learn how to keep the client safe.

#81. 2. Storing flammable liquids (cleaning supplies) and flammable boxes near the emergency oxygen supply is fire hazard.   Ev   Sa/2   1

1. Smoking in the restroom is unhealthy unless it is properly ventilated. However it is not as great a fire hazard as mixing cleaning supplies, boxes, and oxygen.
3. Dust under the beds is not sanitary and may spread infection and cause allergies. However, it is not a significant fire hazard.
4. Stuffed closets can be a safety hazard and could be a fire hazard if a flame was close at hand. This choice is not as great a fire hazard as oxygen and flammable materials.

#82. 2. Reach for Recovery is a self-help group for persons who have had mastectomies. The types of concerns the client has would be best addressed by Reach for Recovery.   Pl   Ps/5   2

1. The concerns this woman has would be better addressed by a support group such as Reach for Recovery.
3. The concerns this woman has would be better addressed by a support group such as Reach for Recovery.
4   The concerns this woman has would be better addressed by a support group such as Reach for Recovery.

#83. 3. The nurse should encourage the client to speak as much as possible.   Pl   Ps/5   1

1. The nurse can speak verbally to this client. The data indicates the client has expressive aphasia, meaning she cannot speak. There is no need for the nurse to write communication. Expressive aphasia may be only verbal communication or it could be verbal and written. The nurse needs to assess this further before asking the client to communicate in writing.

ANSWER	RATIONALE	NP	CN	SA

2. Anticipating the client's needs does not encourage the client to attempt to speak or use other means of communication. It keeps the client dependent.

4. The nurse and the client should develop some type of communication system. This approach creates dependence on family members.

#84. 3. The nurse should reflect on the tone of the client's feelings and not be defensive.   Im   Ps/5   2

1. This response does not focus on the client's feelings.
2. This is a defensive response and not therapeutic.
4. This does not focus on the client's feelings.

#85. 3. This response is most likely to open communication and allow the client to express his/her concerns.   Im   Ps/5   2

1. Introducing the concept of hell to a dying person is not likely to be therapeutic.
2. This answer puts the client off and is nontherapeutic.
4. While it may be appropriate to ask the client at some point if they want to see their clergyman, this answer avoids the question.

#86. 3. Small round burned areas on the abdomen and back are not consistent with a fall. This is more consistent with cigarette burns, which would be abuse.   Dc   Ps/6   4

1. Two visits in a month are not especially indicative of child abuse. This could be a normal pattern. It is also consistent with child abuse.
2. A fall would cause bruises on the arms and legs.
4. A child who is abused may not be affectionate and trusting to the parent, especially if the parent is the abuser.

#87. 1. This response indicates that the client is performing self-injection of insulin. This is the best indicator of acceptance of the diagnosis.   Ev   Ps/5   2

2. This comment indicates denial of the diagnosis.
3. This comment indicates the client expects to get over IDDM. Since IDDM is not a condition from which a person recovers, this comment indicates the client has not accepted the diagnosis.
4. This comment indicates the client has not accepted the diagnosis.

#88. 4. This response opens communication. Initially, the nurse should open communication.   Im   Ps/5   2

1. This response does not open communication.
2. Asking "why" puts the client on the defensive.
3. This response, while true, does not open communication and let the client express feelings.

#89. 3. Persons who are apparently unconscious may be aware when family members are present. Her presence is important for the client and for herself. Notice that the nurse suggests and doesn't tell.   Im   Ps/5   1

1. This statement is not true.
2. The nurse should call if there is any change. However, the client asked if she should visit. The nurse should encourage her to be present.
4. This response ignores the woman's question completely and is nontherapeutic.

#90. 2. Persons who have anorexia and do not eat are in a starvation state and usually have scanty or absent menstruation.   Dc   Ps/6   1

1. The person who has anorexia nervosa has a slow metabolic rate and usually has bradycardia, not tachycardia.
3. Wheezing is not typical of anorexia nervosa.
4. Acne is not typical of anorexia nervosa.

#91. 1. Thiamin deficiency is common in alcoholism. Thiamin is frequently ordered.   Pl   Ps/6   5

2. Antabuse is not likely to be ordered upon admission. Antabuse helps the client abstain from alcohol and is usually ordered close to discharge.
3. Ascorbic acid (vitamin C) is not usually ordered for persons who abuse alcohol.

	4.	Dilantin is an antiseizure medication. The client may be given a drug such as Valium or Ativan to prevent seizures during withdrawal.			
#92.	2.	**Getting lost in familiar territory is a sign of dementia. The other symptoms are not.**	Dc	Ps/6	2
	1.	Being unable to remember dates from the past is not a sign of dementia.			
	3.	Not being able to find a purse is not necessarily a sign of dementia.			
	4.	Not being able to tell the difference between red and green is not a sign of dementia. It is a sign of color blindness.			
#93.	2.	**Behavior modification is based on rewarding desired behavior.**	Pl	Ps/6	2
	1.	Behavior modification is based on rewarding desired behavior, not punishing undesirable behavior.			
	3.	Reminding the client is not behavior modification.			
	4.	Asking the client what she sees as good behavior is not behavior modification.			
#94.	2.	**The client cannot help her need to wash her hands compulsively. The nurse should remind her that lunch is coming soon so the ritual can be performed and she can still make it to the dining room.**	Pl	Ps/6	2
	1.	It is not appropriate to give the client a choice between ritual and eating. The compulsion to perform the ritual is very strong and comes from the unconscious mind.			
	3.	A compulsion is thought to come from the unconscious mind and is not subject to rational thought and control. The client does not know why she washes her hands so often. She probably recognizes that her behavior is not rational but she cannot help it.			
	4.	Prohibiting the client from performing her ritual is likely to put the client into an anxiety attack.			
#95.	1.	**A paper cup is not a hazard and can not be used to injure one's self.**	Pl	Sa/2	2
	2.	A leather belt can be used to hang one's self.			
	3.	A razor can be used to harm one's self.			
	4.	A pillow can be used to smother one's self.			
#96.	2.	**The client is allowed out of bed. It is essential that the nurse lower the bed so the client can safely get out of bed. This must be done before leaving the bedside.**	Im	Sa/2	1
	1.	The nurse should wash hands before leaving the room, but not before leaving the bedside.			
	3.	It is not essential to toilet the client. Lowering the bed is more important.			
	4.	Assessing for pain is not the highest priority.			
#97.	1.	**Several hours is too long to have close contact with someone who has internal radiation. Limiting time with the client and increasing distance from the client reduce radiation exposure.**	Ev	Sa/2	1
	2.	Kissing her is close contact but the time is brief. There is risk but not as much as occurs in response #1. Limiting time with the client and increasing distance from the client reduce radiation exposure.			
	3.	The time period of exposure is brief. Limiting time with the client and increasing distance from the client reduce radiation exposure.			
	4.	The time period of exposure is brief and the cleaning lady is not too close to the client. Limiting time with the client and increasing distance from the client reduce radiation exposure.			
#98.	1.	**An infant who is admitted with severe diarrhea should be in isolation until the cause of the diarrhea has been determined. Many causes of diarrhea are very infectious.**	Pl	Sa/2	4
	2.	The most important criterion is that the child be in a private room for isolation until the cause of the diarrhea is determined.			
	3.	The most important criterion is that the child be in a private room for isolation until the cause of the diarrhea is determined.			

4. The other infant's diarrhea might not be caused by the same thing this child's is. This would put both infants at risk. The most important criterion is that the child be in a private room for isolation until the cause of the diarrhea is determined.

#99. 1. **The nurse should describe the room and the furnishings. The nurse might also have the client walk to the bathroom describing landmarks so the client will feel comfortable ambulating alone.**   Im   Sa/2   1

2. Putting up the siderails is not appropriate unless the client is also confused or unable to get out of bed. The nurse should make the environment safe for the client.

3. Describing the voices of the personnel might be helpful. However, describing the surroundings does more to promote safety.

4. The nurse should place the water pitcher and glass in a position convenient to the client so the client does not have to search for them.

#100. 3. **AIDS is caused by HIV. HIV is spread by body secretions. The razor could come in contact with the client's blood and infect his brother.**   Ev   Sa/2   1

1. Using the same dishes poses no risk of infection.

2. Using the same bathroom as the rest of the family poses no risk of infection.

4. Cooking for the family poses no risk of infection for the rest of the family.

Practice Test Four

1. Which nursing diagnosis is most appropriate for a client who has Cushing's syndrome?
   1. Risk for injury related to osteoporosis
   2. Pain related to cold intolerance
   3. Risk for deficient fluid volume related to excessive loss of sodium and water secondary to polyuria
   4. Risk for injury related to postural hypotension

2. A woman comes into the labor suite stating her water has broken and she is in labor. Which symptoms point to the possible presence of placenta previa?
   1. Sudden knife-like pain in the lower abdomen accompanied by profuse vaginal bleeding
   2. Dark red vaginal discharge that started after she saw the physician this morning
   3. Bright red painless vaginal bleeding
   4. A tender rigid uterine wall and abdomen with no vaginal bleeding evident

3. A 13-month-old is admitted to the pediatric unit with diarrhea and vomiting. The mother tells the nurse that she is worried because her son does not yet walk. She says her other children walked at eight and nine months and asks what could be wrong with this child. How should the nurse respond?
   1. "All babies are different. It is not abnormal that the baby is not yet walking."
   2. "The baby should be walking. I'll let the doctor know he is behind developmentally."
   3. "Your son is probably enjoying being the baby and is not eager to grow up and walk."
   4. "Walking requires complex coordination. Your son is prabably just a little slow to develop this. Don't worry."

4. A woman brings her six-month-old daughter to a clinic for a check-up and immunizations. The mother tells the nurse her infant is cranky, has a bad cold, and has not eaten well the last few days. She asks if the baby will still be able to get her shots. How should the nurse respond?
   1, "There is no problem in giving the shots just because your baby has a cold."
   2. "Your baby will have her check-up, but we will wait until her cold is better before giving her shots."
   3. "The shots often make them a little irritable, so we might as well get it all over with at one time."
   4. "I'm not sure why you came today. We need to reschedule the whole appointment for another day when your baby has no symptoms of a cold."

5. The mother of a two-month-old asks the nurse when she should start her son on

solids. He is taking about 30 ounces of formula per day. How should the nurse respond?
1. "This is a good time to begin."
2. "When he is taking a quart per day."
3. "Babies usually are ready for solids between four and six months of age."
4. "Each baby is different. Some are ready sooner than others."

6. An infant is suspected of having coarctation of the aorta. Which assessment finding is most related to coarctation of the aorta?
1. Respirations are 70 per minute.
2. Blood pressure is higher in the upper extremities than in the lower.
3. There is a heart murmur.
4. Heart rate is 150 per minute.

7. A young child with a history of grand mal seizures is in public school. He is on phenobarbital and hydantoin (Dilantin) to control the seizures. His teacher tells the nurse that he has not had any seizures but he does keep falling asleep in class. What should the nurse include when discussing his drowsiness with the teacher?
1. It is common in children who take barbiturates.
2. It usually occurs after seizures; let him sleep.
3. It is probably not related to his seizure disorder or treatment.
4. It is probably a warning sign that he is about to have a seizure.

8. The nurse is teaching a woman the normal changes of pregnancy. Which statement by the woman indicates correct understanding?
1. "There is decreased oxygen consumption during pregnancy."
2. "There is an increased rate of peristalsis in the GI tract."
3. "I will have a 50% increase in blood volume."
4. "My metabolic rate will decrease."

9. A prenatal client tests positive for chlamydia in her ninth month. She asks why she should be treated since she does not have symptoms. The nurse should tell the client that if she is not treated before delivery there is a risk of which problem?
1. Transplacental infection of the fetus
2. Neonatal ophthalmia
3. Pregnancy-induced hypertension
4. Congenital anomalies

10. A baby is delivered following a pregnancy complicated by gestational diabetes. What should the nurse observe the baby for?
1. Infection
2. Hyperglycemia
3. Acidosis
4. Hypoglycemia

11. A laboring woman who has dystocia is receiving oxytocin. The nurse observes a contraction lasting 90 seconds. What should the nurse do first?
1. Slow down the rate of the oxytocin.
2. Turn the woman on her left side.
3. Give the woman oxygen.
4. Stop the oxytocin.

12. A laboring woman says to the LPN/LVN "My baby is coming! My baby is coming!" She was last checked 15 minutes ago and was 5 cm dilated. What should the LPN/LVN do initially?
1. Have her checked to see if she has progressed.
2. Reassure her she cannot be that far along.
3. Reposition her to begin pushing.
4. Request medication to help her relax.

13. A baby boy is delivered after a rapid labor of three hours. The mother wants him to stay with her for as long as possible before he goes to the nursery. What nursing action takes priority in the immediate newborn period?
1. Suctioning with a bulb syringe.
2. Wrapping the baby in warm blankets.
3. Applying identification bracelets and taking footprints.
4. Assigning an APGAR score.

14. The nurse is talking with a group of young people who are preparing to spend a weekend camping in the woods. Which information is essential to include in the discussion?
1. Wear long pants and long sleeves to prevent tick bites.
2. Sunscreen is not necessary because you will be moving and perspiring.
3. Bring salt tablets to take in case you perspire a lot.
4. Poison ivy is not likely to be contracted unless you have prolonged contact with the plants.

15. The client who is receiving cancer chemotherapy asks why the physician recommended she take it in the evening. The nurse's response should include which information?
1. It is best to have one set time to take it. It really doesn't matter what time.
2. Taking it in the evening means that any nausea that may occur will be during the night when you are asleep and not during meal times.
3. One of the side effects of cancer chemotherapeutic agents is drowsiness. This is less troublesome during the night than during the day.
4. The medication is more effective if you are not active immediately after taking it.

16. The nurse is auscultating the lungs in a post-operative client and hears something

that sounds like a cellophane bag being wrinkled when the client takes in a breath. What nursing care is essential because of the finding?

1. Start emergency oxygen and notify the physician.
2. Have the client take several deep breaths and cough every two hours.
3. Notify the physician and prepare the client for a tracheostomy.
4. Carefully observe the client for cyanosis.

17. A client who had a total thyroidectomy this morning is to be admitted to the surgical floor. What should the nurse have at the bedside when the client arrives?

1. Tracheostomy set
2. Catheterization tray
3. Sterile dressing set
4. Ventilator

18. Iron drops were ordered for a toddler who has iron deficiency anemia. What observation of the child by the nurse indicates the child is receiving the medication?

1. The child is pale and lethargic.
2. The child's skin has brown spots.
3. The child's urine is dark colored.
4. The child has black stools.

19. Which statement made by the parents of a child who has sickle cell anemia indicate understanding of how to reduce the incidence of crises?

1. "I should not let my child play outdoors."
2. "My child should drink lots of fluids every day."
3. "If my child has a fever I should administer aspirin immediately."
4. "We should fly in an airplane rather than taking the child for a long car ride."

20. A person who has psoriasis is seen in the clinic. The lesions are covered with coal tar. Which instruction should the nurse give the client?

1. "Call if you have nausea and vomiting."
2. "Protect the area from sunlight for 24 hours."
3. "Wash off the solution after 6–8 hours."
4. "Call if your skin looks dark during the treatment."

21. The nurse is to observe the client for shock. The client's admitting vital signs are BP 116/70, P 86, R 24. Which finding, if observed, would be most suggestive of shock?

1. BP 140/60
2. Pulse 100
3. BP 114/68
4. Pulse 60

22. A nursing assistant comes to the LPN/LVN and complains that she has more residents to care for than another nursing assistant (NA). She has one more resident assigned to her than the other NA. However, the other NA has more total care residents than the complaining nurse. How should the LPN/LVN handle this situation?

1. Tell the complaining NA that this is the assignment.
2. Promise to give her an easier assignment tomorrow.
3. Discuss with her the needs of her assignment and help her organize her care.
4. Tell her that the other NA will help her as needed.

23. An adult who is being admitted to the medical floor with a bleeding ulcer exhibits all of the following. Which finding suggests the client may be experiencing alcohol withdrawal symptoms?

1. BP 90/60
2. Dizziness
3. Tremors
4. Pallor

24. The client has a prolonged prothrombin time. What question is important to ask the client when interpreting this data?

1. How often do you eat meat?
2. How much alcohol do you drink?
3. Do you take heparin?
4. Have you had a recent injury?

25. The nurse is caring for a newly admitted man who has kidney stones. The man asks if he can get up and take a walk. How should the nurse respond?

1. "It is better for you to remain in bed until the stones pass."
2. "Stay in bed until I check with your physician."
3. "Walking is good for you. Let me help you up."
4. "It is safe for you to ambulate once a day."

26. The nurse is discussing preventive health care with a group of women. Which woman should the nurse advise to have a mammogram?

1. A 20-year-old who says her breasts hurt before her period
2. A 25-year-old who was hit in the breast area by a ball
3. A 32-year-old who has been breastfeeding for 12 months
4. A 52-year-old who has no breast symptoms

27. A 79-year-old asks the nurse if she needs any shots. She reports having had "all the usual shots when I was younger." Which immunization is most important for this person to receive?

1. DPT
2. MMR
3. Pneumovax
4. HIB

28. The LPN/LVN is to assist the school nurse in scoliosis screening. What instructions should be given to the students?

1. Wear a bathing suit under your clothes on the examination day.
2. Bring a urine sample to school.
3. Do not wash your hair the night before the exam.
4. Wash your feet well the morning of the exam.

29. A woman who had a tuberculosis test three days ago reports to the nurse to have the test read. Which finding, if present, indicates a positive result and a need for referral and follow-up?
    1. A red area 12 mm in diameter
    2. A raised area 10 mm in diameter
    3. Itching at the injection site
    4. A rash on the arm near the test site

30. The nurse is to administer a tuberculin skin test. At what angle should the nurse insert the needle?
    1. A 10-degree angle
    2. A 30-degree angle
    3. A 60-degree angle
    4. A 90-degree angle

31. The nurse is discussing child safety with a group of mothers of toddlers. Which statement indicates a need for more instruction?
    1. "My child should be in the back seat in a front-facing car seat."
    2. "My little one needs constant supervision."
    3. "I should keep syrup of ipecac in the house."
    4. "I should put my medicines on a high shelf."

32. Which statement, if made by the client, indicates a possible problem?
    1. "I have a bowel movement every other day."
    2. "My stools recently are black."
    3. "Sometimes I have to strain when I go to the bathroom."
    4. "I usually have three stools a day."

33. The client has recently had a colostomy. The nurse is providing home care and is teaching the client about care of his colostomy. Which comment by the client indicates understanding of the care of his colostomy?
    1. "I will use hot water to irrigate the colostomy."
    2. "If my skin gets red, I will put alcohol on it."
    3. "I will irrigate the colostomy at the same time each day."
    4. "I should do the irrigation while lying in bed."

34. The nurse is doing a pain assessment on the client who has chronic back pain. Which assessment is of greatest value?
    1. Observe the client for grimaces, flinching, and other signs of pain.
    2. Monitor the client's blood pressure.

3. Ask the client to rate his pain on a scale of one to ten.
4. Monitor the client's pulse and respirations.

35. An 80-year-old woman is hospitalized with severe pneumonia. She has been on complete bed rest for several days and receiving complete care. Today she is to be allowed out of bed for the first time. How should the nurse plan the morning care?
    1. Give her a bed bath and then get her out of bed while the nurse makes the bed.
    2. Get her up in a chair and allow her to give herself a bath while the nurse makes the bed.
    3. Give her a bed bath and allow her to rest. Later get her up in the chair while the nurse makes the bed.
    4. Encourage her to give herself a bath while in bed, then get her up in the chair and make the bed.

36. The nurse is caring for a client who had a total gastrectomy performed this morning. When the client returns to the nursing care unit the drainage from the nasogastric tube is red. What is the nurse's best response to this?
    1. Report it immediately to the charge nurse or the physician.
    2. Record the finding and continue to observe.
    3. Immediately apply pressure to the operative site.
    4. Place the client in Trendelenburg's position.

37. The nurse is to administer a nasogastric tube feeding to a client. Which action is essential prior to administering the feeding?
    1. Position the client in supine position.
    2. Aspirate contents from the nasogastric tube and check the pH.
    3. Check the client's vital signs.
    4. Ask the client if she feels full.

38. The nurse is assisting a client with deep breathing and coughing exercises following abdominal surgery. What instruction is most appropriate for the nurse to give the client?
    1. Hold your breath for several seconds and then breathe out forcefully.
    2. Splint your incision while taking in deep breaths and coughing.
    3. Take deep breaths when you are moving in bed.
    4. Deep breathing exercises should be done when you are out of bed.

39. The nurse is caring for all of the following clients. Which is probably at greatest risk for skin breakdown and will need special nursing care measures?
    1. A 75-year-old who is admitted with a broken hip
    2. An 80-year-old who is admitted with angina

3. An 85-year-old who is admitted for diagnostic tests
4. A 78-year-old who is admitted with asthma

40. The nurse is to perform a routine blood glucose check on a diabetic client before administering insulin. Which action is correct?
   1. Puncture the end of the thumb in the middle of the fleshy part.
   2. Puncture the end of the finger on the side.
   3. Draw blood from the antecubital vein in the arm.
   4. Puncture the finger and collect the blood in a vial.

41. A woman is in the clinic complaining of urinary frequency, urgency and pain on urination. Orders include a urine for culture and administration of Gantrisin and pyridium. Which action should the nurse take first?
   1. Obtain a clean catch urine from the client.
   2. Ask the client if she is allergic to sulfa drugs.
   3. Administer the Gantrisin.
   4. Administer the pyridium.

42. An eight-year-old has just had a fiberglass cast applied to his right lower leg following a fractured ankle. The nurse is discussing care of the cast with the parents. Which instruction should be included?
   1. Since water does not dissolve a fiberglass cast, your child may take a bath.
   2. Check the toes on the right leg to be sure they are warm.
   3. Do not cover the cast for two days to allow it time to dry.
   4. Keep the casted leg down for the next two days to promote circulation.

43. The nurse is caring for a woman admitted with thrombocytopenia. Which instruction should the nurse give the client?
   1. Call me when you need to go to the bathroom.
   2. Do not use dental floss or a firm toothbrush.
   3. Wear a mask when you leave the room.
   4. Be sure everyone washes their hands before touching you.

44. At 10:30 A.M., a young woman who has diabetes calls the nurse and says she feels "funny." The nurse notes she is cool to the touch but her skin is moist. When the nurse asks her if she is hungry she responds in an irritable manner that she is hungry. Which initial nursing action is appropriate?
   1. Administer her noon dose of insulin early.
   2. Call the lab to draw a blood glucose.
   3. Have her drink a glass of cola.
   4. Encourage her to drink lots of water.

45. A newborn is to receive phototherapy for hyperbilirubinemia. Which nursing action is essential?
   1. Keep the infant NPO for two hours before the treatment.
   2. Ask the mother to stay away from the infant during the treatment.
   3. Monitor the client's pulse rate very carefully.
   4. Cover the baby's eyes during the treatment.

46. A child at school trips on a shoe lace and falls. Her ankle swells immediately and the child is in a great deal of pain. What is the best initial action for the nurse to take?
   1. Keep the foot down.
   2. Apply a warm compress.
   3. Elevate the foot and apply an ice pack.
   4. Ask the child to try to move her ankle.

47. Oxygen has been ordered for a client who was admitted to the hospital with congestive heart failure. Which assessment finding indicates the oxygen has been effective?
   1. The client no longer complains of pain.
   2. The client's respiratory rate has decreased from 36 to 24.
   3. The client has voided 600 ml of urine in the last three hours.
   4. The client has less ankle edema than was present when admitted.

48. An adult is admitted with meningitis. During the acute phase of the illness, which measure should the nurse include in the nursing care plan to reduce the chance of seizures?
   1. Play the client's favorite music.
   2. Stimulate the client every two hours.
   3. Keep a padded tongue blade at the bedside.
   4. Darken the client's room.

49. The evening nurse caring for an adult who had a partial gastrectomy this morning notes the drainage from the nasogastric tube is bright red. What action should the nurse take?
   1. Chart the drainage amount and color.
   2. Report the findings immediately to the charge nurse.
   3. Disconnect the drainage system.
   4. Immediately apply pressure to the wound.

50. The nurse is caring for a man who had a transphenoidal hypophysectomy earlier today. He says he has to spit a lot. What nursing action is essential?
   1. Ask him to blow his nose.
   2. Do a glucose test on his mouth secretions.
   3. Have him rinse his mouth with water.
   4. Ask him if he needs an antiemetic.

51. A client is admitted with a possible gastric ulcer. Suddenly he calls to the nurse and says, "It hurts so bad." The client is pale and diaphoretic. What should the nurse do initially?

1. Call the physician.
2. Palpate the abdomen.
3. Obtain a stool for guaiac.
4. Place the client in a supine position.

52. A blood transfusion has just been started on an adult. Which assessment is most essential during the first hour?
    1. Temperature
    2. Blood pressure
    3. Respirations
    4. Pulse

53. An adult is admitted in severe hypovolemic shock following an auto accident. A transfusion is ordered. What type of blood is given when the client's blood type is not known?
    1. O positive
    2. O negative
    3. AB positive
    4. AB negative

54. The client has been vomiting for several days. Which blood gas values is he likely to have?
    1. pH 7.32; CO_2 60; HCO_3 30
    2. pH 7.32; CO_2 33; HCO_3 18
    3. pH 7.54; CO_2 28; HCO_3 22
    4. pH 7.54; CO_2 32; HCO_3 34

55. The nurse is caring for an elderly woman who had surgery on her right foot yesterday. The woman had a broken left arm three months ago and has osteo-arthritis. Which type of assistive device will probably be most appropriate for this client?
    1. Quad cane
    2. Crutches
    3. Walker
    4. Tripod cane

56. The nurse administers CPR to an adult male who is found unconscious, has no pulse, and is not breathing. What is the ratio of chest compressions to respirations for one person rescue?
    1. Five chest compressions to one breath
    2. Five chest compressions to two breaths
    3. Fifteen chest compressions to one breath
    4. Fifteen chest compressions to two breaths

57. The nurse is caring for a client who had a portable water seal chest drainage system inserted today. Which observation indicates the client's drainage system is working properly?
    1. There are no bubbles in the water seal bottle.
    2. The suction control chamber has continuous bubbles.
    3. There are bubbles in the drainage chamber.
    4. There is no fluctuation in the fluid in the water seal chamber.

58. What should the nurse do when ambulating a client who has a portable wound drainage system?
    1. Remove the drain during ambulation.

2. Fasten the collection device below the wound.
3. Completely empty the collection device before ambulating.
4. Disconnect the suction apparatus before ambulating.

59. The nurse is discussing positioning with the family of a client who is at home following a total hip replacement a week ago. Which should be included in the discussion?
    1. Keep the client on his unaffected side most of the time.
    2. Position the client to maintain hip flexion.
    3. Keep a pillow between his legs when turning him.
    4. Position the client so the hip is adducted.

60. An 80-year-old woman is having diffculty sleeping. Which nursing action is most appropriate initially?
    1. Ask the physician for an order for a sleeping medication.
    2. Encourage the client to do mild exercises a half hour before going to bed.
    3. Suggest to the client that she not nap during the day.
    4. Recommend the client drink coffee in the evening.

61. The nurse is providing home care to an elderly woman who had a CVA and has right-sided hemiplegia. She is living with her daughter. Which observation indicates that the family needs more instruction?
    1. The client's arms and legs are exercised every day.
    2. The daughter gets her mother out of bed several times a day.
    3. The client is given a shower every other day.
    4. The daughter puts the chair on the right side of the bed when getting her mother out of bed.

62. The family of a 48-year-old woman who has multiple sclerosis and spends most of her time in bed or in a chair asks the nurse why they have been told they should have her take deep breaths and cough frequently. What should the nurse include in the reply?
    1. Deep breathing and coughing will help her to move her secretions so she will not develop pneumonia.
    2. Deep breathing and coughing help to prevent clots from developing in the lung.
    3. When she coughs she increases the amount of oxygen going to the brain, preventing confusion.
    4. Deep breathing increases blood flow to the brain and helps to keep her from getting depressed.

63. An adult is admitted with gastroenteritis. The physician has ordered prochlorperazine (Compazine) 10 mg po tid prn or prochlorperazine (Compazine) 5 mg

suppository every 6 hours prn and loperamide (Imodium) 2 mg po prn. The client has an episode of dairrhea and complains of nausea. What should the nurse administer?

1. Prochlorperazine (Compazine) by mouth
2. Loperamide (Imodium)
3. Prochlorperazine (Compazine) po and Loperamide (Imodium)
4. Prochlorperazine (Compazine) via suppository

64. A clear liquid diet is ordered for an adult following surgery. All of the following are on the client's tray. Which should be removed by the nurse?
1. Ice cream
2. Beef broth
3. Apple juice
4. Iced tea

65. The nurse is administering digoxin to a six-month-old infant. Which finding would cause the nurse to withhold the medication and notify the charge nurse or the physician?
1. Apical heart rate of 85
2. Appears lethargic
3. Circumoral cyanosis
4. Respiratory rate of 38

66. The nurse is teaching a client how to care for a colostomy. Which factor indicates the client needs more instruction?
1. The client says, "I will change the bag as soon as it gets full."
2. The client is observed irrigating the colostomy while sitting on the toilet.
3. The client positions the irrigating solution container at shoulder level.
4. The client places a chlorophyll tablet in the drainage bag.

67. The nurse is caring for a client who has dentures. Which action by the nurse is not appropriate?
1. Place a washcloth in the bottom of the sink before cleaning the dentures.
2. Brush the dentures with toothpaste.
3. Rinse the dentures with hydrogen peroxide.
4. Remove the dentures from the mouth for cleaning.

68. The LPN/LVN is making assignments in a long-term care facility. Staff on duty include another LPN and a new certified nursing assistant.
Which client can most safely be assigned to the nursing assistant?
1. Ms. A., 92 years old, has dementia and advancing congestive heart failure.
2. Ms. B., 83 years old, has Alzheimer's and Parkinson's and is ambulatory with assistance.
3. Mr. C., 76 years old, has just been transferred from an acute care facility

where he had a total hip replacement four days ago.
4. Mr. D., 29 years old, had a closed head injury and is in a semi-vegetative state with a tracheostomy and a gastrostomy.

69. The nurse is caring for a client who is terminally ill. Upon admission the client signed advance directives indicating she does not wish to have any resuscitative measures. The client is now in and out of consciousness. Her daughter comes to the nurse and says "I want everything done for my mother if she stops breathing." How should the nurse respond?
1. Remove the "Do Not Resuscitate" order from the chart.
2. Discuss the client's advance directives with the daughter.
3. Have the daughter sign a consent form since her mother is in and out of consciousness.
4. When the client is conscious ask her again what her wishes are.

70. When explaining Universal Precautions to a client, the nurse should explain that the primary purpose of Universal Precautions is to
1. protect the client with a weak immune system.
2. prevent the spread of AIDS.
3. prevent nosocomial infections.
4. reduce the spread of disease.

71. Upon entering a client's room the nurse sees and smells smoke and flames. What is the best initial nursing action?
1. Attempt to fight the fire.
2. Move the client out of the room.
3. Close the door to the room.
4. Evacuate everyone from the unit.

72. An adult who has liver disease secondary to alcohol abuse has just been told that alcohol is causing his health problems. The nurse expects that the client's initial response will most likely be which of the following?
1. "I don't drink enough to hurt my health."
2. "How could this happen to me? I've always been a good person."
3. "Where can I get help to stop drinking so much?"
4. "I've known for a long time that I drink too much. I guess I really have to stop now."

73. The client is receiving chemotherapy for cancer. Which statement, if made by the client, would indicate that she has accepted the diagnosis and treatment?
1. "I hate getting that treatment."
2. "The doctor isn't sure if I really have cancer."
3. "I have a collection of pretty scarves that I am wearing a lot now."
4. "I don't go anywhere except for my treatments because I look so weird."

74. A hospitalized client asks what is wrong with the person in the next bed. How should the nurse reply?
    1. Ask the client why he wants to know.
    2. Give the client a vague answer.
    3. Tell the client that information is confidential.
    4. Tell the client to ask the head nurse.
75. An adult is being admitted with possible pneumonia. His history indicates he had a tonsillectomy as a child and tuberculosis 10 years ago, which was arrested. Which room assignment is most appropriate?
    1. A room without a roommate
    2. Isolation
    3. A double room with a client who also has pneumonia
    4. A double room with a client who has angina
76. Which activities are appropriate to assign to a certified nursing assistant?
    1. Evaluate vital signs.
    2. Monitor tube feedings.
    3. Assist with activities of daily living.
    4. Discuss discharge insturctions.
77. An adult who recently had an amputation has an above-the-knee prosthesis. Which nursing action will do the most to help the client adjust to the prosthesis?
    1. Adjust the prosthesis for the client.
    2. Offer the client a cane or a walker for ease of movement.
    3. Place an "at risk for fall" sign on the client's door.
    4. Allow the client to manage his own care.
78. The nurse is monitoring a client who is going through barbiturate withdrawal. Which symptom is of most concern to the nurse?
    1. Nausea and vomiting
    2. Anxiety
    3. Hallucinations
    4. Seizures
79. An adult has a substance abuse problem. Which statement, if made by the client, indicates the best understanding of the problem?
    1. "I can never use that drug again."
    2. "When I am off the drug for two years, I will be cured."
    3. "At least I shall be able to go to parties and limit my drugs."
    4. "When I feel upset, I can call the support group."
80. The nurse is caring for a woman whose husband beats her regularly. Which is the most important long-term goal for this woman?
    1. Provide a long-term support group.
    2. Help her feel like a survivor.
    3. Point out the ways she behaved.
    4. Be able to blame the abuser.

81. The nurse has delegated the task of taking the temperature of a client with a new tympanic thermometer to a certified nursing assistant. The nursing assistant says, "This looks easy. I am good at figuring things out." What is the nurse's responsibility?
    1. Allow the nursing assistant to proceed.
    2. Assign the task to another nursing assistant.
    3. Ask another nursing assistant to demonstrate this task to the nursing assistant.
    4. Demonstrate the proper use of the thermometer and observe the nursing assistant.
82. While the nurse is preparing medications a code occurs. One of the nursing assistants offers to help by administering the medications. What is the best response by the nurse?
    1. Allow the nursing assistant to give the medications.
    2. Hold the medications until after the code.
    3. Give the medications and then help with the code.
    4. Ask the nursing assistant when she was checked off on giving medications.
83. The nurse enters the room of a woman who had a vaginal hysterectomy three days ago and finds her crying. What is the best initial approach for the nurse?
    1. Ask her what seems to be troubling her.
    2. Reassure her that feeling depressed is normal after this type of surgery.
    3. Tell her that the nurse will ask the doctor to order hormones for her.
    4. Leave the room so she can work out her feelings.
84. A client who is scheduled for surgery today says to the nurse, "Do you think I'll survive the surgery?" What is the best initial response for the nurse?
    1. "Don't worry, your surgeon is good."
    2. "Tell me about your concerns."
    3. "I can call your clergyman."
    4. "We do a lot of these surgeries here; everything will be okay."
85. The nurse is assessing a client's emotional state and coping strategies. Evidence of which behavior is of most concern to the nurse?
    1. Anxiety
    2. Dysfunctional family unit
    3. Social isolation
    4. Self-mutilation
86. Following a motor vehicle accident the client does not know where he is or what year it is and has short-term memory impairment. Which nursing action is most appropriate?
    1. Offer several choices to the client.
    2. Give simple directions to the client.

3. Give the client the details of the care.
4. Offer written instructions to the client.

87. The nurse is changing a wet to dry dressing. Which action is appropriate?
1. Pouring a sterile solution directly into a sterile container.
2. Removing the old dressings with sterile gloves.
3. Opening the sterile dressings wearing sterile gloves.
4. Packing the wound wearing sterile gloves.

88. The nurse is providing home care for a client who is visually impaired. What safety precautions are most appropriate for this client?
1. Remove scatter rugs.
2. Have hand rails in the bathroom.
3. Have side rails up whenever the client is in bed.
4. Have a bell to call for help.

89. An adult client complains of dizziness when getting out of bed in the morning. Which instruction should the nurse give the nursing assistant regarding care of this client?
1. Have the client wear slippers when getting out of bed.
2. Have the client sit on the edge of the bed for a few minutes.
3. Offer the client some juice before getting out of bed.
4. Tell the client to stay in bed until she is no longer dizzy.

90. An adult had exploratory surgery and post-operatively had an exacerbation of asthma. The client is on a rebreathing mask and seems upset and angry. What is the best nursing approach?
1. Ask the physician for an order for Ativan.
2. Spend some time with the client.
3. Ask the family to have someone stay with the client.
4. Apply wrist restraints.

91. An adult client became incontinent while hospitalized. The client now drinks very little. The nurse understands that this is
1. a coping strategy.
2. a defense mechanism.
3. a way to not bother the nurse.
4. regression.

92. The nurse is evaluating the progress of a client who has had a cerebral vascular accident and realizes there has been limited progress. What should the nurse do?
1. Transfer the client to another caregiver.
2. Reassess the goals with the client.
3. Request a longer hospital stay.
4. Role-play the current plan with the client.

93. The nurse is assessing a client who may be bulimic. What objective finding indicates bulimia?
1. Low self-esteem

2. Loss of tooth enamel
3. Feeling of loss of control
4. Feeling of social inadequacy

94. When caring for an abused client, what is most important for the nurse to do initially?
1. Provide a safe place for the victim.
2. Refer the victim to a long-term support group.
3. Make an appointment with a counselor.
4. Make arrangements for the victim to confront the abuser.

95. The nurse is bathing a client who has contact isolation ordered. The nurse wears gloves. What else is needed?
1. Face mask
2. Sterile gloves
3. Isolation cap
4. Isolation gown

96. The nurse is performing a sterile dressing change. Which action is essential?
1. Touching the corners of the dressing with clean gloves
2. Discussing the wound with the client during the dressing change
3. Irrigating the wound with an antiseptic solution
4. Wearing sterile gloves during the dressing change

97. The nurse is teaching a client who has short-term memory loss how to use the call light. Which factor is least essential for the nurse to assess when teaching this client?
1. Visual status
2. Ambulatory difficulty
3. Orientation to time, place, and person
4. Understanding of the English language

98. An adult asks the nurse why she must have her skin shaved prior to surgery. What is the best nursing response? Reducing the hair by shaving
1. reduces infection by removing hair, which harbors bacteria.
2. provides a clean area on which to operate.
3. disinfects the skin.
4. makes it easier to see the surgical incision.

99. An adult who is undergoing diagnostic tests to diagnose a possible malignancy angrily says to the nurse, "You don't know anything. I want someone competent caring for me." What is the best initial nursing response?
1. "I am a competent nurse. What would you like?"
2. "It must be difficult having all those tests. How can I help you?"
3. "I will get the supervisor who should be able to help you."
4. "I will care for you, but you may not talk to me in that manner."

100. A client who is admitted for surgery reports drinking eight or nine beers everyday. Two days after surgery the nurse notes the client is

shaking and seems disoriented. The nurse's response is based on which understanding of his behavior?
1. The client has probably consumed alcohol since surgery.

2. The client may be having a reaction to the narcotics used for pain control.
3. The client is exhibiting signs of alcohol withdrawal.
4. The client is most likely in severe pain.

Answers and Rationales for Practice Test Four

Answer	Rationale	NP	CN	SA
#1. 1.	**In Cushing's syndrome there are increased amounts of cortisol, which causes osteoporosis. This is an appropriate nursing diagnosis for someone who has Cushing's syndrome.**	Pl	Ph/9	1
2.	Pain related to cold intolerance would be an appropriate nursing diagnosis for someone who has hypothyroidism. Persons with Cushing's syndrome would be more apt to be warm than cold.			
3.	Risk for deficient fluid volume would be an appropriate nursing diagnosis for someone with Addison's disease. The persons with Cushing's syndrome will have high risk for fluid volume excess due to increased amounts of aldosterone, which causes sodium and fluid retention.			
4.	Risk for injury related to hypotension would be an appropriate nursing diagnosis for a person who has Addison's disease. A person with Cushing's syndrome will have hypertension.			
#2. 3.	**Placenta previa is usually painless and the client has bright red bleeding from the vagina.**	Dc	Ph/10	3
1.	Sudden kinfe-like pain in the lower abdomen accompanied by profuse vaginal bleeding is characteristic of abruption of the placenta.			
2.	Dark red vaginal discharge can be normal following a pelvic exam at this point in pregnancy.			
4.	A tender uterine wall and abdomen with no obvious vaginal bleeding is typical of abruption of the placenta.			
#3. 1.	**The normal range for walking is about 7 months to 18 months. Not walking at 13 months is perfectly normal.**	Dc	He/3	4
2.	The normal range for walking is about 7 months to 18 months. Not walking at 13 months is perfectly normal.			
3.	This response is inappropriate. The normal range for walking is about 7 months to 18 months. Not walking at 13 months is perfectly normal.			
4.	This response is not appropriate and is incorrect information. The normal range for walking is about 7 months to 18 months. Not walking at 13 months is perfectly normal.			
#4. 2.	**The mother needs positive reinforcement for bringing the baby in, but the immunizations will be delayed until the baby is well.**	Im	He/3	4
1.	This is not correct. Immunizations are not given when the child has a cold.			
3.	This is an inappropriate response. The shots do make the child irritable, but they are not given when the child has a cold.			
4.	This is poor communication with the parent.			
#5. 3.	**The protrusion reflex disappears around four months of age. Babies are usually ready for solids about this time.**	Im	He/3	4
1.	Two months is too young for solids. The baby still has a stgrong protrusion reflex.			
2.	The baby usually takes a quart of formula a day before the age of four months.			
4.	There may be some truth to this statement but it offers no guidelines to the mother.			

ANSWER **RATIONALE**

#6. 2. **Coarctation of the aorta is a narrowing of the descending aorta that causes a decrease in blood flow to the lower part of the body. The classic sign of coarctation of the aorta is that the blood pressure is higher in the upper extremities than in the lower extremities.** — Dc Ph/10 4

    1. Tachypnea (rapid respirations) is common in heart disease, but is not specific to coarctation of the aorta.

    3. There is no murmur in coarctation of the aorta. A murmur is caused when blood flows somewhere it doesn't usually go. This is not the case with coarctation. Coarctation is a narrowing of the aorta.

    4. Heart rate of 150 per minute is normal for an infant.

#7. 1. **Barbiturates such as phenobarbital frequently cause drowsiness.** — Im Ph/8 5

    2. Drowsiness does occur in the post-ictal phase (after a seizure). However, the question says the child has not had a seizure so this is not the cause of the drowsiness.

    3. The drowsiness is probably related to the phenobarbital used to treat the seizures.

    4. Some persons do have an aura or a sensory experience that usually occurs before a seizure. It is not usually drowsiness. The question says that the child has had no seizures, so this is not likely to be the cause of his drowsiness.

#8. 3. **The blood volume increases by 50 percent by the end of the second trimester.** — Ev He/3 3

    1. Oxygen consumption is increased during pregnancy.

    2. The rate of peristalsis is decreased during pregnancy.

    4. Metabolic rate will increase during pregnancy.

#9. 2. **Chlamydia, the most common sexually transmitted disease, and gonorrhea are the two major cuases of neonatal eye infections which, if untreated, could lead to blindness.** — Im Ph/9 3

    1. Chlamydia is transmitted to the baby during the birth process. It is not transmitted through the placenta. Syphilis and HIV are blood-borne and can be transmitted through the placenta.

    3. Chlamydia infection is unrelated to pregnancy-induced hypertension.

    4. Chlamydia is unrelated to congenital (born with) anomalies. If picked up by the baby during the birth process, the baby can develop an eye infection, which could lead to blindness.

#10. 4. **High blood sugar levels in the mother probably increased pancreatic production of insulin in the infant and he may use his stores of sugar quickly. He now has no influx of sugar from the mother and is at risk for hypoglycemia.** — Dc Ph/9 4

    1. The baby of a diabetic woman is not at increased risk of infection.

    2. The baby of a diabetic woman is not at increased risk for hyperglycemia.

    3. The baby of a diabetic woman is not at increased risk for acidosis.

#11. 4. **The woman may be turned and may receive oxygen, but the most important first action is to remove the source of the tetanic contraction, which is oxytocin.** — Im He/3 3

    1. The nurse should stop the oxytocin. Slowing it down is not sufficient.

    2. The woman may be turned and may receive oxygen, but the most important first action is to remove the source of the tetanic contraction, which is oxytocin.

    3. The woman may be turned and may receive oxygen, but the most important first action is to remove the source of the tetanic contraction, which is oxytocin.

#12. 1. **The nurse should always listen to a laboring mother. This woman needs to be assessed again.** — Dc He/3 3

    2. The nurse should always listen to a laboring mother. After she is checked, it may be appropriate to reassure the woman.

    3. A laboring woman does not push unless it is confirmed that she is fully dilated.

ANSWER	RATIONALE	NP	CN	SA

4. The nurse should initially determine if the woman has progressed in labor. There is no data in the question to indicate the woman needs medication to relax.

#13. 1. Airway takes priority over the other items.   Im   He/3   4

2. The nurse will keep the baby warm, but the highest priority is establishing an airway.

3. The nurse will apply identification bracelets, but the highest priority is establishing an airway.

4. The LPN/LVN does not legally determine APGAR scores.

#14. 1. Long pants and long shirts are the best ways to prevent tick bites. Deer ticks transmit Lyme disease and dog ticks transmit Rocky Mountain spotted fever. Both are serious diseases.   Pl   He/4   1

2. Sunscreen is important to prevent exposure to ultraviolet rays. Prolonged exposure to ultraviolet rays predisposes to the development of skin cancer. If the person perspires and the sunscreen is removed, more should be applied.

3. The most important thing is to replace fluids. The person should bring plenty of water. Salt tablets are not recommended.

4. Sensitive individuals can get severe poison ivy from the slightest exposure to the oils. If clothing rubs against the plant and the person touches the clothing, an allergic reaction can develop.

#15. 2. Most cancer chemotherapeutic agents cause nausea as a side effect. Taking it in the evening means there is less nausea during meal times and awake times. It is often better tolerated.   Im   Ph/8   5

1. It is important to have a regular time to take medication. However, it does matter when the drug is taken. Most cancer chemotherapeutic agents cause nausea as a side effect. Taking it in the evening means there is less nausea during meal times and awake times. It is often better tolerated.

3. Drowsiness is not a major side effect of cancer chemotherapeutic agents. Lack of energy may develop as the bone marrow is depressed and the client has fewer red blood cells. Fatigue due to anemia is not related to the time when the medication is taken.

4. Activity level does not alter the effectiveness of the cancer chemotherapeutic agents.

#16. 2. The client has crackles and is beginning to collect fluid in the air spaces. The best thing for the nurse to do is to deep-breathe and cough the client every two hours. This should resolve the problem. The nurse will also record the findings and nursing actions.   Pl   Ph/9   1

1. The client has crackles and is beginning to collect fluid in the air spaces. The best thing for the nurse to do is to deep-breathe and cough the client every two hours. This should resolve the problem. There is no need to start emergency oxygen. The nurse will record the findings and actions taken.

3. The client has crackles and is beginning to collect fluid in the air spaces. The best thing for the nurse to do is to deep-breathe and cough the client every two hours. This should resolve the problem. The nurse will record the findings and actions. There is no need for an emergency call to the physician and no need for a tracheostomy.

4. The client has crackles and is beginning to collect fluid in the air spaces. The best thing for the nurse to do is to deep-breathe and cough the client every two hours. This should resolve the problem. The nurse will continue to observe the client. This finding does not suggest an immediate risk of cyanosis.

#17. 1. The nurse should have a tracheostomy set at the bedside along with oxygen and suction. The client is at risk for airway obstruction.   Pl   Ph/9   1

2. There is no need for a catheterization tray at the bedside for a thyroidectomy client.

3. There is no need for a sterile dressing set at the bedside for a thyroidectomy client.

4. There is no need for a ventilator at the bedside for a thyroidectomy client.

#18. 4. Iron colors the stools black.   Ev   Ph/8   4

1. The child's color should improve and the energy level should increase if the child is receiving the iron regularly. This observation may indicate the child is not receiving the medication.

2. Oral administration of iron should not cause brown spots on the skin. IM iron could cause brown spots.

3. Iron should not cause dark-colored urine.

#19. 2. Hydration is important to prevent sickling episodes. Dehydration causes a decrease in oxygen tension, which causes sickling. This response indicates that the parents understand how to reduce the incidence of sickling.   Ev   Ph/9   4

1. The child can play outdoors. The child should be adequately hydrated, especially when the weather is hot. This response indicates the parents do not understand how to reduce the incidence of crisis.

3. The child with sickle cell should not receive aspirin. Aspirin is acetyl salycylic acid. Acidosis causes sickling. The child should receive acetaminophen and lots of fluids if he develops a fever. This response indicates the parents do not understand how to reduce the incidence of crisis.

4. Flying is dangerous for the person who has sickle cell. The oxygen saturation is less at high altitudes. Low oxygen saturation can cause sickling. It would be better for the child to ride in a car than fly in an airplane. This response indicates the parents do not understand how to reduce the incidence of crisis.

#20. 2. When coal tar preparations are used the client should protect the areas from sunlight for 24 hours.   Im   Ph/8   1

1. Nausea and vomiting are not frequent side effects of coal tar preparations.

3. The substance stays on for at least 24 hours. It should not be washed off in 6–8 hours.

4. Coal tar is black and may make the skin look dark.

#21. 2. When the client is in shock the pulse rate increases, the blood presure decreases, and the pulse pressure decreases.   Dc   Ph/10   1

1. The BP is higher than the baseline and the pulse pressure is wider. This finding is suggestive of increased intracranial pressure, not shock.

3. This blood pressure reading is so close to the baseline any change is insignificant.

4. A pulse rate of 60 in this client would suggest rising intracranial pressure, not shock.

#22. 3. Rather than responding specifically to the complaint that the assignment is unfair, the nurse should determine what the nursing assistant's real concern is and help her to address that.   Im   Sa/1   1

1. This is a very authoritarian response and does nothing to ease the situation.

2. This approach will not solve the problem and may be impossible to carry out.

4. The charge nurse could assign the other nurse to assist as needed. However, discussing the real issues and concerns is much more appropriate.

#23. 3. Tremors are consistent with alcohol withdrawal. The other signs and symptoms are consistent with blood loss and shock.   Dc   Ph/10   1

1. BP of 90/60 is consistent with blood loss and shock from the GI bleed. It is not symptomatic of alcohol withdrawal.

2. Dizziness is consistent with blood loss and shock from the GI bleed. It is not symptomatic of alcohol withdrawal.

4. Pallor is consistent with blood loss and shock from the GI bleed. It is not symptomatic of alcohol withdrawal.

#24. 2. Heavy alcohol intake can damage the liver and cause a prolonged prothrombin time.　　Dc　Ph/9　1
1. Eating or not eating meat is not likely to affect the prothrombin time.
3. Heparin does not affect prothrombin time. Heparin affects partial thromboplastin time and clotting time.
4. A recent injury should not cause the prothrombin time to be prolonged.

#25. 3. Walking may help the stone to move down through the urinary tract and be passed in the urine. The client who has kidney stones is often more comfortable ambulating.　　Im　Ph/10　1
1. Walking may help the stone to move down through the urinary tract and be passed in the urine. The client who has kidney stones is often more comfortable ambulating.
2. Walking may help the stone to move down through the urinary tract and be passed in the urine. The client who has kidney stones is often more comfortable ambulating.
4. There is no need to limit ambulation to once a day. Walking may help the stone to move down through the urinary tract and be passed in the urine. The client who has kidney stones is often more comfortable ambulating.

#26. 4. The recommendation is that all women age 50 and over have annual mammograms. Symptoms are a late sign of breast cancer.　　Im　He/4　3
1. It is normal for breasts to be tender before the period. She is younger than the age recommended for regular mammography. Mammograms are not indicated for this client.
2. There is no need to do a mammogram for a sports injury. There is a common misconception that a physical injury to the breast causes cancer. This does not appear to be true.
3. There is no need to do a mammogram for a woman who has been breastfeeding. In fact, breastfeeding is thought to help protect a woman from breast cancer.

#27. 3. Older persons are particularly at risk for pneumonia. Pneumovax is highly recommended.　　Dc　He/4　1
1. DPT is diphtheria, pertussis, and tetanus. Pertussis is not given after the age of six. If she hasn't had a tetanus shot in the last 10 years, she may need a booster shot. DPT or pertussis (whooping cough) is not given.
2. MMR is measles, mumps, rubella. Pneumovax is more important than MMR. Most persons in this age group had these diseases as children. The immunization was not available when they were children.
4. HIB is hemophilus influenza B which is given to infants to help prevent meningitis caused by h. influenza B. This is not given to adults.

#28. 1. Preadolescent and early adolescent girls are at the most risk for scoliosis (lateral curvature of the spine). They should be told to wear a bathing suit under their clothing the day of the exam. During the exam they will remove their outer clothing and the nurse will examine them. They will be asked to bend over and hang their arms down so the nurse can assess whether the shoulders and the hips are even.　　Dc　He/4　4
2. Scoliosis is a lateral curvature of the spine. A urine test is not the screening approach.
3. Scoliosis is a lateral curvature of the spine. Hair washing is not related to the assessment process.
4. Scoliosis is a lateral curvature of the spine. There is no examination of the feet when assessing for scoliosis.

#29. 2. Induration or a raised area 10 mm or more indicates a positive reaction and should be referred for follow-up.　　Dc　He/4　1

    1. A red area does not indicate a positive response. A tuberculin skin test should be read with the fingers (feeling a raised area), not the eyes.

    3. Itching does not indicate a positive response to a tuberculin skin test. A tuberculin skin test should be read with the fingers (feeling a raised area), not the eyes.

    4. A rash does not indicate a positive response to a tuberculin skin test. A tuberculin skin test should be read with the fingers (feeling a raised area), not the eyes.

#30. **1.** **A tuberculin skin test is given intradermally, at a 10-degree angle.**   Im   He/4   1

    2. A tuberculin skin test is given intradermally, at a 10-degree angle.

    3. A 60-degree angle is appropriate for a subcutaneous injection. A tuberculin skin test is given intradermally, at a 10-degree angle.

    4. An intramuscular injection is given at a 90-degree angle. A tuberculin skin test is given intradermally, at a 10-degree angle.

#31. **4.** **Medicines should be in a locked cabinet. Toddlers are good climbers. A high shelf is not adequate to prevent curious toddlers from ingesting medicines. This statement indicates a need for more instruction.**   Ev   He/4   4

    1. This statement is correct. Toddlers should be in front facing car seats in the back seat. This statement indicates the mother understands child safety.

    2. Toddlers need constant supervision. This statement indicates the mother understands child safety.

    3. Any household that has toddlers should have syrup of ipecac to administer in case the child accidentally ingests a poison. This statement indicates the mother understands child safety.

#32. **2.** **Black stools can be an indication of upper GI bleeding. The nurse should ask the client if he is taking iron. Iron causes stools to be black.**   Dc   Ph/7   1

    1. A bowel movement every other day is normal for many people.

    3. Sometimes straining at stool is normal. The client should be told to eat more roughage to promote a softer stool.

    4. Three stools a day is normal for many people, especially if they eat a lot of fruits and vegetables.

#33. **3.** **The colostomy should be irrigated at the same time each day. This helps to promote regular function. This answer indicates the client understands the care of his colostomy.**   Ev   Ph/7   1

    1. The client should use warm water, not hot water to irrigate the colostomy. Hot water is too irritating. This answer indicates the client does not understand the care of his colostomy.

    2. Alcohol causes pain if applied to irritated skin. This answer indicates the client does not understand the care of his colostomy.

    4. When possible, the irrigation should be performed in the bathroom in an upright position. This is the normal place and position for moving the bowels. This answer indicates the client does not understand the care of his colostomy.

#34. **3.** **Pain is what the client says it is. Autonomic symptoms such as changes in vital signs are usually not seen in chronic pain.**   Dc   Ph/7   1

    1. Persons with chronic pain often do not exhibit grimaces and other physical signs of pain.

    2. Autonomic symptoms such as changes in vital signs are usually not seen in chronic pain.

    4. Autonomic symptoms such as changes in vital signs are usually not seen in chronic pain.

#35. **3.** **This response best meets her needs for rest and activity. Since she has been very ill and on bed rest for several days, the nurse should increase her activity slowly.**   Pl   Ph/7   1

    1. This option does not allow the client to rest after the bath before getting her out of bed. She has been very ill with a respiratory

condition and has limited oxygenation. Her activities should be spaced.

   2. Having her get out of bed for the first time and bathe herself for the first time is probably too much for this older woman, who has been very ill.

   4. Having her give herself the bed bath and then immediately get up in a chair is probably too much for this older woman, who has been very ill.

#36. 2. **Red drainage in the nasogastric tube immediately following surgery is normal. The nurse should record the amount and color and continue to observe the client.** | Dc | Ph/7 | 1

   1. The drainage as described is normal. There is no need to report this immediately. It should be recorded and the nurse should continue to observe the client.

   3. The drainage is normal. The nurse should not apply pressure to the operative site.

   4. There is no need to place the client in Trendelenburg's position. Bloody drainage in the nasogastric tube during the first few hours after surgery is normal.

#37. 2. **Prior to administering a tube feeding, it is essential for the nurse to be sure the tube is in the stomach. One of the best ways is to aspirate drainage and check the pH. Stomach contents are acid.** | Im | Ph/7 | 1

   1. The client should be positioned in a semi-Fowler's position for a tube feeding. Supine position increases the risk of aspiration.

   3. The nurse may routinely check vital signs. However, checking vital signs is not essential before administering a tube feeding.

   4. The nurse might ask the client if she feels full. However, aspirating the contents is essential. When aspirating the contents to check for proper position of the tube, the nurse will also note the amount of feeding returned. This is a better indication of residual than asking the client if she feels full.

#38. 2. **The nurse should instruct the client to splint (hold) the incision when deep-breathing and coughing to prevent pressure on the suture line.** | Im | Ph/9 | 1

   1. The nurse should instruct the client to take in several deep breaths and then cough while exhaling the last one, then repeat the cycle.

   3. The client needs to take deep breaths when lying in bed. The moving client has less need of deep-breathing exercises than the one who does not move.

   4. Deep-breathing exercises are most needed for those who are confined to bed.

#39. 1. **All of the clients are older. The one who has a broken hip will likely be most immobile and thus most at risk for skin breakdown.** | Pl | Ph/9 | 1

   2. There is no data to suggest that this client is immobile. Most persons with angina are somewhat mobile.

   3. There is no data to suggest that this client is immobile.

   4. There is no data to suggest that the asthma client is immobile.

#40. 2. **A blood glucose check or Accucheck is performed by puncturing the finger on the side.** | Im | Ph/9 | 1

   1. The thumb is not the appropriate place to puncture.

   3. The LPN/LVN does not perform venipunctures for a routine blood glucose check.

   4. Blood is not collected in a vial when a routine blood glucose check is performed.

#41. 1. **The client's symptoms suggest a urinary tract infection. The specimen for culture should be obtained before medications are administered. After getting the specimen for culture, the client will want the pyridium, which is a urinary tract anesthetic.** | Pl | Ph/9 | 1

   2. Gantrisin is a sulfa drug. The nurse should ask the question about allergies before administering the drug. However, the nurse should

initially obtain the clean catch urine for culture to confirm the diagnosis and allow identification of the causative organism.

3. The nurse should initially obtain the clean catch urine for culture to confirm the diagnosis and allow identification of the causative organism. Before administering the Gantrisin the nurse should ask the client if she is allergic to sulfa drugs. Gantrisin is a sulfa drug.

4. Pyridium is a urinary tract anesthetic that is commonly given to clients who have urinary tract infections. The nurse should obtain the clean catch urine first to confirm the diagnosis and identify the causative organism.

#42. 2. The parents should check the toes for warmth. Cold toes would indicate the leg was not receiving adequate blood. The cast may be too tight.   Im   Ph/10   4

1. A fiberglass cast does not dissolve in water. However, the casted extremity cannot be put in water. Water will get under the cast and cause skin damage because it cannot evaporate under a fiberglass cast. To take a bath the child must either keep his leg out of the tub or wrap both ends of the fiberglass cast in plastic to prevent water from getting under the cast.

3. A fiberglass cast dries almost instantly. There is no need to keep it uncovered. This would be necessary for a plaster cast.

4. The casted leg should be kept elevated for the first couple of days to prevent swelling.

#43. 2. Thrombocytopenia is a condition in which the client has too few thrombocytes or platelets. Platelets clot blood. The client is at risk for bleeding and should not use dental floss or a firm bristle toothbrush.   Im   Ph/10   1

1. There is no particular need for the client with thrombocytopenia to call the nurse when going to the bathroom.

3. The client with thrombocytopenia is not infectious and not particularly at risk for infection. Thrombocytopenia is a condition in which the client has too few thrombocytes or platelets. Platelets clot blood.

4. The client with thrombocytopenia is not at great risk for infection. Thrombocytopenia is a condition in which the client has too few thrombocytes or platelets. Platelets clot blood.

#44. 3. The data all suggest the client is hypoglycemic. The appropriate intervention for hypoglycemia is to give something that has sugar in it. Cola has sugar.   Im   Ph/10   1

1. The data all suggest the client is hypoglycemic. Administering insulin would make the client worse. The client needs sugar.

2. The nurse should be able to determine from the client's signs and symptoms that she is hypoglycemic. It would be appropriate for the nurse to do a blood glucose check. It is not necessary for the nurse to call the lab and wait for the results. The nurse should be able to determine the client's condition and act immediately.

4. All the data suggest that the client is hypoglycemic. The client needs sugar, not water.

#45. 4. The baby's eyes should be covered during the time the light is on to prevent damage to the eyes.   Pl   Ph/10   4

1. There is no need to keep the infant NPO before the treatment. The baby needs adequate fluids.

2. There is no need to keep the mother away from the baby. The treatment may be done in the nursery but standard rules would apply. Parents can administer phototherapy at home.

3. The nurse would do routine monitoring of the infant's vital signs, but no special monitoring of pulse rate beyond that is needed.

#46. 3. The data suggest that the child probably has either a sprained ankle or a broken ankle. The nurse should elevate the foot and apply a cold pack to reduce bleeding and swelling at the site.   Im   Ph/10   4

1. The foot should be elevated, not put down. Putting the foot down causes more swelling.
2. Cold, not heat, should be applied to a freshly injured ankle. Heat would encourage bleeding and swelling.
4. The data suggest the child has either a sprain or a break. The nurse does not need to risk further injury by asking the child to move the ankle.

#47. 2. The focus of the question was evaluation of the client's response to oxygen. Oxygen should decrease the client's respiratory rate.   Ev   Ph/10   1

1. The client may have chest pain with congestive heart failure. However, decrease in chest pain may be due to several factors. It is not the best indicator of the effectiveness of oxygen.
3. A person who has congestive heart failure will also be given furosemide (Lasix). A large urine output indicates the Lasix was effective. Oxygen does not increase urine output.
4. A person who has congestive heart failure will also be given furosemide (Lasix). A decrease in edema indicates the Lasix was effective. Oxygen does not decrease edema.

#48. 4. Darkening the client's room reduces stimuli which can cause seizures.   Pl   Ph/10   1

1. Playing the client's favorite music may be appropriate later. To prevent seizures, the client's room should have as few auditory and visual stimuli as possible.
2. The client should have neurological checks periodically, but stimulating the client would be apt to cause seizures, not prevent them.
3. Keeping a padded tongue at the bedside does not prevent seizures. It was formerly used during a seizure. Now, it is no longer recommended that something be put in the client's mouth during a seizure.

#49. 1. Bright red drainage from a nasogastric tube on the day of surgery is normal. The nurse should chart color and amount.   Im   Ph/10   1

2. This finding is normal. There is no need to report immediately to the charge nurse.
3. This finding is normal. The suction system does not need to be turned off.
4. This finding is normal. There is no need to apply pressure to the wound. Bloody drainage in the NG tube on the day of surgery does not mean the client is hemorrhaging from the wound.

#50. 2. A transphenoidal hypophysectomy is the removal of the pituitary gland. The incision is in the mouth above the gum line and goes through the sphenoid sinuses into the brain. Drainage in the mouth could be cerebrospinal fluid. The nurse should test the secretions for glucose. Cerebrospinal fluid tests positive for glucose. If cerebrospinal fluid is leaking out, organisms can enter the brain.   Im   Ph/9   1

1. A person who has had a transphenoidal hypophysectomy recently should not blow his nose. A transphenoidal hypophysectomy is the removal of the pituitary gland. The incision is in the mouth above the gum line and goes through the sphenoid sinuses into the brain.
3. Having the client rinse his mouth is not the essential nursing action.
4. There is no data to suggest that this client needs an antiemetic.

#51. 2. The nurse should initially palpate the abdomen. If the client's ulcer has perforated or ruptured, the client's abdomen will be rigid and board-like. After palpating the abdomen the nurse should call the physician or notify the charge nurse.   Im   Ph/10   1

1. The nurse should call the physician after palpating the client's abdomen.
3. The nurse should call the physician before obtaining a stool for guaiac.

4. The client will be placed in a semi-Fowler's position.

#52. 1. An elevation in temperature is often the first sign of a transfusion reaction. Temperature should be monitored every 15 minutes times 2, then in 30 minutes, and then hourly during the rest of the transfusion. — As — Ph/8 — 1

2. Blood pressure may be monitored, but the most important thing to monitor is the temperature.

3. The nurse may assess respirations, but the most important thing to monitor is the temperature.

4. Pulse may be assessed, but the most important thing to monitor is the temperature.

#53. 2. O negative is the universal donor and can be given to anyone. — Im — Ph/8 — 1

1. O negative is the universal donor and can be given to anyone.

3. O negative is the universal donor and can be given to anyone. AB positive is the universal recipient.

4. O negative is the universal donor and can be given to anyone.

#54. 4. The client who is vomiting will go into metabolic alkalosis. — Dc — Ph/10 — 1

1. These values indicate respiratory acidosis, which might occur with chronic lung disease.

2. These values indicate metabolic acidosis, which might occur with diabetes and diarrhea.

3. These values indicate respiratory alkalosis, which might occur with hyperventilation.

#55. 3. A walker is the best choice for a client who had foot surgery yesterday, had a recent broken arm, and suffers from arthritis, which also is likely to decrease mobility. — Pl — Ph/7 — 1

1. An elderly person who had surgery on her right foot yesterday is probably not ready for a quad cane. A cane is held on the nonaffected side. A recently broken left arm would make using a cane difficult.

2. A client who has had foot surgery and a recent broken arm is not a candidate for crutches. The weight-bearing necessary for crutch walking is likely to reinjure her arm. She will be unable to bear weight on her foot.

4. An elderly person who had foot surgery yesterday is probably not ready for a tripod cane. She will be unable to bear weight on her foot. A cane is held on the nonaffected side. A recently broken left arm would make using a cane difficult.

#56. 4. The ratio of chest compressions to breaths for one-person rescue is fifteen to two. — Im — Ph/10 — 1

1. The ratio of chest compressions to breaths for one-person rescue is fifteen to two. Five to one is the ratio for two-person rescue.

2. The ratio of chest compressions to breaths for one-person rescue is fifteen to two.

3. The ratio of chest compressions to breaths for one-person rescue is fifteen to two.

#57. 2. Continuous bubbles in the suction control chamber indicate the system is functioning correctly. — Ev — Ph/9 — 1

1. There should be bubbles in the water seal chamber. No bubbles in the water seal chamber indicates either that the lung has re-expanded or that there is an obstruction in the tubing. The tube was inserted today. The lung is not likely to have re-expanded.

3. There should not be bubbles in the drainage chamber.

4. The fluid in the water seal chamber should fluctuate slightly with respiration.

#58. 2. Portable wound suction ahould always be maintained below the level of the wound. Otherwise it will not drain. — Im — Ph/9 — 1

1. The drainage device should not be removed until the physician removes it.

3. There is no need to completely empty the collection device before ambulating. If it is full, it could be emptied.

4. The suction apparatus should not be disconnected before ambulating. The physician will remove the device.

#59. 3. The client who has had a hip replacement should keep the hip extended and abducted. A pillow between the legs will keep the hip abducted and prevent adduction.   Im   Ph/7   1

  1. The client should have his position changed frequently (every two hours).

  2. The client who has had a total hip replacement should be maintained in extension.

  4. The client who has had a total hip replacement should be maintained in abduction.

#60. 3. Many older persons nap during the day and then have difficulty sleeping during the night. The client should be encouraged to stay awake during the day to see if this will improve nighttime sleeping.   Im   Ph/7   1

  1. The nurse should initially try nonpharmacologic methods to help the client sleep. If these are not successful the nurse may ask the physician for an order for sleeping medication.

  2. Exercises tend to increase metabolism and keep people awake. Exercises should not be done just before bedtime.

  4. Coffee and other caffeine-containing beverages should not be consumed during the evening as they are stimulants and keep people awake. Many older persons can no longer drink caffeine-containing drinks after noon because it keeps them awake.

#61. 4. The chair should be put on the unaffected side when transferring a hemiplegic to a chair. The daughter's technique is not correct and she needs more instruction.   Ev   Ph/7   1

  1. It is appropriate to exercise the client's arms and legs every day. This does not indicate a need for further instruction.

  2. It is appropriate for the daughter to get her mother out of bed several times a day. This does not indicate a need for further instruction.

  3. It is appropriate to give a shower every other day to an 80-year-old woman. Most older clients do not need a daily shower. This action does not indicate a need for further instruction.

#62. 1. Deep-breathing and coughing expands alveoli and helps the client to move secretions so she will not develop pneumonia.   Im   Ph/7   1

  2. Leg and foot exercises help to prevent deep-vein thrombophlebitis which usually causes blood clots in the lungs. Deep-breathing and coughing expands alveoli and helps the client to move secretions so she will not develop pneumonia.

  3. There may be some truth to this statement. However, the major reason deep-breathing and coughing is encouraged is to expand alveoli and prevent the accumulation of secretions in the lungs.

  4. There may be some truth to this statement. However, the major reason deep-breathing and coughing is encouraged is to expand alveoli and prevent the accumulation of secretions in the lungs.

#63. 3. Compazine is an antiemetic and is given for nausea and vomiting. Because the client has nausea but is not vomiting, the oral route is indicated. Imodium is for diarrhea. The client has had an episode of diarrhea, so the Imodium should be given.   Im   Ph/8   5

  1. The client has nausea but is not vomiting. The prochlorperazine can be given by mouth. The client also has diarrhea and so should be given loperamide.

  2. Loperamide is appropriate. However, the client also has nausea and should receive prochlorperazine as well.

  4. The client is not vomiting and so can probably take the prochlorperazine by mouth. The client also has diarrhea and should receive loperamide as ordered.

#64. 1. Ice cream is a milk product and is not a clear liquid.   Im   Ph/7   6

  2. Beef broth is a clear liquid.

    3. Apple juice is a clear liquid.

    4. Iced tea is a clear liquid.

#65. **1.** **When an infant's apical heart rate is below 100, the nurse should withhold the medication and notify the charge nurse or the physician.**   Dc   Ph/8   4

    2. An infant who needs digoxin may well have little energy and appear lethargic. Lethargy is not a side effect of digoxin.

    3. Circumoral cyanosis is common in infants who have cardiac disease. Digoxin is a heart drug. Circumoral cyanosis is not a side effect of digoxin.

    4. A respiratory rate of 38 is normal for a six-month-old infant.

#66. **1.** **The client should not change the bag each time it gets full. The client should empty the bag when it is half full. This comment indicates incorrect behavior and a need for more instruction.**   Ev   Ph/7   1

    2. The toilet is the ideal place for irrigating a colostomy. This behavior indicates the client understands the procedure.

    3. The irrigating solution container should be placed at shoulder height. This behavior indicates the client understands the procedure.

    4. Chlorophyll tablets are used to prevent odors in the colostomy bag. This behavior indicates the client understands how to care for the colostomy.

#67. **3.** **There is no need to rinse the dentures with hydrogen peroxide. Dentures should be rinsed with water.**   Im   Ph/7   1

    1. A washcloth should be placed in the bottom of the sink to prevent breakage of dentures if they should drop.

    2. Dentures can be brushed with toothpaste.

    4. Dentures should be removed from the mouth for cleaning.

#68. **2.** **A nursing assistant should be able to handle a client who has Alzheimer's and Parkinson's and is ambulatory with assistance.**   Pl   Sa/1   1

    1. The new nursing assistant should probably be able to care for a client who has dementia. However, this client also has advancing congestive heart failure. A new nursing assistant is not likely to have the skills needed to monitor a client who has advancing CHF.

    3. The client is a new client who has had a total hip replacement. The client needs special positioning. A new nursing assistant is not likely to be skilled in caring for this client.

    4. A new nursing assistant is not likely to be skilled in caring for a client who has a tracheostomy and a gastrostomy.

#69. **2.** **The nurse should discuss the client's advance directives with the daughter. Advance directives are the client's wishes and should be followed.**   Im   Sa/1   1

    1. The nurse does not have the authority to change the order. The client's wishes are not to be resuscitated and the physician has written the order.

    3. The purpose of an advance directive is to be sure the client's wishes are followed even when the client is no longer able to make decisions. The nurse cannot simply have the daughter sign away her mother's wishes.

    4. The client made advance directives so she would not have to make decisions at this time. There is no need to bother her with this again. If this is to be discussed with the client at this time, it should be the daughter who does it.

#70. **4.** **The primary purpose of Universal Precautions is to reduce the spread of disease by preventing the mode of transmission of the organism.**   Pl   Sa/2   1

    1. Reverse or protective precautions are used to protect the client who has a weak immune system.

    2. Diseases other than AIDS are prevented by the use of Universal Precautions.

ANSWER	RATIONALE	NP	CN	SA

3. Nosocomial infections are hospital-acquired infections. Universal Precautions will help to prevent nosocomial infections; however, this is not the primary purpose.

#71. 2. The nurse should initially remove the client from the room. Remember RACE (Rescue, Alarm, Contain, Evacuate).   Im   Sa/2   1

   1. The nurse should initially rescue the client and sound the alarm.

   3. The nurse should not close the door to the room until removing everyone from the room.

   4. The nurse should initially remove the client from the room. Remember RACE (Rescue, Alarm, Contain, Evacuate.)

#72. 1. The most common defense mechanism in substance abusers is denial. Denial is also the most common initial response to a bad diagnosis.   Dc   Ps/6   2

   2. Anger response is not usually the initial response to a diagnosis of a serious illness.

   3. Most persons who are confronted with being an alcoholic are not initially going to ask how to get help.

   4. The person who is addicted to alcohol and is confronted with the effects of this addiction is not likely to initially ask for help.

#73. 3. Chemotherapy often causes allopecia (loss of hair). Wearing scarves indicates the client has accepted the side effects of chemotherapy.   Ev   Ps/5   2

   1. This statement does not indicate acceptance of the diagnosis and treatment.

   2. This statement indicates the client has not accepted her diagnosis.

   4. This statement idnciates the client has not accepted her diagnosis.

#74. 3. The nurse should tell the client in a nice way that information about other clients is confidential.   Im   Sa/1   1

   1. The nurse should tell the client in a nice way that information about other clients is confidential.

   2. The nurse should tell the client in a nice way that information about other clients is confidential.

   4. The nurse should tell the client in a nice way that information about other clients is confidential.

#75. 2. A client who has a history of tuberculosis should be isolated when admitted with a respiratory infection. Even after the disease is arrested, the tuberculosis organism is apt to remain walled off in the person's lungs and may activate when the person is under extreme stress or has a respiratory infection. The person should be isolated until sputum cultures prove that tuberculosis has not recurred.   Pl   Sa/1   1

   1. A private room does not protect staff from tuberculosis. A client who has a history of tuberculosis should be isolated when admitted with a respiratory infection. Even after the disease is arrested, the tuberculosis organism is apt to remain walled off in the person's lungs and may activate when the person is under extreme stress or has a respiratory infection. The person should be isolated until sputum cultures prove that tuberculosis has not recurred.

   3. A client who has a history of tuberculosis should be isolated when admitted with a respiratory infection. Even after the disease is arrested, the tuberculosis organism is apt to remain walled off in the person's lungs and may activate when the person is under extreme stress or has a respiratory infection. The person should be isolated until sputum cultures prove that tuberculosis has not recurred.

   4. A client who has a history of tuberculosis should be isolated when admitted with a respiratory infection. Even after the disease is arrested, the tuberculosis organism is apt to remain walled off in the person's lungs and may activate when the person is under extreme stress or has a respiratory infection. The person should be isolated until sputum cultures prove that tuberculosis has not recurred.

#76. 3. Assisting with ADLs is an appropriate activity for the nursing assistant. Pl Sa/2 1
 1. A nursing assistant may take the vital signs, but the nurse is responsible for evaluating them.
 2. Monitoring tube feedings is the responsibility of the nurse.
 4. The discussion of discharge instructions is the responsibility of the nurse.

#77. 4. The nurse should respect the client's dignity and self-esteem. Allowing the client to manage his own care as much as possible will promote self-esteem. Pl Ps/5 1
 1. The nurse should encourage the client to adjust the prosthesis as this is a task he must learn to do by himself.
 2. There is no data to suggest the client needs a cane or a walker.
 3. There is no data to suggest the client is at risk for falls.

#78. 4. Seizures can be life-threatening and are the most dangerous of the symptoms. Dc Ps/6 1
 1. Nausea and vomiting are unpleasant but are not life-threatening symptoms.
 2. Anxiety is unpleasant but is not life-threatening.
 3. Hallucinations can be frightening but are not life-threatening.

#79. 1. Persons who are addicted to a substance should never use that substance again. Ev Ps/6 2
 2. Persons who are addicted to drugs are not cured. Once they are no longer using the substance they must avoid the substance. If they start to use the substance again, the inability to control the use of the substance returns. This response indicates either a lack of knowledge or denial by the client.
 3. Persons who are addicted to drugs are not cured. Once they are no longer using the substance they must avoid the substance. If they start to use the substance again, the inability to control the use of the substance returns. This response indicates the client lacks understanding of the problem.
 4. The client should be participating in the support group on a regular basis, not just when upset.

#80. 2. The most important long-term goal is for the victim to feel as though she has survived the ordeal and can rebuild her self-esteem. Pl Ps/6 2
 1. A long-term support group is helpful but is not the most important long-term goal for this client.
 3. Pointing out her behavior is not helpful to the victim. She needs to rebuild her life.
 4. Blaming the abuser serves no useful purpose. The victim needs to rebuild her life.

#81. 4. The nurse is responsible for assigning and supervising the tasks assigned to the nursing assistant. Im Sa/1 1
 1. Personnel should not be allowed to use equipment if they have not been instructed in how to use it.
 2. The problem is the nursing assistant does not know how to use the new thermometer. The nurse should instruct the staff member on how to use the equipment. There is no data to suggest the need for the temperature is so immediate that another person must be assigned to the task.
 3. Nursing assistants are not responsible for teaching other nursing assistants. Teaching the nursing assistant is the nurse's responsibility.

#82. 2. The code takes priority. The need is immediate. Most medications can safely be administered slightly late. Pl Sa/1 1
 1. The nursing assistant is not qualified or licensed to give medications. Medications should only be administered by the person who prepared them.
 3. The code takes priority over administering medications.

ANSWER	RATIONALE	NP	CN	SA

4. Giving medicatons is not a function of the nursing assistant. Because this is not a task that the nursing assistant can do, it is not possible for the nursing assistant to have been checked off on this procedure.

#83. 1. The nurse should initially assess the client. — Im — Ps/5 — 1

2. This response minimizes the client's feelings and does not help the nurse to determine what the client's problem is.

3. The best initial response is for the nurse to assess the client and allow her to express her feelings.

4. Avoiding the client is not the best initial response. The nurse should initially determine the nature of the client's concerns.

#84. 2. This open-ended comment will allow the client to express thoughts and fears. — Im — Ps/5 — 2

1. This stereotypical response minimizes the fears of the client.

3. Calling the clergyman is not the best initial response. The nurse should explore the client's concerns and then call the clergyman if appropriate for this client.

4. False reassurance is not helpful to the client.

#85. 4. Self-mutilation is a cry for help and needs to be addressed immediately because it shows ineffective coping strategies. — Dc — Ps/5 — 2

1. Anxiety is not as serious a concern as self-mutilation.

2. A dysfunctional family unit is of concern but not as serious a concern as self-mutilation.

3. Social isolation is a cause of concern but not as serious a concern as self-mutilation.

#86. 2. The client may be able to process simple instructions. Too much information is likely to confuse the client further. — Pl — Ps/5 — 1

1. Offering several choices is likely to further confuse the client.

3. The client has short-term memory loss. Giving details of care is likely to cause further confusion.

4. The client may not be able to interpret the written word.

#87. 4. The wound is considered the center of the sterile field. The nurse must wear sterile gloves whenever in contact with the area. — Im — Sa/2 — 1

1. Pouring sterile solution directly into a sterile container is not appropriate. The nurse should pour some solution out of the container first to eliminate bacteria on the lip of the container.

2. There is no need to wear sterile gloves when removing a dressing. The nurse should wear clean gloves to protect the nurse.

3. Wearing sterile gloves to open sterile dressings contaminates the sterile gloves when the unopened packages are touched.

#88. 1. A visually impaired client may have difficulty seeing the rugs and fall. — Pl — Sa/2 — 1

2. Handrails are nice to have, but are not particularly indicated because the client is visually impaired.

3. There is no indication the client is at risk for a fall from the bed.

4. Having a bell is not especially helpful for the visually impaired. They may have difficulty locating the bell.

#89. 2. Sitting on the edge of the bed for a few minutes gives time for the body to adapt to an upright position. This decreases dizziness and reduces the chance the client will fall. — Pl — Sa/2 — 1

1. Wearing slippers when getting out of bed will not help the dizziness. Wearing slippers may be appropriate but is not related to the client's complaint of dizziness when getting up.

3. The client complained of dizziness when getting out of bed in the morning. The most likely problem is orthostatic hypotension. Drinking juice will not help this problem. Drinking juice might be appropriate if the client had low blood sugar.

4. The client complained of dizziness when getting out of bed in the morning. The data does not indicate the client is dizzy before getting up. Staying in bed is not likely to solve the problem and will create additional problems.

#90. 2. Spending time with the client will give the nurse the opportunity to listen to concerns and find the source of the client's anger. — Im — Ps/5 — 1

    1. Chemically restraining the client will not help to identify the problem. Use of chemical restraints is not the first choice.

    3. Having someone stay with the client might be helpful, but it does not help the nurse find out what is bothering the client.

    4. Wrist restraints should only be applied when the client is in danger of hurting himself or others. There is no data to suggest that wrist restraints are necessary. Applying restraints is likely to make the client more upset and angry.

#91. 1. This is a coping strategy on the part of the client. — Dc — Ps/5 — 2

    2. The behavior described is a coping strategy, not a defense mechanism.

    3. The behavior described is a coping strategy. There is no data to suggest what the client is thinking when adopting this coping strategy.

    4. The behavior described is a conscious choice and does not indicate regression—adopting behaviors more appropriate for an earlier age.

#92. 2. The nurse should work with the client to set goals. Sometimes the goals have to be changed or adapted to the progress the client is making. — Ev — Sa/1 — 1

    1. Transferring the client to another caregiver does not solve the problem. There is no data to suggest that the nurse is not giving adequate care.

    3. A longer stay may not be the solution to the problem. The nurse should involve the client in the care plan.

    4. Role-playing the current care plan is not likely to be an effective solution to the problem.

#93. 2. Loss of tooth enamel is an objective sign of bulimia. — Dc — Ps/6 — 1

    1. Low self-esteem is a subjective symptom often associated with bulimia.

    3. Feeling loss of control is a subjective symptom often associated with bulimia.

    4. Feeling social inadequacy is a subjective symptom often associated with bulimia.

#94. 1. The nurse should first provide for the client's safety. — Pl — Ps/6 — 2

    2. Referral to a long-term support group is appropriate, but is not the initial priority. Safety is the initial priority.

    3. Making an appointment with a counselor is appropriate, but is not the initial priority. Safety is the first priority.

    4. Confronting the abuser is dangerous and not an appropriate action.

#95. 4. An isolation gown is needed because the nurse is in direct contact with the client. — Im — Sa/2 — 1

    1. A face mask is indicated for respiratory conditions.

    2. Sterile gloves are not needed for contact isolation. Sterile gloves are used when dealing with open wounds to protect the client from the nurse.

    3. An isolation cap is not needed for contact isolation.

#96. 4. Sterile gloves must be worn during the dressing change. — Im — Sa/2 — 1

    1. Touching the corners of the dressing with clean gloves is a violation of sterile technique and introduces organisms. Sterile gloves should be worn when touching the dressing.

    2. Talking over a sterile field is not appropriate. Bacteria may enter the wound.

    3. Irrigating the wound might be done if ordered by the physician. There is no data in this question to indicate such an order.

#97. 2. The nurse is teaching the client how to use the call light. Problems with ambulation are not relevant. — Dc — Sa/2 — 1

    1. The nurse should assess the client's ability to see the call light.

3. The nurse should assess the client's orientation status as this will help determine the client's ability to learn.

4. The client should be able to understand the instructions.

#98. 1. Hair habors bacteria, which can cause infections.   Im   Sa/2   1

2. There is some truth to this answer. However, the best response is the primary reason for removing hair, which is the removal of a source of bacteria.

3. Removing hair does not disinfect the skin.

4. There is some truth to this answer. However, this in not the best answer because it is not the major reason for removing hair.

#99. 2. The nurse should initially respond with empathy and recognition of the client's feelings. The client's anger is probably stemming from the possible diagnosis and the tests, not the nurse's actions. An empathetic response will help to establish rapport with the client and is appropriate initially.   Im   Ps/5   2

1. The nurse should not initially respond with a defensive reaction. This is likely to escalate the situation. The nurse should recognize that the client's anger is most likely the result of the possible diagnosis and the tests, not the nurse's behavior.

3. Getting the supervisor is not the best initial response. The nurse should recognize that the client's anger is most likely a result of the possible diagnosis and the tests, not the nurse's behavior.

4. Trying to change the client's behavior is not the best initial response. The nurse should recognize that this client's anger is most likely related to the possible diagnosis and the tests, not the nurse's behavior. The client's behavior is not likely to be a deliberate attempt to put the nurse down.

#100. 3. Tremors (shaking) and disorientation are suggestive of alcohol withdrawal. Consuming eight or nine beers daily is evidence the client is an alcoholic. Suddenly stopping alcohol intake will cause withdrawal symptoms.   Dc   Ps/6   1

1. If the client had consumed alcohol since surgery he would not be having symptoms of withdrawal. Shaking and disorientation are symptoms of withdrawal.

2. The symptoms of shaking and disorientation are suggestive of withdrawal, not a reaction to narcotic analgesics.

3. The symptoms of shaking and disorientation are consistent with withdrawal. It may be possible that shaking and disorientation could be due to pain. However, given the history of heavy alcohol abuse, the nurse should consider this option.

Practice Test Five

1. An infant had a repair of a myelomeningocele two days ago. Which assessment is most important to detect a problem commonly seen following myelomeningocele repair?
   1. Bowel sounds
   2. Neuro checks
   3. Blood pressure in all four extremities
   4. Head circumference

2. The mother of a two-year-old tells the nurse she is embarrassed when her child plays with other children because he does not share his toys or even interact with the other children. The nurse's response to the mother is based on the knowledge that a two-year-old usually engages in which type of play?
   1. Solitary
   2. Parallel
   3. Cooperative
   4. Collaborative

3. The parents of a child with Tetralogy of Fallot ask the nurse why it is called a cyanotic heart defect. The nurse responds that it is called a cyanotic heart defect because
   1. It has four separate defects.
   2. It involves left-to-right shunting.
   3. It involves right-to-left shunting.
   4. Blood flow to the lungs is poor.

4. A mother brings her one-month-old son to the clinic for a well-baby visit. The child has a moderately severe hypospadias that was seen by a urologist in the newborn nursery. The mother is upset that the doctors would not circumcise her son before he was discharged. What information should the nurse include when responding to the mother?
   1. The foreskin should not be removed, as it will be used in the repair of the hypospadias.
   2. The child's condition did not allow for elective surgery. It will be done at a later date when he is stronger.
   3. Circumcision is a surgical procedure. Because he will have surgery in the near future, it will be done at the same time to avoid two surgeries close together.
   4. The procedure was not done because circumcision is medically unnecessary, not because he has a hypospadias.

5. An eight-year-old is admitted to the hospital with pneumonia. The child has had frequent respiratory infections. A chloride sweat test is ordered. The nurse knows the reason for this test is to rule out which condition?
   1. Pernicious anemia
   2. Diabetes insipidus
   3. Cystic fibrosis
   4. Glomerulonephritis

6. Written instructions to pregnant women include instructions to perform Kegel's exercises. One of the women asks the nurse why these exercises are important. The nurse should reply that the purpose of these exercises is to
   1. Increase circulation to the uterus.
   2. Strengthen the muscles of the pelvic floor.
   3. Prepare the breasts for nursing.
   4. Condition the pregnant woman for the "work" of childbirth.

7. A 26-year-old woman with a history of heart disease is admitted in labor. She has been on bed rest for four months to prevent dyspnea. During labor this client is likely to receive which of the following?
   1. Extra intravenous fluid to expand her blood volume
   2. General anesthesia
   3. Instruction to push by holding her breath and bearing down
   4. Epidural anesthesia

8. All of the following women are seen in the physician's office. Which is at greatest risk for pre-term labor?
   1. A primigravida who has gained 30 pounds during her pregnancy
   2. A 35-year-old carrying a small baby
   3. A 21-year-old pregnant with twins
   4. A 40-year-old who has four other children

9. A new mother asks the nurse when the baby's umbilical cord will fall off. The nurse replies that it usually takes how many days to detach?
   1. 1–2 days
   2. 3–5 days
   3. 7–10 days
   4. 15–20 days

10. A new mother is two days postpartum, is breastfeeding her infant, and now is preparing for discharge. She states that for contraception she is going to use her diaphragm, which she still has. The nurse's response should be based on which information?
    1. Diaphragms need to be refitted after the birth of a baby.
    2. As long as the diaphragm is in good shape, the client can continue to use it.
    3. Diaphragms are not good contraceptives for postpartal women.
    4. Since the client is breastfeeding, she will not need her diaphragm for four to six months.

11. A laboring woman has been pushing for one hour and is not making progress. The nurse knows that which of the following could

hinder the descent of the fetus in the second stage of labor?
1. A full bladder
2. Paracervical block given during the first stage of labo.
3. Mother placed in a side-lying position
4. Fetus in LOA (left occiput anterior) position

12. The nurse is providing home care to a man who had a transphenoidal hypophysectomy. Which behavior by the client indicates a need for more teaching?
1. He bends over to tie his shoes.
2. He tells the nurse he takes a lot of pills every day.
3. He ambulates daily.
4. He tells the nurse he has ordered a medical identification bracelet.

13. An adult has been diagnosed with Bell's palsy and asks what causes it. The nurse knows that which of the following is correct?
1. Bell's palsy is caused by the chickenpox virus.
2. The cause is unknown.
3. Bell's palsy usually follows a cold or influenza.
4. Trauma to the area brings on the symptoms.

14. Magnetic resonance imaging has been ordered for a client. Which factor should the nurse report to the physician?
1. The client states she had an allergic reaction to iodine.
2. The client has a pacemaker.
3. The client wears a hearing aid.
4. The client takes digoxin.

15. A woman is admitted with Hodgkin's disease. Which does the nurse expect the client to report?
1. Swollen lymph nodes
2. A painful rash
3. Stomach pain
4. Joint pain

16. A client who has congestive heart failure is being admitted. How should the nurse position this client?
1. Supine
2. Sim's
3. Semi-Fowler's
4. Side-lying

17. Which assessment is most essential before administering digoxin to an adult?
1. Ask the client if he has chest pain.
2. Take an apical pulse.
3. Take the client's blood pressure.
4. Ask the client if he is short of breath.

18. The LPN/LVN is caring for an adult who has pneumonia. The nurse should instruct the nursing assistant to report which information immediately?
1. Restlessness
2. Pink-colored skin

3. Nonproductive cough
4. Dry mouth

19. A low-sodium, high-potassium diet is ordered for a client. Which food selection made by the client indicates understanding of the prescribed diet?
1. Orange juice, baked chicken, and a cucumber and tomato salad
2. Milk, roast beef, and spinach salad
3. Iced tea, fish sandwich, and mixed vegetables
4. Cola, fried shrimp, and coleslaw

20. The nurse is teaching unlicensed personnel about preventing the spread of disease in the health care environment. The nurse knows the personnel understand when they state that which is the most important way to prevent the spread of disease?
1. Isolating infected clients
2. Consistently washing hands
3. Wearing a gown when there is a client with a questionable disease
4. Wearing gloves whenever giving care

21. The LPN/LVN is to perform a sterile procedure. Which action will maintain a sterile field?
1. Keeping the sterile field within the line of vision
2. Opening sterile packages with sterile gloves
3. Talking to others over the sterile field
4. Handing the physician medicine over the sterile field

22. A 56-year-old man is visiting the doctor for the first time in seven years for treatment for an infected finger. The office nurse wants him to make an appointment for a physical. The nurse knows he does not understand the importance of a physical when he makes which statement?
1. "I know my blood sugar and weight should be monitored."
2. "I am healthy. If I wasn't, I'd have some problems."
3. "I don't smoke and I exercise daily."
4. "I understand checking my blood pressure is important."

23. The nurse is preparing a client for a KUB (kidney-ureter-bladder x-ray). What is included in the preparation?
1. Keeping the client NPO
2. Explaining the procedure
3. Catheterizing the client
4. Administering an enema

24. The nurse is caring for a client who has a cervical radioactive implant. Which action is not appropriate for the nurse when caring for this client?
1. Post a radioactive symbol on the client's chart and the door to the room.
2. Put on gloves to remove any radioactive implant that may have come out.

3. Wash hands with soap and water after caring for the client.
4. Limit the amount of time with the client.

25. The nurse is preparing a client environment that will reduce the chance of falls. Which action is appropriate?
    1. Keep the side rail down on the side the client gets out of bed.
    2. Keep the lights down since glare bothers some clients.
    3. Call housekeeping to clean up the spilled water.
    4. Make sure that a path is cleared to assist the client when walking.

26. A nurse's aide who had a tuberculosis test planted two days ago has a reddened area 15-mm in diameter. The aide asks the nurse what this means. The nurse understands that the test result is
    1. positive, indicating the aide has been exposed to tuberculosis.
    2. positive, indicating the aide has active tuberculosis.
    3. a false negative and must be repeated.
    4. negative; redness without induration is of no significance.

27. A woman who has emphysema is on continuous oxygen therapy. She appears anxious and short of breath. Her husband increases the oxygen flow to 6 liters/min. The nurse knows this action is most likely to
    1. make breathing easier.
    2. decrease her blood oxygen levels.
    3. have no impact on blood oxygen levels.
    4. cause her to stop breathing.

28. An adult who is waiting for a cardiac catheterization is joking with the staff. The nurse understands that this behavior is most likely
    1. a coping mechanism for the client.
    2. an inappropriate behavior for a serious procedure.
    3. a defense mechanism of denial.
    4. a defense mechanism of rationalization.

29. An adult had an open cholecystectomy and has an open wound. The client refuses to look at the area during the dressing change. What is the most likely reason for this behavior?
    1. Denial of surgery.
    2. Change in body image.
    3. The client fears becoming nauseated at the sight of the wound.
    4. The client does not like the sight of blood.

30. The nurse is supervising an unlicensed person who is giving oral care to an unconscious client. Which observation indicates that the unlicensed person needs further instruction? The client
    1. is in a lateral position with the head turned to the side during oral care.
    2. is positioned in high-Fowler's position.
    3. has a towel placed under the chin.

4. remains in the lateral position for 30 minutes after oral care.

31. Which activity should not be assigned to an unlicensed person?
    1. Record all oral intake.
    2. Measure all output.
    3. Record output on appropriate graphs.
    4. Complete the 24-hour I & O record.

32. The nurse observes a client using a walker. Which observation indicates the client needs more instruction?
    1. The client uses the walker to pull herself out of a chair.
    2. The client moves the walker forward, then takes a step.
    3. The client complains the walker is not waist-high.
    4. The client sometimes does not use the walker.

33. A hearing-impaired client is becoming withdrawn and depressed. He reports that even with a hearing aid he is having increased difficulty hearing. Which suggestion is least likely to be helpful?
    1. Get a hearing guide dog.
    2. Join a social club.
    3. Get a telephone TDD.
    4. Get a closed-caption TV.

34. An adult is taking phenazopyridine hydrochloride (Pyridium) 200 mg PO TID after meals. Which comment by the client indicates a lack of understanding about the medication?
    1. "If I take my medications after meals I avoid upsetting my stomach."
    2. "I am concerned that my urine is bright orange."
    3. "I do not have as great an urge to urinate since I have been on Pyridium."
    4. "I have to let my doctor know if my skin or eyes turn yellow."

35. An adult who is hospitalized with congestive heart failure is receiving an intravenous infusion. The nurse is checking the IV. Which of the following is of greatest concern to the nurse?
    1. The insertion site
    2. The volume infused
    3. The frequency with which the tubing is changed
    4. The presence of a flashback

36. The nurse is working to prevent falls in a restraint-free environment. Which of the following is inappropriate for the nurse to delegate to assistive personnel?
    1. Making sure the bed is in low position
    2. Making sure the bedside table is within reach of the client
    3. Assessing the safety needs of the client
    4. Monitoring client behavior for potential falls

37. Prior to administering a feeding, the nurse checks for placement of a feeding tube. What is the best way to do this?
    1. Check for residual.
    2. Measure the pH of aspirated gastrointestinal fluid.
    3. Inject 10–20 ml of air while auscultating over the epigastric area.
    4. Ask the client to talk or hum.
38. The nurse has assigned a nursing assistant to give the client a bath. Which observation reported by the nursing assistant requires immediate attention by the nurse?
    1. A red area on the back that disappears after it is massaged.
    2. A red area on the hip that does not go away after the area is massaged.
    3. The client's insistence on doing most of the bath.
    4. The indwelling urethral catheter is draining clear, amber urine.
39. The nurse is evaluating how a client who has a halo brace is reacting to this change in his body image. Which statement by the client indicates a need for additional support in adjusting to the brace?
    1. "I shall avoid going out in public since I may bump into people."
    2. "I don't mind that people look at me."
    3. "I told my grandchildren that this looks like a space helmet."
    4. "I like to sleep in the reclining chair that we have."
40. A throat culture is ordered for an adult who has a sore throat. The nurse asks the client if he has taken any medications to treat himself. Which medication, if reported by the client, would be of greatest concern to the nurse?
    1. Aspirin
    2. A throat lozenge
    3. Acetaminophen
    4. An antibiotic
41. The nurse is preparing to give an adult a subcutaneous injection of heparin. What should the nurse check prior to giving the medication?
    1. International Normalized Ratio (INR)
    2. Bleeding time
    3. Prothrombin time
    4. Partial thromboplastin time
42. A young woman has routine blood work done at her prenatal appointment. The results indicate she has a hemoglobin of 10 gm/dl. The nurse explains to her that this result is
    1. high.
    2. insignificant.
    3. low.
    4. normal.
43. The nurse is caring for a client who has congestive heart failure. Which finding indicates her condition is getting worse?
    1. An increase in urine output

2. A decrease in blood pressure
    3. A decrease in heart rate
    4. Warm, moist skin
44. A seventy-two-year-old woman is being treated for pneumonia. Physician's orders include an antibiotic, oxygen PRN for O₂ saturation less than 90, pulse oximetry every 4 hours. The nurse obtains a pulse oximetry reading of 82% on room air. What is the best action for the nurse to take?
    1. Report the finding to the physician.
    2. Report the finding to the registered nurse to get instructions.
    3. Start supplemental oxygen.
    4. Start oxygen and repeat the pulse oximetry in 20 minutes.
45. A fourteen-year-old is going home with a permanent tracheostomy. Which comment by the child's parent indicates to the nurse that the parent needs more instruction?
    1. "I need to ask the doctor how many times a day I can suction my child."
    2. "I will suction if my child cannot effectively cough up sputum."
    3. "I know my child will not need the same amount of suctioning every day."
    4. "I know I should only suction my child if it is really necessary."
46. The nurse is working on a plan to assist an abused client back into the work situation. Which will most likely be most helpful in decreasing the trauma for the client?
    1. Support from significant others.
    2. Support from a counselor.
    3. Support from friends.
    4. Support from coworkers.
47. A ten-year-old child is admitted to the hospital with injuries. Which finding most suggests that additional assessment for child abuse is indicated?
    1. The child asks to have friends visit.
    2. The child asks to have a teacher bring in homework.
    3. The child's parents state that they need to spend some time with the child's siblings.
    4. The child's parents will not leave the child alone while in the hospital.
48. The nurse is to move a client up in bed without any help. Where should the nurse place the client's pillow?
    1. At the bottom of the bed
    2. On the bedside stand
    3. At the head of the bed
    4. Under the client's head
49. The nurse's neighbor complains to the nurse that he feels tired all the time. Which comment suggests to the nurse that the man may have a serious sleep disorder?
    1. "My wife complains because I snore off and on all night."
    2. "I like to nap in the afternoon."
    3. "I wake up early every morning."

4. "My muscles seem to jerk as I fall asleep."

50. A mentally retarded, nonverbal, ambulatory client is found sitting on the floor unable to get up. The LPN/LVN notes the client appears to be in great pain and his right leg is out of alignment. What is the most important action for the nurse to take as the client is readied for ambulance transport?
   1. Give the client pain medication.
   2. Immobilize the leg.
   3. Gather any medical records that need to accompany the client.
   4. Complete the incident report and other documentation.

51. The nurse enters an adult's room to premedicate for surgery. The client says, "You know, nurse, that form I signed said something about a nephrectomy. What does that mean?" How should the nurse respond initially?
   1. "What did your surgeon explain to you about your operation?"
   2. "Don't worry about the technical terms. We'll take good care of you."
   3. "I think you're just nervous about the surgery. This injection will make you feel calmer."
   4. "It is a kidney operation."

52. An insulin-dependent diabetic is admitted with a blood sugar of 415 mg/dL. His wife states, "He always follows his diabetic diet religiously and administers his insulin using a sliding scale twice a day." Upon reviewing his chart, the nurse notes that the client has been hospitalized four times during the past three months for a medical diagnosis of hyperglycemia secondary to noncompliance with medical regimen. When questioned, he says, "It's a little too complicated to keep track of when I need to eat, and when I need to check my blood and take my medicine." Which nursing diagnosis is most appropriate?
   1. Impaired adjustment
   2. Impaired home maintenance
   3. Ineffective therapeutic regimen management
   4. Noncompliance

53. The nurse who is the primary caregiver for an adult client receives a telephone report from the Microbiology Department that the client's blood culture is positive for gram negative rods. The client is not on antibiotics. What should the nurse do first?
   1. Document the result in the appropriate area of the chart.
   2. Inform the client that we now know what is causing his illness.
   3. Place a call to the physician and document the results of the lab work and the notification of the physician in the nurse's notes.
   4. Place the laboratory report on the client's chart as soon as possible.

54. While giving report at 3:15 in the afternoon, the nurse realizes that she/he forgot to chart the client's physical therapy which occurred at 10:30 A.M. Which is the appropriate action for the nurse to take?
   1. Ask the incoming nurse to record it.
   2. Date and time and entry for 3:15 P.M. "Late entry (date: 10:30 A.M.)" before making the addition.
   3. Do not add the information to the chart. Complete an incident report for the omitted charting and forward it to the risk management department.
   4. Because it is already charted by the physical therapists in their progress notes, the nurse does not need to "double chart" the same information. The nurse does not have to do anything.

55. The nurse notes a client has received a medication by mistake. What should the nurse do?
   1. Notify the physician, complete an incident report and make a separate note, in the nursing documentation, of the error, the client's response, and any treatment received by the client due to the medication error.
   2. Complete an incident report and reference it in the nurse's notes.
   3. Make a note of the error and any treatment the client receives because of the error in the nurse's notes.
   4. Report the error to the nursing supervisor and the client's physician and document any treatment prescribed in the nurse's notes.

56. A newly diagnosed diabetic has worked as a manual laborer all his life. He requires teaching so that he can manage his diabetes after discharge. The nurse has given him booklets designed for clients who need an introduction to diabetes. When the nurse evaluates his learning from the booklets, he says he doesn't have his glasses and couldn't read the booklets. When the nurse offers large-print material, he says his wife usually takes care of things at home, and that you should work with her because she prepares all the meals and keeps track of the medicines for both of them. Which understanding of the client's behavior is most likely correct?
   1. He is in denial about his diagnosis.
   2. He is not willing to take responsibility for his own learning.
   3. He cannot read.
   4. He is too anxious about his new diagnosis to be able to process any new information at this time.

57. The nurse is caring for a preschooler who needs stitches resulting from an injury

received during play in the yard. What would be the most appropriate way to prepare the child for the treatment he will receive?

1. Tell the child the nurse and the doctor will "make things all better."
2. Use dolls and explain through play and simulation what will be done.
3. Explain to the child slowly and precisely the steps that will be taken in his treatment.
4. Tell the child that he will have minimal scarring and that any marks will diminish over time.

58. A 76-year-old man living at the long-term care facility has lost 10 pounds in the last two months. He states that although he has had dentures for two years, they have not felt comfortable for the past three or four months so he rarely uses them at mealtime. The nurse's first priority would be to ask the client's physician to do which of the following?

1. Order a mechanical soft or edentulous diet for the client.
2. Order a dental consult to correct the client's problem.
3. Order a dietary consult to assist the client in making educated food choices.
4. Talk to the client regarding the proper use of dentures.

59. A client who has hypokalemia asks the nurse for dietary advice on what foods would help this problem. What should the nurse tell the client?

1. Eggs and cheese
2. Fruits, especially oranges, bananas, and prunes
3. Green leafy vegetables
4. Breads and cereals

60. The client complains of frequent insomnia affecting her ability to rest well. Which of the following factors or lifestyle choices in her assessment history most likely contribute to her inability to sleep?

1. Having a slight snack at bedtime
2. Heart disease prevention of one baby aspirin each day
3. Reading in bed prior to going to sleep
4. Smoking 1 1/2 packs of filtered cigarettes each day

61. The client is unable to adequately bathe himself because he has dressings on his hands that cannot get wet. What is the most appropriate nursing diagnosis for this assessment finding?

1. Risk for infection
2. Deficient knowledge
3. Pain related to specific illness or disease process
4. Self-care deficit (bathing/hygiene)

62. The nurse has delegated care of a client who is very hard of hearing to an unlicensed person. Which of the following would be the least helpful information to give to the unlicensed person to better facilitate communications with the client?

1. Reduce background noise.
2. Adjust the hearing aid.
3. Anticipate what the client may say and finish the statement for the client.
4. Face the client when speaking to the client.

63. The nurse is assessing a 16-year-old mother for potential child abuse. Which factor is most important when assessing potential for child abuse?

1. Age of the mother
2. Marital status
3. Socioeconomic status
4. Abuse as a child

64. An adult is receiving intermittent tube feedings. When the nurse aspirates and measures the gastric contents, the client's wife asks the nurse what she is doing. What information is most important to include in the response? The procedure is done to

1. test that the tube is working.
2. check the placement of the tube.
3. check for gastric emptying.
4. clear the line.

65. Before giving furosemide (Lasix) to an adult, the nurse checks the laboratory report for the last serum potassium level. Which finding would be of concern to the nurse?

1. 3.2 mEq/L
2. 3.7 mEq/L
3. 4.1 mEq/L
4. 4.9 mEq/L

66. A six-year-old was just diagnosed with pediculosis capitis. Which comment by the mother of the child indicates to the nurse in the physician's office that she does not understand how this condition is spread?

1. "I need to wash all his bedsheets in hot water."
2. "I will call the school nurse and tell her."
3. "I think he got this at our neighbor's house, it's very dirty."
4. "I will tell my son not to wear other children's hats."

67. An 85-year-old woman is hospitalized with a fractured hip. She complains to the LPN/LVN that she feels something is wrong and her chest hurts. The nurse notes the client has tachypnea. What should the nurse do immediately?

1. Administer oxygen.
2. Take vital signs.
3. Elevate the head of the bed.
4. Give aspirin.

68. Joan is at lunch in the hospital cafeteria with a nurse coworker. Joan is very allergic to nuts and always carries her anaphylactic kit with her. Joan tells her coworker that there must have been nuts in something she ate as she is

having increasing difficulty breathing. What should the nurse do immediately?
1. Take her to the hospital emergency room.
2. Administer the medication in her friend's anaphylactic kit.
3. Call the floor for help.
4. Monitor the symptoms.

69. A client who had bowel surgery is to be NPO for several days. The nurse anticipates that the client will have an order for
   1. diet therapy.
   2. enteral nutrition.
   3. parenteral nutrition.
   4. nasogastric tube feedings.

70. A client who has mycoplasma pneumonia needs to go to the radiology department for a chest x-ray. What should the client wear?
   1. A face shield
   2. A surgical mask
   3. An N 95 respirator
   4. Gloves and a gown

71. A new client is admitted with a major abscess on her thigh caused by scratching mosquito bites with dirty hands after digging in her garden. She is on isolation precautions in a private room after surgical debridement. The physician changes her dressings daily. What should the nurse wear when providing care for this client?
   1. An N 95 respirator and gloves
   2. Eye protection and a face mask
   3. Gloves and gown
   4. A gown only

72. The nurse is assisting in the attempt to control bleeding from an artery. What personal protection equipment should be worn?
   1. Gloves only
   2. Gown, gloves, mask, and goggles
   3. Mask and gown
   4. None because time should not be wasted

73. A 63-year-old woman is taking digitalis, baby aspirin, K-Dur, and Lasix daily. She complains of multiple symptoms, which include muscle cramps and facial tics. Physical exam reveals positive Chvostek's and Trousseau's signs, hypotension, and confusion. The nurse suspects she has hypomagnesemia. What else should the nurse expect?
   1. Laboratory tests to reveal high serum calcium and potassium levels.
   2. Laboratory tests to reveal low serum calcium and potassium levels.
   3. Altered acid-base balance, which requires administration of $NaHCO_3$ intravenously in addition to treatment for hypomagnesemia.
   4. To monitor cardiac function since hypomagnesemia often causes bradycardia episodes and altered ECG waves.

74. An adult has experienced significant vomiting and diarrhea for the past 24 hours. Her chloride level is 90 mEq/L. What would the nurse expect to find when interpreting her sodium level?
   1. It would be high.
   2. It is impossible to predict the sodium level with this information.
   3. It would be low.
   4. It would be normal.

75. A post-operative client has an NG tube following bowel surgery. The orders read, "acetaminophen 650 PRN for fever above 101°F." The client has a temperature of 101.4°F. What is the most appropriate nursing action?
   1. Administer the acetaminophen by rectal suppository.
   2. Administer the acetaminophen by elixir through the NG tube and turn suction off for 30 minutes.
   3. Administer the acetaminophen by crushing two tablets, giving it through the NG tube, and turning suction off for 30 minutes.
   4. Call the physician and question the order.

76. The nurse is preparing a client with a severe case of inflamed hemorrhoids for a rectal examination by the physician. What is the best position to place her on the examination table?
   1. Dorsal recumbent
   2. Knee-chest
   3. Sim's
   4. Lithotomy

77. The nurse notes that the client has a pulse deficit. What is the most appropriate action for the nurse?
   1. Document this as a normal finding.
   2. Instruct the client to report to the clinic for a weekly re-evaluation.
   3. Report this finding immediately to the client's physician.
   4. Teach the client how to monitor pulse at home.

78. A post-operative client has pain medication ordered PRN for discomfort. During the first assessment, the nurse notes that the client has not received pain medication all day. His vital signs are within normal limits but he is sweating profusely. He smiles at you while speaking and states that he is not hot but is still experiencing some pain and has been since early this morning. What is the most appropriate nursing action?
   1. Administer the largest dose of pain medication allowed because he has been without it all day and then allow him to rest undisturbed.
   2. Administer the minimum dose of medication and reassess his level of pain 30 minutes after administration.
   3. Hold the pain medication because his vital signs are within normal limits and he is

smiling and showing no evidence of being in pain.
4. Encourage the client to continue to do without pain medication so he won't become addicted to the opioid.

79. A woman is scheduled for a biopsy and possible mastectomy in the morning. She is crying and says, "I am so upset because I watched my mother die from ovarian cancer." What is the most appropriate nursing diagnosis?
1. Fear
2. Anxiety
3. Ineffective family coping
4. Spiritual distress

80. Which diagnosis for the client with tuberculosis would have the greatest impact on public health?
1. Ineffective breathing pattern
2. Deficient knowledge
3. Fatigue
4. Ineffective therapeutic regimen management

81. A client comes to the emergency room with complaints of "numbness, tingling, and coldness" of her left leg. She is able to walk. You note that the skin appears pale and is cool to the touch. What should the nurse do first?
1. Ask if she had had a similar condition in her arms or the other leg.
2. Notify the physician immediately.
3. Obtain a detailed nursing health history.
4. Palpate and record the femoral, popliteal, posterior tibial, and dorsalis pedis pulses in the affected leg.

82. The nurse has taken vital signs of a 95-year-old client: oral temperature 98.6°F; pulse 84 with a regular irregularity; respirations 18 and blood pressure 140/86. Which nursing assessment(s) should be done first to obtain more data?
1. Apical pulse for one minute
2. Carotid pulse and temperature
3. Full respiratory system assessment
4. Positional blood pressure readings

83. An adult has returned to the nursing care unit following abdominal surgery. She has an order for meperidine IM prn for severe pain or acetaminophen #3 PO prn for mild to moderate pain. You ask the client if she is experiencing pain now and she states, "Yes, I am." What is the most appropriate initial action for the nurse?
1. Administer the meperidine since she is less than 24 hours post-op.
2. Administer the acetaminophen #3 because meperidine can be given if the acetaminophen doesn't relieve the pain.
3. Assess the client further as to the location and degree of pain using a pain scale.

4. Reposition the client and help her perform some relaxation exercises to reduce her reliance on opioids.

84. The nurse is admitting an adult woman to the ambulatory surgery unit at 6:30 A.M. The assessment reveals that her blood pressure is elevated, her pulse and respirations are rapid, she is diaphoretic, and she has dilated pupils. The nurse attempts to reinforce her pre-operative teaching for today's surgery, but the woman cannot restate anything about her previous instructions. She is wringing her hands and seems to be on the verge of tears. What is the most appropriate initial nursing action?
1. Administer her prescribed pre-operative medication now.
2. Ask her, "How are you feeling right now?"
3. Repeat all her pre-operative instructions slowly.
4. Notify her surgeon of the client's emotional status.

85. The client states, "My discharge plan leaves me with a lot to do. I don't think I can do it. I'm never good at doing things." The nurse knows the client lacks
1. Maturation.
2. Organization.
3. Readiness to learn.
4. Self-efficacy.

86. The nurse is caring for an older client who insists on having a "hot toddy" laced with liquor at bedtime to help her sleep. How should the nurse respond in order to give culturally sensitive and appropriate care?
1. "Is that something you learned from a relative or a friend?"
2. "No one your age should be drinking at bedtime."
3. "That is an old wive's tale. The doctor can prescribe a sleep aid if you need one."
4. "We don't allow alcohol in the hospital."

87. A 55-year-old woman is recovering from a bowel resection. She is receiving epidural analgesia. She lived by herself right up until admission and has no cognitive defects. All of the following interventions will reduce the risk of client falls. Which would be most appropriate for this client?
1. Apply a vest restraint around her so she cannot get out of bed.
2. Make sure someone is always present in her room to prevent her from getting out of bed.
3. Keep the bed in low position and the call bell within her reach.
4. Rearrange the room assignments so that she is in a room directly across from the nurse's station.

88. A nurse prepared the 9:00 A.M. medications for his clients and then was called off the unit briefly before he was able to administer them.

Who may administer the medications to the clients now?
1. Any licensed nurse assigned to the unit and familiar with the clients
2. A pharmacy technician certified to administer medications
3. The nurse who prepared them
4. The nurse manager of the unit

89. In the past twelve-month period, a man has been arrested twice for driving while intoxicated. He is able to perform his activities of daily living without the use of alcohol and restricts his drinking to weekends. This client meets the criteria for which of the following?
    1. Alcohol withdrawal syndrome
    2. Bad judgment syndrome
    3. Substance abuse
    4. Substance dependence

90. A client with a knee injury is scheduled for a MRI examination. The nurse explains the test to the client. Which finding in the client would make the client ineligible for this type of exam?
    1. Presence of a metal plate in the leg from an old fracture
    2. Presence of a ceramic artificial hip
    3. A history of asthma attacks
    4. Allergy to injected dye

91. Which of these clients is at greatest risk for the complications associated with osteoporosis?
    1. A 65-year-old Asian-American man who is sedentary, has a low calcium intake, and takes corticosteroids for chronic obstructive pulmonary disease
    2. A 22-year-old woman with anorexia nervosa who is not having menstrual periods
    3. A 73-year-old postmenopausal woman who has limited mobility due to rheumatoid arthritis, for which she takes corticosteroids, and who drinks a bottle of wine by herself each evening
    4. A 70-year-old woman who takes estrogen therapy, was very athletic in her youth playing tennis and golf, and takes anticonvulsant therapy as a result of a head injury suffered in an auto accident three years ago

92. An adult admitted for surgery also is diagnosed with obsessive-compulsive disorder. The client spends most of her time in the bathroom washing her hands. The client is scheduled for surgery at 8 A.M. and is to be premedicated at 7 A.M. Which nursing action will be most appropriate?
    1. Inform the client at 6:30 A.M. that she will soon be medicated and have to stay in bed after that.

2. When medicating the client, explain to her that she will not be able to get up after receiving the medication.
3. After medicating the client, place a wash basin and wash cloth at the bedside for her use.
4. After medicating the client, assist her in washing her hands at the bedside.

93. A 43-year-old woman with lupus erythematosus expresses frustration about the unpredictable course of her illness and the change in her physical appearance. Which nursing intervention would be most appropriate?
    1. Explore with her the affect the lupus has on her occupation, leisure activities, and personal relationships.
    2. Explain to her that things could be worse, and that she could have a more serious illness, such as terminal cancer, to help her put her situation into perspective.
    3. Help the client reduce conflicts in her personal life.
    4. Teach her what can be expected as the disease progresses.

94. A child's burn is debrided each day with hydrotherapy to remove the eschar. The child's parents ask why this immersion is necessary. What is the most appropriate response for the nurse to make?
    1. "By removing the scab or crusting daily in the special bath, we help prevent infection and then the healthy tissue may be covered by skin grafts."
    2. "By submersion in a whirlpool bath, we can better exercise her limbs to prevent contractures."
    3. "This is a cleansing bath given so that fresh dressings may be applied to the burn areas."
    4. "We decrease her chance of infection by immersion in antibiotic solutions with each debriding bath."

95. The nurse is caring for a client who was admitted for treatment of schizoaffective disorder with visual hallucinations. He tells the nurse that he sees extraterrestrials that are coming to get him. What is the best nursing response?
    1. "You know that extraterrestrials are make-believe."
    2. Call his physician and report this visual hallucination.
    3. Ignore his comment and change the subject.
    4. "You think someone is coming after you?"

96. An adult is almost ready for discharge. She has a complicated care regimen to follow. When conducting client teaching, the nurse notes that the client cannot recall basic information that was discussed the day before. The client also appears distracted.

When asked if she is feeling comfortable about leaving the hospital, she states, "There's just too much to learn. I know I'm going to get home and mess something up." The nurse realizes that the client may be experiencing
1. mild anxiety.
2. moderate anxiety.
3. severe anxiety.
4. panic anxiety.

97. The family of an 88-year-old woman who was admitted with severe dehydration says to the nurse, "Why don't you just tie down her arms so she won't try to get out her IV?" What is the best response for the nurse to make?
1. Ask the physician for an order to restrain the woman.
2. Explain to the family that restraints are not allowed in the hospital unless the doctor orders them.
3. Assess the client's mental status and safety needs.
4. Tell the family that they can restrain the client, but the nurse cannot.

98. An adult client is to have a portable chest x-ray in his room. The client's wife and pregnant daughter are visiting. Which action is essential for the nurse?
1. Ask the pregnant daughter to leave the room and have the wife assist in holding the client.
2. Have the client wear a lead apron over his chest and abdomen.

3. Close the door to the room securely during the x-ray.
4. Ask the wife and daughter to leave the room.

99. The LPN/LVN is providing home care to an elderly widow who has senile dementia. The woman tells the nurse that her daughter hits her and tells her to shut up. The nurse notes one ecchymotic area on the client's right forearm. The daughter seems attentive to the woman when the nurse is present. What action should the nurse take?
1. Immediately call the police.
2. Ask the daughter why she abuses her mother.
3. Ask the physician to order long bone x-rays.
4. Report the woman's remarks and the nurse's findings to the nursing supervisor.

100. A nurse from the float pool is giving medications on a pediatric unit and is to give medications to a two-year-old in room 534, bed B. The child in that room does not have an identification band. What is the best action for the nurse to take?
1. Ask the child what his name is?
2. Give the medication to the child in room 534, bed B.
3. Refuse to give the medication.
4. Ask the adults beside the bed the name of the child in that bed.

Answers and Rationales for Practice Test Five

Answer		Rationale	NP	CN	SA
#1.	4.	**Infants who have had a myelomeningocele repair frequently develop hydrocephalus following the surgery. Increased head circumference is an indication of hydrocephalus.**	Dc	Ph/9	4
	1.	Assessment of bowel sounds is a routine post-operative nursing measure, but it is not related to a common problem seen in these infants.			
	2.	Neuro checks are not a routine post-operative nursing care measure.			
	3.	Blood pressure in all four extremities would be done for infants suspected of having cardiac disease, not surgical repair of myelomeningocele.			
#2.	2.	**A two-year-old usually engages in parallel play. They like to be around others and play the same thing, but do not interact and do not share.**	Im	He/3	4
	1.	Solitary play is characteristic of an infant.			
	3.	Cooperative play is characteristic of a preschool child.			
	4.	Collaborative play is characteristic of preschool and school-age children.			
#3.	3.	**The right side of the heart carries unoxygenated blood. When it passes through defects to the left side of the heart, poorly oxygenated blood is mixed with well-oxygenated blood and gives the cyanotic appearance.**	Im	Ph/10	1

1. Tetralogy of Fallot does have four separate defects: pulmonic valve stenosis, right ventricular hypertrophy, ventricular septal defect, and overriding aorta. However, this does not answer the question, which was why it is called a cyanotic heart defect.

2. Left-to-right shunting takes blood that is in the left side of the heart and has been oxygenated to the right side of the heart and through the lungs again. There is no unoxygenated blood in the systemic circulation and no cause for cyanosis.

4. This is true in Tetralogy of Fallot because of the pulmonic valve stenosis. However, this response does not answer the question. This is not the reason it is called a cyanotic heart defect.

#4. 1. **The extra tissue in the foreskin is used to help repair the hypospadias.**   Im   Ph/9   4

2. This statement is not true. Hypospadias does not put the child in a weakened condition. The foreskin is not removed because it is used in the repair of the hypospadias.

3. This statement is not true. The foreskin is not removed because it is used in the repair of the hypospadias.

4. It is true that circumcision is not medically necessary. However, this is not the reason that the child was not circumcised. The foreskin is not removed because it is used in the repair of the hypospadias.

#5. 3. **The sweat test is a diagnostic for cystic fibrosis. In cystic fibrosis there is a salty taste to the sweat and a high concentration of NaCl. Children with cystic fibrosis usually have frequent respiratory infections as well as malabsorption of nutrients and failure to thrive.**   Dc   Ph/9   4

1. Pernicious anemia is unrelated to the history of respiratory infections and a sweat test.

2. Diabetes insipidus is unrelated to the history of respiratory infections and a sweat test.

4. Glomerulonephritis is unrelated to the history of respiratory infections and a sweat test.

#6. 2. **Kegel's exercises are the tightening and relaxing of the pubococcygeus muscle, which improves the strength of the pelvic floor. It may help prevent cystocele and rectocele.**   Im   He/3   3

1. Kegel's exercises are unrelated to the uterus. They are the tightening and relaxing of the pubococcygeus muscle, which improves the strength of the pelvic floor.

3. Kegel's exercises are unrelated to the breasts. They are the tightening and relaxing of the pubococcygeus muscle, which improves the strength of the pelvic floor.

4. Kegel's exercises are the tightening and relaxing of the pubococcygeus muscle, which improves the strength of the pelvic floor. They are not general conditioning for the work of childbirth.

#7. 4. **Epidural anesthesia decreases blood flow back to the heart from the lower extremities, decreasing the risk of congestive heart failure.**   Pl   Ph/9   3

1. Giving extra intravenous fluid would increase the blood volume to her heart and increase her risk of congestive heart failure.

2. General anesthesia increases the risk of maternal death.

3. Holding her breath and bearing down increases blood volume to the heart and increases risk of congestive heart failure.

#8. 3. **Although there are many unknowns in pre-term labor, a uterus that is overly enlarged by carrying more than one baby is a risk.**   Dc   He/3   3

1. A 30-pound weight gain is normal.

2. A small baby is not a risk factor for premature labor; neither is age.

4. Age and multiparity are not significant risk factors for premature labor.

#9. 3. The average length of time for the cord to detach is 7–10 days. Longer or shorter can be normal as long as the cord is free from signs of infection or bleeding. `Im  He/3  4`

   1. The average length of time for the cord to detach is 7–10 days. Longer or shorter can be normal as long as the cord is free from signs of infection or bleeding.

   2. The average length of time for the cord to detach is 7–10 days. Longer or shorter can be normal as long as the cord is free from signs of infection or bleeding.

   4. The average length of time for the cord to detach is 7–10 days. Longer or shorter can be normal as long as the cord is free from signs of infection or bleeding.

#10. 1. Diaphragms must be refitted after the birth of a baby, an abortion, or weight loss or gain of 15 pounds or more. `Im  He/3  3`

   2. Before continuing to use the diaphragm the woman must be resized. If the fit is okay, the previous diaphragm may be used.

   3. Diaphragms are a very acceptable choice for postpartum contraception.

   4. Breastfeeding should not be relied on for birth control.

#11. 1. A full bladder may prevent descent of the fetus. The mother should be checked. `Dc  He/3  3`

   2. A paracervical block given in the first stage of labor anesthesia will not have an effect in second stage.

   3. Often the side-lying position is helpful when the baby is not descending.

   4. LOA (left occiput anterior) position is a normal position.

#12. 1. Bending over to tie his shoes could raise intracranial pressure. A transphenoidal hypophysectomy is the removal of the pituitary gland. The incision is in the mouth above the gum line and goes through the sphenoid sinuses into the brain. This client has had a brain surgery and is at risk for increased intracranial surgery. This behavior indicates the client does not understand the teaching. `Ev  Ph/9  1`

   2. The person who has had the pituitary gland (master gland) removed will be taking a lot of medicines. This comment indicates the client is taking the medications.

   3. There is no reason the client should not ambulate following a transphenoidal hypophysectomy. Ambulation will help to prevent immobility post-operative complications. This behavior indicates understanding of post-operative care.

   4. The client who has had the pituitary (master) gland removed must have a medical identification bracelet. If the client was in an accident and unable to tell anyone about his medications, he might die. The medications are essential for life. This behavior indicates an understanding of his care.

#13. 2. The cause of Bell's palsy is unknown. `Dc  Ph/10  1`

   1. Shingles is caused by the chickenpox virus.

   3. Guillain-Barré syndrome usually follows a cold or influenza.

   4. The cause of Bell's palsy is unknown. It does not appear to be related to trauma.

#14. 2. A pacemaker is a contraindication for magnetic resonance imaging. `Dc  Ph/9  1`

   1. Iodine is not used during magnetic resonance imaging.

   3. A hearing aid is not a contraindication for magnetic resonance imaging. A hearing aid can be removed during the procedure if needed.

   4. Digoxin is not a contraindication for magnetic resonance imaging.

#15. 1. Hodgkin's disease is cancer of the lymphatic system. The client will have one or more swollen lymph nodes. `Dc  Ph/10  1`

ANSWER	RATIONALE	NP	CN	SA

2. A painful rash is not associated with Hodgkin's disease. The client may have severe itching, but it is not associated with a rash.

3. Stomach pain is not characteristic of Hodgkin's disease.

4 Joint pain is not characteristic of Hodgkin's disease.

#16. 3. Semi-Fowler's position is indicated to make breathing easier for the client.   Im   Ph/7   1

1. Supine position is not appropriate. The client who is in congestive heart failure has shortness of breath and needs to be positioned in semi-Fowler's position.

2. Sim's position is not appropriate. The client who is in congestive heart failure has shortness of breath and needs to be positioned in semi-Fowler's position.

4. Side lying is not appropriate. The client who is in congestive heart failure has shortness of breath and needs to be positioned in semi-Fowler's position.

#17. 2. The nurse should take an apical pulse before administering digoxin.   Im   Ph/8   1

1. Asking the client if he has chest pain is not the most important information for the nurse to obtain from the client before administering digoxin.

3. Taking the client's blood pressure is not the most importation information for the nurse to obtain from the client before administering digoxin.

4. Asking the client if he is short of breath is not the most important information for the nurse to obtain from the client before administering digoxin. This information is nice to know but not most essential.

#18. 1. Restlessness is a sign of hypoxia, which must be further assessed in a person who has pneumonia.   Pl   Sa/1   1

2. Pink-colored skin is a normal finding.

3. A nonproductive cough may occur with pneumonia and should be assessed, but it is not critical and not as significant as restlessness.

4. Dry mouth is commonly seen in clients with pneumonia because most persons with pneumonia are mouth breathers.

#19. 1. Orange juice and tomatoes are high in potassium. Baked chicken is low in sodium.   Ev   Ph/7   6

2. Milk, roast beef, and spinach are all high in sodium.

3. A fish sandwich is high in sodium.

4. Shrimp is high in sodium.

#20. 2. According to the Center for Disease Control, the most effective way to control the spread of disease is consistent hand washing.   Ev   Sa/2   1

1. Isolating infected clients will help. However, most clients are admitted before testing and may not be isolated until after tests have been done and they have been receiving care for some time. The most effective way to control the spread of disease is consistent hand washing.

3. Consistent hand washing is more effective in preventing the spread of disease than occasionally wearing a gown.

4. It is not necessary to wear gloves for *all* care. Consistent hand washing is the most effective way to prevent the spread of disease.

#21. 1. The nurse should keep items above waist level and never turn with the back to a sterile field. The sterile field should always be in the line of vision.   Im   Sa/2   1

2. The outside of a sterile package is contaminated. It may not be opened with sterile gloves because that will contaminate the sterile gloves.

3. Talking over a sterile field may contaminate the field by droplets.

4. Reaching over a sterile field will contaminate the field. The nurse should reach around the field to give another person medicine.

#22. 2. This statement indicates a lack of understanding about health promotion behaviors. Potential health problems can be detected before obvious symptoms are present. Annual physicals are   Ev   He/4   1 recommended for persons over 50 years old whether or not they are experiencing any problems.

1. This response indicates understanding of some health promotion activities. The question asked for a response indicating lack of understanding.
3. This response indicates understanding of some health promotion activities. The question asked for a response indicating lack of understanding.
4. This response indicates understanding of some health promotion activities. The question asked for a response indicating lack of understanding.

#23. 2. The nurse should explain the procedure to the client. There is no special preparation for this procedure. Pl Ph/9 1
1. There is no need to keep the client NPO before a KUB.
3. There is no need to catheterize the client before a KUB.
4. There is no need to give an enema before a KUB.

#24. 2. Dislodged radioactive implants would never be picked up with the hands, even with gloves on. Gloves give no protection against radiation. Any dislodged material should be picked up with long-handled forceps and placed in a lead-lined container. Im Ph/10 1
1. All people caring for the client should be aware of the radiological danger. It is appropriate to label the chart and the door to the room.
3. Washing hands with soap and water is appropriate after caring for any client. This is good care, but not specifically related to the radiation implant.
4. Caregivers, including nurses, should spend as little time as possible with the client while the implant is in place. Radiation is cumulative. Limiting time with and increasing distance from the client will reduce nurse exposure to radiation.

#25. 4. Removing all unnecessary items in the room or hall will reduce the possibility of the client tripping and falling. Pl Sa/2 1
1. The client can use the side rail to assist himself or herself in getting into and out of bed.
2. Decreased lighting increases the chance for the client to fall.
3. All staff members need to take responsibility to clean up wet areas on the floor to prevent falls.

#26. 4. Redness without induration is generally considered to be of no significance when reading the result of a tuberculin skin test. Dc He/4 1
1. The correct procedure is to measure the area of induration, not redness. Lack of induration is a negative test.
2. The correct procedure is to measure the area of induration, not redness. Lack of induration is a negative test. This answer is further incorrect in that a positive test does not mean a person has active tuberculosis.
3. Redness does not indicate the test is falsely negative.

#27. 4. Persons who have chronic obstructive pulmonary disease associated with carbon dioxide retention may become insensitive to carbon dioxide levels to stimulate breathing. Instead, they depend on a low oxygen level to stimulate breathing. Excessive oxygen therapy increases the oxygen level above the set point and decreases the drive to breathe. Im Ph/10 1
1. In persons with emphysema, low-flow oxygen may be beneficial. High-flow oxygen increases the blood level of oxygen and may stop the stimulus to breathe, which is a low oxygen level in persons who have emphysema. The client will no longer breathe and will die if this continues very long.
2. Increased delivery of oxygen will not lower blood oxygen levels. It will raise the oxygen above the level to stimulate breathing.
3. High concentrations of oxygen may increase blood levels.

ANSWER	RATIONALE	NP	CN	SA

#28. 1. **Humor and joking are often ways to handle stress. This should be considered a coping mechanism.**   Dc Ps/5 2

    2. Humor is an appropriate way of coping.

    3. There is no information to suggest that the client is denying the seriousness of the procedure.

    4. The behavior described is not rationalization.

#29. 2. **A surgical wound changes the way the body looks. Some clients are unable to accept the change in body image.**   Dc Ps/5 2

    1. There is no evidence the client is denying the surgical procedure. The client would say, "The doctor didn't really do an operation."

    3. There is no indication that the client fears becoming nauseated. This is an assumption on the part of the nurse.

    4. There is no indication that the client does not like the sight of blood or that there is bleeding at the wound site.

#30. 2. **The unconscious client will not be able to maintain a high-Fowler's position and will fall to the side. The unconscious client should not be placed in this position. This action indicates a need for further instruction.**   Ev Sa/1 1

    1. The unconscious client should be placed in a lateral position with the head turned to the side. This indicates that the unlicensed person is performing the procedure correctly.

    3. Placing a towel under the chin is appropriate during mouth care. It keeps the area clean and dry.

    4. Keeping the client in the lateral position for 30 minutes after oral care prevents pooling of secretions and aspiration of fluids. This action is appropriate and indicates the person understands how to perform the procedure.

#31. 4. **Completing the 24-hour intake and output record requires analysis and assessment. It must be done by the nurse and should not be assigned to unlicensed personnel.**   Pl Sa/1 1

    1. Measuring all oral intake is an activity that may be delegated.

    2. Recording all output is an activity that may be delegated.

    3. Unlicensed personnel may enter data on graphs.

#32. 1. **Walkers are not fixed. Pulling on a walker to get out of a chair is a safety problem. The correct method is to push out of the fixed chair and once standing take hold of the walker.**   Ev Ph/7 1

    2. Moving the walker forward, then taking a step is the correct method for walking with a walker.

    3. The walker should not be waist high. This does not indicate a need for further instruction.

    4. Many clients may not need to use the walker all of the time. This will vary with the reason the client needs a walker and the progress the client is making.

#33. 2. **Joining a social club without addressing the underlying hearing problem may increase his withdrawal and depression.**   Pl Ph/7 2

    1. Getting a hearing guide dog is one possible solution to a severe hearing deficit. This suggestion may be very helpful.

    3. A telephone TDD is likely to be very helpful for a hearing-impaired client.

    4. A closed-caption TV will make it possible for the severely hearing impaired to watch television. This suggestion will be helpful to the client.

#34. 2. **Pyridium turns urine a red-orange color. This is normal and nothing to be concerned about. This statement indicates the client does not understand about the medication.**   Ev Ph/8 5

    1. Pyridium should be taken after meals to avoid stomach upset.

    3. Pyridium is a urinary tract anesthetic and antispasmodic. The reason for giving Pyridium is to reduce the bladder pain and spasms that cause the urgency and frequency.

4. Liver damage is a possible side effect of the drug. The client should inform the health care provider if there is evidence of jaundice.

#35. 2. **Persons who have congestive heart failure are more prone to fluid overload. The volume of fluid infused should be carefully monitored to ensure the client does not receive a volume of fluid greater than intended.**   Dc   Ph/8   1

1. The nurse should always check the insertion site, but this is not the focus of particular concern in the client who has congestive heart failure.

3. The tubing should be changed at regular intervals according to agency policy. This is not the greatest area of concern in a client who has congestive heart failure.

4. The nurse should be aware of a flashback and should report this to the nurse in charge. However, this is not the greatest area of concern for the nurse when the client has congestive heart failure.

#36. 3. **Assessment of safety needs of the client is the role of the nurse and cannot be delegated to assistive personnel.**   Pl   Sa/1   1

1. The bed should be in the low position to prevent falling injuries. This can be delegated to assistive personnel.

2. Falls occur when clients reach for items on the bedside table which are out of reach. Assuring that the bedside table is within reach can be delegated to assistive personnel.

4. Monitoring behavior may be delegated to assistive personnel. Assessment of the behavior and problem solving are the role of the nurse.

#37. 2. **Although all of these methods are used to check placement, the best method is checking pH. If it is acid, it came from the stomach. The pH should be less than five.**   Im   Ph/7   1

1. Checking the residual does not indicate where the fluid came from.

3. Injecting air and listening for the "swoosh" does not indicate exact placement in the gastrointestinal tract.

4. Asking the client to talk or hum is done to determine that there is nothing in the larynx. However, a small-bore feeding tube may not interfere with the client's ability to talk even if it is in the trachea.

#38. 2. **A red area that does not disappear following massage indicates the skin will break down and needs immediate attention.**   Pl   Sa/1   1

1. A red area that disappears with massage is a pressure area that should not break down if the client is turned frequently.

3. Most clients should be encouraged to perform as much self-care as possible. This information is nice to know but does not require immediate action.

4. Clear, amber urine draining from an indwelling urinary catheter is normal. This is nice to know but does not require immediate attention from the nurse.

#39. 1. **There is no safety reason to avoid going out in public. This statement most likely indicates the client has not adjusted to the halo brace.**   Ev   Ps/5   2

2. Stating that he does not mind if people look at him indicates acceptance of the device.

3. Telling his grandchildren that the halo brace looks like a space helmet indicates the use of humor in handling the change in image. This is appropriate.

4. Finding a comfortable way to sleep indicates the client is problem-solving some of the challenges that occur with this brace. This is appropriate.

#40. 4. **A throat culture is done to identify any microorganisms that may be present. Antibiotic use inhibits the growth of microorganisms. The throat culture will not be accurate. Cultures should be taken before any antibiotics are given.**   Dc   Ph/9   4

1. Aspirin does not interfere with a throat culture.

    2. Throat lozenges do not interfere with a throat culture.

    3. Acetaminophen does not interfere with a throat culture.

#41. 4. Partial thromboplastin time (PTT) is the test done to monitor effectiveness of heparin therapy.   Dc   Ph/8   5

    1. INR is a way of reporting prothrombin time, which is used to monitor the effectiveness of coumadin therapy.

    2. Bleeding time is not used to monitor the effectiveness of heparin therapy.

    3. Prothrombin time is used to measure the effectiveness of coumadin therapy.

#42. 3. A hemoglobin result of 10 gm/dl is below the normal hemoglobin, which is 12–16 gm/dl for females and 12–18 gm/dl for males.   Dc   Ph/9   1

    1. The normal hemoglobin for females is 12–16 gm/dl. A result of 10 gm/dl is low, not high.

    2. A hemoglobin result of 10 gm/dl is below the normal hemoglobin, which is 12–16 gm/dl for females. Pregnancy can cause low hemoglobin. Although this is fairly common during pregnancy, the result is significant. The client will likely be treated with an oral iron supplement.

    4. A hemoglobin result of 10 gm/dl is below the normal hemoglobin, which is 12–16 gm/dl for females.

#43. 2. When the heart is not able to pump enough blood, there is a decreased blood flow resulting in a decrease in blood pressure.   Dc   Ph/10   1

    1. Congestive heart failure is characterized by an inability of the heart to pump enough blood. Low cardiac output is indicated by a decrease in blood flow to the kidney, causing a decrease in urine output. If the client's condition were getting worse, the urine output would decrease.

    3. When a client is in congestive heart failure the heart rate increases in an attempt to compensate for the low cardiac output. If the client's condition were getting worse the heart rate would increase.

    4. When a person is in congestive heart failure the skin is usually cool and moist. If the client's condition were getting worse the skin would be cool and moist.

#44. 4. The nurse should start the supplemental oxygen. This action must be followed by a repeat of the pulse oximetry to ensure this measure is effective and determine if further action is needed.   Im   Ph/10   1

    1. The physician has already given an order addressing the action to take in this situation. If the supplemental oxygen does not raise the oxygen saturation to above 90% the physician should be contacted.

    2. The LPN/LVN can carry out a physician's PRN order without first checking with the registered nurse when the parameters are clear; in this case oxygen for an oxygen saturation less than 90%.

    3. Starting oxygen is appropriate, but the best action is to start oxygen and check the pulse oximetry to ensure the client is responding to the oxygen.

#45. 1. This comment suggests the child's mother believes there is a desired or a maximum number of times that the child should be suctioned. Although suction should be used only when necessary, a person should be suctioned when needed. This comment suggests further instruction is needed.   Ev   Ph/10   1

    2. The child should be suctioned when he can not cough up sputum. This comment indicates a correct understanding of indications for suctioning.

    3. Recognizing that the child will not need the same amount of suctioning each day indicates an understanding that suctioning should be done as needed, not on a set schedule.

    4. Stating that she will suction the child only if necessary indicates an understanding that suctioning can be traumatic and should be done only if necessary.

ANSWER	RATIONALE	NP	CN	SA

#46. **1.** **Support from significant others is likely to be most helpful because the significant others will be with the client for the longest periods of time.**   Pl   Ps/6   2

     2. Support from a counselor may be helpful, but time spent with the client is limited.

     3. Support from friends may be helpful, but is probably not the most important.

     4. Support from coworkers is helpful, but these people are there only for a limited time. This is not the most helpful.

#47. **4.** **If abuse has occurred, the abuser often will not leave the child in a situation where the child may talk to a health care worker and tell them what happened. A 10-year-old child will be able to cope with being left by parents, so continuous contact by the parents is not necessary.**   Dc   Ps/6   4

     1. Having friends visit is typical for a 10-year-old. Peer acceptance is important at this age.

     2. School is very important to the 10-year-old who is meeting the developmental stage of industry.

     3. A parent leaving to be with the child's siblings is appropriate. A 10-year-old child can manage in the hospital without constant parental attention. He does not need to be the center of attention and learn how to manipulate the parents.

#48. **3.** **The best place for the pillow is at the head of the bed. This prevents the client's head from striking the top of the bed.**   Im   Ph/7   1

     1. The best place for the pillow is at the head of the bed. This prevents the client's head from striking the top of the bed.

     2. The best place for the pillow is at the head of the bed. This prevents the client's head from striking the top of the bed.

     4. The best place for the pillow is at the head of the bed. This prevents the client's head from striking the top of the bed. Placing the pillow under the client's head increases friction and makes the move more difficult.

#49. **1.** **An on-again, off-again pattern of snoring suggests periods of not breathing—a defining characteristic of sleep apnea.**   Dc   Ph/7   1

     2. Napping alone is not indicative of a serious sleep disorder. Afternoon naps may make it more difficult to fall asleep.

     3. Early rising may be normal or it may suggest depression. It is not a sign of a serious sleep disorder.

     4. Muscle jerking is common during NREM (non rapid eye movement) sleep.

#50. **2.** **The most important action for the nurse to take is to immobilize the leg to prevent further injury. A painful extremity that is out of alignment may be broken.**   Im   Ph/10   1

     1. The nurse might give the client pain medication if ordered. However, the most important nursing action is to immobilize the leg. The findings suggest the leg is broken.

     3. The nurse or someone else should gather client records. However, the priority action is to immobilize the leg. The findings suggest the client may have a broken leg.

     4. At some point the nurse will complete an incident report. However, this is not the priority action. The findings suggest the client may have a fractured leg. Keeping the leg in alignment is top priority.

#51. **1.** **Asking the client what he knows allows the nurse to assess the client's understanding of the procedure about to be done before giving the client pre-operative sedation. If the client does not understand the surgery that was on the consent form, then it is not truly informed consent and the surgeon must be notified. The surgeon may need to discuss the planned operation further with the client to assure that he understands what is to be done. This explanation is not the nurse's responsibility; it is the surgeon's.**   Im   Sa/1   1

2. Telling the client not to worry does not answer the client's question and is patronizing. The nurse needs to assess whether the client actually understands the surgery planned and if informed consent was obtained.

3. Telling the client he/she is nervous does not answer the client's question and is patronizing. The nurse needs to assess whether the client actually understands the surgery planned and if informed consent was obtained. Furthermore, if there is any question about proper consent, no medication should be given until the matter is clarified.

4. This answer is technically correct. However, the client's question indicates the client may not understand the surgery that consent was signed for. The nurse needs to assess whether the client actually understands the surgery planned and if informed consent was obtained.

#52. 3. Ineffective therapeutic regimen management applies when a client has difficulty integrating the treatment plan into his or her activities of daily living. This is the problem the client describes.   Dc   Ph/10 1

1. Impaired adjustment requires the client to verbalize that he doesn't accept his health problem. There is no evidence of that in this case. The client is having difficulty integrating the treatment plan into his ADLs: ineffective therapeutic regimen management.

2. Impaired home maintenance refers to the inability to keep the home clean and safe and the inability to pay for a place to live. There is no evidence of those problems in this case. The client is having difficulty integrating the treatment plan into his ADLs: ineffective therapeutic regimen management.

4. Noncompliance applies when a factor interferes with the client's ability to follow the treatment plan, such as not having transportation to the clinic for follow-up appointments, or not having money to purchase medications. That is not evident in this case. The client is having difficulty integrating the treatment plan into his ADLs: ineffective therapeutic regimen management.

#53. 3. Because the client is not on antibiotics, the physician must be notified immediately so the appropriate antibiotic can be ordered.   Im   Ph/9 1

1. Documenting the results in the chart is not sufficient. Because the client is not on antibiotics, the nurse's first action should be to place a call to the physician, then document the lab results and the call to the physician.

2. Discussing lab results with the client is not a priority. The nurse's first priority is to place a call to the physician and document the call and the lab results.

4. The formal results from the laboratory should be recorded. Because the client is not on antibiotics, the nurse's first action should be to place a call to the physician and document the call and the lab results.

#54. 2. Charting a late entry helps to provide thorough and accurate documentation of the event concerning a client in the nurse's care. You should also sign the entry with your full name and credentials, or as directed by the facility policy.   Im   Sa/1 1

1. Charting should not be delegated to another nurse. Date and time the entry for 3:15 P.M., then write "Late entry (date—10:30 A.M.) before making the addition. The nurse should also sign the entry with full name and credentials, or as directed by the facility's policy.

3. The nurse should never omit information from a chart. This is not a situation requiring an incident report.

4. The information should be recorded in the nursing record as well. Date and time the entry for 3:15 P.M., then write "Late entry (date—10:30 A.M.) before making the addition. The nurse should also sign the entry with full name and credentials or as directed by facility policy.

ANSWER	RATIONALE	NP	CN	SA

#55. 1. **An incident report is required when a medication error occurs. In the nursing documentation, the nurse should record the error, the client's response, and any treatment the client receives as a result of the medication error. An incident report should never be mentioned in the client's record.** Im Sa/1 1

    2. Although the nurse should complete an incident report, the nursing documentation should record the error, the client's response, and any treatment received as a result of the medication error. An incident report should never be mentioned in the client's record.

    3. An incident report is required when a medication error occurs. The nursing documentation should record the client's response, and the physician must be notified.

    4. Although the nursing supervisor and the physician should be notified, an incident report is required when a medication error occurs. The nurse should record the error, the client's response, and any treatment received as a result of the medication error in the nursing documentation.

#56. 3. **Adults who cannot read are often embarrassed about their illiteracy. They devise ways to cover up their disability. Typical explanations are not having glasses and stating that another person "takes care of those things." These statements by the client may mean he is unable to read. The client has worked in a job where he may be able to function without being able to read.** Dc Ph/9 2

    1. There is no evidence the client is in denial. Statements such as "I don't need to learn anything new" would suggest denial. The client is trying to facilitate education by referring the nurse to his wife. It is likely that he cannot read.

    2. There is no evidence that the client is not willing to take responsibility. He is trying to facilitate education by referring the nurse to his wife. It is likely that he cannot read.

    4. There is no evidence that the client is anxious. It is likely that he cannot read.

#57. 2. **Children of preschool age work out learning and anxiety through play.** Pl He/3 4

    1. This child is old enough to conceptualize ideas through play. While this approach might be appropriate for a younger child, this child can be prepared through the use of dolls and through play.

    3. This child is too young to understand a complex explanation, and this might be frightening for him. The best approach is to use play to explain things to the child.

    4. This approach would be more appropriate for a teenager whose physical appearance is very important to his or her self-concept. The best approach is to use play to explain things to this child.

#58. 1. **A mechanical soft or edentulous (without dentures) diet is appropriate for a client who has difficulty chewing. This is the first priority to address the client's immediate nutritional needs and combat his weight loss. Correcting the problem with the dentures can follow.** Pl Ph/7 1

    2. Although a dental consult is indicated to improve the fit of the dentures, the first priority is appropriate nutrition for the client, which can be immediately through a mechanical soft or edentulous diet.

    3. There is no indication that the client does not make educated food choices. He has clearly indicated that dentures and chewing are the main concern. A mechanical soft or edentulous diet is appropriate for a client who has difficulty chewing, to meet his immediate nutritional needs.

    4. Although client teaching about denture use may be indicated, the first priority is the client's nutritional status, which can be met through a mechanical soft or edentulous diet.

#59. 2. Fruits, especially oranges, bananas, and prunes, are high in potassium, which would help correct the potassium deficit of hypokalemia.   Im   Ph/7   6

 1. Eggs and cheese are high in sulfur, which would not help correct the potassium deficit of hypokalemia. Fruits, especially oranges, bananas, and prunes, are the best choice.

 3. Green leafy vegetables are high in magnesium, which would not help correct the potassium deficit of hypokalemia. Fruits, especially oranges, bananas, and prunes, are the best choice

 4. Breads and cereals are not high in potassium. Bread and most cereals contain significant amounts of sodium, which would not help correct the potassium deficit of hypokalemia.

#60. 4. The nicotine in cigarettes is a stimulant and can interfere with sleep.   Dc   Ph/7   1

 1. Eating a large meal before bedtime could interfere with sleep, but a light snack generally does not interfere with sleep. For this client the cause of insomnia is most likely the nicotine in cigarettes.

 2. Some medications, such as those used to treat high blood pressure, asthma, or depression, can cause sleeping difficulties. Aspirin does not have this effect. For this client the cause of insomnia is most likely the nicotine in cigarettes.

 3. A relaxing bedtime ritual, such as reading in bed before going to sleep, can enhance the ability to sleep. For this client the cause of insomnia is most likely the nicotine in cigarettes.

#61. 4. Self-care deficit is the most appropriate nursing diagnosis for this client because of his inability to perform one or more ADLs.   Dc   Ph/7   1

 1. Although not bathing or getting the dressings on his hands wet could increase the risk for infection, self-care deficit is the most appropriate nursing diagnosis for this client because of his inability to perform one or more ADLs.

 2. There is no evidence that the client has deficient knowledge. Self-care deficit is the most appropriate nursing diagnosis for this client because of his inability to perform one of more ADLs.

 3. Although not being able to bathe could be related to pain or a disease process, there is no data to support this. Self-care deficit is the most appropriate nursing diagnosis for this client because of his inability to perform one of more ADLs.

#62. 3. Finishing a statement or thought for a client is rude and can block communication. This action would be least helpful in facilitating communication with the client.   Pl   Sa/1   1

 1. Background noises such as radios and television make it difficult for a client to hear information. Reducing background noise would be helpful in facilitating communication.

 2. Adjusting a hearing aid can help a client hear better. This action would be helpful in facilitating communication.

 4. Facing the client allows the client to read lips and makes words clearer. This action would be helpful in facilitating communication.

#63. 4. Child abuse is a learned behavior. If the mother was abused as a child, she will be more likely to abuse her own child.   Dc   Ps/6   2

 1. Age is not an indicator of potential for child abuse.

 2. Although there is more responsibility and stress for the single mother, this is not the greatest indicator for potential child abuse.

 3. There may be more economic stressors for a 16-year-old mother. However, this is not the greatest indicator for potential child abuse.

#64. 3. Checking gastric contents for residual is the most important information to include. Aspirating gastric contents does give an indication of tube placement. Measuring gastric contents tests for gastric emptying and should be done before giving a feeding.   Im   Ph/7   1

 1. Aspirating gastric contents tests whether there is any left in the stomach. If the nurse can aspirate contents, the tube is patent.

However, this is not the most important information to include when responding.

2. Aspirating gastric contents does give an indication of the placement of the tube. Measuring gastric contents must be done before giving more feeding.

4. Aspirating gastric contents is not done to clear the line.

#65. 1. **The normal serum potassium is 3.5–5 mEq/L. A finding of 3.2 mEq/L is of concern in a person who is taking a potassium depleting diuretic such as furosemide (Lasix).**   Dc   Ph/9   5

2. 3.7 mEq/l is within the normal range of 3.5–5 mEq/L.

3. 4.1 mEq/l is within the normal range of 3.5–5 mEq/L

4. 4.9 mEq/l is within the normal range of 3.5–5 mEq/L.

#66. 3. **Outbreaks of head lice are common in schools and institutions and are not the result of a dirty house.**   Ev   He/4   4

1. Washing bedclothes in hot water indicates understanding of how to prevent spreading of the lice or reinfestation of the child.

2. The school nurse should be notified of this very contagious condition so the other children can be assessed for head lice.

4. Head lice are often spread when children try on each other's hats or use each other's combs or brushes. This response indicates understanding of how the condition is spread.

#67. 1. **Immobilization, advancing age, and hip fracture put this client at high risk for a pulmonary embolism. Tachypnea and chest pain with a sense of impending doom are signs she may be experiencing a severe blockage of the pulmonary artery. One of the immediate actions for this medical emergency is to start oxygen.**   Im   Ph/10   1

2. Taking vital signs is not the best immediate action for the nurse. The nurse should start oxygen and notify the physician. Vital signs can be taken after starting oxygen.

3. Elevating the head of the bed will not assist in the management of a client who has a pulmonary embolism.

4. Although aspirin is both an anticoagulant and an analgesic, it is not the first action the nurse should take when a pulmonary embolism is suspected. The nurse should start oxygen and notify the physician. After establishing an IV line, the client will be treated with morphine to relieve pain and anxiety and IV heparin for anticoagulation. She might be given streptokinase, a thrombolytic agent.

#68. 2. **Symptoms of anaphylactic shock must be recognized early and treatment initiated immediately. Death can occur within minutes if left untreated. Joan is already having dyspnea and must be treated immediately. The nurse should administer the epinephrine in the anaphylactic kit.**   Im   Ph/10   1

1. Joan should be seen by a physician, but treatment should be initiated immediately. After receiving treatment she can be evaluated in the emergency room.

3. Calling for help may be appropriate but the nurse should immediately administer the medications. Calling the floor is a poor choice of help.

4. An anaphylactic reaction is a medical emergency. Joan must be treated, not monitored. Death can occur within minutes if not treated.

#69. 3. **Parenteral nutrition is the infusion of a solution directly into the vein to meet the client's daily nutritional requirements. The client's post-surgical status and the fact that he will remain NPO for only a few days make parenteral nutrition the best choice.**   Pl   Ph/7   6

1. Diet therapy is the treatment of a disease or disorder with a special diet. Parenteral nutrition is the best choice to meet this client's post-surgical nutritional needs.

2. Enteral feedings may be given to a client who cannot take food by mouth. However, this client needs parenteral nutrition to meet his post-surgical nutrition needs for a few days. Clients who have had

bowel surgery must rest the bowel post-op, so enteral feedings would be contraindicated.

4. Although enteral feedings via a nasogastric tube may be given to a client who cannot take food by mouth, this client needs parenteral nutrition to meet his post-surgical nutrition needs for a few days. The client may or may not have a nasogastric tube post-operatively, depending on the surgeon's preference, but it would not be used for feeding, as the bowel must be rested.

#70. 2. This client requires droplet precautions to prevent spreading his disease to others and needs to wear a surgical mask during transport to the radiology department.   Pl   Sa/2   1

1. A face shield would protect the client from splashes or sprays of body fluid from other people. This client requires droplet precautions to prevent spreading his disease to others and needs to wear a surgical mask during transport to the radiology department.

3. An N 95 respirator is used for airborne precautions and is worn by anyone entering the room of a person who has tuberculosis. This client requires droplet precautions to prevent spreading his disease to others and needs to wear a surgical mask during transport to the radiology department.

4. Gloves and gown would not prevent droplet transmission. This client requires droplet precautions to prevent spreading his disease to others and needs to wear a surgical mask during transport to the radiology department.

#71. 3. This client should be on contact precautions, which require the caregiver to wear a gown to protect from wound drainage and to wear gloves to prevent contact with materials such as dressings that may contain infective material. In addition, the nurse should wash hands with antimicrobial soap after glove removal before leaving the client's room.   Pl   Sa/2   1

1. An N 95 respirator is worn to care for a client on airborne precautions. This client should be on contact precautions, which require the caregiver to wear a gown to protect from wound drainage and to wear gloves to prevent contact with materials such as dressings that may contain infective material. In addition, the nurse should wash hands with antimicrobial soap after glove removal before leaving the client's room.

2. Eye protection and a facemask would be worn to protect the caregiver from splashes or sprays of body fluid, which are not expected from this client. This client should be on contact precautions, which require the caregiver to wear a gown to protect from wound drainage and to wear gloves to prevent contact with materials such as dressings that may contain infective material. In addition, the nurse should wash hands with antimicrobial soap after glove removal before leaving the client's room.

4. A gown alone is not sufficient. This client should be on contact precautions, which require the caregiver to wear a gown to protect from wound drainage and to wear gloves to prevent contact with materials such as dressings that may contain infective material. In addition, the nurse should wash hands with antimicrobial soap after glove removal before leaving the client's room.

#72. 2. Gown, gloves, mask, and goggles are all part of standard precautions when there is risk of splashing or spraying of body fluids.   Im   Sa/2   1

1. Gloves alone are not sufficient. Gown, gloves, mask, and goggles are all part of standard precautions when there is risk of splashing or spraying of body fluids.

3. Mask and gown do not provide sufficient protection. Gown, gloves, mask, and goggles are all part of standard precautions when there is risk of splashing or spraying of body fluids.

ANSWER	RATIONALE	NP	CN	SA

4. Gown, gloves, mask, and goggles are all part of standard precautions when there is risk of splashing or spraying of body fluids. Even in emergency situations, proper precautions must be worn. It is essential for the nurse to know where protective equipment is located at all times.

#73. 2. Hypomagnesemia is characterized by low serum calcium and potassium levels. The nurse would suspect low serum potassium levels because the client is taking Lasix, a potassium-depleting diuretic. The nurse would suspect hypocalcemia because the client has hyperreflexia as evidenced by muscle cramps, facial tics, and positive Chvostek's and Trousseau's signs.
Dc Ph/10 5

1. Hypomagnesemia is characterized by low, not high, serum calcium and potassium levels.
3. Altered acid-base balance does not usually occur with hypomagnesemia.
4. ECG changes are not typically associated with hypomagnesemia.

#74. 3. The client has a low chloride level. Normal is 95 to 106 mEq/L. Anions (negative ions) such as chloride are excreted in combination with cations (positive ions) such as sodium during massive fluid losses from the GI tract. This helps maintain osmotic balance. The nurse should suspect a low serum sodium just on the basis of extensive vomiting.
Dc Ph/10 1

1. Chloride and sodium function in combination in this clinical situation to maintain osmotic balance. For example, when the chloride level is high (normal range is 95 to 106 mEq/L), the sodium level is also high. In this scenario, the chloride level is low. The nurse should suspect a low serum sodium just on the basis of extensive vomiting.
2. Sodium level can usually be predicted from chloride level in this clinical setting. Sodium and chloride function in combination to maintain osmotic balance. The nurse should suspect a low serum sodium just on the basis of extensive vomiting.
4. When chloride level is low (normal range is 95 to 106 mEq/L) sodium level is also low in this clinical setting. This is not a normal chloride level. The nurse should suspect a low serum sodium just on the basis of extensive vomiting.

#75. 4. The order is incomplete. It does not contain a route of administration, the dosage units are not specified (milligrams), and the frequency of administration is not specified. The order must be clarified before medication can be administered.
Im Ph/8 5

1. The order is incomplete. It does not contain a route of administration, the dosage units are not specified (milligrams), and the frequency of administration is not specified. The order must be clarified before medication can be administered.
2. The order is incomplete. It does not contain a route of administration, the dosage units are not specified (milligrams), and the frequency of administration is not specified. The order must be clarified before medication can be administered.
3. The order is incomplete. It does not contain a route of administration, the dosage units are not specified (milligrams), and the frequency of administration is not specified. The order must be clarified before medication can be administered.

#76. 3. The Sim's position, with the client lying on her side, relaxes rectal muscles and is the optimal position for examination and client comfort.
Dc He/4 1

1. The dorsal recumbent position is to examine the head, neck, anterior thorax, lungs, breast, axillae, and heart. The Sim's position, with the client lying on her side, relaxes rectal muscles and is the optimal position for examination and client comfort.
2. Although the knee-chest position can be used for rectal examination, it could be very uncomfortable for a client with severe inflammation.

The Sim's position, with the client lying on her side, relaxes rectal muscles and is the optimal position for examination and client comfort.

4.   The lithotomy position is used for examining the female genitalia, rectum, and genital tract and provides maximum exposure of the genital area. However, the Sim's position, with the client lying on her side, relaxes rectal muscles and is the optimal position for examination and client comfort.

#77. 3.   A pulse deficit indicates blood flow too low to initiate a peripheral pulse. This serious finding must be reported to the physician immediately.   Dc   He/4   1

1.   This is not a normal finding. A pulse deficit indicates blood flow too low to initiate a peripheral pulse. This serious finding must be reported to the physician immediately.

2.   A pulse deficit indicates blood flow too low to initiate a peripheral pulse. This serious finding must be reported to the physician immediately.

4.   A pulse deficit indicates blood flow too low to initiate a peripheral pulse. This serious finding must be reported to the physician immediately.

#78. 2.   Due to the unique nature of pain experience, the analgesic regimen needs to be titrated until the desired effect (pain reduction) is achieved. A client must always be reassessed after administering pain medication to see if he experiences relief of his discomfort.   Im   Ph/8   3

1.   Analgesics need to be titrated until the desired effect (pain reduction) is achieved. The most appropriate action would be to administer the minimum dose of medication, reassess his level of pain 30 minutes after administration, and reassess again at the minimal time interval for repeat dosing. A client must always be reassessed after administering pain medication to see if he experiences relief of his discomfort.

3.   Although vital signs are normal, the client reports pain and is sweating, another physiologic indication of pain. The most appropriate action would be to administer the minimum dose of medication, reassess his level of pain 30 minutes after administration, and reassess again at the minimal time interval for repeat dosing. A client must always be reassessed after administering pain medication to see if he experiences relief of his discomfort.

4.   The most appropriate action would be to administer the minimum dose of medication, reassess his level of pain 30 minutes after administration, and reassess again at the minimal time interval for repeat dosing. A client must always be reassessed after administering pain medication to see if he experiences relief of his discomfort. In the post-operative period, addiction should be of no concern.

#79. 1.   Fear is a feeling of emotional distress related to a specific source that can be identified. This client can clearly express that her distress is related to watching her mother die of ovarian cancer. Therefore, fear is the appropriate diagnosis.   Dc   Ps/5   2

2.   Anxiety is a sense of uneasiness to a vague, nonspecific threat. This client can clearly express that her distress is related to watching her mother die of ovarian cancer. Therefore, fear is the appropriate diagnosis.

3.   There is no evidence of lack of support from family members. This client can clearly express that her distress is related to watching her mother die of ovarian cancer. Therefore, fear is the appropriate diagnosis.

4.   In spiritual distress, the client expresses a disturbance in his or her belief system. There is no evidence of that in this scenario. This client

ANSWER	RATIONALE	NP	CN	SA

can clearly express that her distress is related to watching her mother die of ovarian cancer. Therefore, fear is the appropriate diagnosis.

#80. 4. Public health is at risk when infected clients enter the community without proper treatment. Therefore, ineffective therapeutic regimen management, which means the client is not following the treatment plan, presents the greatest risk to public health. — Dc — He/4 — 1

1. Public health is at risk when infected clients enter the community without proper treatment. Therefore, ineffective therapeutic regimen management, which means the client is not following the treatment plan, presents the greatest risk to public health.

2. Public health is at risk when infected clients enter the community without proper treatment. Therefore, ineffective therapeutic regimen management, which means the client is not following the treatment plan, presents the greatest risk to public health.

3. Public health is at risk when infected clients enter the community without proper treatment. Therefore, ineffective therapeutic regimen managementn, which means the client is not following the treatment plan, presents the greatest risk to public health.

#81. 4. Palpating and recording pulses is a key component of assessing a client with numbness and coldness of an extremity. These symptoms suggest poor circulation. Because these symptoms may indicate an emergency situation, this assessment should be done before a comprehensive history is taken. If pulses are absent, the physician should be called immediately. — Dc — Ph/10 — 1

1. Because these symptoms may indicate an emergency situation, a prompt, quick, focused priority assessment of palpating and recording of the femoral, popliteal, posterior tibial, and dorsalis pedis pulses should be done first before a comprehensive history is taken.

2. Because these symptoms may indicate an emergency situation, a prompt, quick, focused priority assessment of palpating and recording of the femoral, popliteal, posterior tibial, and dorsalis pedis pulses should be done. The assessment findings will indicate if a physician is needed immediately. If pulses are absent, the physician should be called immediately.

3. Because these symptoms may indicate an emergency situation, a prompt, quick, focused priority assessment of palpating and recording of the femoral, popliteal, posterior tibial, and dorsalis pedis pulses should be done first before a full history is taken.

#82. 1. If the pulse rhythm is irregular, assessment must occur for 60 seconds rather than 30. An apical pulse provides more information than a radial pulse. — Dc — He/4 — 1

2. Carotid pulse generally assesses cranial circulation. There is no indication from the client's vital signs that cranial circulation is impaired. Temperature is normal. Assessment of the apical pulse takes priority and occurs for 60 seconds because the pulse rhythm is irregular.

3. There is no indication in the client's vital signs of respiratory distress. Assessment of the apical pulse takes priority and occurs for 60 seconds because the pulse rhythm is irregular.

4. The client's blood pressure is within an acceptable range. Assessment of the apical pulse takes priority and occurs for 60 seconds because the pulse rhythm is irregular.

#83. 3. Because the nurse has autonomy in deciding which medication and route have the most efficacy, it is essential for the nurse to gather enough data to make the best decision. In this case, determining the location and degree of pain is essential for choosing the most effective pain medication. Different clients have different levels of pain post-operatively. — Dc — Ph/8 — 5

1. Because the nurse has autonomy in deciding which medication and route have the most efficacy, it is essential for the nurse to gather

enough data to make the best decision. In this case, determining the location and degree of pain is essential for choosing the most effective pain medication. Different clients have different levels of pain post-operatively.

2. Because the nurse has autonomy in deciding which medication and route have the most efficacy, it is essential for the nurse to gather enough data to make the best decision. In this case, determining the location and degree of pain is essential for choosing the most effective pain medication. Different clients have different levels of pain post-operatively.

4. Because the nurse has autonomy in deciding which medication and route have the most efficacy, it is essential for the nurse to gather enough data to make the best decision. In this case, determining the location and degree of pain is essential for choosing the most effective pain medication. Repositioning and relaxation methods may be part of an overall pain control program, but they do not substitute for the administration of pain medications, particularly on the day of surgery.

#84. 2. The client is exhibiting signs of anxiety. Allowing her to talk about her feelings will provide the nurse with additional assessment data about her emotional status. Then the nurse can make the decision about whether the surgeon needs to be notified, or if the client will calm down with nursing interventions.   Im   Ps/5   2

1. The assessment findings are outside the normal limits. Additional assessment is needed before proceeding with care.

3. The client is anxious and will not be able to process any pre-operative teaching at this time. Additional assessment is needed before proceeding with care or teaching.

4. A more extensive nursing assessment needs to be done to determine the cause of the client's anxiety before the surgeon is called.

#85. 4. The response indicates the client lacks self-efficacy, the belief that he or she will succeed.   Dc   Ps/5   2

1. Maturation means the client is developmentally able to learn. There is no indication from the client's response that he lacks sufficient maturation to learn. This response indicates that the client lacks self-efficacy, the belief that he or she will succeed.

2. Organization depends on the nurse who is providing the teaching. He or she should incorporate previously learned information and provide a sequence from simple to complex or familiar to unfamiliar. This response indicates that the client lacks self-efficacy, the belief that he or she will succeed. There is nothing in the question that indicates the client cannot organize his own care at home.

3. Readiness to learn means that the client is able and willing to learn. Some indications of lack of client readiness are anxiety, avoidance, denial, or lack of participation. This client's response does not indicate lack of readiness to learn but a lack of the belief that he will succeed.

#86. 1. This answer is culturally sensitive and allows the client to discuss her tradition.   Im   Ps/5   1

2. Telling the client that no one her age should be drinking at bedtime could be interpreted as a judgmental, ageist response.

3. Dismissing the client's traditions as an old wive's tale is not appropriate.

4. Simply telling the client that alcohol is not permitted in the hospital could be interpreted as culturally insensitive and also would not encourage further communication with the client.

#87. 3. Keeping the bed in low position and the call bell within reach are primary interventions for any client to protect them from the risk of falling. There is no evidence that this client needs any additional   Pl   Sa/2   1 interventions at this time. She has no cognitive defects and is receiving epidural analgesia, which means she is alert.

1. Restraints should be used only as a last resort when other measures have failed to protect the client. This intervention is not the most appropriate for this client, who is alert. She needs to have the bed in low position and access to the call bell so she can call for help if she needs to get up.

2. While it would be nice for a client to always have someone present in the room for assistance, this is unrealistic and not necessary for this client. This client needs to have the bed in low position and access to the call bell so she can call for help if she needs to get up.

4. Rearranging room assignments is done for clients who have a particular risk of falling. This is not the most appropriate intervention for this client, because there is no evidence that this client has a high risk for falling. She needs to have the bed in low position and access to the call bell so she can call for help if she needs to get up.

#88. 3. Guidelines for the safe administration of medications state that medications prepared by one nurse should be administered only by that nurse.   Im   Ph/8   5

1. Guidelines for the safe administration of medications state that medications prepared by one nurse should be administered only by that nurse.

2. Guidelines for the safe administration of medications state that medications prepared by one nurse should be administered only by that nurse.

4. Guidelines for the safe administration of medications state that medications prepared by one nurse should be administered only by that nurse.

#89. 3. Substance abuse is characterized by recurrent ingestion of a substance in situations in which it is detrimental to the client's physical or mental health or the welfare of others. He has been arrested twice for driving while intoxicated.   Dc   Ps/6   2

1. Withdrawal symptoms begin to appear within 6–12 hours of the cessation of long-term drinking. This client has no physical symptoms. This behavior fits the criteria for substance abuse.

2. Bad judgment syndrome is not a substance abuse or dependence category. This behavior fits the criteria for substance abuse.

4. Substance dependence is characterized by increasing use of the substance and withdrawal symptoms if intake is reduced or stopped. Because the client restricts his drinking to weekends, he has not reached this level. He may progress to this level if he begins to drink greater amounts of alcohol more days of the week. His current behavior fits the criteria for substance abuse.

#90. 1. Because the MRI exam uses a powerful magnet, clients with implanted metal devices should have other types of medical imaging exams.   Dc   Ph/9   1

2. Because the MRI exam uses a powerful magnet, clients with implanted metal devices should have other types of medical imaging exams. A ceramic hip would not affect the exam.

3. A history of claustrophobia may make the MRI difficult for some people because the client is placed in a tube. Asthma is not related to complications with MRI. Clients with implanted metal devices should have other types of medical imaging exams.

4. Not every MRI requires dye. Clients with implanted metal devices should have other types of medical imaging exams.

#91. 3. The clients in all of the choices have some risk factors for osteoporosis. This client has the most risk factors (5): advanced age, lack of estrogen, reduced mobility, steroids, and excessive alcohol intake.   Dc   Ph/9   1

ANSWER	RATIONALE	NP	CN	SA

1. Men are at less risk than women are for osteoporosis. This man has three risk factors: decreased activity, low calcium intake, and steroids.

2. This client has two risk factors for osteoporosis: the eating disorder and amenorrhea. Bone strength is at its highest in young adults.

4. This client has two risk factors: advanced age and anticonvulsant therapy. In addition, her active youth helped build bone density.

#92. 1. The client should be informed prior to the time for the medication that she will soon be medicated and will not be able to get out of bed after receiving the medication. This gives the client time to wash her hands. The hand washing ritual helps lessen her anxiety. She should be allowed to do this prior to surgery. Pl Ps/6 2

2. The nurse should inform the client in advance about the need to stay in bed after receiving the medication. This would allow the client time to perform her anxiety-reducing rituals. Informing when giving the medication does not give her time to perform her ritual and is likely to cause great anxiety.

3. It would be better to give the client time to perform her washing ritual before medicating her than to try to accommodate the ritual at the bedside. After receiving pre-operative medication, the client should be encouraged to rest and may go to sleep.

4. It would be better to give the client time to perform her washing ritual before medicating her than to try to accommodate the ritual at the bedside. After receiving pre-operative medication, the client should be encouraged to rest and may go to sleep.

#93. 1. Encouraging the client to discuss the effects of lupus on her lifestyle helps uncover how the unpredictability of the illness and the changes in appearance are affecting the client. By understanding the underlying reasons for the frustration, the nurse can help the client develop adaptive strategies that may alleviate some of the frustration. Im Ps/5 2

2. Explaining to the client that things could be worse is patronizing, blocks communication, and does not constructively assist the client in dealing with her frustration. A more appropriate intervention would be to help uncover how the unpredictability of the illness and the changes in appearance are affecting her day-to-day life so that she can develop adaptive strategies.

3. Frustration with her condition does not mean there are conflicts in her personal life. There are no data to support this intervention. A more appropriate intervention would be to help uncover how the unpredictability of the illness and the changes in appearance are affecting her day-to-day life so that she can develop adaptive strategies.

4. There is no evidence that the client has a lack of knowledge; her problem is frustration with the unpredictability of her disease and her change in appearance. A more appropriate intervention would be to help uncover how the unpredictability of the illness and the changes in appearance are affecting her day-to-day life so that she can develop adaptive strategies.

#94. 1. This information is correct and complete and worded in a way that avoids medical jargon that may be confusing to the child's parents. Im Ph/10 4

2. Debriding in a whirlpool bath is done to prevent infection and tissue sloughing and to keep tissue healthy for skin grafts—not to prevent contractures.

3. Hydrotherapy does not provide complete information about the reasons for debriding, which are to prevent infection and keep tissue healthy for skin grafts. In addition, the wound may or may not be dressed, depending on the individual client's treatment plan.

    4. The debriding bath is not an antibiotic solution. Debriding in a whirlpool bath is done to prevent infection and tissue sloughing and to keep tissue healthy for skin grafts.

#95. 4.   **The response is empathic, and attempts to verify and reflect what the client said. Such responses build trust and rapport between the nurse and client. In addition, this response allows the nurse to assess how much danger the client believes himself to be in and what actions he might be considering to protect himself.**   Im   Ps/6   2

    1. Confronting this client's belief system could cause him to become even more adamant about this belief. The best response would be empathic, verifying or reflecting what the client said, such as "You think someone is coming after you?"

    2. Although the client's response should be documented, calling the physician is not appropriate because this remark is consistent with his admitting diagnosis. The best response would be empathic, verifying or reflecting what the client said, such as "You think someone is coming after you?"

    3. Ignoring the comment or changing the subject could heighten his anxiety or make him even more adamant about this belief. The best response would be empathic, verifying or reflecting what the client said, such as "You think someone is coming after you?"

#96. 2.   **The client is experiencing moderate anxiety, which is characterized by difficulty concentrating and learning new material.**   Dc   Ps/5   2

    1. Clients experiencing mild anxiety are still able to concentrate and focus. This client is experiencing moderate anxiety, which is characterized by difficulty concentrating and learning new material.

    3. While clients with severe anxiety are not able to concentrate, they are also are significantly impaired with pronounced physiological symptoms. This client is experiencing moderate anxiety, which is characterized by difficulty concentrating and learning new material.

    4. Clients with panic anxiety experience psychosis, delusions, and hallucinations. There is no evidence of these symptoms in this client. This client is experiencing moderate anxiety, which is characterized by difficulty concentrating and learning new material.

#97. 3.   **The nurse should assess the client's mental status. She was admitted with dehydration, which can cause disorientation. The family may be observing behaviors that make her a danger to herself.**   Im   Sa/2   1

    1. The nurse should assess the client's need for restraints before contacting the physician.

    2. This is a true statement but does not address the concerns the family has. The nurse should assess the client's mental status and possible need for restraints.

    4. This is not true. The nurse should not tell the client's family to restrain the client.

#98. 4.   **Both the wife and pregnant daughter should be asked to leave the room to prevent exposing them to radiation.**   Im   Sa/2   2

    1. The wife should not be asked to assist in holding the client. This unnecessarily exposes her to radiation. The pregnant daughter should be asked to leave the room.

    2. The client should not be asked to wear a lead apron over his chest when a chest x-ray is done. That would make taking the chest x-ray impossible.

    3. Closing the door to the room during the x-ray might be done for the client's privacy. Closing the door does not significantly reduce radiation exposure to others. This action is not the most important action for the nurse. The nurse should ask the wife and daughter to leave the room to prevent unnecessary exposure to radiation.

ANSWER	RATIONALE	NP	CN	SA

#99. 4. There is not enough data to determine that the woman is being abused. The client's complaints should be taken seriously and should be investigated. Elderly persons bruise easily. One ecchymotic area does not confirm elder abuse. The best action for the nurse is to report the client's remarks and the nurse's findings to the nursing supervisor.   Im   Ps/6   2

    1. There is not enough data to warrant calling the police. A woman with senile dementia has made an accusation that is so far not supported by data.

    2. Asking the daughter why she abuses her mother is making the assumption that the daughter does abuse her mother. This is not justified.

    3. There is not enough data to justify asking the physician to order long bone x-rays.

#100. 4. The best choice in this situation is to ask the adults beside the child's bed the name of the child.   Im   Sa/2   4

    1. A two-year-old child cannot be relied upon to give his name accurately.

    2. Giving the medication to the child in the bed on the medication card without identifying the child is dangerous. Sometimes children get in the wrong bed.

    3. The nurse should make every effort to identify the client before refusing to give medication.

Index

Page numbers in bold indicate figures.

A

A aerogenes, 141
abciximab (ReoPro), 417
abdominal aneurysm, 75
abdomino-perineal resection, 154, 160
abduction, 16, 183
ABO blood groups, 86
abscess, 223
absolutes concept in test taking, 6
abuse, 2, 38–39, 380–381
Acarbose (Precose), 214, 421
Acebutolol (Sectral), 68, 416
acetaminophen (Tylenol), 110, 405, 429
  overdose/poisonings, 307
acetazolamide (Diamox), 131, 430
Acetest, 213
acetone breath, 215
acetyl salicylic acid (see aspirin)
Acetylcholine, 118
acetylcysteine (Mucomyst), 325, 406, 429
acid ash diet, 451
acid base balance, 27–28, 31–32, 34, 166, 451
acid in stomach, 140
acidity of blood, diets to alter, 451
acidosis, metabolic, 28, 171
acidosis, respiratory, 28
acne, 401
acquired immune deficiency syndrome (AIDS), 14, 92–93, 241, 403–404
Actinomycin D (see Dactinomycin)
Activase, 70
activated charcoal, 307
activated partial thromboplastin time (aPTT), 70, 416
active exercise, 15, 185
active immunity, 434
active-passive exercise, 15
active-resistive exercise, 185
activity levels and aging, 35
acute glomerulonephritis (AGN), 180, 347

acute pain, 23
acute renal failure, 171, 177, 179
acyclovir (Zovirax), 225, 231, 239, 403
Addison's disease, 208–209
adduction, 16, 183
adenoidectomy, 322
Adenoside (Adenocard), 70, 416
administration of medication, 393–397
adolescent growth and development, 303
adrenal androgens, 422
adrenal cortex, 204, 207–209, 217
adrenal gland, 118, 165, 204–209
adrenal medulla, 205, 207
adrenalectomy, 216, 219
Adrenalin (see epinephrine)
adrenergic blockers, 210, 412
adrenergic drugs, 412
adrenocorticotropic hormone (ACTH), 203, 421
Adriamycin (see doxorubicin)
Adrucil (see fluorouracil)
adult respiratory distress syndrome (ARDS), 102
afferent nerves, 117
age-related mental disorders, 382–383
ageism, 35
aggression, 376, 390
aggression in children, 311
aging
  changes of, 36–37
  theories of, 35
air embolism, 26–27
Akathisia, 376
albumin, 142–143, 156–157
alcohol consumption, 65
alcohol dependence/abuse, 44, 156, 158, 378–379, 382, 385, 389
Alcoholics Anonymous, 385, 390
Aldactone (see spironolactone)
Aldomet (see methyldopa)
aldosterone, 24, 68, 205
alendronate, 92
alkaline ash diet, 451
alkaline phosphatase, 143, 155, 156

alkalosis, 34
  metabolic, 28
  respiratory, 27, 28
alkylating agents, 55–56, 431
Allegra (see fexofenadine)
allergic reaction, blood transfusion, 87
allografts, 228
allopurinal (Zyloprim), 59–60, 193, 198, 200, 428
alopecia, following chemotherapy, 59–60
alpha adrengeric blockers, 68, 418
alpha agonists, 68, 418
alpha cells of pancreas, 206
alprazolam (Xanax), 368, 408
ALT, 143, 156–157
Altace (see ramipril)
alteplase, 70, 417
aluminum carbonate gel, 212
aluminum containing antacids, 150
aluminum hydroxide (Amphojel), 150, 171, 212, 425
aluminum hydroxide gel, 212
aluminum magnesium antacids, 150
Alupent (see metaproterenol), 324, 412
alveolar ducts, 100
alveoli, 100
alzapam (Ativan), 408
Alzheimer's disease, 138, 382–383
amantadine (Symmetrel), 403
ambenonium (Mytelase), 128, 412
ambulation techniques, 18–19, 31, 185
ambulatory electrocardiogram, 66
Americaine (see benzocaine)
amiloride Hydrochloride (Midamor), 68, 419
amino acids, 142
aminoglutethimide (cytadren), 433
aminoglycosides, 399
aminophylline, 326, 328, 428
amiodarone (Cardarone), 70, 416

cyclophosphamide (Cytoxan),
56, 171, 194, 431–432
cycloplegic eye drops,
131–132, 430
Cyclospasmol (see cyclandelate)
cyclosporine (Sandimmune),
171, 433
cyclopentolate (Cyclogel), 430
cyroprecipitate, 87
cyst, 223
cystic duct, 142
cystic fibrosis, 325–329, 429
cystitis/urinary tract infection
(UTI), 163, 169, 176,
178–181, 346, 348–349, 401
cystoscopy, 168, 176, 179
cytadren (see aminogluethimide)
cytarabine (Ara-C; Cytosaur),
56, 432
cytomegalovirus (CMV), 92, 403
Cytomel (see liothyronine)
Cytosaur (see cytarabine)
Cytovene (see ganciclovir)
Cytoxan (see cyclophosphamide)

D

dactinomycin (Actinomycin D;
Cosmegen), 56, 432–433
Dalmane (see flurazepam)
Danazol (Cyclomen), 238, 423
Dantrolene (Dantrum), 409
dark field examination and
serology (VDRL), 240
Datril (see ibuprofen)
daunorubicin HCl, 433
day of the exam, 7
death and dying, 28–34, 371
infants and children, 306,
309–312
Decadron (see dexamethasone)
decubitus ulcers (see pressure
ulcers)
deep (second degree) burns,
225, **226**
deep vein thrombophlebitis
(DVT), 75–76, **76**, 79, 81
defense mechanisms, 367,
383–384, 388
defibrillation (countershock), 73
deglutition, 139
dehiscence in wound, 49, 51
dehydration, 24, 163
delavirdine (DLV; Rescriptor),
93, 404
delegation of duties, 10–11

delirium tremens (DTs), 379, 390
delirium, 156
Deltasone (see prednisone)
deltoid injection site, **395**
delusions, 376
dementia, 382
Demerol (see meperidine)
denial, 58–59, 367
Denis–Brown splint, 351
Depo-Provera (see medroxy-
progesterone)
Depo-Testosterone (see testosterone)
depression, 39–40, 372–373, 386,
388, 390–391
dermatitis (see contact
dermatitis)
dermis, 221
descending colon, 141
desensitization, 365
desmopressin (DDAVP), 422
dessicated thyroid, 210, 422
Desyrel (see trazodone)
detached retina, 131
detoxification, 379, 385, 389
developmental models, 295,
364–365
dexamethasone (Decadron),
55, 422
dextromethorphan (Benylin DM;
Pertussin), 429
dextrose, 26
DiaBeta (see glyburide)
diabetes insipidus, 216, 218
diabetes mellitus, 170–171,
217–219, 356–358, 419–421
diet for, 452
surgical risk of, 44
Diabinase (see chlorpropamide)
diagonal conjugate pelvis, 235
dialysis, 172
Diamox (see acetazolamide)
diaphoresis, 79–80
diaphragm, in
contraception, 242
diaphragm, in respiration, 100,
244, 246
diarrhea, 32, 146–147, 164, 343
diazepam (Valium), 133, 368, 380,
384–385, 389, 408
Dicumarol (see warfarin)
dicyclomine, 150
didanosine (Videx), 93, 403
Didronel, 92
diencephalon, 116

diet pills, 380
diethylstilbestrol (DES), 56,
423, 432
diets, 443–456
DiGel, 150, 425
digestion, 140
digestive enzymes, 206
digitalis, 65, 72, 82, 413–414
diglycerides, 141
digoxin (Lanoxin), 72, 78–79,
81–82, 320–321, 413–414
digoxin immune FAB, 72
dihydroxy-aluminum sodium
carbonate, 150
Dilantin (see phenytoin)
Dilaudid (see hydromorphone)
diltiazem (Cardizem), 415
dimenhydrinate (Dramamine),
133, 146, 426, 429
dimercaprol, 308
Diodrast, 142
diphenhydramine (Benadryl),
110, 129, 133, 146, 368, 429
diphenoxylate (Lomotil),
147, 425
diplopia, 128
diptheria, tetanus, pertussis
(DTP), 434
disaccharides, 140
disc of vertebrae, 194
disengagement in aging, 35
disopyramide (Norpace), 70, 415
displacement, 367
disseminated intravascular
coagulation (DIC), 90–91
dissociative anesthesia, 45
disulfiram (Antabuse), 379,
385, 390
diuretics, 65, 67, 72, 133, 178,
180, 418–419
Diuril, 78–79, 81
diverticulitis, 153
diverticulosis, 153
dizziness, 19, 136
docusate (Colace; Surfak),
148, 426
Dolophine (see methadone)
Donnazyme (see pancreatin)
dopamine (Dopastat; In-
tropin),128, 412
doppler ultrasonography, 66–67
Doriden, 76
dorsal position, 17
dorsiflexion, 16

thermal burns, 225
thiabendazole, 342
thiamine, thiamine deficiency, 156, 382, 445
thiazide, 65, 67
thiazide diuretics, 158, 418–419
thioguanine, 432
thiopental (Pentothal), 408
thiotepa, 431
thioxanthene, 375
thioxene (Navane), 375
thiridazine (Mellaril), 375, 410
thirst, post-operative, 47
thoracentesis, 102, 110, 112
thoracic aneurysm, 75
thoracic spinal cord injury, 125
thoracic surgery, 109
Thorazine (*see* chlorpromazine)
throat, 101
thrombectomy, 76
thrombin, 65
thromboangiitis obliterans, 415
thrombocytopenia, 55, 86
thrombolytic drugs, 70, 76, 417
thrombophlebitis, 26, 32, 48, 51, 65, 75–76, **76**, 79, 83, 138, 189
thromboplastin, 65
thromboses, 90, 170
thymectomy, 128
thyrocalcitonin, 206
thyroglobulin (Proloid), 210, 422
thyroid antagonists, 423
thyroid cartilage, 184
thyroid gland, 206, 209–211, 422–423
thyroid-releasing factor, 206
thyroid scan, 209
thyroid-stimulating hormone (TSH), 203, 206, 209
thyroid storm, 211
thyroidectomy, 216–218
thyroxin (T4), 206, 219
tic douloureux, 130
ticarcillin, 400
ticlopidine (Ticlid), 417
time allowed for exam, 4
Timentin (*see* ticarcillin)
timolol (Timoptic), 430
tinea (*see* ringworm)
tinnitus, 113, 133, 136, 200, 321, 406
tips for test taking, 4–6
tissue plasminogen activator (tPA), 70

TNM system, staging of oncologic tumors, 54
tobramycin (Nebcin), 399
tocopherol, 445
toddlers, growth and development, 298–299
Tofranil (*see* imipramine)
tonic seizures, 123
tonsillectomy, 322, 326–328
tonsillitis, 322
topical anesthesia, 46
topical antibiotics, 131
topics covered by exam, 2–3
Toradol (*see* ketorolac tromethamine)
total hip replacement, 190–191, **190**, 198, 200
total parenteral nutrition, 145
total protein, 143
Tourette's syndrome, 410
toxoids, 433–435
TPN solution, 145
trachea, 100
tracheal suctioning, 111–114
tracheobronchial suctioning, 103
tracheobronchial tree, 100
tracheoesophageal fistula (TEF), 339, **339**
tracheostomy, 103, 110–112
traction, 187–189, **188**, **189**, 197, 199–200
Trandate (*see* labetalol)
tranquilizers, 133, 380
transesophageal ligation, 157
transfer techniques, 18–19, 31, 33
transient ischemic attack (TIA), 125
transmission-based infection precautions, 14
transphenoidal hypophysectomy, 207, 216–218
transposition of the great vessels, 316–317
transurethral resection of the prostate (TURP), 178
transverse colon, 141
Tranxene (*see* chlorazepate)
tranylcypromine (Parnate), 411
trazodone (Desyrel), 372
tremor, 376
Trendelenburg position, 18, 145
Treponema pallidum, 240
triazolam (Halcion), 368, 408

trichomonas vaginalis, 240, 245
tricuspid atresia, **315**
tricuspid valve, 63
tricyclic antidepressants, 369, 372, 391, 410–411
trifluoperazine, 146
trigeminal neuralgia, 130
triglycerides, 66, 141
trihexyphenidyl (Artane), 129, 409, 413
triiodothyronine (T3), 206
Trilafon, 146
Trimethoprim (Proloprim), 401
triple lumen tube, 157
troglitazone, 214
trophic hormones, 203
troponin, 66, 69
Trousseau's sign, 212
true conjugate pelvis, 235
truncus arteriosus, **315**
Trusopt (*see* dorzolamide)
trypsin, 142, 206
tubal ligation, 243
Tuberculin Skin Test, 109, 304, 434–435
tuberculosis, 109–111, 113, 304, 402, 435
tubocurarine, 46
tubules, 166
tumor classification, 53
Tums (*see* calcium carbonate)
turbinates, 99
Tylenol (*see* acetaminophen)
tympanic membrane, 120
type A/B/O blood, 86
typhoid, 401
tyramine, 373

U

ulcer, 223
ulcerative colitis, 145, 152–153, 401
ulcers (*see* gastric ulcers; peptic ulcer disease; pressure sores)
ultrafiltration in kidney, 166
ultrasound cardiogram, 66
ultrasound, pelvic, 246
umbilical hernia, 151, 342
unconsciousness, 134
undoing, 367
universal asepsis precautions, 13–14

unlicensed assistive personnel (UAP), 30, 33
upper esophageal sphincter (UES), 139, 140
upper GI, 159, 162
upper GI x-rays, 142
upper respiratory infection (URI), 44, 111, 323
urea, 141–142
Urecholine (see bethanechol)
uremia, 171
ureterovesical valve, 166
ureters, 166
urethra, 166, 234
uric acid, 184, 193
uricosuric agents, 193, 200
urinalysis, 45, 167, 176–177
urinary anti-infectives, 399, 402
urinary calculi (see renal calculi)
urinary incontinence, 14, 49
urinary retention, 48–49, 177
urinary tract, 48–49, 118
urinary tract infection (UTI) (see cystitis)
urinary tract surgery, 170–171
urine, 27, 166
urokinase, 417
urolithiasis, 169, 177, 179
urticaria, 164
uterine prolapse, 238
uterus, 234, 238–239
utricle, 121

V

vaccines, 433–435
vagina, 234
vaginal suppositories, 394, **396**
vagus nerve, 140
Valium (see diazepam)
Valsalva maneuver, 73, 145
Valtronol (see ephedrine)
valves of heart, 63
valvular disease of the heart, 72
valvulotomy, 72
vancomycin (Vancocin), 399–400
varicella, 224
varices, esophageal, 157
varicose ulcers, 415
varicose veins, 76, 246
vas deferens, 166–167, 169
vascular disorders, 415
vascular function, post-operative, 48
vascular system, 65
vasectomy, 175–177, 180, 243

vasoconstrictors, 24, 68
Vasodilan (see isoxsuprine)
vasodilation, 81
vasodilators, 68, 133, 415–419
vasomotor instability, 235
vasopressin (Lypressin; Pitressin), 207, 422
Vasospan (see papaverine)
Vasotec (see enlanapril)
vein disorders, 75–83
veins, 65
Velban (see vinblastine)
vena cava filters, 76, **76**
venlafaxine (Effexor), 372
venous thromboembolism, 32, 79, 82
venous thrombosis, 14
ventricle of brain, 117
ventricles of heart, 63
ventricular fibrillation, 70
ventricular septal defect, 314, **315**
ventrogluteal injection site, 393, **395**
venturi mask for oxygen therapy, 103
venules, 65
VePesid (see etoposide)
Verapamil (Calan; Isoptine), 69, 415
Vermox (see mebendazole)
Versed (see midazolam)
vertebrae, 183, 195–196, **195**
vertigo, 133
verucae, 223
very low-density lipids (VLDL), 66
vesicle, 223
vestibular apparatus, 121
vestibule, 234
vestus lateralis injection site, 395, **395**
Vibramycin (see doxycycline)
vidarabine (Vira-A), 432
Videx (see didanosine)
vinblastine (Velban), 56, 432–433
vinca alkaloids, 55–56, 433
vincristine sulfate (Oncovin), 56, 432–433
vindesine sulfate (Eldesine), 433
Viokase (see pancrelipase)
viomycin, 109
Vira-A (see vidarabine)
Viracept (see nelfinavir)
Viramune (see nevirapine)

vision and aging, 40–41
Vistaril (see hydroxyzine)
Vistide (see cidofovir)
vital signs measurement, 12–13, **13**, 30
Vitamin A, 445
Vitamin B$_1$, 156, 445
Vitamin B$_2$, 445
Vitamin B$_6$, 111, 445
Vitamin B$_{12}$, 88, 95–96, 141, 445
Vitamin C, 153, 445
Vitamin D, 212, 445
Vitamin E, 445
Vitamin K, 65–66, 80, 153, 157, 445
vitamins, 141, 445–446
vitreous humor, 120
Vivactil (see protripyline)
vocal cords, 100
voice box, 100
voluntary admission, psychiatric, 383
vomiting, 133, 146, 156–158, 164, 307, 426–427
post-operative, 47, 50–51
VP-16 (see etoposide)
vulva, 234

W

walkers, 185
warfarin (Coumadin; Dicumarol), 65, 70, 76, 80–81, 416
water-soluble vitamins, 445–446
weight management
hypertension and, 68–69
cancer and, 60
Wellbutrin (see buproprion)
Wernicke–Korsakoff syndrome, 156, 378, 382
wheal, 223
wheezing, 72
Whipple's Procedure, 159
white blood cells, 86
white blood count (WBC), 54, 58, 60
white cell disorders, 91
whole blood, 86
Wilm's tumor, 347–350
windpipe, 100
worms, parasitic, 342–345, 401
wound care, 49

X

x-ray, 66, 101, 109, 168, 184

Xanax (*see* alprazolam)
xenografts, 228
Xylocaine (*see* lidocaine)

Y

yeast infections, 240, 404
yellow bone marrow, 85, 183

Z

Z track injection, 95–96, 393, **395**
Zantac (*see* ranitidine)
Zerit (*see* stavudine)
Zestril (*see* lisinopril)
zidovudine (AZT; Retrovir), 93, 403
Zinacef (*see* cefuorxime)

zinc, 448
Zocor (*see* simvastin)
Zofran (*see* ondansetron)
Zoladex (*see* goserelin)
Zoloft (*see* sertraline)
Zovirax (*see* acyclovir)
Zyloprim (*see* allopurinal)
Zyprexa (*see* olanzapine)

License Agreement for Delmar Learning, a division of Thomson Learning, Inc.

Educational Software/Data

You the customer, and Delmar, a division of Thomson Learning, incur certain benefits, rights, and obligations to each other when you open this package and use the software/data it contains. BE SURE YOU READ THE LICENSE AGREEMENT CAREFULLY, SINCE BY USING THE SOFTWARE/DATA YOU INDICATE YOU HAVE READ, UNDERSTOOD, AND ACCEPTED THE TERMS OF THIS AGREEMENT.

Your rights:

1. You enjoy a non-exclusive license to use the software/data on a single microcomputer in consideration for payment of the required license fee (which may be included in the purchase price of an accompanying print component), or receipt of this software/data, and your acceptance of the terms and conditions of this agreement.

2. You acknowledge that you do not own the aforesaid software/data. You also acknowledge that the software/data is furnished "as is" and contains copyrighted and/or proprietary and confidential information of Delmar Learning, a division of Thomson Learning, Inc. or its licensors.

There are limitations on your rights:

1. You may not copy or print the software/data for any reason whatsoever, except to install it on a hard drive on a single microcomputer and to make one archival copy, unless copying or printing is expressly permitted in writing or statements recorded on the diskette(s).

2. You may not revise, translate, convert, disassemble or otherwise reverse engineer the software/data except that you may add to or rearrange any data recorded on the media as part of the normal use of the software/data.

3. You may not sell, license, lease, rent, loan, or otherwise distribute or network the software/data except that you may give the software/data to a student or an instructor for use at school or, temporarily, at home.

Should you fail to abide by the Copyright Law of the United States as it applies to this software/data your license to use it will become invalid. You agree to erase or otherwise destroy the software/data immediately after receiving note of Delmar Learning, a division of Thomson Learning, Inc. terminating of this agreement for violation of its provisions.

Delmar Learning, a division of Thomson Learning, Inc. gives you a LIMITED WARRANTY covering the enclosed software/data. The LIMITED WARRANTY follows this License.

This license is the entire agreement between you and Delmar Learning, a division of Thomson Learning, Inc., interpreted and enforced under New York law.

This warranty does not extend to the software or information recorded on the media. The software and information are provided "AS IS." Any statements made about the utility of the software or information are not to be considered as express or implied warranties. Delmar Learning, a division of Thomson Learning, Inc. will not be liable for incidental or consequential damages of any kind incurred by you, the consumer, or any other user.

Some states do not allow the exclusion or limitation of incidental or consequential damages, or limitations on the duration of implied warranties, so the above limitation or exclusion may not apply to you. This warranty gives you specific legal rights, and you may also have other rights which vary from state to state. Address all correspondence to: Delmar Learning, a division of Thomson Learning, Inc., Executive Woods, 5 Maxwell Drive, Clifton Park, NY 12065-2919 Attention: Technology Department

LIMITED WARRANTY

Delmar Learning, a division of Thomson Learning, Inc., warrants to the original licensee/purchaser of this copy of microcomputer software/data and the media on which it is recorded that the media will be free from defects in material and workmanship for ninety (90) days from the date of original purchase. All implied warranties are limited in duration to this ninety (90) day period. THERE-AFTER, ANY IMPLIED WARRANTIES, INCLUDING IMPLIED WARRANTIES OF MERCHANTABILITY AND FITNESS FOR A PARTICULAR PURPOSE, ARE EXCLUDED. THIS WARRANTY IS IN LIEU OF ALL OTHER WARRANTIES, WHETHER ORAL OR WRITTEN, EXPRESS OR IMPLIED.

If you believe the media is defective, please return it during the ninety day period to the address shown below. Defective media will be replaced without charge provided that it has not been subjected to misuse or damage.

This warranty does not extend to the software or information recorded on the media. The software and information are provided "AS IS." Any statements made about the utility of the software or information are not to be considered as express or implied warranties.

Limitation of liability: Our liability to you for any losses shall be limited to direct damages, and shall not exceed the amount you paid for the software. In no event will we be liable to you for any indirect, special, incidental, or consequential damages (including loss of profits) even if we have been advised of the possibility of such damages.

Some states do not allow the exclusion or limitation of incidental or consequential damages, or limitations on the duration of implied warranties, so the above limitation or exclusion may not apply to you. This warranty gives you specific legal rights, and you may also have other rights which vary from state to state. Address all correspondence to: Delmar Learning, a division of Thomson Learning, Inc., Executive Woods, 5 Maxwell Drive, Clifton Park, NY 12065-2919 Attention: Technology Department

Set-Up Instructions for Delmar's NCLEX-PN® Review

1. Double click My Computer.
2. Double click the Control Panel icon.
3. Double click Add/Remove Programs.
4. Click the Install button and follow the on screen prompts from there.

System Requirements

Processor: Pentium required, recommend Pentium II or better
Hard Disk: 50MB free disk space
Memory: 16MB required, 32MB RAM or better recommended
OS: Windows 98, Windows 2000, Windows XP
CD-ROM drive for installation
Graphics: 800 × 600 resolution w/256 color capabilities